GASTROINTESTINAL BLEEDING

GASTROINTESTINAL BLEEDING

Choichi Sugawa, M.D.
Professor of Surgery
Department of Surgery
Wayne State University
Detroit, Michigan

Bernard M. Schuman, M.D.
Professor of Medicine
Department of Medicine
Section of Gastroenterology
Medical College of Georgia
Augusta, Georgia

Charles E. Lucas, M.D.
Professor of Surgery
Department of Surgery
Wayne State University
Detroit, Michigan

Igaku-Shoin New York • Tokyo

Published and distributed by

IGAKU-SHOIN Medical Publishers, Inc.
One Madison Avenue, New York, N.Y. 10010

IGAKU-SHOIN Ltd.,
5-24-3 Hongo, Bunkyo-ku, Tokyo

Library of Congress Cataloging-in-Publication Data

Gastrointestinal bleeding / [edited by] Choichi Sugawa, Charles E. Lucas, Bernard M. Schuman.
p. cm.
Includes bibliographical references and index.
1. Gastrointestinal hemorrhage. I. Lucas, Charles E., 1937–
II. Sugawa, Choichi, 1935– . III. Schuman, Bernard M.
[DNLM: 1. Gastrointestinal Hemorrhage—diagnosis.
2. Gastrointestinal Hemorrhage—therapy. WI 143 G2553]
RC840.H44G37 1992
616.3′3—dc20
DNLM/DLC
for Library of Congress 92-1468
CIP

ISBN: 0-89640-221-5 (New York)
ISBN: 4-260-14221-6 (Tokyo)

Printed and bound in the U.S.A.

10 9 8 7 6 5 4 3 2 1

Dedication

To the residents in surgery and the fellows in gastroenterology who have so diligently participated with us in the management of patients with gastrointestinal bleeding.

PREFACE

The information explosion during the past generation has revolutionized many phases of the health care delivery system. Nowhere is this phenomenon more apparent than in the diagnosis and treatment of gastrointestinal problems, especially gastrointestinal bleeding. To meet the challenge of gastrointestinal hemorrhage, the patient care team requires a very well organized and efficient multidisciplinary approach to diagnosis and treatment. This complex clinical problem, for which quick and correct decisions are needed, can come to a happy resolution if there is a convergence of physicians with expertise in the important elements of therapy of gastrointestinal bleeding.

Successful management of gastrointestinal bleeding mandates a thorough understanding of many clinical syndromes, the relevant pathology, and the consequent physiologic responses to bleeding and shock. For specific types of bleeding, a thorough knowledge of epidemiology and pharmacology is required to facilitate appropriate decision making. Much of the data base, upon which appropriate diagnostic studies and therapeutic intervention depend, has been generated in just the last twenty years. The editors believe that this book will bring pieces of information together in a way that will build a bridge of intercommunication for the many specialists providing care to patients with gastrointestinal hemorrhage. The organization of chapters and the approach to different aspects of bleeding are presented so that the emergency room physician, the internist, the gastroenterologist, the family physician, and the surgeon will find relevant guidance from authors with medical or surgical proficiency in their day-to-day encounters with bleeding from the gastrointestinal tract.

The editors wish to thank our distinguished contributors, all of whom are internationally recognized in their fields of expertise. The reader should know that each chapter is written by the specialist who was first called upon by a member of the editorial team. Each chapter reflects the extraordinary time and effort put forth by each of the contributors who, by dint of their exertion, made it possible for the editors to fulfill the interdisciplinary objective of this book. We hope the reader will concur that this goal has been met.

The editors also thank Mrs. Joyce Campbell and Mrs. Doris Hoag for their dedicated and skillful editorial assistance.

Choichi Sugawa
Bernard M. Schuman
Charles E. Lucas

CONTRIBUTORS

Jamie S. Barkin, M.D.
Professor of Medicine
Chief, Division of Gastroenterology
University of Miami School of Medicine
Mount Sinai Medical Center
Miami Beach, Florida

Talmadge A. Bowden, Jr., M.D.
Professor of Surgery
Chief, Section of Gastrointestinal Surgery and Surgical Endoscopy
Medical College of Georgia
Augusta, Georgia

Ross M. Bremner, Jr., M.D.
Research Associate
Department of Surgery
University of Southern California School of Medicine
Los Angeles, California

Robert J. Cowan, M.D.
Professor of Radiology
Director of Nuclear Medicine
Department of Radiology
Bowman Gray School of Medicine
Winston-Salem, North Carolina

W. David Curtis, M.D.
Assistant Professor of Medicine
Section of Gastroenterology
Medical College of Georgia
Augusta, Georgia

Tom R. DeMeester, M.D.
Professor and Chairman
Department of Surgery
University of Southern California School of Medicine
Los Angeles, California

Philip E. Donahue, M.D.
Professor of Surgery
Chairman, Division of General Surgery
Cook County Hospital
University of Illinois
Chicago, Illionis

Gregory L. Eastwood, M.D.
Professor of Medicine and
Dean, School of Medicine
Medical College of Georgia
Augusta, Georgia

Karl T. Esrason, M.D.
Senior Fellow in Gastroenterology
The Scripps Clinic & Research Foundation
La Jolla, California

Joseph F. Fitzgerald, M.D.
Professor of Pediatrics
Director, Gastrointestinal/Liver Disease Section
James Whitcomb Riley Hospital for Children
Indiana University School of Medicine
Indianapolis, Indiana

David E. Fleischer, M.D.
Professor of Medicine
Chief of Endoscopy
Georgetown University
Washington, D.C.

Kenneth A. Forde, M.D.
Professor of Clinical Surgery
Columbia University
College of Physicians and Surgeons
New York, New York

David Fromm, M.D.
Penberthy Professor and Chairman
Department of Surgery
Wayne State University Health Center
Detroit, Michigan

David W. Gelfand, M.D.
Professor of Radiology
Department of Radiology
Bowman Gray School of Medicine
Winston-Salem, North Carolina

Frederick L. Greene, M.D.
Professor of Surgery
Director of Surgical Endoscopy
University of South Carolina School of Medicine
Columbia, South Carolina

Joseph W. Griffin, Jr., M.D.
Professor of Medicine
Acting Administrative Chief, Section of Gastroenterology
Medical College of Georgia
Augusta, Georgia

Pradeep K. Gupta, M.D.
Fellow in Gastroenterology
Department of Medicine
Georgetown University
Washington, D.C.

Frank J. Harford, M.D.
Associate Professor of Surgery
Stritch School of Medicine
Loyola University
Maywood, Illinois

William S. Haubrich, M.D.
Senior Consultant Emeritus in Gastroenterology
The Scripps Clinic & Research Foundation
La Jolla, California
Clinical Professor of Medicine
University of California
San Diego, California

Yasuo Idezuki, M.D.
Professor and Surgeon-in-Chief
Second Department of Surgery
University of Tokyo
Tokyo, Japan

Dennis M. Jensen, M.D.
Professor of Medicine
Division of Gastroenterology
UCLA Center for the Health Sciences
West Los Angeles Veterans Administration Medical Center
and the Center for Research and Education (CURE)
UCLA School of Medicine
Los Angeles, California

Loren A. Laine, M.D.
Associate Professor of Medicine
Director of Endoscopy
Division of Gastrointestinal and Liver Diseases
University of Southern California School of Medicine
Los Angeles, California

Alexander T. Lalos, M.D.
Fellow in Hepatology
Department of Medicine
Center for Liver Diseases
University of Miami School of Medicine and
Veterans Administration Medical Center
Miami, Florida

Anna M. Ledgerwood, M.D.
Professor of Surgery
Wayne State University Medical Center
Detroit, Michigan

Blair S. Lewis, M.D.
Assistant Clinical Professor of Medicine
Mount Sinai Medical Center
Mount Sinai School of Medicine (CUNY)
New York, New York

Charles E. Lucas, M.D.
Professor of Surgery
Wayne State University Medical Center
Detroit, Michigan

C. Lawrence Lutcher, M.D.
Professor of Medicine
Chief, Section of Hematology/Medical Oncology
Medical College of Georgia
Augusta, Georgia

Francis C. Pettigrew, M.D.
Research Fellow
Department of Surgery
University of South Carolina School of Medicine
Columbia, South Carolina

David A. Peura, M.D.
Associate Professor of Medicine
Division of Gastroenterology
Director of Clinical Services
University of Virginia Health Sciences Center
Charlottesville, Virginia

Jack Pickleman, M.D.
Professor of Surgery
Chief, Division of General Surgery
Loyola University
Stritch School of Medicine
Maywood, Illinois

J. Loren Pitcher, M.D.
Professor of Medicine
Chief Medical Officer
Associate Dean for Clinical Affairs
University of New Mexico School of Medicine
Albuquerque, New Mexico

Jeffrey M. Rank, M.D.
Assistant Professor of Medicine
Division of Gastroenterology, Hepatology and Nutrition
University of Minnesota
Minneapolis, Minnesota

Ernest J. Ring, M.D.
Professor of Radiology
Chief, Angiography/Interventional Radiology
University of California Medical Center
San Francisco, California

William D. Routh, M.D.
Assistant Professor of Radiology
Head, Cardiovascular Interventional Section
Bowman Gray School of Medicine
Winston-Salem, North Carolina

Eugene R. Schiff, M.D.
Professor of Medicine
Chief, Division of Hepatology
University of Miami School of Medicine
and Veterans Administration Medical Center
Miami, Florida

Theodore R. Schrock, M.D.
Professor of Surgery
University of California Medical Center
San Francisco, California

Bernard M. Schuman, M.D.
Professor of Medicine
Section of Gastroenterology
Director, Special Procedures/Endoscopy Unit
Medical College of Georgia
Augusta, Georgia

Stephen E. Silvis, M.D.
Professor of Medicine
University of Minnesota
Staff Physician in Gastroenterology
Veterans Administration Medical Center
Minneapolis, Minnesota

Michael V. Sivak, Jr., M.D.
Chairman, Department of Gastroenterology
Cleveland Clinic Foundation
Cleveland, Ohio

Christopher Steffes, M.D.
Bovill Research Fellow
Department of Surgery
Wayne State University Medical Center
Detroit, Michigan

Choichi Sugawa, M.D.
Professor of Surgery
Wayne State University Medical Center
Detroit, Michigan

C. Paul Swain, M.D.
Consultant Gastroenterologist and Senior Lecturer in Medicine
The Royal London Hospital
Whitechapel, London, United Kingdom

Jeremiah G. Turcotte, M.D.
Professor of Surgery
Director of Transplant Center and Liver Transplant Program
University of Michigan Medical Center
Ann Arbor, Michigan

John J. Vargo, II, M.D.
Assistant Professor of Medicine
Uniformed Services University of the Health Sciences
Division of Gastroenterology
National Naval Medical Center
Bethesda, Maryland

Jack A. Vennes, M.D.
Professor of Medicine
Division of Gastroenterology, Hepatology and Nutrition
University of Minnesota
Minneapolis, Minnesota

Jerome D. Waye, M.D.
Clinical Professor of Medicine
Mount Sinai School of Medicine (CUNY)
Chief, Gastrointestinal Endoscopy Unit
Mount Sinai Hospital
Chief, Gastrointestinal Endoscopy Unit
Lenox Hill Hospital
New York, New York

Frederick H. Weber, Jr., M.D.
Senior Fellow
Department of Medicine
Division of Gastroenterology
University of Virginia Health Sciences Center
Charlottesville, Virginia

Jeffrey S. Wenger, M.D.
Senior Fellow
Department of Medicine
Division of Gastroenterology
University of Miami School of Medicine
Miami Beach, Florida

Robert B. Williams, M.D.
Research Fellow
Department of Surgery
University of South Carolina School of Medicine
Columbia, South Carolina

CONTENTS

I

GENERAL CONSIDERATIONS

1

UPPER GASTROINTESTINAL BLEEDING: THE MAGNITUDE OF THE PROBLEM

Frederick L. Greene, M.D.
Robert B. Williams, M.D.
Francis C. Pettigrew, M.D.

"Disease is very old and nothing about it has changed. It is we who change as we learn what was formerly imperceptible."

Charcot

UPPER GASTROINTESTINAL BLEEDING: THE OVERALL PROBLEM

Upper gastrointestinal bleeding has been recognized as a worldwide problem during the past several decades, and will continue to be a cause of morbidity and mortality in the United States and throughout the world during the 1990s and beyond. Although the etiology of bleeding may have changed because of prophylactic intervention (e.g., a reduction of stress gastritis during recent years), the introduction of new drugs (e.g., nonsteroidal anti-inflammatory agents [NSAIDs]) and the ability to "learn what was formerly imperceptible" by endoscopy, bleeding from the upper GI tract continues to be important as a contributor to morbidity and mortality.

In August 1980, the first Consensus Development Conference on Gastrointestinal Endoscopy was convened. It reported[1] the current magnitude of upper gastrointestinal bleeding and the impact of early diagnosis with fiberoptic endoscopy. Prior to the widespread use of newer endoscopic technology, identification of proximal gastrointestinal bleeding was possible only with contrast studies or rigid endoscopy. Both the sources and the frequency of upper gastrointestinal bleeding were better classified by the use of emergent flexible endoscopy. Early reports by Palmer in the late 1960s[2] showed an overall rate of ulcer bleeding of 43%, with gastric ulcer bleeding accounting for 12.6% of the total. By the end of the 1970s, a survey undertaken by the American Society for Gastrointestinal Endoscopy[3] revealed that 21.9% of 2,097 patients were bleeding from gastric ulcers. In 1985, this increase was further reflected in the rising rate of hospitalization due to bleeding gastric ulcers of 25 per 100,000 population per year versus a rate

TABLE 1.1. Aging Trends in Patients with Upper Gastrointestinal Bleeding

Date of Series	*Patients > 60 Years (%)*
1921–1936	6–17
1932–1947	24–38
1953–1973	40–48

Source: Ref. 6.

of fewer than 22 per 100,000 for bleeding duodenal ulcer.[4] Despite the aggressive use of emergent flexible endoscopy in the 1980s, the 5–12% mortality rate associated with upper gastrointestinal bleeding has not changed in several decades.[5] In view of the greater risk of bleeding in the older population, this plateau of mortality may indicate that the death rate is actually being reduced, since elderly patients currently make up a greater proportion of the bleeding population[6] and are at greater risk of dying with associated diseases (Table 1.1).

Failure of medical therapy for proximal gastrointestinal bleeding can be associated with patient age, other illnesses, and total transfusion requirements. Studies have shown at least a 10-fold increase in mortality from nonvariceal bleeding in patients above 60 years of age.[7] Associated illnesses including congestive cardiac failure, chronic obstructive airway disease, chronic renal failure, and preexisting malignant disease add to the overall mortality rate. Rates of rebleeding, once the initial episode is medically controlled, are greater in patients older than 60 who have endoscopic evidence of a visible vessel.[8] These rebleeding episodes result in at least a sixfold increase in the overall mortality rate.[9] Deaths in patients with proximal gastrointestinal bleeding are generally not due to exsanguination, but are related to the consequences of cardiovascular complications resulting in impaired tissue perfusion. These complications are associated with the total volume of blood loss, although the rate of blood loss continues to be the critical factor, rather than the total volume of blood loss consequent to the bleeding episode.

Specific data relative to population-based estimates of the frequency of upper gastrointestinal bleeding are difficult to ascertain. Epidemiological studies from three or four decades ago reveal annual rates ranging from 48 to 144 hospital episodes per 100,000 population[9-12] (Table 1.2). To derive meaningful data, all underlying disorders known to contribute to proximal gastrointestinal bleeding must be reviewed. These include esophageal and gastric varices, peptic ulcer disease, esophagitis, Mallory-Weiss syndrome, gastritis, duodenitis, angiodysplasias, drug-induced bleeding, malignancy, and undiagnosed causes.

TABLE 1.2. Incidence of Upper Gastrointestinal Bleeding*

Source	*Nation*	*Incidence*
Herner et al., 1965 (11)	Sweden	145
Jones et al., 1973 (9)	Scotland	116
Schiller et al., 1973 (12)	England	48
Cutler and Mendeloff, 1973–1976 (10)	USA	150

*Per 100,000 population.

One method of deriving data is to use diagnostic codes currently in vogue for assigning discharge diagnoses. The 10th revision of the *International Classification of Disease, Clinical Modification* (*ICD-9CM*) is one such vehicle.[13] Although the *Clinical Modification* is specific for some conditions, universal data regarding rates of associated bleeding are not available. Additional epidemiological information may be obtained from the Hospital Discharge Survey of the National Center for Health Statistics.[10] This survey only abstracts discharge data from 400 of the approximately 7,000 hospitals with an average length of stay of 30 days or less and includes just 200,000 discharges per year. Additional information may be obtained from statistics generated from the Department of Veterans Affairs hospitals,[10] although these data are not comparable to those of the Hospital Discharge Survey. Finally, national mortality data may reflect the overall magnitude and eventual outcome in patients diagnosed with upper gastrointestinal bleeding. These data, however, generally reflect the underlying disease process and may not list patients who have bled from these causes.

Cutler and Mendeloff[10] estimated 1.081 million discharges from nonfederal hospitals in 1978 in which one or more conditions related to upper gastrointestinal bleeding were diagnosed. These authors found an additional 7,045 discharges from Veterans Administration hospitals attributed to proximal gastrointestinal tract bleeding. In the nonfederal hospitals, the discharge rate for patients having upper gastrointestinal bleeding translated to 503.6 per 100,000 population. Many of these discharges involved diagnoses not specified as bleeding and, therefore, represent an overestimate of the problem.

In 1988, Kurata and Corboy[14] reviewed data from the National Hospital Discharge Survey and the Commission on Professional and Hospital Activities. This study represents more than 750 nonfederal, short-term U.S. hospital stays and over 400,000 patient records yearly. The authors analyzed trends in gastric, duodenal, and nonspecified ulcers. Hospitalizations for peptic ulcer disease were noted to decrease by 25% over the 15-year interval from 1970 to 1985. This decrease was primarily attributed to a greater than 50% reduction in admissions for uncomplicated duodenal ulcers. Of note is that hospital rates for bleeding duodenal ulcers declined only slightly during the first nine years and, thereafter, remained fairly stable. This trend can be attributed to the introduction of improved medical therapy, specifically the introduction of H-2 antagonists. Conversely, a 20% increase in hospitalizations for gastric ulceration was found and can be attributed to a greater than 100% increase in bleeding gastric ulcers noted between 1980 and 1985. Kurata and Corboy noted no increase in gastric perforation and reported a decline in hospitalizations for uncomplicated gastric ulcers. The increased bleeding rate might be attributed to the concomitant increase in the use of NSAIDs, while H-2 antagonists may be the major factor accounting for the reduction in uncomplicated cases. Gilbert's review[4] of these data appropriately noted that this may underestimate the problem in that federal hospitals were not included.

When estimates for bleeding associated only with peptic ulcer disease are derived, a total of 114,000 discharges, or 53.5 per 100,000, are reported. Since the proportion of bleeding attributed to peptic ulcer disease is approximately 35%, a total estimate of discharges for bleeding in 1978 equated to 322,000, or 150.4 per 100,000.[10] Specific rates of upper gastrointestinal bleeding may be derived for gender and age. Males show a consistently higher rate (two- or threefold) of bleeding which is directly related to patient age.

Additional data may be derived by reviewing the use of endoscopy in the diagnosis of upper gastrointestinal tract bleeding (Table 1.3). During the past decade, esophagogas-

TABLE 1.3. ASGE Bleeding Survey (1978–79)

Diagnosis	*Incidence (%)*
Gastric erosions	29.6
Duodenal ulcer	22.8
Gastric ulcer	21.9
Varices	15.4
Esophagitis	12.8
Erosive duodenitis	9.1
Mallory-Weiss tear	8.0
Neoplasm	3.7
Esophageal ulcer	2.2
Stomal ulcer	1.9
Osler-Rendu-Weber syndrome	0.5

Source: Ref. 3.

troduodenoscopy (EGD) has been used more aggressively by surgeons and gastroenterologists in the early evaluation of patients with bleeding. This use has been documented in community-based,[15] academic,[16] and federally supported[17] institutions. Larson et al.[16] utilized endoscopic confirmation of bleeding sites in all patients within 24 hours of presentation. While they were unable to derive hospitalwide bleeding rates from this study, the contribution of specific processes to the total bleeding problem was evident in the 115 patients examined. Gastritis was the leading cause of bleeding (41%), followed by gastric ulcers (16%), duodenal ulcers (13%), varices (11%), and Mallory-Weiss tears (5%). Thirty percent of these patients had two or more endoscopic findings during their acute evaluation. In addition, the incidence of bleeding lesions in this series may have reflected the specific population of patients treated (i.e., a greater incidence of bleeding gastritis seen in association with trauma care) and may not adequately reflect global trends.

Further indicators of the current magnitude of problems associated with proximal gastrointestinal bleeding may be revealed in well-designed studies utilizing early endoscopic identification. Accuracy rates of 90% or higher may be currently achieved in classifying patients according to their bleeding site. These findings may also give more reliable data by following outcomes prospectively in these patients in relation to rebleeding rates, surgical intervention, transfusion requirements, or death. Poor outcome, judged by endoscopically derived studies, is related to older age and associated medical illnesses including hepatic or pulmonary dysfunction. Pimpl et al.[18] reported a 71% mortality rate when bleeding was associated with four or more associated illnesses. These authors showed a 1.2% mortality rate in patients without these complicating factors.

The mortality outcome remains lower in patients who stopped bleeding within 48 hours of detection. While upper gastrointestinal bleeding will cease spontaneously in 75% of patients, the 25% who continue to bleed actively have a 30% or higher overall mortality. A similar increase in mortality is seen in patients who begin bleeding while hospitalized because of associated diseases.

Although the need for emergent surgical intervention continues to diminish in the treatment of most causes of proximal gastrointestinal tract bleeding, 15–30% of patients

TABLE 1.4. Underlying Disease Versus Mortality—ASGE Bleeding Survey

	With a History (%)	*Without a History (%)*
Renal (*n* = 170)	29.4	9.4
Liver (*n* = 488)	24.6	6.9
Neoplasm (*n* = 173)	24.3	9.6
CNS lesion (*n* = 307)	23.5	8.7
Lung (*n* = 394)	22.6	8.2

Source: Ref. 3.

will need operative control.[19] The mortality and morbidity attributed to operative intervention may only reflect the increased age and comorbidity of patients who continue to bleed and in whom operative control is attempted as a last resort (Table 1.4).

Epidemiology of Peptic Ulcer Bleeding

Proximal gastrointestinal tract bleeding from ulceration of the stomach secondary to both gastric and duodenal ulcer disease continues to cause hospitalization in 150 per 100,000 population in the United States yearly, with a death rate of 10–15%. Although only 10–15% of patients require surgical management of their bleeding, the presentation of complicated and chronic ulcer-related problems has remained unchanged even in the era of drugs which selectively block histamine release of gastric acid.

A number of retrospective and prospective studies have championed the benefits of early endoscopy in both the identification and localization of ulcer-related bleeding. This very select diagnostic modality, which is more accurate than barium contrast studies, has had an epidemiological impact in showing that peptic ulceration may have multiple sites, may include gastric and duodenal locations synchronously, and may be characterized by gross features which indicate a greater risk of rebleeding. In one such study, Larson and co-workers[16] showed that age at the time of a peptic ulcer bleed is a significant factor in predicting the eventual outcome. This translates into a future increase in the magnitude of this problem as the general population ages.

Surgical intervention for the traditional complications of peptic ulcer disease has been dramatically reduced in the age of aggressive medical management. This decline becomes particularly evident when reviewing the reduction in the number of gastric resections for benign disease performed by surgical residents over the past 10–15 years. A problem created by this apparently beneficial trend is the realization that massive uncontrolled bleeding continues to occur in approximately 5% of patients who present with peptic ulcer bleeding. Gastrointestinal surgeons must continue to remain adept at resection and reconstructive techniques in order to treat this critically ill group of patients.

Hemorrhage is the most frequent complication in peptic ulcer disease, occurring in 20–30% of patients. These bleeding episodes manifest as either hematemesis or melena, and are dependent on the source of bleeding in the upper tract and on the rate of bleeding. Gastric ulcers account for approximately 10–20% of bleeding episodes, while duodenal ulcers are reported as a cause of upper gastrointestinal bleeding in 20–40% of reported series. Results of an international survey[20] of over 4,000 patients in 21 countries showed that peptic ulceration was the most frequent cause of upper gastrointestinal bleeding

(36.7%). Incidence of bleeding from peptic ulcers varied from 6% to 78%, depending on the location of the center. Such variation supports worldwide difference in both the incidence of peptic ulcer disease and the rate of bleeding once the process is established. While bleeding peptic ulcer disease is more frequent in males, evidence suggests a slightly higher predilection for bleeding ulcers in females.

Using aggressive, early endoscopic evaluation, stigmata of recent hemorrhage such as a visible vessel, oozing, or adherent clot represent the greater likelihood of rebleeding from the ulcerated process. American and European studies have shown that 15–30% of patients with bleeding peptic ulcers demonstrate persistent or recurrent bleeding following the index bleed. Most rebleeding is noted within 48 hours; this risk drops to less than 5% at 72 hours. Clinical factors that predict further bleeding include hemodynamic instability or shock at presentation, severe anemia, and bright red blood per nasogastric tube after resuscitation.[21] Although previous reports suggest that higher rates of both ulceration and bleeding occur in patients with blood group O, subsequent data have cast doubt on this association.[22] Seasonal variation has been reported in studies of peptic ulcer disease showing an increased incidence of duodenal ulcer in winter months, with a greater likelihood of bleeding during these times.[23]

Stress Gastritis: Ulcer

Stress ulceration or bleeding is traditionally found in patients with associated underlying diseases. These comorbid conditions include sepsis, multiple trauma, pulmonary failure, hepatic disease, renal failure, major surgical intervention, burns, and head injury. Recent aggressive use of mucosal cytoprotection with antacids, prostaglandin analogs, and H-2 antagonists has reduced the overall incidence of these lesions.[24] Acute erosions remain common in patients treated in critical care settings, and are frequently manifested by hematemesis and melena. These lesions occur in the body of the stomach and are often multiple.

Mucosal ischemia is often cited as the common denominator in the development of stress erosions. Frequently, an episode of shock secondary to one of the previously mentioned comorbid conditions precedes the development of these erosions. It has been hypothesized that impaired energy metabolism with a reduction of mucosal adenosine triphosphate (ADP) during periods of ischemia may predispose gastric tissue to injury.[24] Additionally, back diffusion of hydrogen ions likely contributes to gastric insult.

Drug-Induced Bleeding

Ingestion of salicylates and NSAIDs results in erosions or acute ulcers which are prone to bleeding or perforation. These complications have been related to patient age and female gender and indicate the importance of physician knowledge of the potential complication when prescribing these medications.[25] There is no evidence that upper gastrointestinal tract bleeding is more likely to occur as a result of using any specific NSAID.

Several studies report that patients hospitalized with acute gastrointestinal tract bleeding are more likely than control patients to have ingested aspirin in the preceding 48 hours. With respect to NSAIDs, Somerville et al.[26] have shown an increased risk of bleeding from both gastric and duodenal ulcers in patients over 60 years. These drugs are estimated to cause bleeding from peptic ulceration in 20% of the patients in this age group. Armstrong and Blower[27] reported that in 235 consecutive patients presenting with bleeding and perforation from peptic ulceration, 60% were ingesting NSAIDs compared to 10% of the control group. Alcohol may potentiate the effect of both aspirin and NSAIDs as a cause of acute upper gastrointestinal tract bleeding.

Mallory-Weiss Syndrome

In 1929, Mallory and Weiss[28] described upper gastrointestinal bleeding from a mucosal tear at the gastroesophageal junction. A single linear laceration usually occurs in the long axis of the proximal lesser curvature of the stomach and may extend to the esophageal mucosa. Bleeding arises from the plexus of arteries and veins located in the submucosal layer. Mallory-Weiss tears are a cause of bleeding in 1–3% of patients presenting with hematemesis and melena but may occur in 15% of alcoholic men presenting with upper gastrointestinal bleeding. Ten percent of patients may present with melena alone. Most patients do not require transfusion, and less than 10% require operative control. Mortality has been reported to be under 5% in a large series.[29]

Esophageal and Gastric Varices

Upper gastrointestinal tract bleeding is a frequent complication in patients who develop portal hypertension from alcoholic and nonalcoholic causes. Varices in the distal 5 cm of the esophagus tend to be more superficial and more likely to bleed than those in other sites.[30] As many as 30% of patients with known varices presenting with upper gastrointestinal bleeding may be bleeding from nonvariceal sites. Mortality is related to the magnitude of the bleed, as well as the severity of hepatic disease, usually cirrhosis. Approximately 30–40% of patients die as a consequence of their initial bleed, and an additional one-third will rebleed within 6 weeks of their initial presentation. The remaining one-third survive for at least one year but eventually have sequelae of their disease in the form of rebleeding or hepatic failure.[31]

Bleeding occurs in advanced liver disease from varices because of a portal venous pressure above 12 mm Hg, the increasing size of varices, and an associated coagulopathy. Bleeding may be further induced by drugs such as aspirin, NSAIDs, or alcohol. Epidemiological studies show that bleeding varices account for 5–15% of admissions due to acute upper gastrointestinal hemorrhage in Europe and the United States.

Upper Gastrointestinal Tract Tumors

Classically, tumors of the upper gastrointestinal tract are associated with chronic blood loss, but they may cause acute gastrointestinal tract hemorrhage in 2–4% of patients presenting with acute blood loss. Gastric carcinoma and leiomyoma account for most of these lesions, while lymphoma of the stomach makes up a small portion.[32] Benign entities such as pancreatic rests or polyps of the stomach and duodenum may also present with acute hemorrhage.

Vascular Abnormalities

As a result of the aggressive use of endoscopy in the assessment of upper gastrointestinal tract bleeding, identification of vascular lesions of the mucosal lining of the gastrointestinal tract has become more common. While angiodysplasias account for the bulk of these lesions and may be found in the stomach, duodenum, and proximal small bowel, these account for fewer than 1% of presentations with acute upper gastrointestinal tract bleeding. Patients may present with chronic, recurrent gastrointestinal blood loss or acute, exsanguinating hemorrhage. These lesions are often multiple, are usually less than 5 mm in diameter, and are associated with an older age group. Angiodysplasias of the upper gastrointestinal tract are frequently associated with similar lesions of the colon, which emphasizes the importance of studying the entire gastrointestinal tract in these patients.[33]

Hereditary lesions such as those which occur in the Rendu-Osler-Weber syndrome may cause overt or chronic upper gastrointestinal tract bleeding. Inherited as an autosomal dominant defect, these lesions occur throughout the gastrointestinal and respiratory tract mucosa, range from 1 to 3 mm in diameter, and cause gastrointestinal tract bleeding in 20% of affected patients.

CONCLUSION

The transition in the management of peptic ulcer disease from surgical to medical modalities will occur in many areas of the world as levels of health care and economic status improve. One unfortunate result of the Westernization of populations is the development of disease processes previously foreign but indigenous to Western cultures. This has been seen especially when incidence levels of peptic ulcer disease, breast cancer, and carcinoma of the large bowel have been recorded. Such "evolution" of disease phenomena ensures that proximal gastrointestinal bleeding will appear in socioeconomic groups who are achieving lifestyles incorporating the stresses and diets currently seen in Western Europe, North America, and Japan.

The magnitude of the problem of acute upper gastrointestinal tract bleeding remains essentially unchanged worldwide. Although new technology and methods of bleeding control have gained popularity, overall outcome indicators relating to operative intervention, morbidity, and eventual mortality remain essentially the same. While specific processes such as peptic ulcer disease have been drastically changed in character, the rates of gastrointestinal tract bleeding requiring operative therapy remain high. As new drugs are introduced which affect esophageal and gastric mucosae adversely, gastrointestinal bleeding will remain a problem. Finally, as people live longer with increased associated rates of cardiovascular and pulmonary disease, mortality from acute gastrointestinal tract bleeding will increase and continue to challenge the ingenuity and skill of the physician.

REFERENCES

1. Roth HP: Endoscopy. What is its role in upper GI bleeding? *Dig Dis Sci* 26 (Suppl 7):1–5, 1981.

2. Palmer ED: The vigorous diagnostic approach to upper gastrointestinal tract hemorrhage: A 23-year prospective study of 1400 patients. *JAMA* 207:1477–1480, 1969.
3. Silverstein FE, Gilbert DA, Tedesco FJ, et al: The national ASGE survey on upper gastrointestinal bleeding. I. Study design and baseline data. *Gastrointest Endosc* 27:79–89, 1981.
4. Gilbert DA: Epidemiology of upper gastrointestinal bleeding. *Gastrointest Endosc* 36 (Suppl 5):8–13, 1990.
5. Pitcher JL: Therapeutic endoscopy and bleeding ulcers: Historical overview. *Gastrointest Endosc* 36 (Suppl 5):2–7, 1990.
6. Allan R, Dykes P: A study of the factors influencing mortality rates from gastrointestinal hemorrhage. *QJ Med* 180:533–550, 1976.
7. Silverstein FE, Gilbert DA, Tedesco FJ, et al: The national ASGE survey on upper gastrointestinal bleeding. II. Clinical prognostic factors. *Gastrointest Endosc* 27:80–93, 1981.
8. Matthewson K, Pugh S, Northfield TC: Which peptic ulcer patients bleed? *Gut* 29:70–74, 1988.
9. Jones PF, Johnston SJ, McEwan AB, et al: Further hemorrhage after admission to hospital for gastrointestinal hemorrhage. *BR Med J* 3:660–664, 1973.
10. Cutler JA, Mendeloff AI: Upper gastrointestinal bleeding. Nature and magnitude of the problem in the U.S. *Dig Dis Sci 26* (Suppl):90–96, 1981.
11. Herner H, Kallgard B, Lauritzen G: Hematemesis and melena from a limited reception area during a five year period. *ACTA Med Scand* 177:483–492, 1965.
12. Schiller KFR, Truelove SC, Williams DG: Hematemesis and melena with special reference to factors influencing the outcome. *Br Med J* 2:7–14, 1970.
13. *The International Classification of Diseases, Clinical Modification,* 10th revision. Ann Arbor, Mich., Commission on Professional and Hospital Activities, 1991.
14. Kurata JH, Corboy ED: Current peptic ulcer time trends. An epidemiological profile. *J Clin Gastroenterol* 10:259–268, 1988.
15. Johnston JH: Endoscopic risk factors for bleeding peptic ulcer. *Gastrointest Endosc* 36 (Suppl 5):16–20, 1990.
16. Larson G, Schmidt T, Gott J, et al: Upper gastrointestinal bleeding: Predictors of outcome. *Surgery* 100:765–772, 1986.
17. Greene FL, Howard ML: The status of gastrointestinal endoscopy by surgeons in the Veterans Administration health care system: A survey. *Am Surg* 55:77–80, 1989.
18. Pimpl W, Boeckl O, Waclawiczek HW, et al: Estimation of the mortality rate of patients with severe gastroduodenal hemorrhage with the aid of a new scoring system. *Endoscopy* 19:101–106, 1987.
19. Branicki FJ, Coleman SY, Pritchett CJ, et al: Emergency surgical treatment for nonvariceal bleeding of the upper part of the gastrointestinal tract. *Surg Gynecol Obstet* 172:113–120, 1991.
20. Morgan AG, Clamp SE: OMGE international upper gastrointestinal bleeding survey, 1978–1986. *Scand J Gastroenterol* 23 (Suppl 144):51–58, 1988.
21. Bornman PC, Theodorou NA, Shuttleworth RD, et al: Importance of hypovolemic shock and endoscopic signs in predicting recurrent hemorrhage from peptic ulceration: A prospective evaluation. *Br Med J* 291:245–247, 1985.
22. Lam SK, Sircus W: Studies and duodenal ulcer. *QJ Med* 44:369–373, 1975.
23. Gardiner GC, Pinsky W, Myerson RM: The seasonal incidence of peptic ulcer activity—fact or fancy? *Am J Gastroenterol* 45:22–26, 1966.
24. Brooks FP: The pathophysiology of peptic ulcer disease. *Dig Dis Sci* 30 (Suppl):15–29, 1985.

25. Guess HA, West R, Strand, LM, et al: Fatal upper gastrointestinal hemorrhage or perforation among users and nonusers of nonsteroidal anti-inflammatory drugs in Saskatchewan, Canada 1983. *J Clin Epidemiol* 41:35–45, 1988.
26. Somerville K, Faulkner G, Langman M: Nonsteroidal anti-inflammatory drugs and bleeding peptic ulcer. *Lancet* 1:462–464, 1986.
27. Armstrong CP, Blower AL: Non-steroidal anti-inflammatory drugs and life-threatening complications of peptic ulceration. *Gut* 28:527–531, 1987.
28. Mallory GK, Weiss S: Hemorrhages from lacerations of the cardiac orifice of the stomach due to vomiting. *Am J Med Sci* 178:506–530, 1929.
29. Sugawa C, Benishek D, Walt AJ: Mallory-Weiss syndrome. A study of 224 patients. *Am J Surg* 145:30–36, 1983.
30. Spence RAJ: The venous anatomy of the lower esophagus in normal subjects and in patients with varices: An image analysis study. *Br J Surg* 71:739–742, 1984.
31. Shearman DJC, Finlayson NDC, Carter DC (eds): *Diseases of the Gastrointestinal Tract and Liver,* ed 2. Edinburgh, Churchill Livingstone, 1989, pp 281–310.
32. Skudder PA, Schwartz SI: Primary lymphoma of the gastrointestinal tract. *Surg Gynecol Obstet* 160:5–8, 1985.
33. Boley SJ, Sammartano R, Brandt LJ, et al: Vascular ectasias of the colon. *Surg Gynecol Obstet* 149:353–360, 1979.

2

LOWER GASTROINTESTINAL BLEEDING: THE MAGNITUDE OF THE PROBLEM

Kenneth A. Forde, M.D.

"Always he kept on asking: where did that blood come from?"
Carl Sandburg: *Ossawatomie*

INTRODUCTION

The passage of blood, old or fresh, from either end of the gastrointestinal tract is always a cause of anxiety for the patient. For the physician, bleeding represents both a challenge and a frustration. Continued or recurrent bleeding may threaten life, and delay in identification of the specific cause may lead to empiric and difficult management with a guarded prognosis. This chapter presents an overview of lower gastrointestinal bleeding, with emphasis on incidence, clinical patterns, and predictors of increased mortality.

Lower gastrointestinal bleeding refers to overt or occult bleeding emanating from the area between the duodenum and the anus. Hematochezia is not always bright red blood, nor does rectal bleeding necessarily imply that the bleeding site is the colorectum. Attempts to identify the origin of bleeding by the appearance of the passed blood have been unsatisfactory. Blood exiting from the rectum may be pink, bright red, mahogany, maroon, port wine, black, or invisible (occult). Bleeding may also be one component of a broader symptom complex which may include diarrhea, weight loss, or pain. However, attempts to predict the source of rectal bleeding through association with particular clinical signs and symptoms have been highly inaccurate.[1]

Gastrointestinal tract bleeding is so common that its true incidence is difficult to define unless the bleeding is severe. Many patients never tell a physician of the occasional drop of blood seen at defecation, and the search for occult hemoglobin in the stool is not common. Nevertheless, gastrointestinal tract bleeding accounts for approximately 8% of hospital admissions.[2] One study reported that 21% of 286 patient admissions for gastrointestinal bleeding during a five-year period had colorectal lesions identified as the cause.[3] Our experience at an urban academic medical center includes 178 patients seen over 10 years with a discharge diagnosis of acute lower gastrointestinal bleeding.[4] There was no gender preference, and the mean age was 64 years (range, 4 months to 95 years).

TABLE 2.1. Significant Lower Gastrointestinal Bleeding: Etiology By Age Group

Infants, children	Meckel's diverticulum Juvenile polyps Inflammatory bowel disease
Adolescents, young adults	Meckel's diverticulum Inflammatory bowel disease Juvenile polyps
Adults up to age 60 years	Diverticulosis Inflammatory bowel disease Polyps Carcinoma Arteriovenous malformations (vascular ectasias)
Elderly (over 60 years) patients	Diverticulosis Arteriovenous malformations or vascular ectasias Carcinoma

Bleeding from the gastrointestinal tract presupposes mucosal disruption; a variety of conditions, some of them iatrogenic, may be at fault. Their incidence, detection, severity, and management depend to some extent on the age group in which they occur. For this reason, the following discussion of these diseases is presented in chronologic groupings[5] (Table 2.1).

AGE GROUPS

Infants and Young Children

The common causes of lower gastrointestinal tract bleeding in infants and young children include anal fissures, Meckel's diverticula, and juvenile polyps. Bleeding from fissures is usually bright red, is small in amount, and rarely causes anemia. In contrast, bleeding from a Meckel's diverticulum is often severe enough to require hospitalization, transfusion, and emergency surgical intervention.[6] Bleeding from juvenile polyps may also present as severe hypovolemia but more commonly results in anemia from chronic slow blood loss. Habr-Gama of Brazil evaluated 42 children for rectal bleeding and found 59 polyps in 32 of them.[7] Excluding 13 schistosomal polyps in one child and an adenoma in another from a family with a history of polyposis, all polyps were of the juvenile (hamartomatous) type.

Adolescents and Young Adults

The common causes of minor intermittent bleeding in adolescents and young adults include hemorrhoids, fissures, and nonspecific proctitis. When these entities become chronic, anemia may occasionally result. Inflammatory bowel disease and Meckel's diverticula, however, can cause serious bleeding in this age group.[6,8] Although rare, most severe episodes of enigmatic bleeding in this age group arise from small bowel lesions, particularly some types of arteriovenous malformations.[9]

Middle-Aged Adults

Minor rectal bleeding in middle-aged individuals is due most commonly to fissures, hemorrhoids, or benign polyps. All three conditions tend to result in intermittent hemorrhage, although a ruptured internal hemorrhoid may result in significant but self-limited bright red bleeding. The leading causes of serious hemorrhage is this age group, in contrast, are diverticulosis, inflammatory bowel disease, and carcinoma.[5] The bleeding from diverticulosis may be life-threatening, whereas inflammatory bowel disease or cancer seldom presents with hemorrhagic shock.

The Elderly

The most common causes of serious lower gastrointestinal tract hemorrhage in the elderly are diverticulosis and angiodysplasia.[5] The bleeding from gut ischemia and carcinoma in this age group is usually not massive or life-threatening.[10] Other common causes of bleeding in the elderly are polyps and hemorrhoids. Less common causes include inflammatory bowel disease, radiation colitis, fissures, and rectal ulcers.[5]

MESENCHYMAL NEOPLASMS

Although small bowel leiomyomas and leiomyosarcomas are rare causes of gastrointestinal bleeding, they are usually not discovered until a late stage, when local extension of benign disease or unresectable malignant spread is present.[11] Akwari et al.[12] found that bleeding was the most common presenting symptom in 108 primary leiomyosarcomas treated at the Mayo Clinic. Bright red rectal bleeding was noted in 30% of jejunal and ileal lesions, in 33% of colon tumors, and in 31% of rectal leiomyosarcomas. Only 48% of these sarcomas were surgically resectable for anticipated cure. With increased use of enteroscopy, enteroclysis, and intraoperative total endoscopy, it is hoped that more leiomyomas will be detected earlier, when they are smaller (Figure 2.1 and Plates 1, 2). Concomitant with surgical extirpation of the mesenchymal tumor, other sites of cryptic bleeding should be ruled out by total endoscopy.[13]

MEDICAL DISORDERS

Certain medical disorders cause or are associated with lower gastrointestinal tract bleeding in all age groups.[14] These include systemic diseases such as bacillary, viral, or fungal infections; lymphoproliferative diseases; chronic renal failure; connective tissue disorders; and amyloidosis. Other system disorders include altered hemostasis due to congenital (e.g., hemophilia) or iatrogenic (radiation, antibiotic, or other drug-induced) defects in the clotting cascade or in platelet function. Therapy with anticoagulants, antiplatelet activation agents and drugs, and chemotherapeutic agents (e.g., vincristine) have been implicated as causes of significant hemorrhage. Recognizing these drug-related disorders of coagulation enhances the likelihood of successfully reversing the primary disorder or discontinuing the drug which caused the hemorrhagic diathesis.

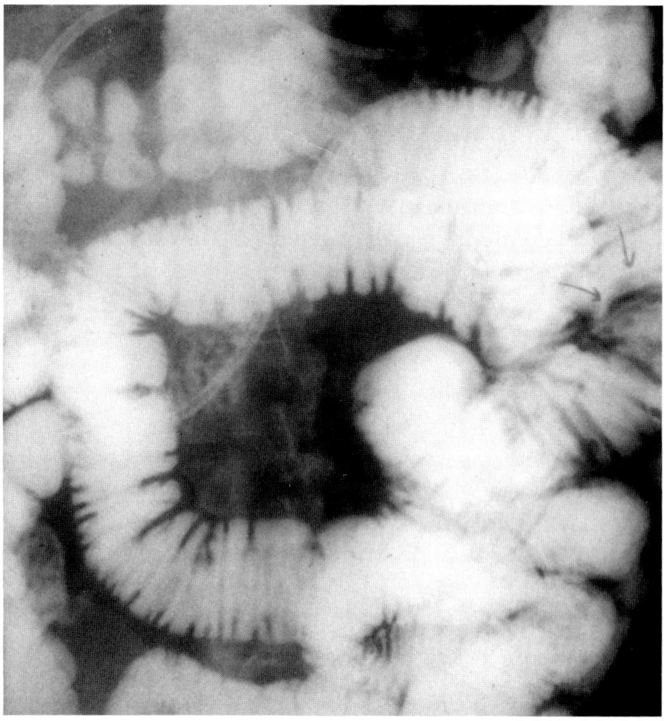

Figure 2.1. Proximal jejunal lesion in a patient with a 30-year history of enigmatic gastrointestinal bleeding (also see Plates 1 and 2).

Infectious Enterocolitides

Rectal bleeding in all of these infectious conditions is usually part of a general symptom complex which may include diarrhea, pain, fever, and other constitutional symptoms. Rectal bleeding has been commonly reported with pseudomembranous colitis, campylobacter enteritis, typhoid fever, tuberculosis, amebiasis, shigellosis, gonococcal proctitis, and herpes simplex proctitis.[15] The latter three conditions are more common in the male homosexual population. The bleeding in most of these conditions is usually not severe, although massive hemorrhage has been described in typhoid fever[16] as well as tuberculosis.[17]

Chronic Renal Failure

Frequently encountered in chronic renal failure, lower gastrointestinal bleeding ranges from minimal to massive. The causes of bleeding in this patient group range from coagulation abnormalities such as platelet dysfunction with thrombocytopenia and prolonged bleeding time to structural or anatomical problems such as diverticulosis or angiodysplasia. This is a particularly challenging group of patients to manage. The incidence of significant lower gastrointestinal hemorrhage in over 4,000 renal transplant patients we reviewed[18] is low (0.9%), but the mortality rate of nonoperative management of transplant patients with significant rectal bleeding is 80%. Causes of bleeding in these patients include opportunistic infection; pseudomembranous, ischemic, and uremic colitis; and idiopathic colonic and rectal ulcers.

Hemophilia

Patients with hemophilia experience an 8–25% incidence of gastrointestinal bleeding, which is rarely fatal. Most gastrointestinal bleeding in these patients arises proximal to the jejunum (53%), whereas 32% of patients bleed from unknown sites. Some of these latter patients may bleed from the distal bowel.[19] Most hemophiliac patients have a precipitating factor such as the ingestion of alcohol or the use of nonsteroidal anti-inflammatory drugs. The etiological role of these agents in lower gastrointestinal bleeding is uncertain.

CLINICAL PRESENTATION

The clinical importance of the different forms of bleeding relate to the short- or long-term threat they pose to the patient. Thus, severe bleeding, whether recent, continuing, or recurrent, poses the greater threat and will be discussed in further detail.

Diverticulosis

Diverticulosis, usually without diverticulitis, was formerly thought to be the most common cause of massive lower gastrointestinal hemorrhage. Boley et al.[20] and others have drawn attention to vascular ectasias, which are now recognized as a common cause of significant bleeding in the elderly. Clearly, the prior primacy of diverticulosis among the causes of lower gastrointestinal tract bleeding was established when barium studies were the main means of diagnosis. Prior to the use of selective mesenteric angiography and emergency colonoscopy, the diagnosis was often made by exclusion. The diagnostic tools of the time were rigid sigmoidoscopy, barium enema, and exploratory celiotomy. A diverticulum spurting blood during rigid sigmoidoscopy is a rare sight, and a barium enema can document the presence of diverticulosis but cannot verify the presence of bleeding. Furthermore, the surgeon can seldom demonstrate the bleeding point in either a closed or an open segment of colon filled with blood. Even the pathologist is usually unable to substantiate the specific site of hemorrhage in diverticulosis except, like the radiologist, by excluding other sources. Colon resections for massive bleeding are often necessary at night or on weekends, when injection studies, even if customarily done at the particular institution, are not available. Since selective mesenteric angiography may show both extravasation of contrast medium and the specific angiographic architecture (Figure 2.2) of both angiodysplastic lesions and diverticulosis, the diagnosis of bleeding from a diverticulum is more secure with this modality. Since the bleeding rate has to be equal to or greater than 0.5 ml per minute for visual extravasation, only the more active bleeding episodes will be angiographically demonstrable. Given these constraints, recent angiographic series in the 60- to 70-year age group[21,22] demonstrate a comparable incidence of diverticulosis and arteriovenous malformations as the cause of significant rectal bleeding. Right-sided diverticula are seen to bleed on angiographic studies more commonly than left-sided lesions.[23]

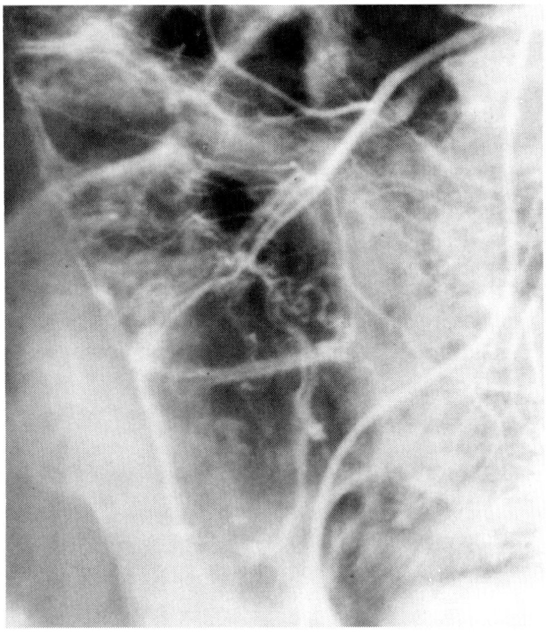

A

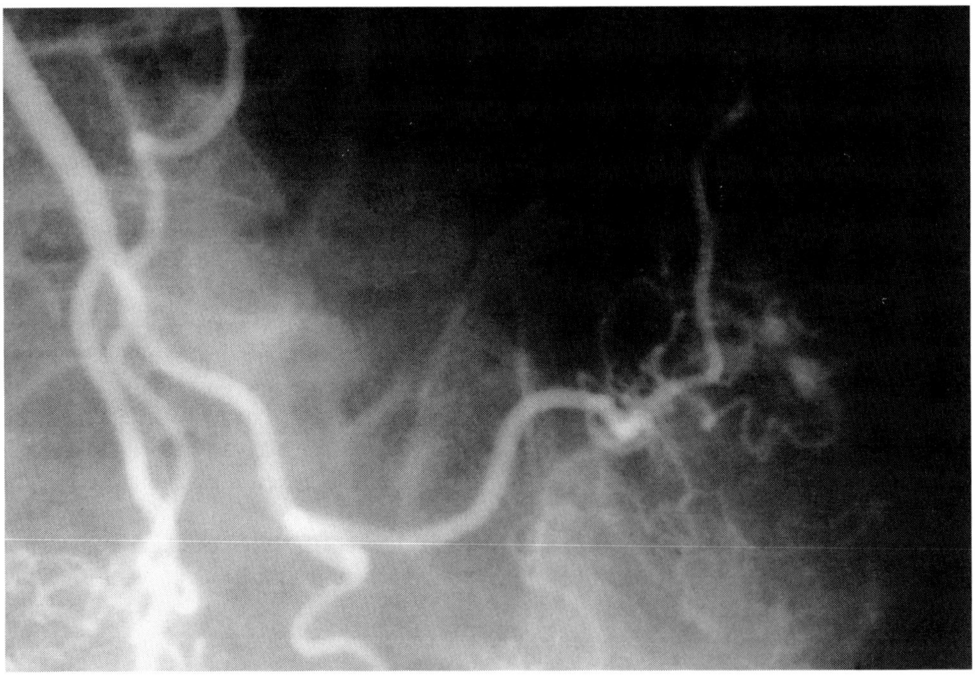

B

Figure 2.2. Selective angiographic studies. (*A*) Bleeding angiodysplasia of the ileocecal region. Note the early filling vein. (*B*) Bleeding left colon diverticulum. Note the extravasation into the bowel lumen but the absence of an early filling vein.

Most endoscopists with experience in emergency colonoscopy for bleeding agree that successful visualization of bleeding sites is more likely than angiographic visualization in patients with less rapid bleeding rates (Plate 3). Diverticulosis has been more commonly seen than vascular malformations on endoscopic visualization of a bleeding site.[10,24] In contrast to angiographic studies, left-sided diverticula are more commonly identified as the bleeding site on colonoscopy.[10,24] Emergency colonoscopy has confirmed that bleeding from both diverticulosis and vascular ectasias is sporadic even when the bleeding episode has been massive. Consequently there are windows in time permitting certain forms of diagnosis and therapy (e.g., endoscopy) that, at other times, are not feasible.

Mayers et al.[25] and Baer[26] showed that the pathogenesis of bleeding from colonic diverticula involves erosion or rupture of the vasa recta which penetrate the colonic wall through the connective tissue septa, resulting in sudden massive arterial bleeding, which usually stops spontaneously. Approximately 25–30% of patients have a second bleeding episode,[27] and 50% of these patients with recurrent bleeding have additional episodes of significant bleeding. Earlier workers believed that diverticulosis was a common cause of chronic, mild, intermittent lower gastrointestinal bleeding. This view was based on the process of exclusion. During the more than 15 years that colonoscopy has been actively practiced, endoscopists have rarely reported small amounts of blood at diverticular orifices, even after vigorous bowel cleansing.[28] Clearly, some other cause of intermittent low-grade bleeding needs to be ruled out even in the patient whose barium enema reveals only diverticulosis[29,30-35] (Table 2.2). Steger et al.[13] emphasized that lower gastrointestinal tract bleeding may arise simultaneously from multiple sources in the same patient. Therefore, patients who recover from an acute bleeding episode are candidates for elective interval total colonoscopy at a later date.

Angiodysplasia

Much controversy centers on the various vascular malformations seen in the gastrointestinal tract with respect to nomenclature, microscopic pathology, incidence, and distribution. These lesions have been referred to as *vascular ectasias, angiodysplasias,* or *arteriovenous malformations*. Some are true angiomas or lymphangiomas.[36-38] The strongest advocates of a "unified theory" have been Boley et al.[20] and Brandt,[29] who

TABLE 2.2. Rectal Bleeding with Barium Enema Negative Diverticula

			Colonoscopic findings			
Reference	*No. of Patients*	*% with Pathology*	*CA*	*POLYPS*	*IBD*	*AVM*
Tedesco, Waye et al.[30]	258	41.5	29	39	19	17
Waye[31]	93	50	15	14	10	4
Hunt[32]	561	42	62	78	54	—
Teague et al.[33]	215	41	27	29	26	2
Swarbrick et al.[34]	239	40	23	39	24	—
Guillem et al.[35]	106	48	8	29	7	5

Abbreviations: CA, cancer; IBD, inflammatory bowel disease; AVM, arteriovenous malformation.

require pathological confirmation for the vascular ectasias which they believe are confined to the cecum or proximal right colon. These lesions are often associated with aortic stenosis and are estimated to occur in up to 25% of patients over age 60. Ischemic necrosis of the endothelium overlying these ectatic vessels is thought to be the pathogenesis of their bleeding. However, there are many types of abnormalities in vascular anatomy and proliferation[22,37] which may present in both the small and large intestines. Consequently the breadth of the problem challenges the managing clinician. Since bleeding from diverticulosis is usually arterial and that from vascular ectasias is venous, one would expect that bleeding from the former would be more massive and catastrophic, while bleeding from the latter would be less severe and more self-limited. This expectation has not been borne out in large clinical studies. Both disorders have the capacity for massive hemorrhage. Although both entities are prone to spontaneous cessation, the vascular ectasias appear to have a greater tendency toward recurrent bleeding. Fortunately, the first episode of massive lower gastrointestinal tract bleeding (assumed to be diverticular in the old literature) has a 70% likelihood of spontaneous cessation.[27] After the second bleeding episode, however, the propensity for continued bleeding is remarkably increased.

Vascular ectasias do not always bleed massively. In fact, their manner of clinical presentation may vary from intermittent occult blood in the stool to iron deficiency anemia, melena, or even bright red hematochezia. Some patients require multiple transfusions over many years. Factors implicated in recurrent bleeding from vascular ectasias include failure to discover and treat all lesions, especially those in the upper gastrointestinal tract; the intermittent appearance of some lesions; and the development of new lesions over time. Angiodysplastic lesions, especially in the younger age group, may be part of the syndrome of hereditary hemorrhagic telangiectasia (Osler-Weber-Rendu disease),[39] a diffuse disorder involving mucous membranes from the nose and mouth to the anus. This widespread disease process makes control of the syndrome difficult when only one area of involvement is recognized and treated.

Other conditions with which vascular ectasias have been associated are chronic renal failure, cirrhosis, radiation therapy, and collagen vascular disorders. Because some acquired arteriovenous malformations or vascular ectasias are associated with aortic stenosis,[40] control of the bleeding problem has even been reported after valvular replacement.[41]

Inflammatory Bowel Disease

While overt bleeding occurs in both ulcerative colitis and Crohn's disease, it is not usually severe.[8] Profuse bleeding occurs with about equal frequency in both disorders (1–6%). While spontaneous cessation led to conservative management in the past, recent experience with massive rebleeding has prompted consideration of more aggressive surgical intervention with the first episode.[8]

Neoplasms

Adenomas and carcinomas of the colon usually bleed intermittently or not at all. Although overt or occult gastrointestinal tract bleeding, especially in groups at high risk for the development of carcinoma, should prompt a search for neoplasms, failure to discover blood loss in the gastrointestinal tract is by no means assurance of their absence. Sometimes evidence of bleeding which prompts the search for neoplasms has been instigated by the administration of a drug (Plate 4). Experience has demonstrated that one should rule out a neoplasm in the susceptible individual even if bleeding stops on cessation of the drug or anemia is corrected with iron. A cancer may be overlooked by the failure to investigate even minor episodes of gastrointestinal bleeding. Lessons from the endoscopic literature (Tables 2.1, 2.2) have shown the extent of lesions which can cause bleeding per anum. One of the hidden statistics of mortality from nonmassive lower gastrointestinal tract bleeding is the carcinoma missed through failure to investigate bleeding in such patients aggressively (Plate 5).

Radiation Proctitis

Radiation proctitis is an uncommon but important cause of lower gastrointestinal tract bleeding. Approximately 5–15% of patients having radiation therapy develop some form of enteritis or colitis. Men who have undergone radiation therapy for a prostatic or bladder cancer and women who have had similar treatment for pelvic visceral malignancy often experience bright red rectal bleeding. Endoscopically, the process is usually limited to the rectum and distal sigmoid. While these episodes of intermittent (sometimes separated by intervals of several years) bleeding are unpredictable and cause much anxiety, they are usually self-limited or, at most, manageable by medical measures.[42] Occasionally, however, bleeding is severe enough to require transfusion and endoscopic or formal surgical therapy.

Ischemia

Intestinal ischemia is another rare cause of lower gastrointestinal tract bleeding. Rectal bleeding, usually self-limited, may be one of the presenting forms of large bowel ischemia. This may result from loss of the blood supply of the inferior mesenteric artery due to aortoiliac vascular disease or resection.[43,44] Sometimes the inferior mesenteric artery must be sacrificed during aneurysmectomy or aortoiliac reconstruction.[44] Significant colon ischemia from this cause is seen in about 1% of aneurysmectomy patients and can be suspected on the basis of bright red rectal bleeding, with or without acidosis, within the initial four days after aneurysmectomy. The diagnosis is confirmed by endoscopy.[44]

Rare Causes

Still more rare causes of gastrointestinal tract bleeding (minor or massive) include carcinoid tumor of the ileum, colonic varices, cytomegalovirus, solitary cecal and rectal ulcers, aortoenteric fistulas, ruptured splenic artery aneurysm, lymphoma, and postischemic colonic ulcers. Direct trauma, either self-inflicted or otherwise induced, may cause anal bleeding. These injuries should be suspected in patients with a history compatible with rectal penetration.

ENIGMATIC BLEEDING

Despite the vast array of diagnostic tools and strategies currently available, approximately 5% of patients with gastrointestinal tract bleeding (many of them in the lower tract) have no identifiable source of blood loss.[45,46] These patients, although few in number, account for a disproportionately large amount of medical resources and time, often over many years, since recurrent bleeding is very common in these patients.[3] The diagnostic yield in this group has improved in recent years through the use of intraoperative total gastrointestinal endoscopy,[45] small bowel enteroscopy,[46] and occasionally intraoperative mesenteric angiography, with or without dye injection.[47,48] The most common lesions identified in these patients have been areas of angiodysplasia,[49] usually in the small bowel, as well as leiomyomas of the small intestine.

MORTALITY

The mortality rate for all patients with lower gastrointestinal hemorrhage has been reported to be as high as 11.4%. The mortality rates for massive bleeding in surgical series have ranged from 17% to 21%.[21] Factors which contribute most to high mortality include age and its multiple associated degenerative disorders and increased vulnerability to surgical intervention. Systemic diseases such as chronic renal failure or refractory coagulopathy, inaccurate diagnosis, and immunosuppression from cancer chemotherapy or acquired immune deficiency syndrome also increase the chance of dying from massive bleeding. Blind partial or subtotal colectomy has been well documented as a prelude to a greater postoperative mortality. Concomitantly, the decreased morbidity and mortality associated with guided selective resection or avoidance of surgery altogether have been clearly demonstrated.[23,27,50,51] Selective angiography has played a major role in the reduction of mortality when bleeding detected by angiography can be stopped by the use of intra-arterial vasopressin. Even if the cessation of bleeding is only temporary, it allows stabilization of the patient and better preparation for surgery, if needed, diminishing the anticipated risk.[27,52] At times angiographic control of bleeding is definitive, thus averting an operation altogether.

CONCLUSION

Lower gastrointestinal tract bleeding, a problem that previously was handled with difficulty, can now be managed with more confidence and less empiricism because the diagnosis can be conducted with modern diagnostic facilities. It is hoped that newer medical and surgical therapies, many of them endoscopic, will permit even more directed, less invasive therapy which will further decrease mortality in these patients.

REFERENCES

1. Mant A, Bakey EL, Chapus PH, et al: Rectal bleeding: Do other symptoms aid in diagnosis? *Dis Colon Rectum* 32:191–196, 1989.

2. Johnson SJ, Jones PF, Kyle J, et al: Epidemiology and course of gastrointestinal hemorrhage in North East Scotland. *Br Med J* 3:655–660, 1973.
3. Spiller RC, Parkins RA: Recurrent gastrointestinal bleeding of obscure origin: Report of 17 cases and a guide to logical management. *Br J Surg* 70:489–493, 1983.
4. Colacchio TA, Forde KA, Patsos TJ, et al: Impact of modern diagnostic methods on the management of active rectal bleeding: Ten year experience. *Am J Surg* 143:607–610, 1982.
5. Berry AR, Campbell WB, Kettlewell MGW: Management of major colonic hemorrhage. *Br J Surg* 75:637–640, 1988.
6. Benson CD, Linkner LM: The surgical complications of Meckel's diverticulum in infants and children. *Arch Surg* 73:393–398, 1956.
7. Habr-Gama A: Paediatric colonoscopy, in Hunt RH, Waye JD (eds): *Colonoscopy—Techniques, Clinical Practice and Colour Atlas.* London, Chapman and Hall, 1981, pp 395–399.
8. Robert JR, Sachar DB, Greenstein AJ: Severe gastrointestinal hemorrhage in Crohn's disease. *Ann Surg* 213:207–211, 1991.
9. Richardson JD, Max MH, Flint LM Jr, et al: Bleeding vascular malformations of the intestine. *Surgery* 84:430–436, 1978.
10. Forde KA: Colonoscopy in acute rectal bleeding. Gastrointestinal bleeding. *Gastrointest Endosc* 27:219–220, 1981.
11. Silberman H, Crichlow RW, Caplan HS: Neoplasms of the small bowel. *Ann Surg* 180 (2):157–161, 1974.
12. Akwari OE, Dozois RR, Weiland LH, et al: Leiomyosarcoma of the small and large bowel. *Cancer* 42:1375–1384, 1978.
13. Steger AC, Galland RB, Hemingway A, et al: Gastrointestinal hemorrhage from second source in patients with colonic angiodysplasia. *Br J Surg* 74:726–727, 1987.
14. Schlesinger PK, Rubenstein HA: Medical causes of intestinal bleeding. *Prob Gen Surg* 4:377–395, 1987.
15. Corman ML: *Colon and Rectal Surgery*. Philadelphia, JB Lippincott Co, 1984, pp 734–759.
16. Wig JD, Malik AK, Khanna SK, et al: Massive lower gastrointestinal bleeding in patients with typhoid fever. *Am J Gastroenterol* 75:445–448, 1981.
17. Verna P, Kapur BML: Massive bleeding due to intestinal tuberculosis. *Am J Gastroenterol* 71:217–219, 1979.
18. Stylianos S, Forde KA, Benvenisty AI, et al: Lower gastrointestinal hemorrhage in renal transplant patients. *Arch Surg* 123:739–744, 1988.
19. Mittal R, Spero JA, Lewis JH, et al: Patterns of gastrointestinal hemorrhage in hemophilia. *Gastroenterology* 88:515–522, 1985.
20. Boley SJ, DiBiase A, Brandt LJ, et al: Lower intestinal bleeding in the elderly. *Am J Surg* 137:57–64, 1979.
21. Leitman IM, Paull DE, Shires GT III: Evaluation and management of massive lower gastrointestinal hemorrhage. *Ann Surg* 209:175–180, 1989.
22. Browder W, Cerise EJ, Litwin MS: Impact of emergency angiography in massive lower gastrointestinal bleeding. *Ann Surg* 204:530–536, 1986.
23. Casarella WJ, Kanter IE, Seaman WB: Right sided colonic diverticula as a cause of acute rectal hemorrhage. *N Engl J Med* 286:450–453, 1972.
24. Vellacoff KD: Early endoscopy for lower gastrointestinal hemorrhage. *Ann R Coll Surg Engl* 68:243–244, 1986.
25. Meyers MA, Alonso DR, Gray DFJ: Pathogenesis of bleeding colonic diverticulosis. *Gastroenterology* 71:577–583, 1976.

26. Baer JW: Pathogenesis of bleeding colonic diverticulosis: New concepts. *CRC Crit Rev Diag Imaging* 11:1–20, 1978.
27. McGuire HH Jr, Haynes BW Jr: Massive hemorrhage from diverticulosis of the colon: Guidelines for therapy based on bleeding patterns observed in 50 cases. *Ann Surg* 175:847–855, 1972.
28. Madsen PER, Bekker C, Yde S, et al: Diverticulosis coli: Not a common cause of minor bleeding. *Lancet* 1:298–299, 1983.
29. Brandt LJ: *Gastrointestinal Disorders of the Elderly*. New York, Raven Press, 1984, pp 290–296.
30. Tedesco FJ, Waye JD, Raskin JB, et al: Colonoscopic evaluation of rectal bleeding. *Ann Intern Med* 89:907–909, 1978.
31. Wayne JD: Colonoscopy in rectal bleeding. *S Afr J Surg* 147 (3):143–149, 1976.
32. Hunt RH: Rectal bleeding. *Clin Gastroenterol* 7:719–740, 1978.
33. Teague RH, Manning AP, Thornton JR, et al: Colonoscopy for investigation of unexplained rectal bleeding. *Lancet* 1:1350–1352, 1978.
34. Swarbrick ET, Hunt RH, Fevre DI, et al: Colonoscopy for unexplained rectal bleeding. *Gut* 17:823, 1976.
35. Guillem JG, Forde KA, Treat MR, et al: The impact of colonoscopy on the early detection of colonic neoplasms in patients with rectal bleeding. *Ann Surg* 206:601–611, 1987.
36. Camilleri M, Chadwick VS, Hodgson JF: Vascular anomalies of the gastrointestinal tract. *Hepatogastroenterology* 31:149–153, 1984.
37. Britt L, Warren L, Moore O: Selective management of lower gastrointestinal bleeding. *Am Surg* 49:121–125, 1983.
38. Baum S, Anthanasoulis CA, Waltman AC, et al: Angiodysplasia of the right colon: A cause of gastrointestinal bleeding. *Am J Roentgenol* 129:789–794, 1977.
39. Vase P, Grove O: Gastrointestinal lesions in hereditary hemorrhagic telangiectasia. *Gastroenterology* 91:1079–1083, 1986.
40. Weaver GA, Alpern MD, Davis JS, et al: Gastrointestinal angiodysplasia associated with aortic valvular disease, part of a spectrum of angiodysplasia of the gut. *Gastroenterology* 77:1–11, 1979.
41. Cappell MS, Lebwohl O: Cessation of recurrent bleeding from gastrointestinal angiodysplasia after aortic valvular replacement. *Ann Intern Med* 105:54–57, 1986.
42. Tannenbaum GA, Forde KA: Radiation enteritis and colitis: General considerations in medical and surgical management. *Surg Rounds,* May 1986, pp 42–56.
43. Hagihara PF, Ernst CB, Griffen WO Jr: Incidence of ischemic colitis following abdominal aortic reconstruction. *Surg Gynecol Obstet* 149:571–573, 1979.
44. Forde KA, Lebwohl O, Wolff M, et al: Reversible ischemic colitis: Correlation of colonoscopic and pathologic changes. *Am J Gastroenterol* 72:182–185, 1979.
45. Bowden TA: Intraoperative endoscopy of the gastrointestinal tract, in Dent TL, Strodel WE, Turcotte JG, et al (eds): *Surgical Endoscopy*. Chicago, Year Book Publishers, 1985, pp 167–188.
46. Lewis BS, Wayne JD: Chronic gastrointestinal bleeding of obscure origin: Role of small bowel enteroscopy. *Gastroenterology* 94:1117–1120, 1988.
47. Anthanasoulis CA, Moncure AC, Greenfield AJ, et al: Intraoperative localization of small bowel bleeding sites with combined use of angiographic methods and methylene blue injection. *Surgery* 87:77–84, 1980.
48. Hines JR, Stryker SJ, Nieman HL, et al: Intraoperative angiography in intestinal angiodysplasia. *Surg Gynecol Obstet* 152:453–459, 1981.

49. Thompson JN, Salem RR, Hemingway AP, et al: Specialist investigation of obscure gastrointestinal bleeding. *Gut* 28:47–51, 1987.

50. Gianfrancisco JA, Abcarian H: Pitfalls in the treatment of massive lower gastrointestinal bleeding with "blind" colectomy. *Dis Colon Rectum* 25:441–445, 1982.

51. Drapanas T, Pennington DG, Kappleman M, et al: Emergency subtotal colectomy: Preferred approach to management of massive bleeding diverticular disease. *Ann Surg* 177:519–526, 1973.

52. Wright HK: Massive colonic hemorrhage. *Surg Clin North Am* 60:1297–1304, 1980.

3

PATHOLOGY OF THE BLEEDING LESIONS

C. Paul Swain, M.D.

Close observation of the pathology of gastrointestinal bleeding can offer insights into the causes of the bleeding and its recurrent nature, as well as the potential and limitations of various therapies for this common medical emergency.

PEPTIC ULCER BLEEDING

Pathology

Peptic ulcer bleeding is usually due to the chance erosion of an ulcer into an artery. This was established by comprehensive studies of morbid anatomy conducted in Paris and Vienna in the first half of the nineteenth century. The Parisian pathologist Cruveilhier (Figure 3.1) in 1829 described the appearance of a vessel protruding from the floors of gastric ulcers in patients dying of gastrointestinal bleeding as follows:

> At the level of the lesser curve there is a deep ulceration. The edge and floor of the ulcer are cicatrised, excepting at a point where there is a clot of blood elevated like a nipple; a stylet introduced into the coronary (left gastric) artery of the stomach and directed toward the end of the vessel pushes the clot out and enters the cavity of the stomach; but on withdrawing the stylet a little, and pushing it in the same direction, it can be made to reenter the vessel, which was not completely severed but only cut about three quarters of its circumference.[1]

Rokitansky, whose huge personal series of postmortem examinations in Vienna formed the basis of his comprehensive three-volume textbook of pathological anatomy, published between 1842 and 1846,[2] described patients dying from bleeding duodenal ulcers which had penetrated the gastroduodenal artery. He made it clear that these chronic ulcers had penetrated a vessel that was outside the serosal surface of the duodenum.

Since the time of Cruveilhier and Rokitansky, many pathological series, including

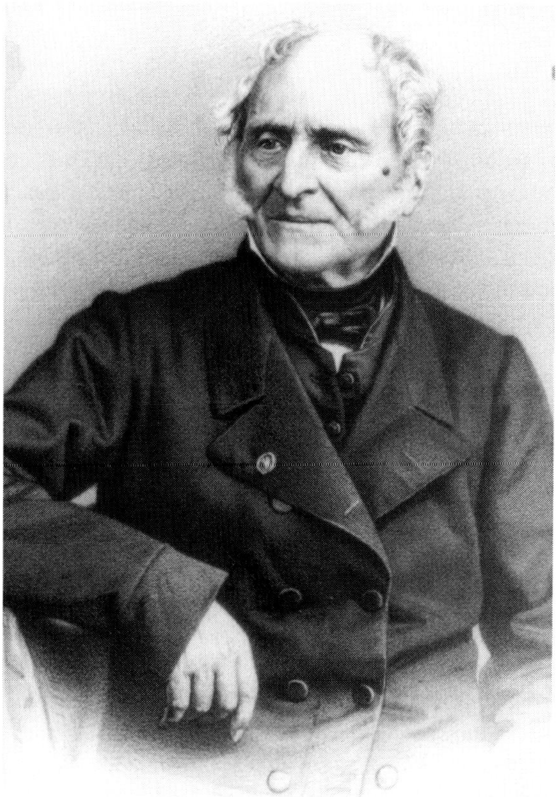

Figure 3.1. Jean Cruveilhier, 1840. An engraving from a daguerrotype.

those of Dieulafoy,[3] Bolton,[4] Tixier, and Clavel,[5] Meulengracht,[6] Osborne,[7] and Chalmers et al.,[8] have stressed that the finding of an exposed and eroded artery in the floors of ulcers in patients dying of gastrointestinal bleeding indicates the source and cause of major bleeding from ulcers.

A recent investigation attempted to examine in detail the source of the bleeding in a consecutive series of 27 patients whose gastric ulcers were removed at urgent gastrectomy because of recurrent bleeding.[9] Erosion of a single artery in the floor of the gastric ulcer was found to be the significant source in all but one patient; this patient was found to be bleeding from a duodenal ulcer that was not included in the specimen. In 4 patients with bleeding ulcers, the accompanying vein as well as the artery was breached; in 10 patients, small vessels (<0.1 mm) were also found to have been eroded. These small vessels and veins were not thought to have contributed significantly to the blood loss. As first pointed out by Rokitansky in 1842,[2] bleeding arteries in gastric and duodenal ulcers are frequently serosal, i.e., on the outside of the stomach or duodenum because the ulcerating process has completely destroyed the submucosa and muscularis propria. Nearly one-half of gastric ulcers were found to have eroded a serosal artery; in the other half the artery was submucosal, with an intact muscularis propria.

Vascular Anatomy of Bleeding Peptic Ulcer

Site of the Bleeding Ulcer and Artery: Anatomy of Ulcer Bleeding

Severe bleeding from ulcers in the duodenum and stomach is common at two sites. In the duodenum the proximal inferoposterior duodenal bulb[10] and in the stomach the high posterior lesser curve are the common sites of severe recurrent bleeding. It is probably not accidental that these sites are close to the largest arteries related to the stomach and duodenum; the gastroduodenal artery runs under the duodenal bulb at the first site, and the left gastric artery runs down behind the lesser curve close to the second site. Vessels are commonly eroded a few branch points from the main trunk, but particularly severe bleeding can ensue if the main branch is eroded. The main trunk of the gastroduodenal artery, a branch of the hepatic artery, is large (3–6 mm),[11] larger than arteries that are usually eroded by gastric ulcers. Measurements of the eroded vessel in patients with fatal bleeding from duodenal ulcers suggest a bimodal distribution, with one-third of the vessels being larger than 1 mm (up to 3.45 mm).[10] Erosion of the gastroduodenal artery may explain why the results of treatment in drug trials and trials of therapeutic endoscopy appear to suggest that duodenal ulcers respond less well to such treatment than gastric ulcers (Plate 6).

The duodenal bulb, i.e., the first 1.5 inches of the duodenum, receives its blood supply from two main sources.[12] The inferoposterior surface of the bulb, which is the common site of severe bleeding, is supplied chiefly by small branches from the gastroduodenal artery given off as that vessel passes behind the bowel. The anterosuperior surface is supplied from an artery called the *supraduodenal artery,* which can arise from either the gastroduodenal or the hepatic artery.[13] Mayo[14] and Mall[15] have observed that the duodenal mucosa close to the pylorus is relatively poorly vascularized.

The capillaries of the stomach mucosa are supplied by long mucosal arteries (mean length, 120 μm)[16] which cross the submucosa obliquely to penetrate the muscularis mucosae and reach the mucosal layer. Although arteries of this caliber are frequently breached by bleeding gastric ulcers,[9] they are probably too small to account for major bleeding from ulcers. There is a wide connection of the mucosal arteries throughout the stomach by their free anastomosis as they approach the muscularis mucosae and again on the glandular side of that muscle layer.[17-21] There are no anatomical end arteries in the stomach.[16] In the anterior and posterior walls of the body of the stomach arise an extensive branching plexus of larger arteries within the stomach wall, but these originate outside the stomach wall from the arterial chain on the greater and lesser curves.[12,16,22–24] The erosion of an ulcer into one of these arteries, either on the submucosal side in acute ulcers or on the serosal side in chronic ulcers, is the usual cause of major bleeding.[1-10,25,26] The left gastric artery divides into two branches as it turns down the lesser curve, one running anterior and the other posterior to the midpoint of the lesser curve, and both vessels lie within the lesser omentum. One or both of these branches, usually the anterior, joins directly with the small right gastric artery to complete the arterial chain of the lesser curve.[16]

There are minor anatomical variations which may affect the pattern of bleeding. On the lesser curve, which is the most common site of major bleeding from gastric ulcers, the mucosal arteries may not arise from a plexus of vessels within the stomach wall but rather outside the stomach, directly from the right and left gastric arterial chains.[23]

In the pyloric antrum, the plexus in the submucosa is formed of smaller vessels[16,19,23] than at other sites, which may explain the lower incidence of significant bleeding and rebleeding from antral ulcers.[14]

A Stochastic Theory of Ulcer Bleeding: Big Artery, Big Bleed Theory

One might argue that a statistical (stochastic) approach based on the chance erosion of arteries of different sizes could explain the wide range of clinical patterns of ulcer bleeding.[27,28] Most ulcers erode only small vessels, which bleed trivially. When some ulcers erode into medium-sized vessels, they produce manifest bleeding, but normal mechanisms of thrombosis and healing prevent recurrent bleeding. Erosion of larger arteries exceeding the capacity of normal mechanisms of hemostasis produces the clinical patterns of recurrent or continuous hemorrhage.

Trivial bleeding from ulcers is probably very common. Endoscopists frequently observe stigmata of recent hemorrhage, i.e., blood adherent to ulcers in patients without evidence of manifest bleeding.[29] They know that trivial trauma of granulation tissue on the edge of an ulcer can cause minor bleeding, while similar trauma of normal mucosa does not. Bleeding severe enough to cause hematemesis or melena is usually due to the ulcerating process pathologically eroding a single artery of moderate size in the floor of the ulcer crater (Plate 7).

The size of the artery that is accidentally eroded by the ulcer is probably an important determinant of the pattern and the outcome of ulcer bleeding. Flow and, therefore, the potential rate of blood loss vary with the fourth power of the internal diameter of the vessel. Increasing the vessel's diameter by only 1.2 times doubles the flow; if the diameter is doubled, the flow increases by 16-fold.

Theoretical Model of Blood Loss

To illustrate the dynamics of blood loss that can be inferred from these measurements, a simplified model (Table 3.1) for estimating the rate of blood loss from a bleeding gastric artery was constructed based on radiographic and histological measurements. It assumes that the artery branches at three points into three branches of equal cross-sectional area on the way from the aorta to the bleeding point, and that the distances between the branch points are equal.

Using Poiseuille's formula for deriving flow rate in a cylinder, if the mean internal diameter of a bleeding gastric artery is 0.3 mm,[9] the average rate of calculated blood loss would be 67 cc/hr (Table 3.1). Because flow increases with the fourth power of the internal diameter, a 1.2 times increase in the internal diameter of the artery would double the flow from a bleeding artery. Blood flow from a vessel with an internal diameter of 0.6 mm can be 1,066 cc/hr if the other parameters are not altered.

Clinical data which may support this stochastic theory of the cause of gastrointestinal bleeding include the observation that large ulcers are significantly more likely to be associated with bleeding than small ulcers,[30] since there is a greater chance that a large ulcer will erode into a vessel of significant size. Wara's[31] observation of a lower incidence of rebleeding from a visible vessel in an antral ulcer than in a high lesser curve or

TABLE 3.1. Estimate of the Rate of Blood Loss From a Typical Bleeding Gastric Artery Based on Radiographic and Histological Measurements

Data:

Blood viscosity, μ = 2.70 centipoises

Blood pressure = 120/80 = 100 mm Hg mean

Length of individual vessels $L/4$ = 3.5 cm

Cross-sectional area of bleeding vessel $A/4 = 7.1 \times 10^{-2}$ mm^2

If pressure difference P = 100 mm Hg

Length of vessel	$L1$	$= L2$	$= L3$	$= L4$
Cross-sectional area of vessel	$A1$	$= 3A2$	$= 9A3$	$= 27A4$
Flow rate	$Q1$	$= 3Q2$	$= 9Q3$	$= 27Q3$
Pressure difference	ΔP	$= \Delta P1 + \Delta P2 + \Delta P3 + \Delta P4$		

Poiseuille has shown that

$$\text{Flow rate } Q = \frac{\pi d4 \times \Delta p \pi}{128\ \mu l}$$

$$\text{Blood loss } Q4 = \left(\frac{1}{1 + 1/3 + 1/9 + 1/27}\right)\left(\frac{A^2}{4}\right)\Bigg| \times \Delta P$$

$$= 67 \text{ cc/hr}$$

Source: Swain et al.[9]

duodenal ulcer would also be explainable by the smaller size of the arteries found in this area.[16,19,23]

Drabig in 1937[32] suggested that major bleeding might be due to ulcer erosion into unusually large submucosal arteries but quoted Djorup[24] in regard to normal arterial diameter: 1.0 mm in the cardia and 0.5 mm in the fundus of the stomach. The arteries in his cases were at the upper limit of this normal diameter. Voth in 1962[25,26] also hinted that ulcer bleeding might be due to the ulcer's eroding into an abnormally large vessel but ultimately suggested that the eroded artery is at the upper limit of normal. There is limited information on size variations in arteries in the human stomach and duodenum.

Size of the Bleeding Artery

Measurements of the size of bleeding arteries in gastric ulcers in 27 patients requiring urgent gastrectomy because of recurrent bleeding varied from 0.1 to 1.8 mm, with a mean external diameter of 0.7 mm.[9] Measurements of the size of bleeding arteries in 29 patients with fatal duodenal ulcer bleeding showed that the bleeding artery varied in size from 0.1 to 3.45 mm, with a mean external diameter of 0.9 mm.[10]

Pathology of the Bleeding Vessel: Rotten Artery, Recurrent Bleed Theory

The artery is usually rotten at the bleeding point, and the pattern of the rot may affect the clinical pattern of bleeding.

Arteritis

Arteritis with a polymorphonuclear infiltrate and fibrinoid necrosis was observed in more than three-quarters of the eroded arteries in bleeding gastric ulcers[9] (Plate 8) and in 60% of the eroded arteries in bleeding duodenal arteries.[10] This arteritis is presumably chemical, being caused by acid digestion of tissue in the ulcer. Arteritic degeneration is focal, being more severe on the side of the arterial wall closest to the ulcer floor, as is clearly seen in Plate 9. Although the opposite wall of the bleeding artery is sometimes inflamed, it is always intact. This extensive arteritis leading to necrosis of the vessel wall (Plate 9) produces a hole in the side of the vessel wall closest to the ulcer floor, which not only causes bleeding but may prevent vascular mechanisms of hemostasis such as vessel contraction from occurring and expose clot formed by intravascular thrombosis to the effects of acid and proteolytic enzyme digestion.

In one-quarter of the cases, the vein accompanying the eroded artery is also involved. Rarely, erosion of a vein is the main cause of bleeding from a peptic ulcer (Plate 10).

Aneurysmal Dilatation

More surprisingly, aneurysmal dilatation of the artery, always placed eccentrically, with the dilatation directed toward the ulcer crater and often protruding into it, is observed at the bleeding point in half of these bleeding arteries in gastric ulcers (Plates 11 and 12). Aneurysmal dilatation was found less commonly (14%) on eroded vessels in bleeding duodenal ulcers.

Thrombus and Recanalization

Thrombus above or within the bleeding vessel is very common, being seen in 89% of gastric and 59% of duodenal bleeding arteries. This indicates that clot-forming mechanisms were activated but were inadequate to staunch the bleeding.

Recanalized thrombus is seen in about one-quarter of such cases. This suggests that in these cases the artery had bled, stopped bleeding as normal clotting mechanisms became effective, but rebled when recanalization occurred.

Pathological Processes and Further Bleeding

The extensive nature of the chemical arteritis leading to necrosis of the vessel wall might explain why normal mechanisms of intravascular thrombosis or repair are inadequate to prevent further bleeding. In any case, thrombosis is inefficient in the presence of an acid environment.[33] Erosion of one side of the vessel wall without rupture of the artery prevents retraction/contraction mechanisms by which most severed arteries of the size that are involved in ulcer bleeding (about 0.7 mm in the stomach and 1.0 mm in the duodenum) usually stop bleeding. The presence of true or false (clot-covered) aneurysms at the bleeding point may explain the common clinical pattern of intermittent but severe bleeds as the aneurysm holds for a while and then ruptures. Successful drug-induced healing of an ulcer around a protruding aneurysm (Plate 12) may not prevent a further catastrophic bleed. Thrombosis and recanalization suggest another mechanism for the common intermittent pattern of ulcer bleeding and the endoscopic observation that about three-quarters of patients at risk for further bleeding do not bleed at their initial urgent endoscopy.

The Arteriosclerotic Artery as a Rare Cause of Further Bleeding

Because elderly patients are at high risk of death from bleeding ulcer, it has sometimes been suggested that arteriosclerotic change in the wall of arteries of patients with ulcer bleeding is a factor which can splint the eroded artery, preventing vasospasm and healing and explaining the poor outcome in elderly patients.[34-36]

This view is incorrect. The arteriosclerotic and atheromatous changes frequently seen in medium-caliber vessels in the branches of the cerebral and coronary arteries in elderly patients are rarely encountered in the gastric and duodenal arteries. Frank[37] has reviewed the literature on arteriosclerosis and gastric bleeding, gathering the very few cases in which this finding was substantiated. He analyzed submucosal arteries of the stomach in 100 postmortem examinations and found only 2/100 instances of moderate arteriosclerosis. In 35 cases, minimal or moderate arteriosclerosis was seen in the submucosal ramifications of the gastric arteries. In Frank's view, this was of doubtful functional significance. These data are supported by those of Osborne,[7] who found 0/58 cases of atheroma/arteriosclerosis in patients dying of bleeding gastric ulcer and by Swain,[28] who recorded 0/27 cases of atheroma in patients having gastric resections for bleeding ulcer and 1/29 in patients dying of bleeding duodenal ulcer. Atheromatous plaques are sometimes found in larger vessels from which the vessels supplying the stomach and duodenum are derived. Brooks[38] found macroscopic arteriosclerotic lesions in the branches of the celiac axis in 19/368 postmortem examinations. Maljatzakaja[39] reported relatively little arteriosclerotic change in the large branches of the left gastric and gastroduodenal arteries in a systematic study of this process in 85 cases. In the gastroduodenal artery he described uniform, diffuse thickening of intima and elastic lamellation in 16/85 cases, which, if present, was associated with severe aortic arteriosclerosis.

Rarely, patients have been found at postmortem or resection to have bled repeatedly from large and apparently arteriosclerotic arteries in the submucosa.[32,37,40-43]

True or false aneurysms are found fairly commonly in arteries that have bled in the base of gastric ulcers (50%),[9] as well as duodenal ulcers (14%)[17] (Plate 12). Aneurysms not due to peptic ulceration rarely occur on arteries adjacent to the stomach and duodenum. These may either rupture into the peritoneum or erode through to bleed into the stomach or duodenum.[44-47]

Acid-Pepsin and Recurrent Ulcer Bleeding

The recurrent nature of peptic ulcer bleeding may be due to the highly acidic nature of gastric juice, which prevents effective hemostasis by acting adversely on various pH-dependent aspects of the coagulation cascade and platelet function.[33]

Is recurrent bleeding from peptic ulcers more common than expected? It is possible to list other causes of troublesome recurrent bleeding where pH is not relevant. For example, recurrent bleeding from subarachnoid hemorrhage[48,49] occurs with roughly the same frequency (20-30%) as peptic ulcer bleeding and recurrent bleeding from aortic aneurysm occurs even more frequently.

One would also predict that recurrent bleeding would be far more common at sites of low pH in the gastrointestinal tract, i.e., the stomach and duodenum, than at other sites if pH were important as a cause of recurrent bleeding. It is, of course, true that most gastrointestinal bleeding episodes are due to a gastric or duodenal cause, but recurrent anemia from peptic ulcers or gastric carcinoma is not more common than that from colonic or esophageal ulcers or cancer. Indeed, some patients with gastric carcinoma may be protected by achlorhydria. Recurrent bleeding from telangiectasia is not obviously more of a problem in the stomach than in the colon, although a gastric source for gastrointestinal bleeding is more likely with hereditary hemorrhagic telangiectasia, perhaps because that is where the largest gastrointestinal telangectasias tend to congregate. There is no evidence that low pH is important in the recurrence of bleeding from esophageal varices, since the esophagal pH is usually about 8.

A major difficulty with the hypothesis that pH is important in the pathogenesis of recurrent bleeding is that therapy directed at reducing pH has not been convincingly effective in improving the outcome. For example, the Collins and Langman[50] meta-analysis of 27 published studies of cimetidine and ranitidine, randomizing a total of 2,500 patients in the treatment of bleeding peptic ulcer, showed that the rebleeding rates in treated and untreated patients with bleeding duodenal ulcer were identical. A recent randomized study of high-dose omeprazole in 1,154 patients has also failed to demonstrate a reduction in further bleeding or improvement in endpoints in patients with gastrointestinal bleeding.[51] Omeprazole-treated patients had equal or nonsignificant lower rates than placebo-treated patients for recurrent bleeding (14.7% vs. 14.7%), transfusion requirements (48% vs. 55%), and the need for surgery (10.6% vs. 11.1%), while omeprazole-treated patients had a statistically nonsignificant higher mortality [40 vs. 30 (20 vs. 6 after surgery)].

Another study by Peterson et al.[52] compared sustained achlorhydria using intravenous cimetidine infusion and nasogastric infusion of antacid with cimetidine alone in 70 patients. Rebleeding occurred in 6/35 (17%) of the cimetidine plus antacid group and in 4/35 (11%) of the cimetidine alone group. This difference was not statistically significant.

Implications for Drug and Endoscopic Therapy of Bleeding Ulcer

If a burst waterpipe were to flood your kitchen, would you call a plumber or a pharmacologist? If severe ulcer bleeding is conceived as being due to holes in necrotic, often aneurysmally dilated, large arteries, it is difficult to expect miracles from H-2 blockers or other ulcer-healing drugs. Healing the ulcer and reducing the pH may not be sufficient to promote effective thrombosis or healing of an aneurysmally dilated artery. Certainly, if the ulcerating process is not reversed, the ulcer may erode further into the same vessel or into another vessel. Most rebleeds occur within 48 hours, whereas the time scale of effective ulcer healing is much longer.

There may be some logic in the use of antifibrinolytic drugs to discourage the dissolution of a clot. However, a protruding clot over an eroded vessel in an ulcer floor will be removed by repair mechanisms at some stage, leaving the surface of the vessel that bled dangerously exposed. Antifibrinolytic drugs seem to offer limited protection against further bleeding from aneurysms.

The presence of aneurysm may encourage clinicians still interested in drug therapy for peptic ulcer bleeding to consider using agents that lower systolic blood pressure while maintaining circulating volume, in imitation of current medical therapy for aneurysm at other sites.

There are implications for clinicians interested in endoscopic therapy for bleeding ulcers. The majority of these bleeding arteries are less than 1 mm in diameter. Lasers and endoscopic electrode systems are effective in coagulating arteries up to 1 mm in diameter in animal models, but these thermal methods become less effective as the vessel diameter increases above 1 mm. Arteries greater than 1 mm are occasionally encountered as a source of bleeding, and reliable endoscopic means to deal with such vessels need to be developed.

The presence of aneurysm or vessel necrosis at the bleeding point may explain why endoscopic coagulation therapy directed at the vessel sometimes causes arterial bleeding and lends support to the empirically derived method of treating around the circumference of an exposed vessel in order to increase the chance of thermally coagulating the normal vessel without disturbing the aneurysm.

DIEULAFOY'S ULCER (OR EROSION) (EXULCERATIO SIMPLEX)

A currently popular and arguably mythical cause of rare gastrointestinal bleeding is the eponymous entity ascribed to Dieulafoy. Dieulafoy, in his excellent article in 1889,[3] described 11 cases of acute gastric ulcers of the high lesser curve confined to the submucosa which bled from a vessel visible in the floor of the ulcer and titled his article "Exulceratio Simplex" ("From a Simple Ulcer"). The name of Dieulafoy has now become associated with bleeding from a large vessel protruding from an ulcerated area less than 5 mm in diameter (i.e., endoscopically an erosion)[32,53] or, mythically, as argued by Bolton,[4] from an area without ulceration. Perhaps Dieulafoy might feel that it is better to be misquoted than not quoted at all. Dieulafoy, by the way, is humorously depicted as a marvelously smooth private practitioner in Proust's great novel *Remembrance of Things Past.*[54]

Review of the 101 cases included by Veldhuyzen Van Zanten[53] in the quite large literature of causes of bleeding ascribed to the Dieulafoy exulceratio simplex suggests that this is a mixed bag with an unconvincing label. The cases can be grouped as follows:

1. An erosion, i.e., an ulcerated area of less than 5 mm with a protruding, eroded vessel.[4,26,53,55-67] This type includes the majority of cases. It seems likely that some evolve as bleeding from a conventional ulcer, and the ulcer heals around the bleeding vessel.
2. Aneurysms of uncertain cause on submucosal gastric arteries.[68-76]
3. Unusual, sometimes acquired, vascular anomalies. Louwerens et al.,[77] for example, suggest that their case was a vascular anomaly with a large anastomosis between superior and inferior mesenteric arteries secondary to a blockage at the origin of celiac and superior mesenteric arteries. Various "malformations" are claimed for Dieulafoy, mostly arterial (i.e., aneurysmal or "abnormally large"), by Fixa et al.,[78] Richter,[79] and Gough,[80] but some are described as arteriovenous malformations,[81]

distinctive arteriovenous malformations,[82] or hemangioma.[83] An interesting recent fashion has been to suggest that "caliber-persistent artery of the stomach" with an (artifactually) convoluted, abnormally large, nontapering artery may be the cause of the bleeding,[84] but most of these cases conform to my definition of an ulcer with a vessel, i.e., a break in the mucosa greater than 0.5 cm with an eroded artery in or protruding from the ulcer floor. Eidus et al.[85] have suggested that the apparent convolution was not artifactual in their case.

4. Cases in which major bleeding occurred and was seen at endoscopy to be coming from the proximal stomach but which could not be located at operation, gastrectomy, or postmortem, e.g., case 5 of Veldhuyzen Van Zanten et al.[53]

Dieulafoy[3] made it clear that he was describing an ulcer, not an erosion. His ulcers were described as being the size of a sous, a coin which in 1898 measured 10 mm in diameter.

Some authors suggest that Gallard's early description (1884) of "Aneurysmes miliares de l'estomac, donnant lieu a des hematemeses mortelles"[68] is the first description of the entity that they are describing. An even earlier report from Murchison[55] at the Middlesex hospital in 1870, "Two Cases of Fatal Haematemesis from Very Minute Ulcers Perforating a Small Artery in the Coats of the Stomach," gives a more convincing account of this entity than many recent descriptions.

Some authors try to distinguish this as a specific pathological entity on the grounds that (1) the lesion is characteristically high on the lesser curve within 6 cm of the cardia, but this area is the most common site for massive bleeding from ulcers; (2) the vessel is larger than normal, but large vessels are often found to be eroded as a source of bleeding from acute ulcers and, in any case, measurements of normal arterial size in the stomach are not available; (3) there is a specific arteriovenous vascular anomaly capable of bleeding, with little or no break in the mucosa, but the majority of accounts which include assessable histology reveal an eroded artery deep to the muscularis mucosae or aneurysm; and (4) there is little or no ulceration or inflammation, but the distinction between an erosion and an ulcer is an artificial one based on size, while inflammation in an ulcer may clear as the ulcer heals.

GASTRIC EROSIONS

Major bleeding from an artery eroded by a single erosion, usually on the high lesser curve of the stomach, was discussed in the previous section.

Erosions are a common finding in patients with gastrointestinal bleeding but are an unusual cause of massive bleeding. Sometimes multiple erosions are seen, many with stigmata of recent hemorrhage. Although it is probable that a small amount of blood has been lost from each erosion with stigmata of recent hemorrhage, the vessels eroded are probably too small, singly or in combination, to cause massive bleeding, and that when massive bleeding does occur, it is due to the erosion of a single medium-sized artery. Bolton[4] has argued eloquently against the concept of *gastrorrhagia,* or diffuse bleeding from multiple bleeding sites, and for the theory of a single eroded vessel as the cause of gastrointestinal bleeding. Several endoscopic series have suggested that erosions are a common cause of gastrointestinal bleeding. For example, the survey of 2,097 patients contributed by 277 members of the American Society for Gastrointestinal Endoscopy suggested that bleeding was secondary to the endoscopic finding of erosions in 30% of cases.[86] There is a problem in that erosions are a common finding in endoscopic studies in the absence of bleeding.[87-89] Laine and Weinstein[90] have pointed out that erosions are an uncommon cause of major bleeding. In their prospective study of 329 patients who had gastrointestinal bleeding with hemodynamic instability or who required blood transfusion, only 3% had endoscopic erosive gastritis as the only significant endoscopic finding. Jensen[91] reported significant bleeding from erosions in 2% of patients admitted for severe upper gastrointestinal bleeding. In my own series of 725 endoscopies for gastrointestinal bleeding, erosive gastritis was described in 31%, stigmata of hemorrhage adherent to the erosions in 28% of these patients, but only 11 patients had further bleeding and 3 came to gastrectomy (Plates 13 and 14).

Linear Erosions and Hiatus Hernia

Cameron and Higgins[92] described linear erosions positioned on the crests of folds at the diaphragmatic impression in one-third of 109 patients with large hiatus hernia and suggested that these erosions were caused by the mechanical trauma of folds rubbing together during diaphragmatic movement with breathing. Some patients were anemic, perhaps due to blood loss from these erosions.

PROLAPSE GASTROPATHY

Prolapse gastropathy is a syndrome characterized endoscopically by a focal area with subepithelial hemorrhage and, occasionally, erosions within a few centimeters of the cardioesophageal junction. This mucosal area may be seen to form the apex of a knuckle of gastric mucosa which prolapses into the distal esophagus during retching. These patients often give a history of retching prior to hematemesis.[93-96] Shepherd et al.[96] described the histological appearance following endoscopic biopsy in 21 cases of prolapse gastropathy. They reported inflammation in 85%, submucosal hemorrhage in 38%, and superficial ulceration in 10%.

"CONGESTIVE GASTROPATHY," VASCULAR ECTASIA, AND PORTAL HYPERTENSION

McCormack et al.[97] and Quintero et al.[98] suggested that portal hypertension can produce a vascular abnormality which may be associated with bleeding. In the McCormack et al. series, half of the patients with varices and abnormal-appearing gastric mucosa had mucosal vascular ectasia at endoscopic biopsy, and all seven who came to surgery had both mucosal and submucosal vascular ectasia. Quintero et al. reported that mucosal vascular ectasia was present on antral endoscopic biopsy in 8 of 11 cirrhotic patients bleeding from red spots in the antrum. They also suggested that hypergastrinemia and low levels of pepsinogen 1 might explain these findings.

Francavilla[99] found that erosions occurred significantly more frequently in cirrhotics

(35% of 237 patients) than in noncirrhotics (5% of 1,142 patients; $p < 0.001$) and were observed more frequently in patients with large, long variceal cords. Erosions were no more common in alcoholic than in nonalcoholic cirrhotics.

ANGIODYSPLASIA

Although endoscopic biopsy is often disappointing, operative histological examination preceded by careful injection of the vascular system is more frequently rewarding.[100-103]

The characteristic abnormality is the presence of significantly dilated submucosal venous channels (up to twice the normal diameter),[102] as well as tortuous, thin-walled, endothelium-lined venules and veins. The crypt architecture is not altered, and there is little or no inflammation in the lamina propria. Since the main abnormality is located in the submucosa, superficial, mainly mucosal endoscopic biopsies may not show any microscopic abnormality. The vessels of angiodysplasia are not true malformations, as are some congenital lesions, but resemble ordinary venules and capillaries, apart from their increase in size and concentration.

Large angiodysplasia may show additional microscopic pathology. The mucosa may have abnormal, dilated, and tortuous capillaries and venules, causing distortion and compression of the crypts. Hypertrophy of the intima is sometimes seen, as in true arteriovenous malformation.[104] Submucosal arteries are occasionally dilated, may be sclerotic, and rarely contain atheromatous (cholesterol) emboli.[105,106]

Cannulation of the artery and vein of resected specimens at surgery is done by flushing heparinized saline, with subsequent injection of radiopaque silicone rubber[100,102,107,108] or colloid barium sulfate[109] into the arterial system for radiological and histological demonstration of the presence of angiodysplasia.

The cause of gastrointestinal angiodysplasia has yet to be established. Boley et al.[110] persuasively argued that colonic angiodysplasias are caused by a degenerative aging process in which dilatation of submucosal veins occurs as a result of repeated obstruction by muscular contraction where the veins penetrate the muscular layer of the colon. This may cause dilatation and ectasia of the associated venules, with the consequent appearance of arteriovenous shunts.

REFERENCES

1. Cruveilhier J: *Anatomie pathologique du corps humaine.* Paris, Balliere, 1829, p 42.
2. Rokitansky CF von: *Handbuch der allgemeinen pathologischen Anatomie.* 3 vols. Vienna, Braunmuller and Seidel, 1842–1846. Vol 3, pp 193–194. For the English translation, see Rokitansky CF von: *A Manual of Pathological Anatomy,* 4 vols. London, Sydenham Society, 1839–54, vol 2, pp 33–34. Translated from the German by Edward Sieveking.
3. Dieulafoy G: Exulceratio simplex. *Bull Acad Med* 39–40:49–82, 1898.
4. Bolton C: *Ulcer of the Stomach.* London, Edward Arnold, 1913.
5. Tixier L, Clavel C: *Les grandes hemorrhagies gastroduodenales.* Paris, Masson et Cie, Libraire de l'Academie de Medecin, 1933, p 27.
6. Meulengracht E: Fifteen years experience with free feeding of patients with bleeding peptic ulcer: Fatal cases. *Arch Intern Med* 80:697–708, 1947.

7. Osborne GR: The pathology of gastric arteries with special reference to fatal haemorrhage from peptic ulcer. *Br J Surg* 41:585–589, 1954.
8. Chalmers TC, Zamcheck N, Curtens GW, et al: Fatal gastrointestinal haemorrhage. Clinico-pathological correlations in 101 patients. *Am J Clin Pathol* 22:634–645, 1952.
9. Swain CP, Storey DW, Bown SG, et al: Nature of the bleeding vessel in recurrently bleeding gastric ulcers. *Gastroenterology* 90:595–608, 1986.
10. Swain P, Kalabakas A, Grandison A, et al: Size and pathology of vessel and ulcer in patients with fatal bleeding from duodenal ulcer. *Gastroenterology* 96:A133, 1990.
11. Michels NA: *Blood Supply and Anatomy of Upper Abdominal Organs with a Descriptive Atlas.* Philadelphia, Lippincott, 1955.
12. Reeves TB: A study of the arteries supplying the stomach and duodenum and their relation to ulcer. *Surg Gynecol Obstet* 30:374–385, 1920.
13. Wilkie DPD: The blood supply of the duodenum. *Surg Gynecol Obstet* 13:399–405, 1911.
14. Mayo WJ: Anaemic spot on the duodenum which may be mistaken for ulcer. *Surg Gynecol Obstet* 6:600–601, 1908.
15. Mall FP: The vessels and walls of the dog's stomach. *Johns Hopkins Hosp Rep* 1:1–36, 1896.
16. Barlow TE, Bently FH, Walder DN: Arteries, veins, and arteriovenous anastomoses in the human stomach. *Surg Gynecol Obstet* 93:657–671, 1951.
17. Arnold F: *Handbuch der Anatomie des Menschen,* Freiburg, 1847, pp 115–118.
18. Barclay AE, Bentley FH: The vascularisation of the human stomach. *Br J Radiol* 22:62–67, 1949.
19. De Busscher G: Les anastomoses arterio-veneuses de l'estomac. *Acta Neerl Morphol* 6:87–105, 1948.
20. Clara M: Die *Arterio Venoesen Anastomosen.* Leipzig: J A Barth, 1937.
21. Disse J. Ueber die Blutgefasse der menschlichen Magenschleimhaut besonders ueber Arterien derselben. *Arch Mikro Anat* 63:512–531, 1904.
22. Hoffman L, Nather K: Zur anatomie der Magenarterien. *Arch Klin Chir* 115:650, 1921.
23. Jatrou ST: Ueber die arterielle Versorgung des Magens und ihre Beziehung zum Ulcus ventriculi. *Dtsch Z Chir* 159:196–220, 1920.
24. Djorup F: Untersuchungen ueber die feinere topographische Verteilung der Arterien in den verschiedenen Schichten des menschlichen Magens. *Z Anat Entw* 64:279–347, 1922.
25. Voth D: Zur Pathogenese ungewohnlicher, arterieller Magenblutungen. *Med Welt* 19:1095–1097, 1962.
26. Voth D: Das architeconische Prinzip der Magenarterien in seiner Bedeutung fur die Magenblutung. *Zentralbl Allg Pathol* 103:553–554, 1962.
27. Swain CP: When and why do ulcers bleed and what can be done about it? *Aliment Pharmacol Therap* 1:455S–467S, 1987.
28. Swain CP: Pathophysiology of bleeding lesions. *Gastrointest Endosc* 36:S21–22, 1990.
29. Kalabakas A, Xourgias B, Karamanolis D, et al: Incidence and significance of stigmata of recent haemorrhage in ulcer patients without clinical evidence of recent bleeding. *Gut* 31: A1206, 1990.
30. Matthewson K, Pugh S, Northfield T: Which peptic ulcer patients bleed? *Gut* 29:70–74, 1988.
31. Wara P: Endoscopic prediction of major rebleeding—a prospective study of stigmata of hemorrhage in bleeding peptic ulcer. *Gastroenterology* 88:1209–1214, 1985.
32. Drabig F: Uber zwei todlicher Magenblutung aus arrodierten submucosaen Magen arterien. *Virchows Arch* 300:487–494, 1937.

33. Green FW, Kaplan MM, Curtis LE, et al: Effect of acid and pepsin on blood coagulation and platelet aggregation. *Gastroenterology* 74:38–43, 1978.
34. Anderson WAD: *Pathology*. London, Henry Kempton, 1948.
35. Burger M: *Altern und Krankheit*. Leipzig, Georg Thieme, 1947, p 268.
36. Jones FA: *Modern Trends in Gastroenterology*. London, Butterworth, 1952, pp 423–441.
37. Frank W: Hematemesis associated with gastric arteriosclerosis. *Gastroenterology* 7:231–240, 1946.
38. Brooks H: A preliminary study of visceral arteriosclerosis. *Am J Med Sci* 131:778–786, 1906.
39. Maljatzakaja MI: Uber die Atherosklerose der Bauch arterien. *Beitr Z Pathol Anat* 94:81–110, 1934.
40. Hirschfeld H: Ein Fall von todtlicher Magenblutung in Folge miliaren Aneurysmas einer Magenschleimhaut-arterie. *Berl Klin Wochenschr* 41:584–587, 1904.
41. Lewin AM: Zur lehre der Arteriosklerose des Magens. *Arch Verdauungsk* 14:114–122, 1908.
42. Buday KV: Uber die Sklerose der Magenarterien. *Beitr Pathol Anat* 44:327–348, 1908.
43. Antonie T: Arteriosclerosis of the arteries of the stomach. *Med J Aust* 48:210–211, 1961.
44. Crile G, Newell ET: Abdominal apoplexy. Spontaneous rupture of a visceral vessel. *JAMA* 114:1155, 1940.
45. Green WT, Powers JH: Intra-abdominal apoplexy. *Ann Surg* 93:1070–1074, 1931.
46. Monaci M: Una rara complicazione dell arterio-sclerosi gastrica: Rottura dell'arteria gastrica sinestra e conseguente ematoma gastrico intramurale e sottosieroso. *Arch ''De Vecchi'' Anat Patol* 12:1067–1069, 1959.
47. Taylor CE: Ruptured anastomotic aneurysm of gastric arteries. Case report and review of literature. *Am J Surg* 68:258–260, 1945.
48. McKissock W, Richardson A, Walsh L: Posterior communicating aneurysms: A controlled trial of the conservative and surgical treatment of ruptured aneurysms of the internal carotid artery at or near the point of origin of the posterior communicating artery. *Lancet* 1:1203–1206, 1960.
49. Winn HR, Richardson AE, Jane JA: The long term prognosis in untreated cerebral aneurysms: The incidence of late hemorrhage: A 10 year evaluation of 364 patients. *Ann Neurol* 1:358–370, 1977.
50. Collins R, Langman M: Treatment with histamine H2 antagonists in acute upper gastrointestinal hemorrhage: Implications of randomised trials. *N Engl J Med* 313:660–666, 1985.
51. Daneshmend TK, Hawkey CJ, Langman MJS, et al: Omeprazole v. placebo for acute upper gastrointestinal bleeding: A randomized double blind controlled trial in 1154 patients. *Gut* 31:A1206, 1990.
52. Peterson WL, Hartless K, Meadows T: Prevention of recurrent ulcer bleeding: Double blind, randomized trial of a regimen designed to produce sustained achlorhydria. *Gastroenterology* 98:A106, 1990.
53. Veldhuyzen Van Zanten SJO, Bartelsman JFWM, Schipper MEI, et al: Recurrent massive haematemesis from Dieulafoy vascular malformation—a review of 101 cases. Progress report. *Gut* 27:213–222, 1986.
54. Proust M. *Remembrance of Things Past,* Vol 2, *The Guermantes Way* (trans. Scott Monrieff CK, and Kilmartin T). Penguin Books, pp 349, 354–355. (Originally published 1921; English translation published 1981.)
55. Murchison C: Two cases of fatal haematemesis from very minute ulcers perforating a small artery in the coats of the stomach. *Trans Pathol Soc Lond* 21:162–166, 1870.
56. Juler GL, Labitzke HG, Lamb R, et al: The pathogenesis of Dieulafoy's gastric erosion. *Am J Gastroenterol* 79:195–200, 1984.

57. Saur K: Die solitare Exulceratio simplex (Dieulafoy) als Ursache einer schweren akuten Magenblutung. *Chirurg* 44:293–299, 1973.

58. Chapman I, Lapi N: A rare cause of gastric hemorrhage. *Arch Intern Med* 112:347–351, 1963.

59. Rossi NP, Green EW, Pike JD: Massive bleeding of the upper gastrointestinal tract due to Dieulafoy's erosion. *Arch Surg* 97:780–797, 1968.

60. Roding H: Zur Behandlung der Exulceratio simplex Dieulafoy des Magens. *Zentralbl Chir* 7:253–256, 1963.

61. Markby C: Massive haemorrhage from superficial gastric erosions. *Br J Surg* 52:685–691, 1965.

62. Katano M, Fujii Y, Muto Y, et al: A case of Exuleratio simplex (Dieulafoy). *Jpn J Surg* 10:63–66, 1980.

63. Streicher HJ: Die solitaire Exulceratio Simplex (Dieulafoy) als Ursache massiver Intestinalblutungen. *Dtsch Med Wochenschr* 91:991–995, 1966.

64. Magriter R, Weinman S, Reidler L, et al: Die Exulceratio simplex Dieulafoy. *Leber Magen Darm* 7:353–356, 1977.

65. Broberg A, Ihre Th, Pyk E, et al: Exulceratio simplex as a conceivable cause of massive gastric hemorrhage. *Surg Gynecol Obstet* 154:186–188, 1982.

66. Cornelius HV: Zur Pathogenese der sogenannten akuten solitaren Magenerosion (Dieulafoy). *Frankfurter Z Pathol* 63:582–588, 1952.

67. Mallory T: Case 32402. *N Engl J Med* 235:524–527, 1946.

68. Gallard T: Aneurysmes miliares de l'estomac, donnant lieu a des hematemeses mortelles. *Bull Soc Med Hop Paris* 1:84–91, 1884.

69. Donaldson GA, Hamlin E: Massive hematemesis resulting from rupture of a gastric artery aneurysm. *N Engl J Med* 243:369–373, 1950.

70. Goldman RL: Submucosal arterial malformation (aneurysm) of the stomach with fatal hemorrhage. *Gastroenterology* 46:589–594, 1964.

71. Hoelzer H: Uber einer todliche Verblutung aus einem miliaren Aneurysma einer Magenschleimhautarterie. *Zentralbl Chir* 61:1996–1999, 1936.

72. Albrich W: Ein Fall von Verblutung aus einem Aneurysma einer Magenarterie. *Wien Med Wochenschr* 41:792–793, 1951.

73. Millard M. Fatal rupture of gastric aneurysm. *Arch Pathol* 59:363–371, 1955.

74. Bailey ME: Rupture of a gastric artery aneurysm. *J Can Med Assoc* 75:131–133, 1956.

75. Helliwell M, Irving JD: Haemorrhage from gastric artery aneurysms. *Br Med J* 282:460–461, 1981.

76. Tanner NC: The diagnosis and management of massive haematemesis. *Br J Surg* 300:1411–1413, 1964.

77. Louwerens JWK, Gratama S, Zwaan A, et al: Dieulafoy erosion in the stomach as a result of an intra-abdominal vascular anomaly (case report). *Br J Surg* 75:489–490, 1988.

78. Fixa B, Komarca O, Devorakova I: Submucosal arterial malformation of the stomach as a cause of gastrointestinal bleeding. *Gastroenterologia* 105:357–365, 1966.

79. Richter RM: Massive gastric hemorrhage from submucosal arterial malformation. *Am J Gastroenterol* 64:324–326, 1975.

80. Gough MH: Submucosal arterial malformation of the stomach as the probable cause of recurrent severe haematemesis in a 16-year-old girl. *Br J Surg* 64:522–524, 1977.

81. Sherman L, Shenoy S, Satchidand SK, et al: Arteriovenous malformation of the stomach. *Am J Gastroenterol* 72:160–164, 1979.

82. Mortensen NJ, Mountford RA, Davies JD, et al: Dieulafoy's disease: A distinctive arteriovenous malformation causing massive gastric haemorrhage. *Br J Surg* 70:76–78, 1983.

83. Bongiovi JJ, Duffy JL: Gastric hemangioma associated with upper gastrointestinal bleeding. *Arch Surg* 95:93–98, 1967.

84. Miko TL, Thomazy VA: The caliber persistent artery of the stomach: A unifying approach to gastric aneurysm, Dieulafoy's lesion, and submucosal arterial malformation. *Hum Pathol* 19:914–921, 1988.

85. Eidus LB, Rasuli P, Manion D, et al: Caliber persistent artery of the stomach (Dieulafoy's vascular malformation). *Gastroenterology* 99:1507–1510, 1990.

86. Gilbert DA, Silverstein FE, Tedesco FJ, et al: The national ASGE survey on upper gastrointestinal bleeding. III. Endoscopy in upper gastrointestinal bleeding. *Gastrointest Endosc* 27:94–102, 1981.

87. Sauerbruch T, Schreiber MA, Schussler P, et al: Endoscopy in the diagnosis of gastritis. *Endoscopy* 16:101–104, 1984.

88. Nesland AA, Berstad A: Erosive prepyloric changes in persons with and without dyspepsia. *Scand J Gastroenterol* 20:222–228, 1985.

89. Green PHR, Fevre DI, Barrett PJ, et al: Chronic erosive (verrucous) gastritis. A study of 108 patients. *Endoscopy* 9:74–78, 1984.

90. Laine L, Weinstein WM: Subepithelial hemorrhages and erosions of human stomach. *Dig Dis Sci* 33:490–501, 1988.

91. Jensen D: Endoscopic control of gastrointestinal bleeding with non-laser devices, in Fleischer D, Jensen D, Bright P, et al (eds): *Therapeutic Laser Endoscopy in Gastrointestinal Disease*. Boston, Martinus Nijhoff, 1983, pp 39–49.

92. Cameron AJ, Higgins JA: Linear gastric erosion. A lesion associated with large diaphragmatic hernia and chronic blood loss anemia. *Gastroenterology* 91:338–342, 1986.

93. Axon ATR, Clarke A: Haematemesis: A new syndrome? *Br J Med* 1:491–492, 1975.

94. Young GP, Thomas RJS, Wall AJ: Retrograde gastric mucosal prolapse as a cause of haematemesis. *Med J Aust* 2:488–489, 1976.

95. Thomas E, Khatak KG: Hemorrhage due to retrograde prolapse of the stomach. *Am J Gastroenterol* 71:477–480, 1979.

96. Shepherd HA, Harvey J, Jackson A, et al: Recurrent retching with gastric mucosal prolapse: A proposed prolapse gastropathy syndrome. *Dig Dis Sci* 29:121–128, 1984.

97. McCormack TT, Sims J, Eyre-Brook I, et al: Gastric lesions in portal hypertension: Inflammatory gastritis or congestive gastropathy? *Gut* 26:1226–1232, 1985.

98. Quintero E, Pique JM, Bombi JA, et al: Gastric mucosal vascular ectasias causing bleeding in cirrhosis. A distinct entity associated with hypergastremia and low serum levels of pepsinogen 1. *Gastroenterology* 93:1054–1061, 1987.

99. Francavilla A: The role of portal hypertension in gastric erosions of cirrhotics: Possibilities and limits. *Endoscopy* 19:253–254, 1987.

100. Aldabagh SM, Trujillo YP, Taxy JB: Utility of specimen angiography in angiodysplasia of the colon. *Gastroenterology* 91:725–729, 1986.

101. Hartford WV: Gastrointestinal angiodysplasia: Clinical features. *Endoscopy* 20:149–151, 1988.

102. Shah IA: Angiodysplasia: Morphological diagnosis. *Endoscopy* 20:149–151, 1988.

103. Gilmore PR: Angiodysplasia of the upper gastrointestinal tract. *J Clin Gastroenterol* 10:386–394, 1988.

104. Holman E: Contributions to cardiovascular physiology gleaned from clinical and experimental observations of arteriovenous communications. *J Cardiovasc Surg* 3:48–63, 1962.

105. Margolis AR, Galdabini JJ: Case records of the Massachusetts General Hospital (Case 36-1974). *N Engl J Med* 291:569–575, 1974.

106. Mitsudo SM, Boley SJ, Brandt LJ, et al: Vascular ectasias of the right colon in the elderly: A distinct pathologic entity. *Hum Pathol* 10:585–600, 1979.

107. Reynolds DG: Injection techniques in the study of intestinal vasculature under normal conditions and in ulcerative colitis, in Boley SJ, Schwartz SS, Williams LF (eds): *Vascular Disorders of the Intestine*. New York, Appleton-Century-Crofts, 1971, pp 383–395.

108. Reed DK, Porter LE, Zajiko AB, et al: Pre- and intraoperative localization of small bowel arteriovenous malformation. *J Clin Gastroenterol* 8:166–170, 1986.

109. Moore JD, Thompson NW, Appleman HD, et al: Arteriovenous malformations of the gastrointestinal tract. *Arch Surg* 111:381–389, 1976.

110. Boley SJ, Brandt LJ, Mitsudo SM: Vascular lesions of the colon. *Adv Intern Med* 29:301–326, 1984.

Color Plates

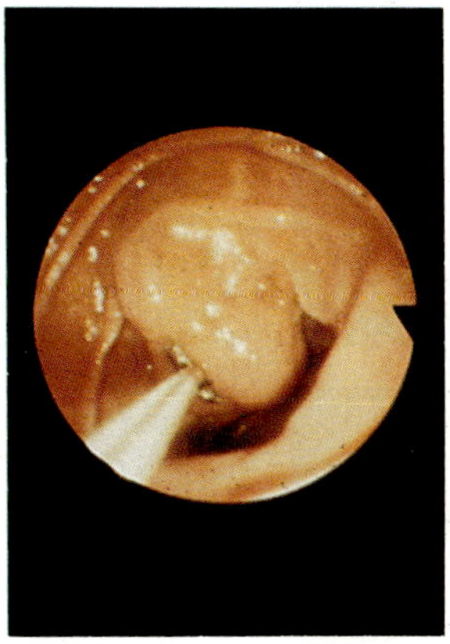

Plate 1. Gastrointestinal bleeding. Endoscopic view of a submucosal lesion (see also Figure 2.1).

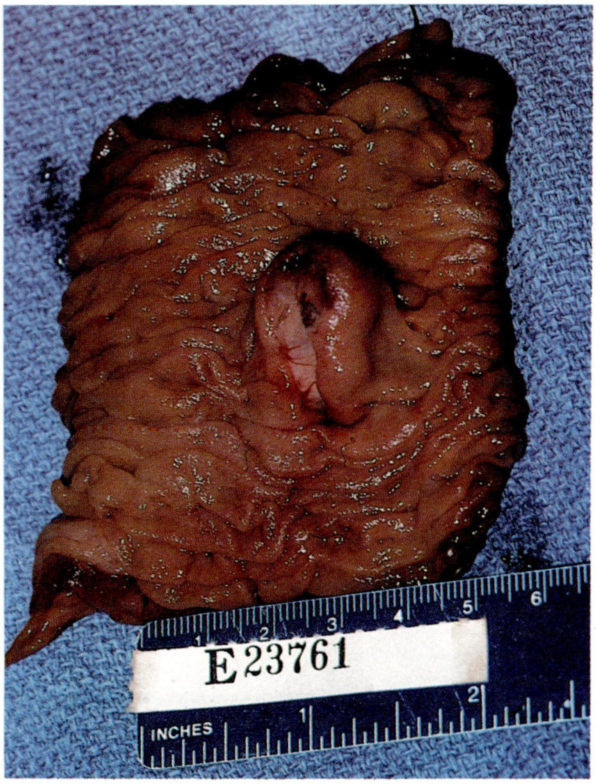

Plate 2. Resected segment of jejunum with leiomyoma.

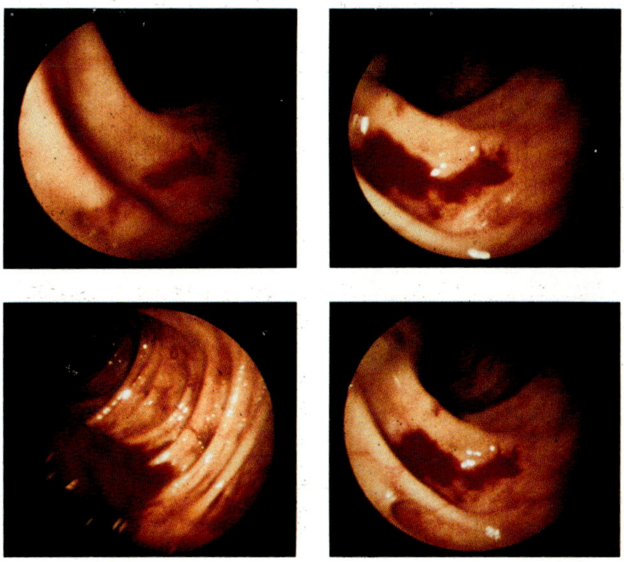

Plate 3. Colonoscopic view of an actively bleeding right colon diverticulum.

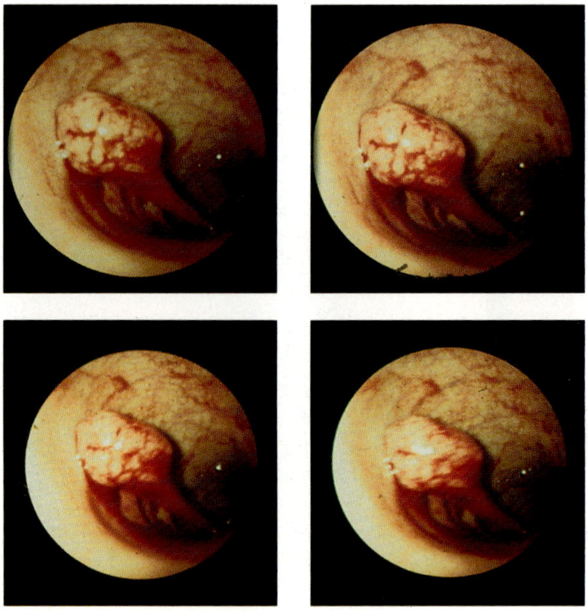

Plate 4. Colonoscopic view of an actively bleeding polyp in a chronically anticoagulated patient.

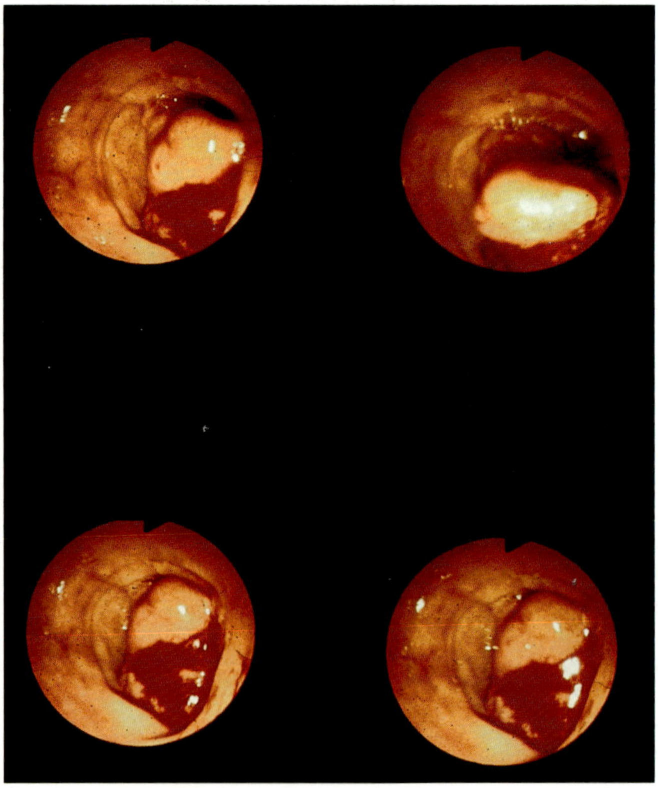

Plate 5. Colonoscopic view of an actively bleeding polypoid carcinoma.

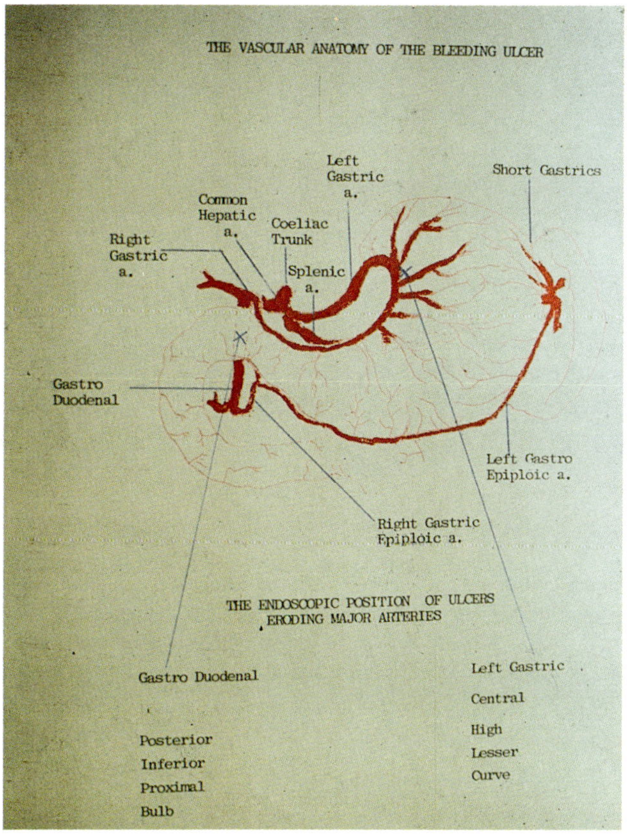

Plate 6. Vascular anatomy of the bleeding ulcer.

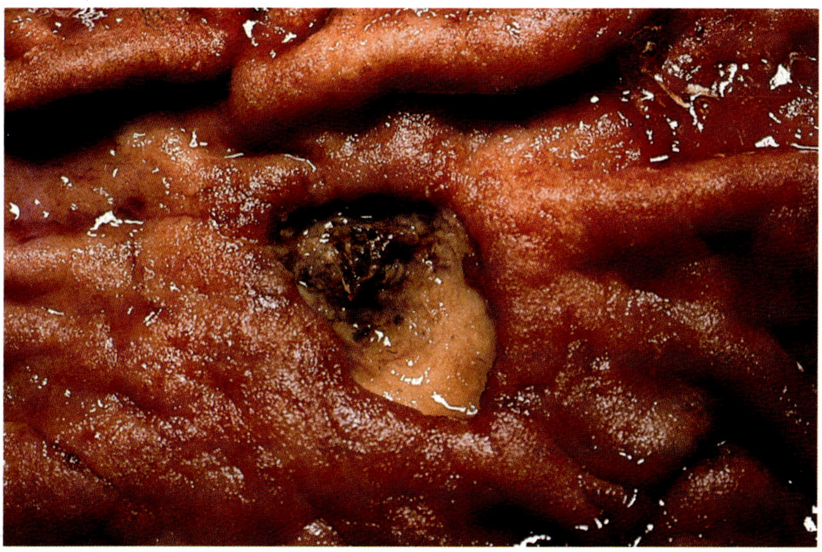

Plate 7. A resected bleeding gastric ulcer with a prominent vessel in the floor.

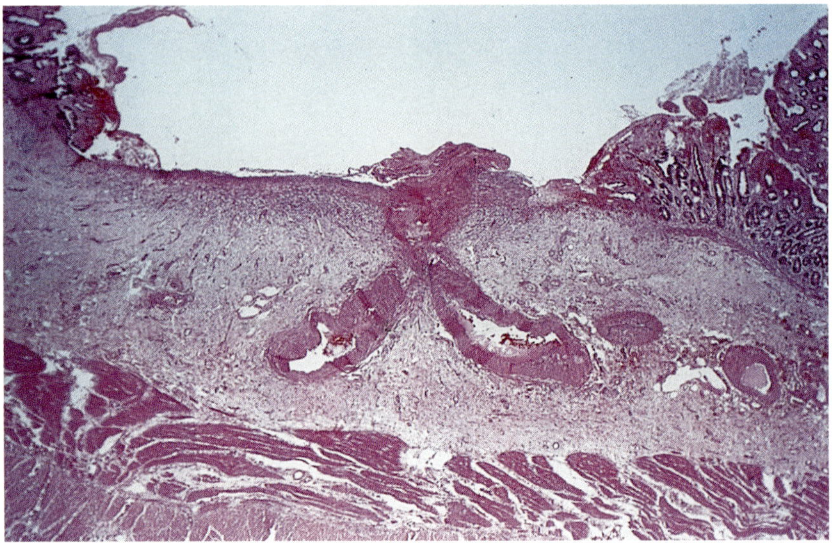

Plate 8. A resected bleeding gastric ulcer. This is an acute ulcer with an intact muscularis propria. The submucosal vessel curves up toward the ulcer floor, is aneurysmally dilated at the bleeding point, and then curves back down to run on in the submucosa. The material protruding above the surface of the ulcer is adherent clot forming a pseudoaneurysmal roof to the bleeding vessel.

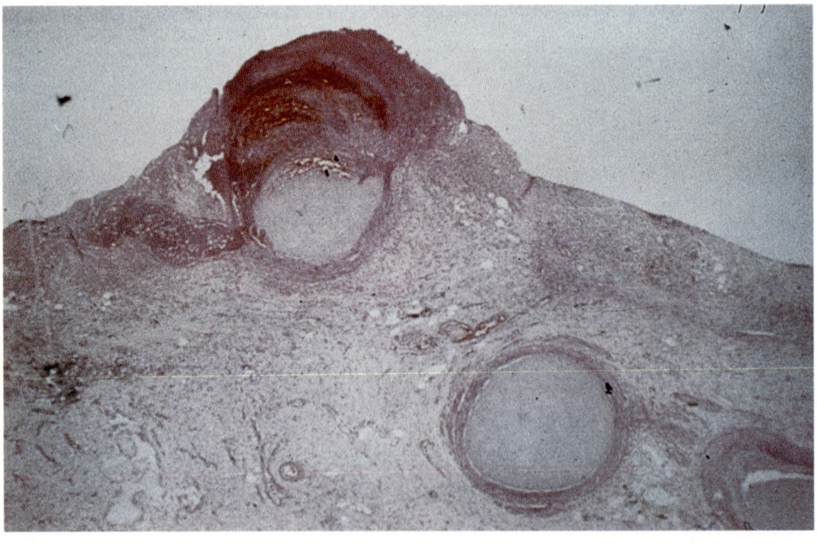

Plate 9. The structure protruding above the ulcer floor is the bleeding artery. The undersurface of the vessel is intact, but the surface protruding into the stomach is badly damaged and shows an acute focal arteritis with fibrinoid necrosis.

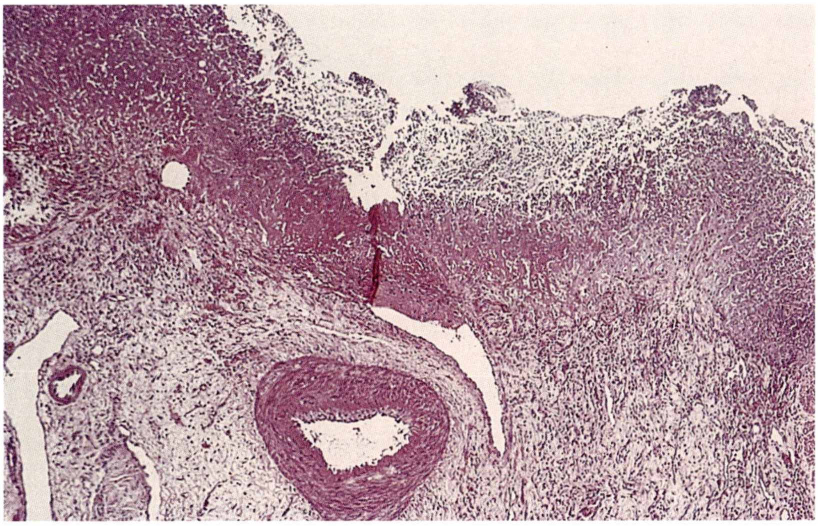

Plate 10. Most series emphasize erosion of an artery as the cause of ulcer bleeding. The accompanying vein is also commonly eroded. In this unusual case in which a patient had a surgically removed gastric ulcer for recurrent bleeding, the artery was found to be intact but the large accompanying vein was eroded and was the cause of the bleeding.

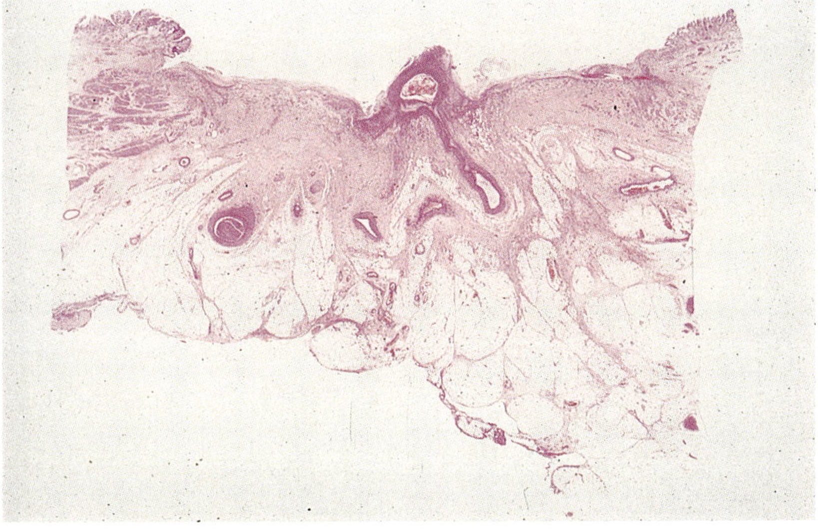

Plate 11. This is a chronic ulcer that has bled. The muscularis propria has been replaced by scar tissue. The eroded vessel is of serosal origin and has been pulled up by the ulcerating and scarring process into a V configuration. The vessel protrudes into the ulcer crater and is aneurysmally dilated.

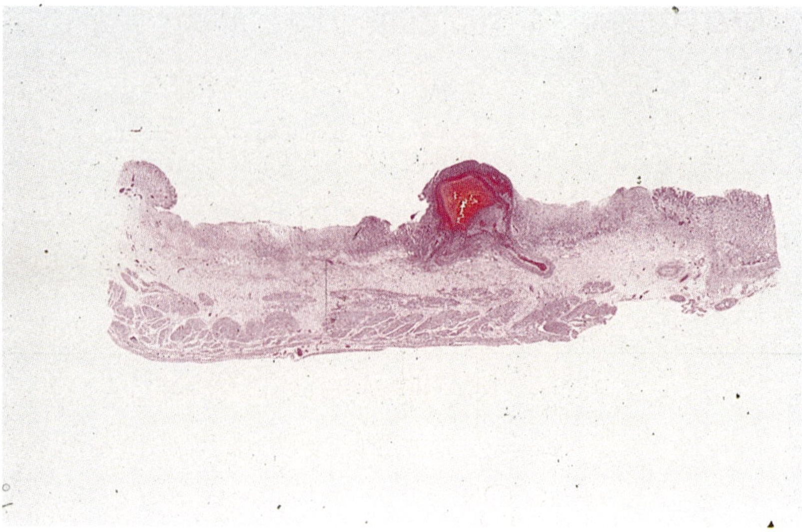

Plate 12. A large (3.2-mm) aneurysm produced in response to the ulcerating process has formed on a medium-sized (0.6-mm) submucosal artery. This is an acute ulcer with an intact deep muscle layer. This ulcer is epithelializing (healing) well. It illustrates that healing of the ulcer is unlikely to influence recurrence of bleeding from this aneurysm.

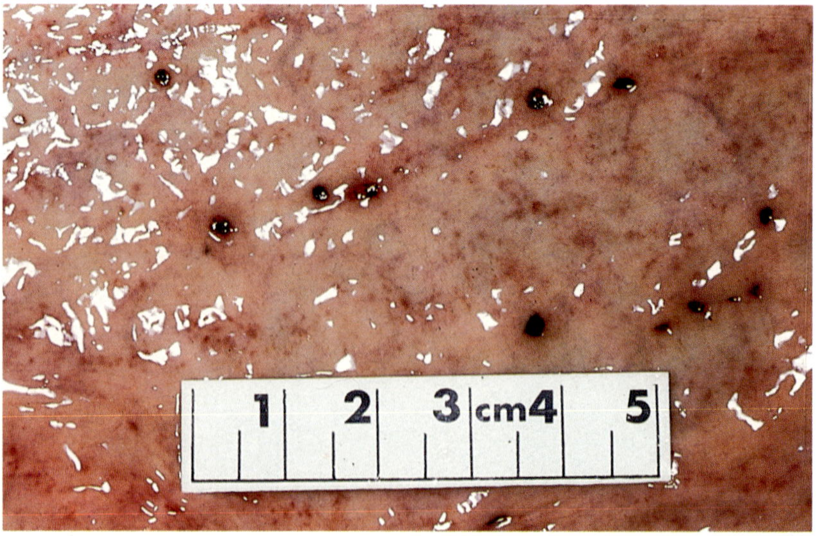

Plate 13. Multiple erosions are an uncommon cause of major gastrointestinal bleeding. In this patient who had taken nonsteroidal anti-inflammatory medication and had had a gastrectomy for recurrent bleeding, multiple punched-out erosions measuring 2–3 mm each with stigmata of recent bleeding can be seen.

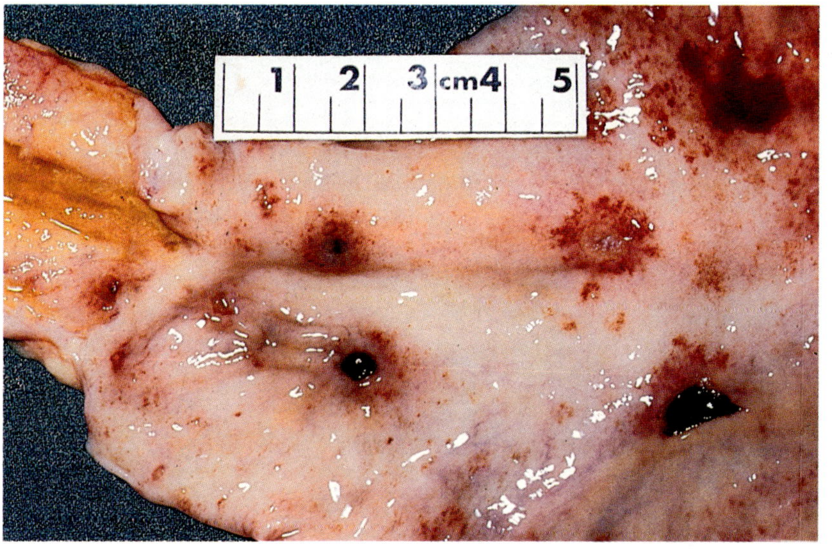

Plate 14. In the same specimen in the antrum, the erosions are larger and three are ulcers, i.e., greater than 0.5 mm in diameter.

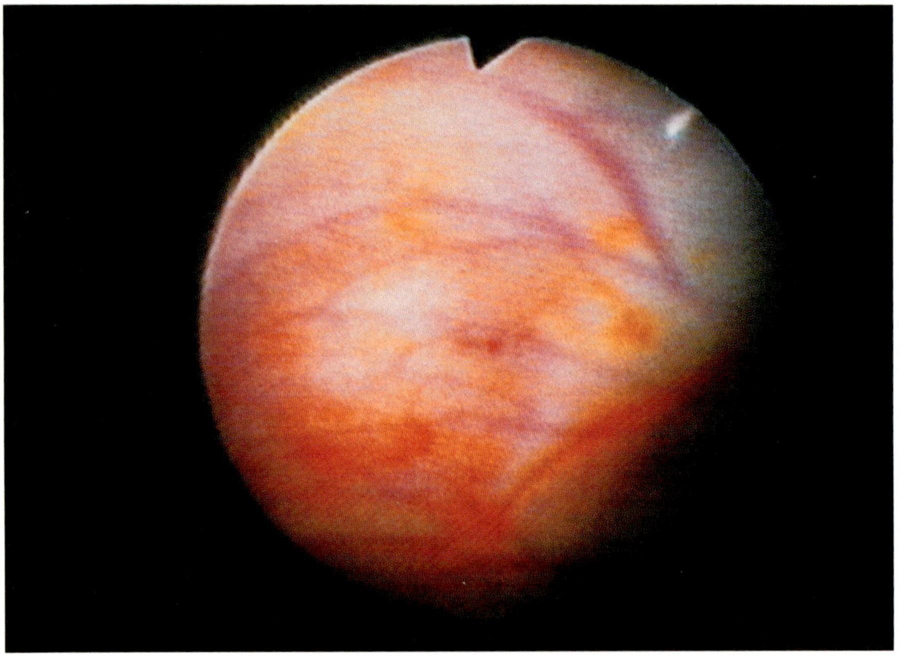

Plate 15. Colonic telangiectasia in a one-month-old infant with persistent hematochezia.

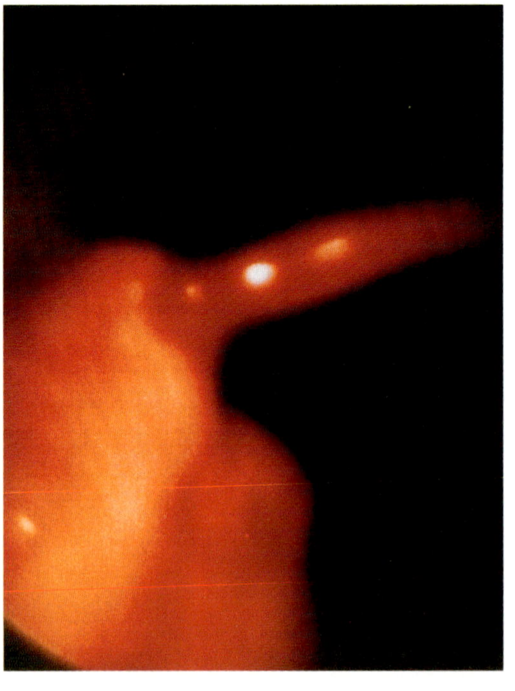

Plate 16. Bleeding varix in a 15-year-old girl with cirrhosis secondary to autoimmune chronic active liver disease.

4

GASTROINTESTINAL BLEEDING IN INFANTS AND CHILDREN

Joseph F. Fitzgerald, M.D.

Gastrointestinal (GI) bleeding occurs not infrequently in infants and children, although it is a much less common event than in adults. The sight of blood in vomitus or in the stool of a pediatric patient generates great anxiety in a parent, and subsequently in the physician of the infant or child. The bleeding may be small in amount and from a cause of relatively little significance (e.g., an anal fissure), or it may be massive and the initial presentation of portal hypertension, peptic ulcer disease, or fulminant ulcerative colitis. Early reviews of GI hemorrhage in infancy and childhood indicated that no site or cause of bleeding was found in 15–30% of cases.[1,2] Technical advances in fiberoptic instrumentation and imaging techniques now allow the identification of a bleeding site in virtually all infants and children who experience a significant bleed. The problem of chronic occult bleeding generates less concern in the pediatric population, where malignant disease of the gastrointestinal tract is rare to nonexistent.

The site of the bleeding lesion is suggested by the characteristics of the bleeding episode, as in adult patients. The vomiting of bright red blood, denatured blood, or a combination of both strongly suggests that the site of bleeding is proximal to the ligament of Treitz. The passage of black, sticky stool (melena), which is blood denatured from the actions of various secretions entering the GI tract, indicates a lesion high in the gastrointestinal tract. The presence of maroon clots in the stool suggests a bleeding site in the distal small bowel or proximal colon. Bright red blood mixed with the stool (hematochezia) places the bleeding point(s) in the distal half of the colon. Blood mixed with mucus suggests an inflammatory process, either infectious or nonspecific (e.g., inflammatory bowel disease), and ''currant jelly'' stools accompany vascular congestion and hyperemia, as is seen with an intussusception. Frank hematemesis indicates massive bleeding and is associated with a high likelihood of recurrence.[3] Diffuse mucosal disease is suggested by the passage of loose stool or blood without stool. The finding of bright red blood coating a formed stool, or in the toilet water or on the cleansing tissue following the passage of formed stool, strongly points to an anorectal lesion.

Acute GI hemorrhage, manifested by sudden onset of hematemesis or hematochezia, may be accompanied by only an abrupt onset of weakness and listlessness. Chronic GI bleeding usually presents as iron deficiency anemia, often accompanied by the subjective complaint of progressive fatigue. Patients who suffer intermittent episodes of bleeding experience intermittent hematochezia. Their stools are negative for occult blood between episodes.

Many substances that resemble blood arising from the GI tract cause undue parental panic. Red food coloring, as in Kool-Aid, various gelatin preparations, liquid medications, and certain fruits and fruit juices (e.g., tomato and cranberry juices, beets, and clingstone peaches), resemble blood when vomited or expelled in a diarrheal stool. Dark stools which resemble melena may follow the ingestion of spinach and chocolate, and may follow the consumption of bismuth and iron preparations. Over 30 years ago, Longino and Holder[4] correctly advised that the first step in the approach to GI bleeding in infants and children was to confirm the presence of blood by a guaiac test. The examining physician must always entertain the possibility that the blood that is vomited or apparently passed in the stool may have its origin outside of the GI tract. The blood may actually be the result of vigorous epistaxis, hemoptysis, hematuria, and, in the pubertal female, the onset of menarche.

CAUSES OF GI BLEEDING IN INFANTS AND CHILDREN

In the First Month of Life (Table 4.1)

Most episodes of bleeding in this period are minor and self-limited, allowing nonemergent evaluation and management. Significant GI bleeding in a newborn, however, is of great concern since neonates have a small circulating blood volume and an impaired ability to compensate for the bleeding. Animal studies indicate that newborns have an immature sympathetic-adrenal response to hypovolemia manifested by persistent bradycardia, a delay in peripheral vascular response, and a sustained reduction in myocardial blood flow.[5] Impairment of myocardial contractility may persist after fluid resuscitation.

TABLE 4.1. Causes of GI Bleeding in Neonates

Ingested maternal blood
Peptic disease, including ulcer, gastritis, and esophagitis
Traumatic injury to the esophagus or stomach
Hemorrhagic disease of infancy
Vascular malformations (telangiectasias, arteriovenous malformations, and hemangiomas)
Necrotizing enterocolitis
Allergic colitis
Infectious colitis
Small bowel volvulus
Anal fissure

Swallowed maternal blood accounts for 30% of the cases of GI bleeding in newborns.[6] Hemorrhagic disease of infancy is very uncommon today but may be seen when the mother is receiving medications such as warfarin sodium, promethazine, and phenytoin. Peptic disease, including ulceration and gastritis, may occur in newborns, especially in association with neonatal asphyxia. Ulceration of the esophagus may complicate nasogastric intubation in this age group.

Hematochezia in the neonatal period is most commonly associated with an allergic colitis. This diagnosis can be established at this age, after the exclusion of active anal disease, by the careful performance of fiberoptic proctosigmoidoscopy with rectal biopsy. The inflamed, edematous mucosa becomes normal within 72 hours of withdrawal of the offending antigen. One must consider the high likelihood that an infant who has developed colitis from the ingestion of cow milk formula is likely to develop similar manifestations when offered a soy-isolate protein formula.[7,8] The offending protein can often be reintroduced as early as 4 months of age, and virtually always by 18 to 24 months of age.

Patients with bacterial colitis usually appear ill, with fever and bloody, mucoid stools. Microscopic examination of the stool reveals abundant fecal leukocytes, often in sheets. Appropriate stool studies provide the diagnosis. Fiberoptic endoscopy of the lower GI tract is rarely necessary and, when performed, usually reveals asymmetric areas of inflammation and edema with occasional superficial ulcerations. Necrotizing enterocolitis occurs primarily in the prematurely born and in the stressed infant after the initiation of feeding. The presence of occult or gross lower GI bleeding is often accompanied by the development of abdominal distention and feeding intolerance in these patients. The diagnosis is supported by the detection of pneumatosis intestinalis on abdominal radiographs. GI vascular malformations are suggested when similar lesions are observed on the patient's skin and when a thrill or bruit is either palpated or auscultated on abdominal examination (Plate 15).

One Month to Three Years (Table 4.2)

Many of the causes of GI bleeding seen in neonates are also seen in infants. Additional diagnoses include Mallory-Weiss tear,[9] bleeding esophageal varices associated with extrahepatic portal hypertension, intussusception, Meckel diverticulum, enteric duplication, benign nodular lymphoid hyperplasia, and inflammatory bowel disease.

Portal vein atresia with compensatory cavernous transformation of the periportal vessels presents as isolated splenomegaly in the first year of life and/or with hematemesis or melena during the second year of life. The bleeding stops abruptly following decompression of the portal system, which prevents severe hemodynamic instability. Ascites is conspicuously absent. Intussusception frequently complicates an acute infectious enteritis. This occurs suddenly, with spasms of abdominal pain, often accompanied by vomiting. The passage of currant jelly stool indicates compromise of the normal enteric blood flow. The infant with a bleeding Meckel diverticulum or enteric duplication painlessly passes maroon and bright red blood per rectum. Benign nodular lymphoid hyperplasia ranks behind anal fissure and allergic colitis as a cause of bright red lower GI tract bleeding in infants less than one year of age.[10] The author has diagnosed ulcerative colitis in four patients who were less than two years old; Crohn's disease also has been reported in infants.[11]

TABLE 4.2. Causes of GI Bleeding in Infants Up to Three Years of Age

Peptic disease
Mallory-Weiss tear
Swallowed blood during epistaxis
Vascular malformation
Esophageal varices associated with cavernous transformation of the portal vein
Trauma
Intussusception
Meckel diverticulum
Enteric duplication
Volvulus
Infectious/allergic enterocolitis
Benign nodular lymphoid hyperplasia
Inflammatory bowel disease
Pseudomembranous colitis
Juvenile polyp
Anal fissure

Children Over Three Years of Age (Table 4.3)

Children with severe esophagitis may present with anemia associated with hemoccult-positive stool. Dysfunction of the lower esophageal sphincter, with resultant exposure of the esophagus to gastric peptic juices, often complicates the course of patients with collagen vascular diseases such as scleroderma and dermatomyositis.[12] These patients often develop atypical esophageal ulcers. Hemobilia and *hematochylia* should be considered in the child who has experienced closed abdominal trauma within days or weeks of presentation with intermittent hematemesis accompanied or immediately preceded by epigastric or right upper quadrant pain.[13,14] Henoch-Schonlein syndrome, a small vessel vasculitis of undetermined etiology characterized by purpura, spasmodic abdominal pain, and arthralgia/arthritis, is often accompanied by gross or occult GI bleeding. Occasionally, hemorrhage can be massive.[15] This disease complex may be complicated by profound hypoprothrombinemia, which can result in bleeding into extraintestinal organs such as the brain, lungs, and testes.[16,17] Upper GI endoscopic investigation of eight pediatric patients with Henoch-Schonlein purpura revealed erosive gastritis in one, hemorrhagic-erosive duodenitis in four, and both findings in one patient.[18] Severe inflammatory changes and angiitis were noted on the biopsy specimens obtained from the duodenum. The vascular abnormalities were histologically identical to those found in the skin of patients with anaphylactoid purpura.[18]

A bleeding Meckel's diverticulum or enteric duplication should be considered in the patient who is passing a large volume of both dark and bright red blood per rectum and who has normal findings on upper GI fiberendoscopy. Children with hemolytic uremic syndrome may present with bloody diarrhea hours to days before the appearance of chemical azotemia.[19] The relative thrombocytopenia should suggest this diagnostic possibility, since most causes of GI tract bleeding are associated with a thrombocytosis rather

TABLE 4.3. Causes of GI Bleeding in Children and Adolescents

Swallowing blood (e.g., with epistaxis)
Esophagitis
Peptic disease
Esophageal varices
Traumatic hematobilia or hematochylia
Anaphylactoid purpura
Meckel diverticulum
Duplication cyst
Infectious colitis
Inflammatory bowel disease
Hemolytic uremic syndrome
Neurofibromatosis
Antibiotic-associated colitis
Hereditary hemorrhagic telangiectasia
Primary nonspecific ileal ulcers
Gastrointestinal bleeding in the immunocompromised child

than a thrombocytopenia. There is now compelling evidence that hemolytic uremic syndrome is initiated by a shiga-like toxin produced by several enteric pathogens, including *Escherichia coli* and *Shigella dysenteriae*, and perhaps also by *Campylobacter jejuni*.[20,21] GI neurofibromatosis associated with persistent hemoccult-positive stools is a rare cause of chronic anemia.[22] Severe antibiotic-associated colitis with pseudomembrane formation may present with blood-tinged, malodorous diarrhea. Other signs usually include fever, leukocytosis, vomiting, abdominal distention, and abdominal tenderness.[23] Colonoscopy allows the diagnosis of hereditary hemorrhagic telangiectasia in children presenting with lower GI tract bleeding in the first decade of life, before they develop either skin or nasal lesions.[24] Rarely, primary nonspecific ileal ulcers have been found in children with recurrent passage of mixed dark and bright red blood. Complete upper and lower GI fiberendoscopic studies revealed no pathology in our most recent patient. Small bowel scintigraphy was unrewarding, but a very faint "blush" was noted in the distal ileum angiographically. The ulcer found in this patient was identical to those previously described in the literature.[25] The ulcer was solitary and sharply demarcated, and there was no obvious surrounding inflammation.

GI bleeding in the immunocompromised child presents a new set of diagnostic considerations to the clinician.[26] Aggressive efforts are needed to diagnose opportunistic infections leading to mucosal injury in all areas of the GI tract, stress ulcerations, and neutropenic colitis ("typhlitis") in these patients, whose ranks have increased significantly at major children's hospitals with active organ transplantation programs.[27]

ASSESSMENT

The major immediate concern in the actively bleeding infant or child is restoration and maintenance of cardiovascular stability. Communication between the gastroenterologist, surgeon, and intensivist greatly facilitates the care of the aggressively bleeding, hemodynamically unstable patient. The finding of an *age-matched* tachycardia associated with orthostatic hypotension suggests a volume deficit of 25–35% and dictates that the vascular compartment be expanded as rapidly as possible with a volume expander such as lactated Ringer solution and/or colloid (e.g., plasmanate). The insertion of one or more large-bore venous catheters is necessary to accomplish volume restoration. Blood replacement should be accomplished as rapidly as possible, and it is prudent to maintain one calculated blood volume in the blood bank available for transfusion as needed until the hemorrhagic crisis has resolved.

The patient's *medical history* should be obtained immediately from the patient or from a parent. Questions regarding the patient's general health; medical history, including information regarding serious illnesses and previous surgical procedures; history of an abnormal bleeding tendency; family history of bleeding disorders; medication history; and, in the older female, menstrual history provide valuable information. A description of the bleeding episode (e.g., hematemesis, melena, or hematochezia) will help to localize the bleeding site and allow the clinician to generate a statistically probable differential diagnosis. I have found the parental estimation of blood loss to be of limited value. The consistency of the stool and a history of painful defecation is worthwhile information in the evaluation of the patient with lower gastrointestinal tract bleeding.

A complete *physical examination* should be performed once the patient is judged to be cardiodynamically stable. The general appearance, with attention to pallor, dehydration, trauma, and the appearance of chronic illness, allows insight into diagnostic considerations. The heart rate and blood pressure should be measured in the supine and sitting (and upright when possible) positions to determine orthostatic changes. Thorough examination of the skin may uncover ecchymoses and petechiae suggestive of a bleeding diathesis, stigmata of polyp syndromes, signs of chronic liver disease, telangiectasias, and neurofibromas. Thorough abdominal examination may detect abdominal distention, hepato- and/or splenomegaly, masses, bruits, friction rubs, and focal areas of tenderness. Thorough anorectal examination will uncover perianal disease and intrarectal and pararectal masses and will allow examination of the stool for gross or occult blood. Expelled gastric fluids can be tested for blood using the Gastroccult (Smith Kline Diagnostics, Sunnyvale, CA 94086).

Apt and Downey in 1955[28] described a simple bedside test which differentiates adult from fetal hemoglobin in the vomitus or stool of newborn infants and allows detection of swallowed maternal blood. Adult hemoglobin is denatured by alkali to yellow-brown globin hematin, while fetal hemoglobin is unaffected by the addition of alkali. The test is performed by adding one part stool or gastric content to five parts water in a test tube. The supernatant hemoglobin solution is filtered or decanted after centrifugation at 2,000 rpm for one to two minutes. One ml of 0.25 N sodium hydroxide is then added to 5 ml of the hemoglobin solution, and the color change is noted after two minutes. Again, the color turns to yellow-brown if it is adult hemoglobin but remains pink if it is fetal hemoglobin. Blood from the newborn should be used as a control. The test should not be performed with melenic stool or coffee-ground gastric contents, since the blood is already denatured in those substances and will falsely indicate adult hemoglobin.

Blood should be obtained for a complete blood count, platelet count, reticulocyte count, prothrombin time, partial thromboplastin time, fractionated serum bilirubin, serum aminotransferase and gamma glutamyl transferase activities, blood urea nitrogen, electrolytes, and blood glucose. Urine should be examined for gross and occult blood.

Evaluation from this point is outlined in Figure 4.1. The *passage of a nasogastric tube* allows gentle aspiration and the examination of gastric contents. Irrigation of the stomach with either water or saline at room temperature will provide information on the site of bleeding. Recent bleeding has not originated in the nasopharynx, esophagus, or stomach if the aspirate is clear. A clear aspirate, however, does not exclude a bleeding duodenal lesion. The nasogastric tube should be removed if there is no evidence of active bleeding during this probing maneuver. It is my practice to pass a larger-diameter tube through the mouth when fresh blood is encountered in the stomach. The stomach should be distended with saline or tap water at room temperature and then irrigated with 10- to 30-ml aliquots, depending on the patient's size. Iced water or saline lavage has been abandoned in small infants because of the risk of clinically significant hypothermia and, more recently, in patients of all ages in light of the fact that cooling may impair coagulation.[29] The goal of gastric lavage is the evacuation of blood and blood clots to allow endoscopic examination of the upper GI tract. Continued aggressive bleeding precludes optimal endoscopic evaluation. Intravenous vasopressin (5.5 mU/kg/min) is effective in reducing the degree of hemorrhage, thereby allowing endoscopic examination. The infusion of vasopressin reduces cardiac output, and both systemic and splanchnic blood flow. Complications include myocardial ischemia and cardiac arrhythmia,[30,31] as well as hypertension, hyponatremia, oliguria, and seizures related to the antidiuretic hormone effect. A simultaneous nitroglycerin infusion (0.6 μg/kg/min) may reverse the detrimental cardiac side effects of vasopressin while preserving the beneficial effects.[32]

Upper GI fiberendoscopy should be performed when the infant or child vomits

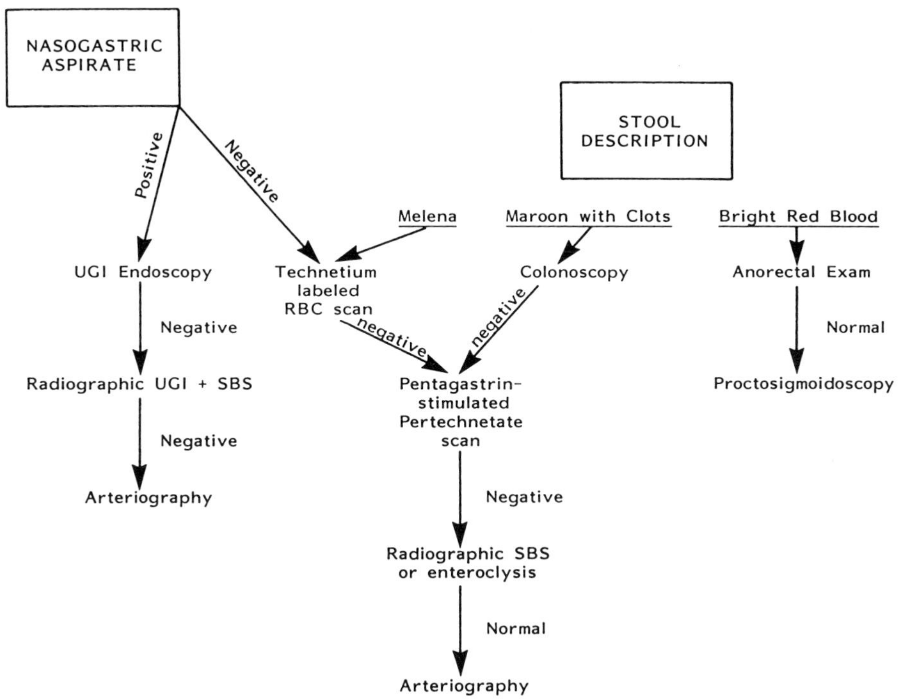

Figure 4.1. Evaluation of the infant or child with GI bleeding. (From Fitzgerald JF, Clark JH: *Manual of Pediatric Gastroenterology*. Churchill Livingstone, New York, 1988, p. 113.)

blood, or when the nasogastric aspirate is positive for blood, after the patient is hemodynamically stable and the aspirate has cleared sufficiently to allow adequate examination. All children less than 10 years of age are examined under general anesthesia in our endoscopy suite, which is located in the operating room area. The patient's status is carefully and linearly monitored by the pediatric anesthesiologist, as well as by the gastroenterologist and, when indicated, the pediatric surgeon. Endoscopy allows identification of bleeding sites and pathology from the oral cavity through the third portion of the duodenum. Frequently, we can examine the entire duodenum and proximal jejunum in younger children. Direct therapy of the bleeding lesion can be performed at this time (see below). A fiberoptic bronchoscope can be used to examine the esophagus, stomach, and proximal duodenum of the neonate and the young, small infant. This instrument has only two-way deflection of its tip and a small suction channel which limits its usefulness. It does prevent tracheal compression, which can lead to CO_2 retention and alteration of cardiorespiratory function.

From 20 to 50% of bleeding sites remained unidentified in the preendoscopic era[2,6] compared to less than 20% at the present time.[33] We have experienced extremely few complications over the past 23 years during more than 3,000 pediatric upper GI examinations. These have included four cases of aspiration pneumonia and the occasional complaint of sore throat, which is usually short-lived. We have experienced no perforations, procedure-related bleeding, infections, or deaths.

Contrast radiography of the small bowel is considered when no lesion is found on upper GI endoscopy to account for the bleeding. A recurrence of bleeding in the face of negative endoscopic and imaging studies of the upper GI tract and small bowel should lead to the performance of *arteriography,* searching for a primary or secondary vascular anomaly.[13,34-36]

A *technetium(Tc)-99M-labeled red blood cell scan* may identify an actively bleeding lesion.[37,38] This technique has been found to be accurate and sensitive in the detection of both acute and chronic-intermittent bleeding sites located distal to the ligament of Treitz. In animal studies it is possible to detect bleeding rates as low as 0.5 ml/min.[37] A sample of the patient's blood is obtained, and the red blood cells are labeled with Tc-99M and then reinjected. Gamma camera images are obtained every 5 minutes for 30 to 60 minutes and at regular intervals for as long as 24 hours when the initial study fails to demonstrate active bleeding.[38] Surgical management usually follows the definitive demonstration of a bleeding lesion on a Tc-99M-labeled red blood cell scan at our institution when a solitary lesion is suspected. A negative Tc-99M-labeled red blood cell scan is followed by a *pentagastrin-stimulated sodium pertechnetate* scan in the hope of identifying a collection of aberrant gastric mucosa in a Meckel diverticulum or a duplication cyst.[39] The latter can be located at any level of the gastrointestinal tract. Pentagastrin, in a dosage of 6 μg/kg body weight, is injected subcutaneously after a fast of approximately eight hours. The Tc-99M sodium pertechnetate is administered intravenously 15 minutes later. The sensitivity of this test can be increased further by inhibiting gastric secretion with oral administration of cimetidine (10 mg/kg) one hour before the injection of pentagastrin (Figure 4.2). False-positive scans can be seen in patients with ureteral obstruction or a sacral meningomyelocele.

Colonoscopy is the first diagnostic test performed in patients with hematochezia. We have performed colonoscopy in approximately 1,200 children and have experienced four perforations. Two occurred in patients with severe Crohn colitis, and the other two occurred during polypectomies. Limited colonoscopy (i.e., to the mid-transverse colon)

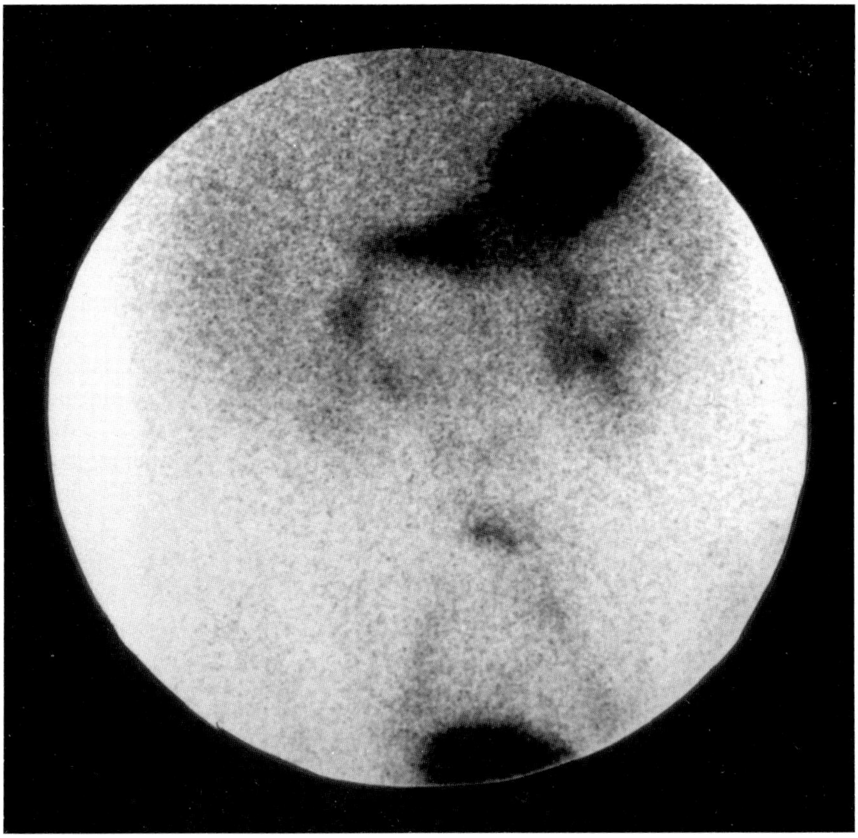

Figure 4.2. Pentagastrin-stimulated, cimetidine-blocked sodium pertechnetate scan revealing ectopic gastric mucosa in the lower midabdomen (*Meckel diverticulum*) in an 11-year-old male with intermittent abdominal pain and lower GI tract bleeding.

can be accomplished in infants at any age using a pediatric endoscope designed for examination of the upper GI tract. The limitation of this instrument is its reduced suction channel. These fiberoptic instruments allow biopsy, polypectomy, and electrocautery. We examine virtually all children under the age of 10 in our endoscopy suite with general anesthesia. The colon is prepared preferably by the administration of a poorly absorbable electrolyte solution (e.g., NuLytely; Braintree Laboratories, Inc., Braintree, MA 02184) in a dosage of 100 ml/kg. The cleansing solution is ingested in a chilled state as rapidly as the patient can tolerate. The patient who is unable to tolerate the polyethylene glycol-electrolyte solution is prepared by the provision of a clear liquid diet for 72 hours, administration of a cathartic (e.g., magnesium citrate or Dulcolax tablets) on the day prior to the examination, and phosphosoda enemas the night before and the morning of the procedure. The older child can be examined readily with appropriate parenteral sedation.

The exclusion of pathology in the colon places the lesion in the small bowel. Colonoscopy is then followed by a *pentagastrin-stimulated sodium pertechnetate scan*. *Contrast radiographic imaging* of the small bowel, preferably an enteroclysis study, is performed if the pentagastrin-stimulated sodium pertechnetate scan is negative. If no pathology is found on contrast imaging of the small bowel, *arteriography* searching for a vascular anomaly should be considered. We have performed *intraoperative endoscopy* successfully on rare occasions during the past 20 years. Upper GI fiberendoscopy is performed in the usual way, followed by surgical celiotomy. The surgeon telescopes the small intestine over the endoscope, allowing simultaneous external and internal examination of the small intestine. The distal small bowel can also be examined from below intraoperatively if the colon is adequately prepared beforehand.

Careful anorectal examination will usually provide important clues to the etiology of the passage of bright red blood per rectum. The blood is small in amount and appears on the stool or tissue following a bowel movement. The blood may be noted in the toilet water. Pain with the passage of stool strongly suggests an anal fissure. Bleeding hemorrhoids are virtually nonexistent in the pediatric age group. A pedunculated polyp is often palpated on careful rectal examination. The passage of bright red blood per rectum is rarely an emergency, and rigid proctosigmoidoscopy or fibersigmoidoscopy can be performed on an elective basis. We perform the latter examination under anesthesia in younger patients after limited distal colon preparation.

THERAPY

Esophageal varices should be suspected when a patient with splenomegaly has evidence of upper GI tract bleeding. The endoscopist should be prepared to perform sclerotherapy if bleeding varices are found (Plate 16). We inject the varices with 5% sodium morrhuate. I initially injected 0.5-ml aliquots into the varices, moving cephalad in counterclockwise rotation from the esophagogastric junction. I subsequently found it more effective to inject 1-ml aliquots into the dilated veins at or near the esophagogastric junction only. We have successfully obliterated esophageal varices in more than 40 pediatric patients to date. Some have, however, suffered renewed bleeding, with subsequent formation of new varices. We have not experienced a perforation to date; one patient has developed a modest stricture. Another patient was found to have an esophageal ulcer following initial injection which resolved without sequelae. One patient developed acute respiratory failure following injection sclerosis with 5% sodium morrhuate. This patient had symptoms and signs suggestive of adult respiratory distress syndrome. Animal studies following injection of sodium morrhuate suggest that this agent may cause severe, though transient, pulmonary hypertension which is associated with increased lymph flow.[40] We have found injection sclerosis of esophageal varices a safe and effective procedure in infants and children. It is our practice to prescribe oral propranolol, 5 mg/kg every six hours, adjusted to reduce the baseline heart rate by 25%, until the esophageal varices have been obliterated.[41]

Isolated bleeding lesions in the upper and lower GI tracts can be successfully controlled by the injection of epinephrine in a 1:10,000 dilution, in 0.5-ml aliquots, into and around the bleeding point. A recent randomized study reported a 96% success rate in the initial control of bleeding using this technique.[42] The epinephrine is injected with a sclerotherapy needle, which can be inserted through the biopsy channel of even the smaller pediatric endoscopes.

We have stopped bleeding in both the upper and lower GI tracts using electrocoagulation. Initially, we used the monopolar probe, which involves the risk of perforation due to the deep path that the electric current takes through the tissue. Also, tissue may adhere to the probe, reducing its efficacy. We have used it successfully, however, on many occasions. The BICAP probe (ACMI, Stamford, CT 06904) completes an electric circuit between two electrodes which are only 1 to 2 mm apart. The path taken through the tissue by the electrical current is shallow, which reduces the risk of perforation. Pressure can be applied on the lesion as electrocoagulation is being accomplished. The heater probe, used successfully in the management of acute bleeding in adults, does not fit through the smaller pediatric endoscopes, limiting its use in pediatrics. Colonic polyps are removed with polyp snares using monopolar or BICAP electric current.

Peptic mucosal injury may be managed with a high-potency antacid (0.5 ml/kg every two hours) to maintain a gastric pH above 4.0. Intravenously administered H-2 receptor blockers may augment the effect of the antacid in protecting the mucosa from ongoing injury. Cimetidine can be administered intravenously in a dosage of 5 mg/kg every six hours; ranitidine in a dosage of 1.2 to 1.9 mg/kg every eight hours; and famotidine in a dosage of .04 mg/kg every eight hours. I have not found sucralfate to be effective in treating this condition.

CONCLUSION

Bleeding is not an uncommon cause for referral to a pediatric gastroenterologist. Rapid initial assessment allows the generation of an age-matched differential diagnosis. The employment of techniques and technology similar to those used in the evaluation of adults with acute GI bleeding allows one to arrive promptly at the diagnosis, which permits the application of proper management. The author strongly suggests an aggressive approach to the diagnosis and management of GI tract bleeding in infants and children.

REFERENCES

1. Brayton D, Norris WJ: Gastrointestinal hemorrhage in infancy and childhood. *JAMA* 150:668–671, 1952.
2. Spencer R: Gastrointestinal hemorrhage in infancy and childhood: 476 cases. *Surgery* 55:718–734, 1964.
3. Northfield TC, Smith T: Haematemesis as an index of blood loss. *Lancet* 1:990–991, 1971.
4. Longino LA, Holder TM: Rectal bleeding in infants and children. *Pediatr Clin North Am* 6:1153–1161, 1959.
5. Horton JW, Coln D: Cardiovascular functions and fluid compartments in newborn canine hemorrhagic shock. *Am J Physiol* 248:R724–731, 1985.
6. Sherman NJ, Clatworthy HW: Gastrointestinal bleeding in neonates: A study of 94 cases. *Surgery* 62:614–619, 1967.
7. Halpin TC, Byrne WJ, Ament ME: Colitis, persistent diarrhea and soy protein intolerance. *J Pediatr* 91:404–407, 1977.
8. Powell GK: Milk- and soy-induced enterocolitis of infancy. *J Pediatr* 93:553–560, 1978.
9. Powell TW, Herbst CA, Ulshen M: Mallory-Weiss syndrome in a 10-month-old infant requiring surgery. *J Pediatr Surg* 19:596–597, 1984.
10. Kaplan B, Benson J, Rothstein F, et al: Lymphonodular hyperplasia of the colon as a patho-

logic finding in children with lower gastrointestinal bleeding. *J Pediatr Gastroenterol Nutr* 3:704–708, 1984.

11. Chong SKF, Blackshaw AJ, Morson BC, et al: Prospective study of colitis in infancy and early childhood. *J Pediatr Gastroenterol Nutr* 5:352–358, 1986.
12. Flick JA, Boyle JT, Tuchman DN, et al: Esophageal motor abnormalities in children and adolescents with scleroderma and mixed connective tissue disease. *Pediatrics* 82:107–111, 1988.
13. Hawes DR, Franklin EA Jr, Fitzgerald JF, et al: Traumatic hematobilia. *Am J Dis Child* 125:130–131, 1973.
14. Bismuth H: Hemobilia. *N Engl J Med* 288:617–619, 1973.
15. Weber TR, Grosfeld JL, Bergstein J, et al: Massive gastric hemorrhage: An unusual complication of Henoch-Schonlein purpura. *J Pediatr Surg* 18:576–578, 1983.
16. Clark JH, Fitzgerald JF: Hemorrhagic complications of Henoch-Schonlein purpura. *J Pediatr Gastroenterol Nutr* 4:311–315, 1985.
17. Bryn JR, Fitzgerald JF, Northway JD, et al: Unusual manifestations of Henoch-Schonlein syndrome. *Am J Dis Child* 130:1335–1337, 1976.
18. Tomomasa T, Hsu JF, Itoh K, et al: Endoscopic findings in pediatric patients with Henoch-Schonlein purpura and gastrointestinal symptoms. *J Pediatr Gastroenterol Nutr* 6:725–729, 1987.
19. Craner GE, Burdick GE: Acute colitis resembling ulcerative colitis in the hemolytic-uremic syndrome. *Dig Dis* 21:74–76, 1976.
20. Kaplan BS, Cleary TG, Obrig TG: Recent advances in understanding the pathogenesis of the hemolytic-uremic syndromes. *Pediatr Nephrol* 4:276–283, 1990.
21. Chamovitz BN, Hartstein AI, Alexander SR, et al: *Campylobacter jejuni*-associated hemolytic-uremic syndrome in a mother and daughter. *Pediatrics* 71:253–256, 1983.
22. Buntin PT, Fitzgerald JF: Gastrointestinal neurofibromatosis. *Am J Dis Child* 119:521–523, 1970.
23. Fitzgerald JF: Antibiotic-related diarrhea, in Lebenthal E (ed): *Textbook of Gastroenterology and Nutrition in Infancy,* ed 2. New York, Raven Press, 1989, pp 1153–1157.
24. Cynamon HA, Milov DE, Andres JM: Multiple telangiectases of the colon in childhood. *J Pediatr* 112:928–930, 1988.
25. Grosfeld JL, Schiller M, Weinberger M, et al: Primary nonspecific ileal ulcers in children. *Am J Dis Child* 120:447–450, 1970.
26. Berry R, Perrault J: Gastrointestinal bleeding, in Walker WA, Durie PR, Hamilton JR, et al (eds): *Pediatric Gastrointestinal Disease.* Philadelphia, BC Decker, 1991, pp 111–131.
27. Bodey GP, Fainstein V: Infections of the gastrointestinal tract in the immunocompromised patient. *Annu Rev Med* 37:271–281, 1986.
28. Apt L, Downey WS: "Melena" neonatorum: The swallowed blood syndrome, a simple test for the differentiation of adult and fetal hemoglobin in bloody stools. *J Pediatr* 47:6–12, 1955.
29. Waterman NG, Walker JL: The effect of gastric cooling on hemostasis. *Surg Gynecol Obstet* 137:80–82, 1973.
30. Beller BM, Treviso A, Urban E: Pitressin-induced myocardial injury and depression in a young woman. *Am J Med* 51:675–679, 1971.
31. Kelly KJ, Stang JM, Mekhjian HS: Vasopressin provocation of ventricular dysrhythmia. *Ann Intern Med* 92:205–206, 1980.
32. Groszmann RJ, Kravetz D, Bosch J, et al: Nitroglycerin improves the hemodynamic response to vasopressin in portal hypertension. *Hepatology* 2:757–762, 1982.

33. Ament ME, Berquist WE, Vargas J, et al: Fiberoptic upper endoscopy in infants and children. *Pediatr Clin North Am* 35:141–155, 1988.
34. Allison DJ, Hemingway AP, Cunningham DA: Angiography in gastrointestinal bleeding. *Lancet* 2:30–33, 1982.
35. Meyerovitz MF, Fellows KE: Angiography in gastrointestinal bleeding in children. *AJR* 143:837–840, 1984.
36. Afshani E, Berger PE: Gastrointestinal tract angiography in infants and children. *J Pediatr Gastroenterol Nutr* 5:173–186, 1986.
37. Markisz JA, Front D, Royal HD, et al: An evaluation of 99^{M} Tc-labeled red blood cell scintigraphy for the detection and localization of gastrointestinal bleeding sites. *Gastroenterology* 83:394–398, 1982.
38. Gupta S, Luna E, Kingsley S, et al: Detection of gastrointestinal bleeding by radionuclide scintigraphy. *Am J Gastroenterol* 79:26–31, 1984.
39. Treves S, Grand RJ, Eraklis AJ: Pentagastrin stimulation of technetium-99M uptake by ectopic gastric mucosa in a Meckel's diverticulum. *Radiology* 12:711–712, 1978.
40. Monroe P, Morrow CF, Millen JE, et al: Acute respiratory failure after sodium morrhuate esophageal sclerotherapy. *Gastroenterology* 85:693–699, 1983.
41. Ozsoylu S, Kocak N, Yuce A: Propranolol therapy for portal hypertension in children. *J Pediatr* 106:317–321, 1985.
42. Chung SCS, Leung JWC, Sung JY, et al: Injection or heat probe for bleeding ulcer. *Gastroenterology* 100:33–37, 1991.

5

APPROACH TO CHRONIC GASTROINTESTINAL BLEEDING

Jack A. Vennes, M.D.
Jeffrey M. Rank, M.D.

INTRODUCTION

Gastrointestinal bleeding is considered *chronic* when it is low grade but persistent and arises from a source in the gut. *Overt* bleeding is visible as melena, hematemesis, or red rectal bleeding. *Occult* gastrointestinal bleeding is characterized by iron deficiency anemia or by positive tests for occult blood in stools. This chapter addresses the discovery of chronic blood loss when it is (1) occult and continuous or (2) overt and intermittent. Some causes of chronic bleeding are also responsible for acute hemorrhage; these are dealt with in other chapters.

Pursuing a precise diagnosis of a bleeding site is possible in 95% of patients using modern techniques.[1] The presence of blood loss is generally detected easily as anemia, hemoccult-positive stool examinations, or overt bleeding. Locating the site of bleeding is necessary for making management decisions. This is typically accomplished with endoscopic techniques. Isotope studies, angiography, and radiography are important in selected clinical circumstances. Historical data and, to a lesser degree, physical findings are somewhat helpful in the initial evaluation of patients and in choosing specific diagnostic studies.

HISTORY

The history can be of value in the initial evaluation of patients with chronic gastrointestinal bleeding. The nature of the blood loss can be established by the presentation. If the patient has not noted hematochezia or hematemesis and blood loss is suspected because of routine screening tests, the evaluation will proceed much differently than if the patient presents with maroon stool and shock. Hematemesis, of course, predicts an upper source proximal to the first part of the jejunum.[2] The presence of melena or hematochezia helps to predict the site of bleeding[3] but must be evaluated in the context of the overall clinical situation. In the patient with hemodynamic instability, the presence of hematochezia does not rule out an upper source. Conversely, melena may rarely appear following slow bleeding from the right colon.[4]

The quantity of blood loss may be poorly estimated by the patient, and is best evaluated by physical examination and laboratory testing. However, some crude quantitation can be made by asking about discoloration of the toilet water (red or pink), the presence of clots, and whether blood is limited to coating normal stool. It is important to determine if previous episodes of bleeding have occurred and with what frequency. A history of epistaxis or menorrhagia clearly will change the course of future evaluations.

Although early care usually will not change greatly because of the patient's history, if standard evaluations fail to yield a source of bleeding, further testing may be guided by this information. Obviously, one must identify medications which may exacerbate gastrointestinal bleeding. Aspirin and other nonsteroidal anti-inflammatory agents, warfarin, and subcutaneous heparin alter hemostasis, potentially converting undetectable bleeding into significant hemorrhage. Similarly, a history of increased clotting time for small lacerations, bleeding following dental brushing, and easy bruising warrant examination of coagulation times and platelet counts. Von Willebrand's disease should be considered when a patient has a history of abnormal clotting and intermittent gastrointestinal bleeding.[5]

A history of gastric or intestinal surgery is important, as bleeding may be found at anastomotic sites. Known liver disease and portal hypertension should alert the diagnostician to the possibility of bleeding varices, including gastric, small bowel, and mesenteric varices. If the patient or members of the family have a history of polyposis, the possibility of small bowel adenomas or hamartomas should be considered. A known history of peptic disease will increase the necessity of investigating the upper gastrointestinal tract.

Recent weight loss, fever, chills, or night sweats are symptoms which require consideration of inflammatory diseases, including Crohn's disease, systemic vasculitis, and malignancy. Abdominal pain may direct attention to the possibility of ischemia or peptic disease, depending upon its location, quality, and duration. Chronic blood loss secondary to amebic colitis should be considered in patients from tropical South America and Asia and in homosexual males. Hookworm infestation is common worldwide and can lead to profound iron deficiency.[6] A *Strongyloides* infestation is an occasional cause of chronic blood loss.[7] Patients at risk for these infections should have their stool examined for ova, parasites, and appropriate treatment prior to further evaluation.

PHYSICAL EXAMINATION

Physical findings are only occasionally helpful in directing the endoscopic search for bleeding sources. The vascular lesions of hereditary hemorrhagic telangiectasia are usually present on the face and on the buccal, nasal, and oropharyngeal mucosa. Skin lesions of the blue rubber bleb syndrome[8,9] and acquired telangiectasia of the CREST syndrome are discernible in the same locations. The angiodysplasias frequently found in the proximal colon of elderly patients do not have helpful visible cutaneous counterparts. Pigmented macular lesions on the lips, hands, and feet suggest chronic blood loss from

Peutz-Jeghers hamartomas anywhere in the gut. Pigmented velvety plaques in the axilla or groin (acanthosis nigricans) may herald the presence of adenocarcinoma, most frequently in a hollow viscus.

Spider nevi, hepatosplenomegaly, and Dupuytren's contractures all direct attention to probable portal hypertension. An auscultatory finding of aortic stenosis increases the probability of cecal angiodysplasias. Purpuric skin lesions of Henoch-Schoenlein purpura or thrombocytopenia will also be found in the gut.

CHRONIC OCCULT GASTROINTESTINAL BLEEDING

Indications for Study

The pursuit of a specific diagnosis of occult bleeding can be a frustrating endeavor. Symptoms may be absent or nonspecific, such as fatigue. Laboratory evidence of anemia or occult blood in the stool may be fortuitously discovered in the course of attention to other medical problems. Discovery of abnormalities on routine tests mandates further testing to find the specific cause. Therefore testing for occult blood in the stool should be limited to those patients in whom a positive test would make it likely that significant disease exists. For example, younger patients on aspirin therapy might have positive stools for occult blood, and the probability of finding a clinically important source is low, making the cost effectiveness of this diagnostic test very low.

Relatively large amounts of blood can be passed with apparently normal stools. Melena may not appear until at least 100 ml/day of blood is passed.[10] Normal persons lose no more than 5 ml of blood per 100 g of feces per day. Therefore, a test to determine excessive or abnormal blood loss should not be unduly sensitive. The hemoccult tests presently used will predictably detect twice the normal daily blood loss. False-positive reactions are found in only 1% of examinations even if a meat-free diet is not used.

Evaluation of iron deficiency anemia requires a more thorough evaluation of the gastrointestinal tract, whether or not occult blood is currently present. Occult blood loss may occur intermittently and therefore avoid detection.

Before embarking on an expensive and perhaps trying evaluation, it is important to be certain that the patient is indeed iron deficient. A definitive diagnosis can be made in over 90% of patients with iron deficiency anemia. The presence of microcytic indices or hypochromasia is not diagnostic. Diagnostic requirements include iron saturation of less than 12%, elevated iron-binding capacity, and low serum ferritin. For those with obvious sources of blood loss, such as the menstruating or pregnant woman, a trial of oral iron replacement is reasonable, with deferment of a definitive gastrointestinal evaluation. Anemia may be microcytic and hypochromic in the absence of iron deficiency when the true diagnosis is chronic disease or hypothyroidism. Conversely, the microcytic, hypochromic indices of iron deficiency may be masked by concomitant deficiencies of vitamin B_{12} and folate.

Colonoscopy

Colonic lesions are the most frequent source of occult blood in the stool;[11] therefore, viewing the entire colon is the minimum evaluation of positive stools in appropriate patients. Colonoscopy is a better choice than radiographic examination, since flat mucosal lesions are visible only endoscopically.[12-14] Single-column barium studies are grossly inadequate. If colonoscopy is not available or cannot be completed, an air contrast barium enema in combination with flexible sigmoidoscopy may be substituted. The combination is necessary for adequate viewing of the sigmoid colon.

If potential bleeding sites are not seen on colonoscopy, further evaluation is indicated, provided that specific symptoms or signs are present and the patient is iron deficient. In the asymptomatic patient with adequate iron stores, it may be reasonable and cost effective to end the evaluation after colon pathology is ruled out. Routine colonoscopic screening for colon cancer detection should be continued as pertinent.

Like patients having a positive fecal occult blood test, those with iron deficiency anemia also require an examination of the colon. Benign or malignant neoplasms and vascular anomalies comprise the majority of colonic lesions responsible for chronic blood loss. Angiodysplasias may not be visualized when hemoglobin levels of less than 10 g % are present. Iron repletion or transfusion of red blood cells may be necessary for adequate visual assessment. In addition, naloxone reversal of narcotic analgesics that may induce vessel spasm upon reaching the cecum with colonoscopy may improve visualization of angiodysplasias. An attempt should be made to traverse the ileocecal valve to assess for the presence of ileal vascular malformations or Crohn's disease.

Clearly, benign or malignant neoplasms of the colon should be removed by endoscopic or surgical methods. Later follow-up negative occult blood testing will determine that the polyp or mass was indeed the source of bleeding. Other colonic lesions presenting with blood loss are infrequent, and treatment of these disorders must be individualized. Inflammatory bowel disease may present with iron deficiency anemia due to chronic blood loss and malabsorption of iron. While improvement may occur with standard pharmacological intervention (steroids), chronic oral iron repletion may be necessary. Radiation injury may be associated with significant chronic blood loss and is difficult to treat effectively. Surgical excision of the affected colon is hazardous for multiple reasons and should be reserved for patients in whom iron repletion is not effective.[15]

Angiodysplasia

Angiodysplasia has become so important as a cause of acute or chronic blood loss in recent reported experience[16-19] that a brief recap is in order. Unlike other vascular lesions, angiodysplasia of the colon is not associated with vascular abnormalities in other systems. Pathogenesis of angiodysplasia lesions is unknown. The coincidence with aortic stenosis has been noted for a long time;[20] more recently, patients with chronic renal failure were noted to have an increased incidence of angiodysplasia in the gastrointestinal tract,[21] but the pathogenic basis for it is lacking.[22] Two-thirds of the patients with angiodysplasias are over 70 years of age.[11] Lesions are usually found in the cecum and proximal ascending colon, and are multiple and small, less than 5 mm in diameter. Bleeding is intermittent and may be minimal or massive. Angiographically, ectasias appear as densely opacified, tortuous intramural veins which empty contrast slowly. The late-emptying vein is present in more than 90% of patients.[19] An early-filling vein sign is also found in a majority of older people with ectasias. Colonoscopic electrocautery or photocoagulation can be used to ablate angiodysplasia lesions in the right colon. The coagulation is directed at the circumference of the lesions initially and then is applied to the center. These lesions can be satisfactorily ablated with lower power settings than are used for application of these techniques to bleeding sites elsewhere. This is fortunate because the thin-walled cecum is at greater risk for perforation. Lesions may recur, and follow-up surveillance for recurrent blood loss and/or colonoscopy is indicated. An alternative therapeutic pathway in patients with very active, massive bleeding includes angiography for diagnosis and embolic therapy or surgical resection for large lesions and significant continued active hemorrhage. The response of vascular ectasias to endoscopic laser or thermal probe application is variable. If the anemia can be corrected and ongoing blood loss is slow enough to allow iron repletion, the decision to forgo therapeutic maneuvers to correct angiodysplastic lesions is a rational option.

Upper Gastrointestinal Endoscopy

The decision to progress with further evaluations following colonoscopy must be weighed against the costs and likelihood of benefits to the patient. If iron deficiency is present, an extensive approach is justified. Although chronic occult bleeding as a presenting feature may represent a small proportion of patients with disorders of the esophagus, stomach, and duodenum, these disorders are so common that investigation of this area is often fruitful. Again, because of the ability of the endoscope to view virtually the entire mucosa, to obtain tissue samples, and to provide therapeutic intervention, this mode of examination is preferable to radiologic tests.

In addition to the colon, vascular abnormalities may occur anywhere in the gastrointestinal tract; again, it is wise to ensure an adequate preendoscopic hemoglobin level to allow visualization. Esophageal lesions associated with chronic blood loss include ulcerations and erosions, especially in the presence of Barrett's esophagus. Tumors of the esophagus may present with anemia, but this is rare without dysphagia, pain, or weight loss. Esophageal diverticula may also be associated with erosions and chronic blood loss. Interestingly, varices and Mallory-Weiss tears have been associated with chronic occult blood loss.

Nearly all common gastric and duodenal lesions occasionally present with chronic occult blood loss. Erosions within a hiatal hernial pouch not uncommonly present with iron deficiency anemia. Tumors of the stomach, both benign and malignant, usually bleed slowly, leading to anemia prior to other symptoms. Linear antral vascular ectasia, the so-called watermelon stomach, is a recently reported lesion that often presents with iron deficiency anemia.[23] This lesion should be specifically looked for during gastroscopy, as it is correctable and often missed.

Disorders of the small bowel potentially responsible for occult blood loss and within the view of the standard fiberoptic endoscope include all peptic lesions, vascular anomalies, and several rare conditions (Table 5.1). Distortions of the duodenum suggesting extrinsic lesions such as duplication cysts or pancreatic pseudocysts may be noted during endoscopy.

The bulk of iron absorption occurs across the duodenal and jejunal mucosa, and significant disruption of iron delivery may occur with surgical bypass of the duodenum, as seen in the Billroth II anastomosis. Disorders which affect duodenal mucosal integrity may also result in iron deficiency. Celiac sprue often will selectively disturb duodenal mucosa early in the disease and iron deficiency anemia may be the first manifestation.

TABLE 5.1. Sources of Chronic Bleeding

I. Occult
- A. Mucosal erosion, benign
  1. Esophagitis: acid—peptic reflux, Barrett's esophagus, pill esophagitis
  2. Gastritis: postgastrectomy stomatitis, postgastrectomy bile reflux, antritis—nonsteroidal anti-inflammatory drugs
  3. Duodenitis—acid peptic
  4. Radiation proctitis: chronic ulcerative colitis, Crohn's disease, ischemic colitis, Henoch-Schöenlein purpura
- B. Focal structural abnormalities
  1. Polyps, benign: adenoma, leiomyoma, hamartoma (Peutz-Jeghers disease), hemangioma
  2. Malignancy—any hollow viscus
  3. Blue rubber bleb syndrome
  4. Whipple's disease
- C. Vascular abnormalities
  1. Angiodysplasia
  2. Telangiectasia (Rendu-Osler-Weber syndrome)
  3. Hemangioma
  4. Watermelon stomach
  5. CRST syndrome
  6. Portal hypertension

II. Overt, intermittent
- A. Ulceration: benign, mucosal, peptic
  1. Esophageal
  2. Gastric
  3. Duodenal
  4. Stercoral—colon
  5. Ulcerative jejunitis
  6. Amyloid
- B. Focal structural abnormalities
  1. Hemorrhoids
  2. Diverticula—duodenum, colon
  3. Meckel's diverticulum
- C. Vascular abnormalities
  1. Hemobilia—source
     - Aneurysm of a splenic or hepatic artery
     - Hepatic adenoma
     - Pancreatic pseudocyst
     - Pancreatic or biliary tumor

Note: Some causes of chronic bleeding belong in either the occult or the overt category. In reading this table, it is helpful to consider their *usual* pattern.

If lesions with the potential to cause chronic blood loss are not seen during endoscopy, it is reasonable to obtain multiple biopsy specimens from the third portion of the duodenum prior to extubation to rule out mucosal abnormalities.

Most of the small bowel is beyond the diagnostic capabilities of standard endoscopic methods. Radiographic studies may detect gross lesions in the small bowel. Enteroclysis is the most sensitive examination in the detection of small bowel diverticula, including Meckel's diverticulum,[24] and offers increased sensitivity over the standard small bowel barium follow-up test in locating small bowel tumors.

If no diagnosis has emerged following colonoscopy, upper gastrointestinal endoscopy, small bowel biopsy, and standard radiographic views of the small bowel, the decision to continue investigations must be geared to the individual patient. A decision to observe the patient and follow the efficacy of iron replacement at this stage is an option. If iron replacement is ineffective or if the patient develops symptoms, further diagnostic measures are indicated. Other methods to evaluate gastrointestinal blood loss further include angiographic, enteroscopic, and nuclear medicine techniques. These studies are usually directed at the evaluation of *active* bleeding and are therefore included in the discussion of overt intermittent bleeding.

OVERT INTERMITTENT BLEEDING

Clinical Examples

Not all chronic bleeding occurs as slow, sustained seepage. In diagnosis and management, it is helpful to recognize that chronic blood loss may occur as repeated episodes of overt bleeding interspersed with periods when bleeding is absent. The periodicity and severity of acute blood loss depend on the clinical activity of the underlying process. Unreplaced blood loss may be cumulative, resulting in iron deficiency and anemia. Table 5.1 depicts a dichotomy between occult and overt bleeding. It is useful for diagnosis and management, although there are many clinical conditions which belong in both lists.

Peptic ulcer of the stomach is a notable example of chronic bleeding in some clinical states compared to acute overt bleeding in others. Both can be evaluated endoscopically but require different management—replacement of acute blood loss with endoscopic control of arterial bleeding emergently versus an orderly evaluation of anemia.

Conversely, ulcerative colitis typically undergoes exacerbation and remission, most frequently with occult bleeding. Overt bleeding suggests severe activity, occurring as hematochezia or blood mixed with mucus. Accurate diagnosis can be made by means of flexible sigmoidoscopy, although specific mucosal changes may rarely involve the rectum.

Hemorrhoids are the most frequent source of intermittent lower gastrointestinal bleeding. Finding bright red blood on the outside of formed stool or toilet tissue is the rule, with considerable diagnostic certainty as to the site of bleeding. Hemorrhoidal bleeding is chronic and intermittent, and infrequently obscure.

Painless intermittent overt bleeding from a Meckel's diverticulum is often truly obscure, presenting as intermittent hematochezia. Diagnosis of the diverticulum is sought by small bowel enteroclysis. A Tc-99 pertechnetate scan may detect a Meckel's diverticulum by showing concentration of the isotope in ectopic gastric mucosa.[25,26]

Chronic overt intermittent bleeding occurs relatively frequently from colonic diverticula, most often affecting elderly patients.[11] Diagnostic obscurity often applies here as well, and proof of the diverticular bleeding source is hard to come by either endoscopically or angiographically. Bleeding is seldom associated with diverticulitis. In occasional patients with diverticulosis, overt painless bleeding abruptly ensues, stopping spontaneously in 80% of patients. In the remaining 20% of patients, angiography is a preferred method of investigation. Although most diverticula are situated in the left colon and sigmoid, most diverticular bleeding discovered by angiography arises from the right colon.[27]

Investigation of the Small Bowel

Active bleeding whose source remains obscure following standard endoscopic techniques presents a new challenge. Further evaluation of the small bowel is accomplished by direct endoscopy to or beyond the ligament of Treitz, preferably using a pediatric colonoscope.[28] This is called *push-type enteroscopy* for no very good reason. Insertion is facilitated by fluoroscopic control. Passage into the proximal jejunum is usually possible and well tolerated. Diagnostic and therapeutic options are available, as in routine upper endoscopy.

Similarly, the terminal ileum can usually be evaluated by push-type retrograde colonoscopes entering at the ileocecal valve. This can be especially helpful in evaluation of bleeding from Crohn's disease.

Sonde-type enteroscopy is under active investigation.[29] The endoscope is carried into the deep duodenum by a pediatric colonoscope. The 5-mm enteroscope is released, a balloon is inflated, and the tube is carried down to the ileocecal valve, usually in six hours. The enteroscope is slowly withdrawn to visualize the sources of blood loss. The technique is tedious and uncomfortable, with marginal visibility at times. Nonetheless, bleeding, most often from angiodysplasia, may be discovered within the small bowel. At present, there are no therapeutic options.

Intraoperative endoscopy can be spectacularly successful in detecting vascular malformations as bleeding sources.[30,31] A pediatric colonoscope has the best combination of length and a diameter small enough to get past the endotracheal tube and pass into the small bowel. The endoscope is gently passed, traversing the small bowel as the surgeon and endoscopist work together to telescope the bowel over the endoscope, always under direct vision. During retrieval of insufflated bowel, operating room lights are dimmed and the bowel is transilluminated, with good viewing externally and endoscopically. Despite gentle handling, variable edema of the small bowel ensues. The effect, if any, on postoperative ileus has not been measured.

Radiographic studies during transit of barium through the small bowel are indicated when other methods have failed to detect a bleeding source. Some variant of enteroclysis in which high-density contrast or methyl cellulose is instilled via a tube passed to the jejunum is increasingly being chosen.[24] Double-contrast fluoroscopic visualization is sequentially accomplished with compression radiographs as needed. Enteroclysis methods have added a new and accurate dimension to the discovery of Meckel's diverticula, Crohn's disease, lymphoma, and neoplasms as sources of blood loss.

Radionuclide scanning is used mainly to confirm that bleeding is actively occurring.[25] 99m-Tc sulfur colloid and 99m-Tc-labeled red blood cells are useful to identify the anatomical level of bleeding. Labeled erythrocytes remain in the circulation for up to 24 hours, permitting sequential scanning for focal bleeding sites.

OBSCURE BLEEDING SOURCES

Throughout this chapter, we have stressed the everyday sources of chronic blood loss and their routine discovery. The dictum is true that "common things occur commonly." However, when a diagnosis is not forthcoming despite the usual measures, we would do well to consider more obscure causes of chronic blood loss. Amyloidosis of the gastrointestinal tract is associated with chronic blood loss in one-half of reported patients.[32,33] We were surprised recently to learn that Whipple's disease[34] may be associated with chronic blood loss. Both of these obscure sources may be discovered on mucosal biopsy.

Diseases which occur rather commonly may become obscure in the search for chronic bleeding because the bleeding is unusual or infrequent. Examples include portal gastropathy in patients with portal hypertension[35,36] or multiple gastrointestinal tumors in neurofibromatosis.[37] The diagnostic challenge never ends.

CONCLUSION

Chronic blood loss takes many clinical forms; most of them are discoverable with persistence, skill, and an array of diagnostic methods. In the interests of cost effectiveness and good patient care, it is important to be certain of the indications before initiating a workup. Chronic blood loss is most accurately evaluated by endoscopic methods. This blood loss is most often colonic in origin. Therefore, full colonoscopy is the usual first endoscopic procedure. However, upper gastrointestinal endoscopy is initially indicated for obvious upper gastrointestinal symptoms or melena.

There is a rational sequence of evaluation for each patient. Individual variables are active components of decision making, including the skills and diagnostic tools available locally. These variables are more important than algorithms.

When chronic blood loss occasionally defies specific diagnosis and treatment, it is usually good practice to look again for a likely common source of bleeding or persistent anemia.

REFERENCES

1. Rosen AM, Fleischer DE: Upper GI bleeding in the elderly. *Geriatrics* 44:26–40, 1989.
2. Northfield TC, Smith T: Haematemesis as an index of blood loss. *Lancet* 1:990–991, 1971.
3. Schiller KFR, Truelove SC, Williams DG: Haematemesis and melena with special reference to factors influencing the outcome. *Br Med J* 2:7–14, 1970.
4. Luke RG, Lees W, Rudick J: Appearances of the stools after the introduction of blood into the cecum. *Gut* 5:77–79, 1964.
5. Moroose R, Hoyer LW: Von Willebrand factor and platelet function. *Annu Rev Med* 37:157–163, 1986.

6. Blumenthal DS: Intestinal nematodes in the United States. *N Engl J Med* 297:1437–1439, 1977.
7. Bhatt BD, Cappell MS, Smilow PC, et al: Recurrent massive upper GI hemorrhage due to *Strongyloides* infection. *Am J Gastroenterol* 85:1034–1036, 1990.
8. Sandhu KS, Cohen H, Radin R, et al: Blue rubber bleb nevus syndrome presenting with recurrences. *Dig Dis Sci* 32:214–219, 1987.
9. Morris SJ, Kaplan SR, Tedesco FJ: Blue rubber bleb nevus syndrome. *JAMA* 239:1887–1889, 1978.
10. Schiff L, Stevens RJ, Shapiro N, et al: Observations on the oral administration of citrated blood in man. *Am J Med Sci* 203:409–412, 1942.
11. Reinus JF, Brandt LJ: Upper and lower gastrointestinal bleeding in the elderly. *Gastroenterol Clin North Am* 19:293–318, 1990.
12. Hogan WJ, Stewart ET, Geenen JE, et al: A prospective comparison of the accuracy of colonoscopy vs. air-barium contrast exam for detection of colonic polypoid lesions. *Gastrointest Endosc* 23:230–233, 1977.
13. Tarin D, Allison DJ, Modlin IM, et al: Diagnosis and management of obscure gastrointestinal bleeding. *Br Med J* 2:751–754, 1978.
14. Tedesco FJ, Waye JD, Raskin JB, et al: Colonoscopic evaluation of rectal bleeding. *Ann Intern Med* 89:907–909, 1978.
15. Appelmen RM, Beahres OH: Surgical management of gastrointestinal hemorrhage from an undetermined source. Proc staff meet. *Mayo Clin Proc* 40:121–126, 1965.
16. Richter JM, Hedberg SE, Athanasoulis CA, et al: Angiodysplasia: clinical presentation and colonoscopic diagnosis. *Dig Dis Sci* 29:481–485, 1984.
17. Gilmore PR: Angiodysplasia of the upper gastrointestinal tract. *J Clin Gastroenterol* 10:386–394, 1988.
18. Hemingway AP: Angiodysplasia as a cause of iron deficiency anaemia. *Blood Rev* 3:147–151, 1989.
19. Casarella WJ, Galloway SJ, Taxin RN, et al: Lower gastrointestinal hemorrhage. New concepts based on arteriography. *AJR* 121:357–368, 1974.
20. King RM, Pluth JR, Giuliani ER: The association of unexplained gastrointestinal bleeding with calcific aortic stenosis. *Ann Thorac Surg* 44:514–516, 1987.
21. Marcuard SP, Weinstock JV: Gastrointestinal angiodysplasia in renal failure. *J Clin Gastroenterol* 10:482–484, 1988.
22. Cappell MS, Lebwohl O: Cessation of recurrent bleeding from gastrointestinal angiodysplasias after aortic valve replacement. *Ann Intern Med* 105:54–57, 1986.
23. Gostout CJ, Ahlquist DA, Radford CM, et al: Endoscopic laser therapy for watermelon stomach. *Gastroenterology* 96:1462–1465, 1989.
24. Maglinte DDT, Lappas JC, Kelvin FM, et al: Small bowel radiography: How, when, and why? *Radiology* 163:297–305, 1987.
25. Thrall JH, Swanson DP: Diagnostic interventions in nuclear medicine. *Curr Probl Diagn Radiol* 18:9–37, 1989.
26. Treves S, Grand RJ, Eraklis AJ: Pentagastrin stimulation of technetium-99m uptake by ectopic gastric mucosa in a Meckel's diverticulum. *Radiology* 128:711–712, 1978.
27. Casarella WJ, Kanter IE, Seaman WB: Right-sided colonic diverticula as a cause of acute rectal hemorrhage. *N Engl J Med* 286:450–453, 1972.
28. Parker HW, Agayoff JD: Enteroscopy and small bowel biopsy utilizing a peroral colonoscope. *Gastrointest Endosc* 29:138–139, 1983.

29. Lewis BS, Waye JD: Chronic gastrointestinal bleeding of obscure origin: Role of small bowel enteroscopy. *Gastroenterology* 94:1117–1120, 1988.
30. Bowden TA: Endoscopy of the small intestine. *Surg Clin North Am* 69:1237–1247, 1989.
31. Whelan RL, Buls JG, Goldberg SM, et al: Intra-operative endoscopy, University of Minnesota experience. *Am Surg* 55:281–286, 1989.
32. Brandt K. Cathcart ES, Cohen AS: A clinical analysis of the course and prognosis of forty-two patients with amyloidosis. *Am J Med* 44:955–969, 1968.
33. Jarnum S: Gastrointestinal haemorrhage and protein loss in primary amyloidosis. *Gut* 6:14–18, 1965.
34. Feldman M, Price G: Intestinal bleeding in patients with Whipple's disease. *Gastroenterology* 96:1207–1209, 1989.
35. Sarfeh IJ, Tarnawski A: Gastric mucosal vasculopathy in portal hypertension. *Gastroenterology* 93:1129–1131, 1987.
36. Wenger J, Huffman RT, Landry MS: Persistent blood loss from the stomach of patients with cirrhosis and esophageal varices. *South Med J* 63:560–566, 1970.
37. Cox JGC, Royston CMS, Sutton DR; Multiple smooth muscle tumours in neurofibromatosis presenting with chronic gastrointestinal bleeding. *Postgrad Med J* 64:149–151, 1988.

6

LIVER DISEASE IN GASTROINTESTINAL BLEEDING

Alexander T. Lalos, M.D.
Eugene R. Schiff, M.D.

INTRODUCTION

The association of cirrhosis with gastrointestinal bleeding was originally described by Banti over 150 years ago.[1] Since then, despite major advances in medical and surgical treatment, gastrointestinal bleeding continues to be a leading cause of death in cirrhosis, which is not surprising when one considers the deleterious effect that hepatic dysfunction has on essentially all organ systems of the body.[2] The management of liver disease in this setting continues to be difficult but has become more important now that long-term survival after orthotopic liver transplantation is possible.

The goals of this chapter are three. First, we will review the important clinical features of liver disease as they may appear on initial evaluation of the patient. Second, we will discuss the differential diagnosis of gastrointestinal bleeding. Finally, we will outline the medical management of the major complications of hepatic insufficiency which may develop as a consequence of gastrointestinal bleeding. For the most part, we will focus primarily on chronic liver disease, making reference to acute or fulminant hepatic failure as deemed appropriate.

CLINICAL EVALUATION OF LIVER DISEASE

Identifying liver disease in a patient with acute gastrointestinal bleeding may be an easy task in the face of massive ascites and a history of ethanol abuse or chronic viral hepatitis. However, it takes an astute clinician to suspect cirrhosis when bleeding is the initial manifestation of the underlying disease. In these cases, much can be learned by paying careful attention to the history, the physical examination, and the results of routine laboratory tests.

In obtaining the history, the clinician must be very familiar with the epidemiology of chronic liver disease, which is influenced by the geographic location and type of medical practice. In the United States and most Western countries, the leading cause of cirrhosis is chronic ethanol abuse. A detailed history of alcohol use, obtained from the patient and family or friends, is needed to determine whether the level of ingestion is in the hepatotoxic range. A daily consumption of 80 g of ethanol for a period of 5–10 years can result in alcoholic liver disease in males; females appear to be at risk with daily dosages of 40 to 60 g. It is possible that lower levels of intake may also be harmful if coexistent hepatic diseases such as hepatitis C infection are present. For unknown reasons, perhaps related to genetic predisposition, only 15–20% of all people who ingest alcohol at these levels will develop clinically apparent liver disease. Therefore, one cannot attribute liver disease to alcohol from the history alone or assume the presence of liver disease given a history of heavy ethanol use.

Chronic viral hepatitis, due to hepatitis B or the recently described hepatitis C, is also a leading cause of cirrhosis in the United States and worldwide. Hepatitis B infection is common in patients with intravenous drug abuse and in sexually promiscuous populations, including heterosexuals and homosexuals, with the acquired immunodeficiency syndrome. Hepatitis B infection is also endemic in the Far East, and a significant number of patients who originate from this area may be chronic hepatitis B virus carriers. Hepatitis C infection is usually seen as a result of previous blood transfusion or intravenous drug abuse. The risk of sexual transmission of hepatitis C is not clearly determined at this time and, if present, appears to be infrequent.[3] Cases of chronic viral hepatitis due to non-A, non-B, and non-C viruses probably exist and may be more definitely characterized in the future.

Other causes of chronic liver disease may be cryptic and undiagnosed on presentation. A background of autoimmune disease in a young woman with signs of hepatic dysfunction should raise the possibility of chronic autoimmune hepatitis. A history of inflammatory bowel disease suggests sclerosing cholangitis, while thyroid disease and pruritus in a middle-aged female may indicate primary biliary cirrhosis. The long-term use of some medications, such as nitrofurantoin or alpha-methyldopa, has been associated with the development of chronic active hepatitis and cirrhosis in some patients, while oral contraceptive use may predispose the patient to developing Budd-Chiari syndrome. Excessive dietary supplements of vitamin A or niacin may cause hepatic failure, with the former manifesting clinically as chronic liver disease with ascites and portal hypertension and the latter as acute hepatocellular failure.

Family history is also important, as genetic factors are involved in the development of alcoholic liver disease, as well as metabolic disorders such as Wilson's disease or hemochromatosis. Occupational history may reveal exposure to hepatotoxic chemicals such as carbon tetrachloride or a needle stick injury in a health care worker with chronic hepatitis.

Physical examination should be focused on identifying signs of cirrhosis. In advanced liver disease, the general appearance of the patient may be one of cachexia; however, some individuals with early cirrhosis may appear to be well built or even obese. The skin examination may reveal spider angiomas, particularly on the chest, neck, and back, or increased skin pigmentation from hemochromatosis or long-standing cholestasis, as seen in primary biliary cirrhosis. Digits may be clubbed if the hepatopulmonary syndrome is present and nail beds may be white, a condition known as *leukonychia*. Palmar erythema is also commonly noted. On abdominal exam, bulging flanks or shifting dullness indicates the presence of ascites. The abdominal wall may have prominent veins which fill from the umbilicus toward the periphery, and in some cases the classic "caput medusa" may be seen. In chronic liver disease, the spleen may become significantly enlarged over time; however, massive splenomegaly should alert the clinician to the possibility of underlying myeloproliferative syndrome or thrombosis of the portal or splenic vein. The liver in advanced cirrhosis is often small and shrunken; however, it may be enlarged and palpable in the setting of active alcohol abuse or infiltrative and vascular obstructive disorders. A careful neurological exam should include an evaluation for the presence of asterixis, as well as a formal assessment of mental status such as the number connection test.[4] Upon the completion of a thorough history and physical exam, the diagnosis of liver disease may be suspected and/or diagnosed with certainty.

Careful review of routine laboratory test results can also help in the diagnosis of liver disease. The complete blood cell count often reveals a mild anemia, usually macrocytic, particularly in the setting of alcohol abuse. Nutritional deficiency of folate or acanthocytosis with hemolytic anemia may also contribute to macrocytosis. Thrombocytopenia is almost always present and may be due to bleeding, hypersplenism, and bone marrow depression from alcohol. Low white blood cell counts may result from hypersplenism, although leukocytosis with a left shift is seen in cases of infection or alcoholic hepatitis.

Serum electrolytes will often reveal hyponatremia, which may be severe. Hypokalemia is also seen as as result of increased aldosterone activity, as well as vomiting and diarrhea from gastrointestinal bleeding. A low serum carbon dioxide level does not imply acidosis but is usually a response to chronic respiratory alkalosis that is common in cirrhotic patients. Blood urea nitrogen (BUN) values may be low unless there is an active or recent hemorrhage causing elevation. Of course, if renal failure has ensued, the BUN and creatinine values will both be elevated.

The most important laboratory values are those which measure the integrity and function of the liver. The aminotransferases, aspartate aminotransferase (AST) or serum glutamic-oxaloacetic transaminase (SGOT) and alanine aminotransferase (ALT) or serum glutamic-pyruvic transaminase (SGPT), are released from damaged or dying hepatocytes. ALT is predominantly of liver origin, whereas AST appears in various other tissues, such as muscle and brain, and is less specific for hepatic damage. A ratio of AST to ALT above 3:1 is highly suggestive but not diagnostic of alcoholic liver disease as long as the overall elevation is not above 500 units.[5] Otherwise, aminotransferase elevations are nonspecific, and the absolute levels do not correlate with functional hepatic reserve or degree of acute liver damage. Alkaline phosphatase is elevated in chronic obstructive or cholestatic disorders of the liver but may also be increased because of bone destruction. Modest elevations of this enzyme may be seen in alcoholic liver disease and with the onset of hepatocellular carcinoma in a cirrhotic liver.

A more accurate reflection of liver function is the synthetic capability of the liver. Since most coagulation factors are synthesized in the liver, with some having half-lives as short as a few hours, the prothrombin time is a convenient and dynamic measurement of hepatocellular function. One must remember that levels of coagulation factors may fall quickly during hemorrhage when there is underlying hepatic dysfunction; therefore, a normal initial prothrombin value should not rule out liver disease in the mind of the clinician. Conversely, on the basis of hemodilution, even patients with normal hepatocellular function may have elevated prothrombin times following massive bleeding and rapid transfusion. Albumin levels also reflect hepatic function, but clearance of this protein occurs over a period of 21 days, so levels may be normal in the setting of acute liver failure. Again, massive transfusion, as well as renal or enteric losses of protein, will lead to low albumin levels and should not erroneously suggest underlying liver disease.

A detailed review of the laboratory workup for the etiology of liver disease is beyond the scope of this chapter. The basic laboratory evaluation should include serological testing for viral hepatitis, including the newly described hepatitis C. Autoimmune liver disease should be screened for by obtaining an antinuclear antibody, anti–smooth muscle antibody, and quantitative immunoglobulins (Igs) looking for an increased total of IgG. When primary biliary cirrhosis is suspected, an antimitochondrial antibody test should also be obtained; it will be positive in approximately 90% affected of patients. The evaluation should also include iron and iron-binding capacity studies to rule out hemochromatosis and a ceruloplasmin level to screen for the presence of Wilson's disease, a rare but devastating illness if undetected.

In the last two decades, there have been major advances in noninvasive imaging of the liver. Patients with gastrointestinal bleeding who are suspected of having liver disease should have either an ultrasound or computed tomography (CT) scan of the abdomen. Either of these studies may demonstrate irregularity or nodularity of the liver surface suggestive of cirrhosis, as well as any mass lesions that may be present. Addition of a Doppler examination to ultrasound can determine the patency of the hepatic and portal veins, aiding the workup of portal hypertension.[6] CT scanning with contrast can provide the same information and may also identify retroperitoneal or intraperitoneal variceal structures. Both ultrasound and CT examinations will readily diagnose the presence of ascites and allow guided paracentesis if this is necessary. In the clinical setting of acute bleeding, ultrasound has the advantage of being portable and of not requiring a potentially nephrotoxic contrast agent. Magnetic resonance imaging is an effective way to evaluate the hepatic parenchyma and its vascular structures; however, its role in the routine workup of patients in the clinical setting is not as cost effective.

Despite all the advances in laboratory and radiological evaluation of liver disease, the etiology and extent of the underlying hepatic dysfunction can still be best assessed by liver biopsy. Biopsy can be performed by the percutaneous approach using a Menghini or Jamshidi needle with the aspiration technique, or with the Tru-cut or Vim-Silverman needle under laparoscopic guidance. The latter technique has the advantage of allowing direct visualization of the liver and will help in the diagnosis of cirrhosis when percutaneous biopsy yields a fragmented specimen or inconclusive results. We do not recommend liver biopsy in a patient who has had recent gastrointestinal bleeding until after the patient has been unequivocally stabilized.

DIFFERENTIAL DIAGNOSIS OF GASTROINTESTINAL BLEEDING IN LIVER DISEASE

The etiology of gastrointestinal bleeding in patients with chronic liver disease may be elusive even after a thorough endoscopic evaluation. Differentiating variceal from nonvariceal bleeding has significant therapeutic and prognostic implications. Familiarity with the potential bleeding sites in these patients and the relationship of each of the lesions to the underlying disease is important in making the correct diagnosis and guiding appropriate therapy.

Gastroesophageal varices are the most common and clinically significant cause of gastrointestinal bleeding in liver disease. Gastroesophageal varices form from preexisting anatomical communications which join the coronary and short gastric veins with the esophageal and azygous veins. They enlarge because of increased flow from the higher-pressure portal venous system to the lower-pressure systemic venous system and eventually rupture from a combination of hemodynamic and mechanical factors that have been defined.[7]

Prior to the advent of fiberoptic endoscopy, varices were identified radiologically, and when they were seen in the setting of gastrointestinal bleeding, they were assumed to be the cause. Surprisingly, early endoscopic series in patients with portal hypertension revealed that varices were the source of bleeding in less than half of the cases of acute hemorrhage.[8-10] What was not appreciated at that time was the intermittent nature of variceal bleeding,[11] and in the absence of active hemorrhage from varices at the time of endoscopy, co-existing pathological lesions such as erosive gastritis or peptic ulcer were often felt to be the bleeding source. Recent studies now show that in patients with portal hypertension and bleeding, the etiology proves to be variceal in approximately 90% of patients.[12,13]

Treatment of acute or recurrent bleeding for gastroesophageal varices is a complex topic and will be addressed elsewhere in this textbook. As hepatologists and nonendoscopists, we will focus on the important points in the clinical assessment of the patient who presents with variceal bleeding. Initial evaluation should proceed as outlined in the preceding section. After this evaluation is complete, several key questions must be answered.

1. Does the patient in fact have liver disease?

Variceal bleeding results from portal hypertension, of which cirrhosis is one cause. Extrahepatic obstruction of the portal or splenic vein may cause gastroesophageal varices in the absence of liver disease. Various noncirrhotic hepatic diseases such as schistosomiasis, congenital hepatic fibrosis, or nodular regenerative hyperplasia may cause portal hypertension without evidence of hepatocellular dysfunction. Likewise, post-hepatic obstruction of the hepatic veins or inferior vena cava can cause portal hypertension and lead to the formation of varices. Noncirrhotic patients with variceal bleeding have a better prognosis because of their preserved hepatocellular function, and require different medical and surgical treatment than cirrhotic patients.

2. What precipitated the bleeding?

Variceal bleeding may occur as a consequence of advancing liver disease, but sometimes a precipitant factor may be identified. Of particular importance is hepatocellular carcinoma, which can cause an increase in portal hypertension by increased arteriovenous shunting through the tumor or direct invasion of the portal vein. This can be ruled out by obtaining appropriate radiological evaluation of the liver and an alpha fetoprotein level. Elevation of this tumor marker above 400 ng/ml is fairly specific for the diagnosis of hepatocellular carcinoma.[14]

Obstruction of the portal vein without hepatocellular carcinoma may be seen in some cirrhotic patients as hepatopetal flow diminishes. In addition, underlying alcoholic pancreatitis may cause splenic vein thrombosis in a patient who already has alcoholic liver disease.

3. What is the prognosis of the patient?

The modified Child's score based on clinical parameters should be determined in every patient with chronic liver disease. The Child's score (Table 6.1) plays two important roles with respect to variceal bleeding. First, it serves as an important predictor of future hemorrhage in cirrhotic patients who have never bled from esophageal varices.[15] This is of particular importance when patients are being considered for prophylactic therapeutic trials to prevent variceal bleeding. A recent study by the North Italian Endoscopic Club revealed that the risk of developing variceal bleeding was increased from 17% to 39% in Child's C as opposed to Child's A cirrhotics.[13] Similarly, the Child's score has been found to correlate with increasing size of esophageal varices and the presence of "red signs," both of which are endoscopically defined risk factors for bleeding.[16] Second, more important than its role in predicting bleeding, the Child's score has both a short- and a long-term influence on the survival of cirrhotic patients who have had variceal bleeding.[17] To a large extent, this allows the clinician to match the appropriate medical, endoscopic, or surgical treatment to each patient.

4. Is or will the patient be a candidate for liver transplantation?

The patient with cirrhosis is likely to develop varying degrees of functional and mechanical complications. In the absence of ascites, encephalopathy, or variceal bleeding, cirrhosis is said to be compensated and carries a relatively good outlook, with a documented 47% 10-year survival.[18] However, by definition, once variceal bleeding has occurred, cirrhosis is said to be decompensated and the prognosis worsens significantly. The initial episode of variceal hemorrhage is associated with a 40% mortality, and only approximately 30% of patients who bleed will be alive in one year.[19] Although the

TABLE 6.1. Prognostic Indexes: Child-Turcotte Classification (Pugh's Modification)*

	Points		
	1	*2*	*3*
Encephalopathy (grade)	0	1–2	3–4
Ascites	None	Slight	Moderate
Bilirubin (mg/dl)	1–2	2–3	>3
Albumin (g/dl)	>3.5	2.8–3.5	<2.8
Prothrombin time (secs. prolonged)	1–4	4–10	10

Grade	Total Score (Pts.)
A	5 or 6
B	7–9
C	10–15

*Original index used malnutrition in place of prothrombin time.

bleeding patient usually has entered an advanced stage of the underlying disease and the possibility of liver transplantation should be considered, some patients have relatively good functional reserve, and management should focus on prevention of recurrent bleeding rather than transplantation.

Liver transplantation candidacy depends on many factors, including psychosocial profile, financial and social support, the significance of any coexisting medical disease, and, to an extent, the etiology of the underlying liver disease. If necessary, a transplantation physician should be consulted regarding this matter. Whether or not transplantation is a present or future option in the individual patient may greatly affect the approach to variceal bleeding. Which of these patients should have liver transplantation is a question which will be addressed in a later section.

The clinical assessment outlined above is dynamic and should be undertaken periodically in the stable patient who has had variceal bleeding, as many of these factors may change over time.

Congestive Gastropathy

As stated previously, erosive gastritis was a frequent source of gastrointestinal bleeding in early endoscopic studies of patients with portal hypertension. The etiology of this lesion was questioned by Sarfeh et al., who noted that rebleeding was common in patients with erosive gastritis and could be prevented by portal decompressive surgery.[20] McCormack et al. performed biopsies of gastritis in patients with portal hypertension and found that dilation and tortuosity of the submucosal veins, in the absence of inflammation, was a constant finding.[21] The term *congestive gastropathy* was coined. Papazian et al. subsequently characterized the endoscopic appearance of this entity as erythema seen primarily in the gastric fundus with a superimposed yellowish network resembling a "mosaic."[22]

Portal hypertension alone may not be the cause of this disorder, as wedged hepatic vein pressure has been found to be similar in portal hypertensive patients with or without endoscopic evidence of gastropathy.[21] Also, congestive gastropathy has been noted in the absence of esophageal varices in cirrhotic patients.[16] It has been suggested that gastropathy may result because portal hypertension makes the gastric mucosa susceptible to irritants, particularly alcohol.[23] Consistent with this theory is that congestive gastropathy is rare in India, where alcoholic cirrhosis is a less common cause of portal hypertension.[24] Helicobacter pylori does not appear to be a factor in pathogenesis.[25,26]

From a clinical standpoint, congestive gastropathy primarily causes chronic gastrointestinal blood loss, resulting in iron deficiency anemia.[26] Overt gastrointestinal hemorrhage with melena or hematemesis is less usual, but not rare, and it may not always be clear whether congestive gastropathy or varices is the cause of a recent gastrointestinal bleed. Treatment is not well established but appears to depend on reducing portal pressure by medical or surgical means, as therapy directed toward acid-peptic disease has not been shown to be effective for congestive gastropathy.[26]

Ectopic Varices

Portal hypertension promotes the development of collaterals throughout the portal-splanchnic complex. As a result, varices can develop and bleed at sites other than the gastroesophageal junction. Bleeding from these "ectopic varices" is rare but the mortality is high, perhaps because the diagnosis is often delayed or not suspected.

Cappell and Price have recently reviewed 62 cases in the literature of small and large intestinal varices.[27] Underlying cirrhosis was the cause of portal hypertension in 45 patients. The most frequent site of ectopic varices was the rectosigmoid region of the colon, presumably developing from the hemorrhoidal plexus. The next most frequent site was an ileal stoma in patients with sclerosing cholangitis who had undergone colectomy for ulcerative colitis. Varices were also found in the cecum, right colon, ileum, and jejunum. Duodenal varices have also been reported by others.[28]

Why ectopic varices develop and bleed in only some patients with portal hypertension is not clear. There is a reported association with previous sclerotherapy of esophageal varices, which theoretically increases portal venous blood flow through other existing portosystemic shunts.[29] Previous abdominal surgery of any kind also appears to be a risk factor for the development of ectopic varices, perhaps related to local venous obstruction from mesenteric adhesions.[27,28]

Diagnosis requires a high degree of suspicion. The clinical setting is usually massive or recurrent gastrointestinal bleeding in the cirrhotic patient with no obvious esophageal or upper tract source. Angiography is the most helpful examination in identifying ectopic varices, although they do not bleed actively in the venous phase.[27] Upper endoscopy and colonoscopy are useful primarily in ruling out other lesions. Sclerotherapy is not an option in most cases, and portal decompressive surgery is usually required to control bleeding. Selective shunts such as the distal splenorenal shunt may not decompress small or large intestinal varices. Of course, before any surgical intervention is undertaken in any bleeding patient with cirrhosis, the question of planned or future liver transplantation must be addressed.

Peptic Ulcer Disease

The prevalence of peptic ulcer disease, with or without bleeding, is believed to be increased in cirrhosis. Older data, obtained primarily from radiological studies and autopsy examinations, placed the risk of peptic ulcer in this group of patients at between 10% and 15%, or five times that of the population at large.[30] Early endoscopic series in patients with liver disease and gastrointestinal bleeding similarly reported a prevalence of peptic ulcer between 11% and 16%.[8-10] Recently, peptic ulcer was found in 8.7% and 21% of nonbleeding patients undergoing liver transplantation evaluation at the University of Pittsburgh and the Mayo Clinic, respectively; these figures are consistent with the previous data.[31,32]

It is not known why there is an increased risk of peptic ulcer in liver disease. Acid production is known to be reduced in cirrhosis, making it likely that a decreased gastric mucosal defense is more important in the pathogenesis.[33] The susceptibility of the gastric mucosa to gastric irritants such as alcohol and aspirin has been demonstrated in portal hypertensive animal models.[23] The role of alcohol itself in ulcer disease is not clearly defined, and most studies suggest that it is not a causative factor.[34] However, Rabinovitz et al. have shown that duodenal ulcer is more common in alcoholics undergoing evaluation for transplantation than in any other group of patients with end-stage liver disease.[31] The role of tobacco use, a known risk factor for developing peptic ulcer, has not been evaluated in cirrhosis.

Medical treatment of peptic ulcer in individuals with liver disease is no different from that of other patients. However, cirrhotics who develop complications of peptic ulcer are generally not candidates for elective surgery to prevent recurrence and should be maintained on prophylactic antiulcer therapy. In addition, hospitalized patients with fulminant hepatic failure should receive prophylactic antiulcer therapy with H-2 receptor antagonists or sucralfate to prevent stress-related gastric mucosal lesions that are the cause of significant morbidity and mortality in this setting.

Mallory-Weiss Syndrome

Gastrointestinal bleeding caused by linear tears in the mucosa of the gastroesophageal junction is known as the Mallory-Weiss syndrome. These lesions are the presumed source of gastrointestinal bleeding in a minority of patients examined endoscopically.[35] The syndrome is associated with a history of recurrent vomiting, alcohol abuse, and the use of aspirin or nonsteroidal anti-inflammatory drugs.

Recently, Paquet et al. reported an increased incidence of Mallory-Weiss syndrome in patients with portal hypertension.[36] In their series of 339 patients with portal hypertension and gastrointestinal bleeding, gastroesophageal tears were found in 16% of patients overall and in 30% of Child's class C cirrhotics. Sclerotherapy injection directed at the bleeding site was uniformly successful in arresting hemorrhage. These results suggest that portal hypertension may play a role in the pathogenesis of the Mallory-Weiss syndrome. It is likely that the common precipitants of this syndrome initiate the tear but that the bleeding is driven by the underlying elevated venous pressure in the gastroesophageal mucosa. This is supported by the observation in the above study that the gastroesophageal tears were more common when the etiology of portal hypertension was alcoholic cirrhosis as opposed to extrahepatic portal venous obstruction. Regardless, it appears that the Mallory-Weiss syndrome is probably more common in patients with chronic liver disease than was previously appreciated, and when it is seen, underlying chronic liver disease or portal hypertension should be excluded.

MEDICAL PROBLEMS COMPLICATING GASTROINTESTINAL BLEEDING IN LIVER DISEASE

Disorders of Hemostasis

Bleeding diathesis is common, if not the rule, in patients with liver disease. It may not be the inciting event in most cases of gastrointestinal bleeding, but its presence complicates control of hemorrhage and subsequent medical or surgical management. In this section, we will review the various defects in coagulation and discuss the available treatment options.

Thrombocytopenia is common in cirrhosis of any etiology. This is due primarily to hypersplenism as a result of portal hypertension, although immune destruction may also play a role in autoimmune hepatitis and possibly in alcoholic liver disease. Alcohol itself, being the most common etiological factor in liver disease, also contributes to thrombocytopenia in many cases by a primary bone marrow depressant effect. Eighty percent of alcoholic patients with or without liver disease requiring hospitalization will present with thrombocytopenia, but their platelet counts will often increase within 48–72 hours of cessation of drinking and will reach supranormal levels within two weeks, even in the absence of a correctable nutritional deficiency.[37] In addition to reduced numbers of platelets, there is evidence of qualitative dysfunction. Ingeberg et al. have demonstrated abnormal in vitro platelet aggregation and impaired release of procoagulants in cirrhotics.[38] Others have suggested that platelet dysfunction results from reduced availability of arachidonic acid for prostaglandin production as a consequence of the altered cholesterol:phospholipid ratio seen in liver disease.[39] In the clinical setting, one must also remember that the use of nonsteroidal anti-inflammatory agents or aspirin may be responsible for platelet dysfunction. The bleeding time, a test that can be rapidly and easily done at the bedside, can be used to assess the adequacy of platelet function.

Coagulation defects are also very common in cirrhosis since, except for factor VIII or Von Willebrand factor, the necessary clotting factors, including prothrombin and fibrinogen, are synthesized in the liver. Once production of these factors becomes deficient, an increased prothrombin time will be noted. Therefore, the presence of any coagulopathy in the steady state implies moderate to severe hepatic dysfunction. An exception is the readily reversible hypoprothrombinemia secondary to vitamin K deficiency seen in cholestatic liver disease. In addition to the reduced factor levels in cirrhosis, there is dysfibrinogenemia, or qualititatively abnormal fibrinogen, resulting in increased thrombin times.[40] This abnormal fibrinogen appears to be synthesized from regenerating hepatocytes and differs from normal fibrinogen in its level of sialic acid content.

Enhanced fibrinolysis may also be seen in liver disease and is caused by disseminated intravascular coagulation (DIC) or coagulation changes which accompany hepatic failure. The latter are characterized by decreased hepatic synthesis of coagulation factor regulators and inhibitors such as protein S and anti-thrombin III, which result in consumptive coagulopathy. The two entities can be differentiated by the D-dimer test, which is positive only in true DIC.[41] Clinically, the importance of identifying the presence of fibrinolysis is that the prothrombin time is used as a reliable measure of hepatic function and is a major prognostic factor in both fulminant hepatic failure and acute alcoholic hepatitis. In these cases, the contribution of fibrinolysis to the prothrombin elevation must be determined so that hepatocellular function is not underestimated. Since factor VIII is not made in the liver, a depletion of this factor, along with factor V, would suggest a consumptive coagulopathy as opposed to pure hepatic failure.

Aggressive treatment of bleeding disorders is essential in cirrhotic patients with hemorrhage. On admission, all alcoholics should be given parenteral folate and thiamine to correct any nutritional deficiency contributing to thrombocytopenia. Otherwise, platelet transfusions are the mainstay of therapy for severe thrombocytopenia, with levels of at least 60,000 being desirable in the setting of active bleeding, although lower levels may be acceptable once bleeding has ceased. When platelets are given, the number of transfusions should be guided by the general rule that replacement of 8–10 units of blood, or one body volume, will be accompanied by a reduction of the platelet count by approximately 50% in noncirrhotic patients.[42] Therefore, in cirrhotic patients with initial low counts, platelet transfusions may be required after four to six units of packed red blood cells have been replaced. Of course, serial complete blood count determinations will aid in guiding therapy.

There are recent studies to suggest that qualitative platelet dysfunction in cirrhosis can be treated effectively with desmopressin or (DDAVP), a vasopressin analog. Burroughs et al. demonstrated a reduction in bleeding time from an average of 11 to 6 minutes in nine cirrhotic patients given desmopressin intravenously at a dose of 3 μg/kg prior to liver biopsy.[43] A similar reduction in bleeding time in cirrhotic patients with DDAVP infusion has been documented by others.[44] Unfortunately, the half-life of DDAVP is short, approximately 55 minutes, and tachyphylaxis may be a problem after serial injections. As a result, its role as therapy in active gastrointestinal hemorrhage is undefined.[45] DDAVP appears to function by increasing levels of factor VIII or Von Willebrand factor in the serum, levels which, surprisingly, are not reduced at baseline in liver disease.

Patients admitted with prolonged prothrombin times should be given 10 mg of vitamin K by subcutaneous or intramuscular injection on each of the first three days of hospitalization. This may be particularly efficacious in patients with cholestatic liver disease and secondary fat malabsorption or those receiving intravenous antibiotics, both of which may induce vitamin K deficiency. Unfortunately, vitamin K will not correct the prothrombin time if the reduced synthesis of coagulation factors is due entirely to hepatic failure.

Bleeding patients with liver disease whose prothrombin time is elevated will require transfusions of fresh frozen plasma. These should be given primarily when there is active hemorrhage, although prophylactic transfusion may be required in acute liver failure, where increased prothrombin times exceeding 30 seconds may be seen. In general, correction of the prothrombin time to less than 15 seconds is probably unnecessary and may be dangerous in variceal bleeding or fulminant liver failure, where the increased intravascular volume may have the undesirable effect of elevating either portal or intracerebral pressure. When fresh frozen plasma is transfused, the quantity needed should be guided by the general rule that two units will be required for every four units of packed red blood cells transfused. As stated previously, a normal prothrombin time in a compensated cirrhotic may rise quickly during active hemorrhage and should be closely monitored.

In fulminant hepatic failure, the safe and rapid replenishment of clotting factors may be accomplished with therapeutic exchange plasmapheresis. Munoz et al. treated 19 such patients with plasmapheresis and fresh frozen plasma replacement and achieved a drop in the prothrombin time from an average of 28.3 seconds to 17.7 seconds in one or two sessions.[46] The ability to correct coagulopathy in these patients is necessary to facilitate the placement of central lines, pulmonary artery catheters, and intracerebral pressure monitoring devices.

Finally, the appearance of fibrinolysis and consumptive coagulopathy in liver disease is usually an ominous occurrence associated with a poor prognosis. It can be treated only with repeated transfusions of fresh frozen plasma or liver transplantation, as the empiric use of heparin is unproven and is not recommended.

Hepatic Encephalopathy

Hepatic encephalopathy is a complex neuropsychiatric disorder seen in acute and chronic liver disease that is characterized by marked neural inhibition. Theories concerning the pathogenesis of this syndrome include (1) impaired hepatic clearance of neurotoxins such as ammonia, mercaptans, and short-chain fatty acids; (2) an increase in the serum ratio of aromatic to branched chain amino acids, resulting in the accumulation of false neurotransmitters in the central nervous system; and (3) increased plasma and central nervous system levels of the neuroinhibitor gamma-amino-butyric acid (GABA) and endogenous benzodiazepine-like ligandins. Speculation persists as to the validity and importance of each of these hypotheses.

There are multiple precipitating factors for hepatic encephalopathy, but gastrointestinal bleeding is one of the most common. This is not surprising, since many of these cerebrotoxins can be derived from the degradation of blood in the intestinal tract. Christensen et al. have recently shown that when hepatic coma complicates variceal bleeding in cirrhotic patients, the mortality during hospitalization increases from approximately 10% to 50%.[47] This may be due to complications of encephalopathy such as sepsis and pulmonary aspiration, or it may reflect a poor underlying hepatic reserve in these patients. Regardless, aggressive treatment and correction of precipitating factors is required to optimize the outcome. The first step in the treatment of encephalopathy precipitated by gastrointestinal bleeding, besides arresting hemorrhage, is to remove the potentially digestible blood from the gastrointestinal tract through nasogastric suction. Blood itself is a cathartic and may induce rapid intestinal transit when hemorrhage is massive. When bleeding is more moderate or has ceased, lactulose, a nonabsorbable carbohydrate, can be given in doses of 30 cc every six hours or as needed to promote three or four bowel movements in a 24-hour period. Lactulose works by causing an osmotic diarrhea and has the added effect of acidifying the intestinal contents and suppressing ammonia absorption from the gut. Caution should be taken to avoid dehydration and hypernatremia that may result from overzealous therapy. When oral treatment is not possible, as in acute gastrointestinal bleeding, lactulose can be effectively given in serial retention enemas of 250 cc in 500 cc of tap water. Recently, a more palatable, less expensive, nonabsorbable carbohydrate, lactitol, has been developed and may prove to be an alternative to lactulose, particularly in the outpatient setting.[48]

If the clinical circumstances preclude enteral feeding, total parenteral nutrition is required. Erikkson and Conn recently reviewed most published clinical trials of branched-chain amino acid solutions in acute encephalopathy and found that the efficacy of this treatment has not been unequivocally proven, largely because of the difficulties involved in performing studies of this type.[49] Nevertheless, reversal of abnormal branched-chain amino acid to aromatic amino acid ratios has been shown to occur after infusion of these solutions, and we continue to use them on an empiric basis. Intralipids, because of the potential neurotoxicity of short-chain fatty acids, should be avoided in severe acute encephalopathy or fulminant hepatic failure until this form of nutritional replacement has been proven to be safe and effective in these settings. Once enteral feeding is possible, a low-protein diet may be given, as well as the branched-chain amino acid enteral supplements which are now available.

Paramount in the management of hepatic encephalopathy is the identification and treatment of all precipitating factors. Metabolic disturbances such as hypokalemia and metabolic alkalosis that result from vomiting and nasogastric suction, as well as diuretic use, should be corrected. Infection, particularly spontaneous bacterial peritonitis, must be ruled out or treated aggressively if present. Azotemia, which exacerbates hepatic encephalopathy, may respond to volume expansion or hemodialysis if the latter is appropriate.

Of critical importance, particularly in the setting of fulminant hepatic failure, is the avoidance of central nervous system depressants such as hypnotic or narcotic agents which may deepen and prolong hepatic encephalopathy. Of course, sedation is necessary to perform upper endoscopy and other invasive procedures safely or to treat alcohol withdrawal. Benzodiazepines are often used in these settings but are believed to cause neural inhibition at the same receptor site as GABA, leading to worsening of the underlying encephalopathy.[50] To complicate matters, patients with liver disease may be particularly sensitive to even routine doses of these medications because of reduced protein binding, decreased metabolism, and a small volume of distribution, which cause a marked increase in half-life. For instance, the half-life of diazepam, a common premedicating sedative, may reach 100 hours in cirrhosis.[51] Recently, midazolam, a short-acting benzodiazepine with a half-life of two hours in normal patients, has become popular for sedation in endoscopy. Even this agent has been shown to have a doubling of the half-life in cirrhosis, with some patients having significant blood levels up to 12 hours after injection.[52] Because of its short half-life, midazolam is still the most appropriate agent for temporary sedation in patients with liver disease; however, smaller and less frequent doses than usual should be given. Oxazepam, a benzodiazepine with a half-life unchanged by the presence or absence of liver disease, is the most reasonable agent to use in controlling alcohol withdrawal where prolonged therapy is required.

Some physicians are in the habit of using narcotic agents for sedation, either alone or in combination with benzodiazepines. Narcotics such as morphine were originally believed to have normal metabolism in cirrhosis, but recent reports have shown that the half-life of these agents may be prolonged two or three times in advanced liver disease.[53] Therefore, clinicians must be aware that narcotics may accumulate in the cirrhotic when they are given at the usual dosing intervals. Similarly, if naloxone, a narcotic antagonist, is required to reverse narcotic effects, it may need to be given serially if there is any question of narcotic contribution to a patient's prolonged coma.

Ascites and Renal Failure

The initial goal of therapy in gastrointestinal bleeding is to restore the patient's intravascular volume and blood oxygen-carrying capacity with a combination of crystalloid solutions and blood products. In patients with liver disease, this may result in the development or exacerbation of ascites. Subsequent efforts to mobilize this fluid may then precipitate functional renal failure or the hepatorenal syndrome. In order to avoid this scenario, the clinician must understand the forces behind ascites formation and be familiar with the basic concepts of fluid management in these patients.

For many years, researchers debated whether ascites formed because of "overflow" or "underfill" of the intravascular space. At present, the theory most widely accepted for ascites formation combines both of these concepts. It is now believed that peripheral vasodilation is the initiating event leading to decreased effective arterial blood flow.[54] Increased levels of plasma renin, aldosterone, norepinephrine, and vasopressin concentrations follow, giving rise to renal vasoconstriction with sodium and water retention. The result is plasma volume expansion, but because of portal hypertension, some of this volume begins to sequester in the peritoneal space, forming ascites. As hepatic function deteriorates, vasodilation becomes severe and ascites becomes massive, which results in a decrease in the effective arterial volume to the point where renal failure or the hepatorenal syndrome is precipitated.

Hemodynamically significant gastrointestinal bleeding accelerates the above clinical events in the following way. The acute loss of 1 liter of blood, for instance, results in approximately a 20% loss of effective arterial volume. The neurohumoral mechanisms already favoring salt and water retention are intensified. Volume replacement with saline will increase total body sodium, much of which leaves the intravascular space. After an initial drop in the portal venous pressure, vasoconstriction will occur and, together with volume replacement, the portal pressure may rise to approximately 20% above the prehemorrhage level, further favoring ascites formation.[55] The clinician may then have an impression of volume overload, but low systolic blood pressure and unreliable central venous pressure monitoring encountered in the setting of advanced liver disease will be confusing. Subsequent institution of diuretic therapy will lead to further reductions of arterial blood volume and possibly to the hepatorenal syndrome.

The management of ascites and renal failure in the bleeding patient with liver disease begins with a careful clinical assessment. The patient should be screened for underlying cardiac diseases, such as alcoholic cardiomyopathy, that may also complicate volume management. Underlying renal disease, particularly in diabetics, hemodialysis patients, or renal transplant recipients, should be identified. If the patient has recently been hospitalized, the use of a nephrotoxic agent such as iodinated dye for radiological studies or aminoglycoside antibiotics should be ascertained. Of particular importance is the recent use of nonsteroidal anti-inflammatory agents, which are known to precipitate functional renal failure in stable cirrhotic patients.[56] The physical examination should be thorough; however, one must realize that assessing the volume status is extremely difficult in patients with liver disease.

Laboratory examinations should include BUN and creatinine determinations, with the caveat that both of these levels may overestimate the glomerular filtration rate in cirrhotics. Urine sodium and osmolality, as well as urinalysis, should be obtained. These may help in differentiating hepatorenal syndrome from acute tubular necrosis, but not from prerenal azotemia, a common dilemma (Table 6.2). If ascites is present, a diagnostic paracentesis should be performed. This can be safely done with a 21-gauge needle, even in the presence of moderate coagulopathy. The fluid should be sent for a cell count and immediately inoculated into blood culture bottles to rule out spontaneous bacterial peritonitis. A total neutrophil count above 300 is consistent with infection. This condition should be treated empirically before culture results are available. A striking elevation in the neutrophil count above 10,000 suggests a secondary bacterial peritonitis and should initiate a search for an occult intra-abdominal process such as a ruptured viscus. In addition, total protein and albumin determinations of the ascitic fluid should be obtained. A gradient between the serum and ascitic fluid albumin level of greater than 1.1 g/dl is consistent with underlying portal hypertension as the etiology for the ascites.[57] A high total protein level (above 3 g/dl) may be seen with a high albumin gradient and is consistent with an extrahepatic postsinusoidal cause of portal hypertension such as Budd-Chiari syndrome or right-sided heart failure.[58] A high total protein in the setting of a low albumin gradient is seen with peritoneal carcinomatosis or an inflammatory process involving the peritoneum.

Volume replacement following hemorrhage should begin with packed red blood cells if anemia is present or if the acute blood loss is massive. A hematocrit of 30% in a hemodynamically stable patient should be the goal of therapy. Transfusion to higher

TABLE 6.2. Differential Diagnosis of Acute Azotemia in the Patient with Liver Disease

	Important Differential Urinary Findings		
Biochemical Characteristics	*Prerenal Azotemia*	*Hepatorenal Syndrome*	*Acute Failure (Acute Tubular Necrosis)*
Urine sodium concentration (mEq/liter)	<10	<10	>30*
Urine:plasma creatinine ratio	<30:1	>30:1	<20:1
Urine osmolality	At least 100 mOsm > plasma osmolality	At least 100 mOsm > plasma osmolality	Equal to plasma osmolality
Urine sediment	Normal	Unremarkable	Casts, cellular debris

*It has recently been appreciated that radiocontrast agents and sepsis may lower the urinary sodium concentration in the patient with acute tubular necrosis.

Source: Reprinted with permission from Epstein MD, *The Kidney in Liver Disease*, ed 3. Baltimore, MD, Williams and Wilkins Co, 1988.

hematocrit levels to serve as a "buffer" against recurrent bleeding may cause a dangerous increase in portal pressure, because of the rebound phenomena noted earlier, and may precipitate or perpetuate bleeding of portal hypertensive etiology. If volume expansion alone is required, solutions which are oncotically active should be given (e.g., albumin infused as a 25% or 5% solution). Fresh frozen plasma may be more appropriate if coagulopathy is present, but this carries the risk of transmitting viral hepatitis. Adequacy of volume replacement should be assessed clinically by following the urine output and vital signs; however, a pulmonary artery catheter may be required to assess left ventricular filling pressures accurately.

When ascites develops, treatment should initially be conservative. If the patient is taking enteral feedings, sodium should be restricted to less than 2 g/day. Fluid restriction is not needed unless there is coexistent hyponatremia to less than 130 mEq/dl. Initially, particularly in the setting of fulminant hepatitis or severe alcoholic hepatitis, it is best to avoid the use of diuretics, as they precipitate metabolic disturbances, hepatic encephalopathy, and renal failure.[59] When confronted with symptomatic ascites, therapeutic large-volume paracentesis is the quickest and most efficient way to remove fluid. Some physicians have remained reluctant to use this method due to the fear of precipitating hypotension or renal failure, beliefs which were once widely held. Many reports characterizing the hemodynamic and renal parameters following large-volume paracentesis show it to be both safe and effective. Gines et al., in a series of 58 patients with ascites randomized to either diuretics or large-volume paracentesis, found a lower rate of hepatic encephalopathy, hyponatremia, and renal impairment in the group receiving paracentesis.[60] Originally, it was believed that 5 liters were the maximal amount of ascites that could be removed safely with each paracentesis, but Tito et al. have shown that withdrawal of up to 25 liters without renal impairment is possible.[61] Studies with large-volume paracentesis have usually involved infusing 5–10 g of albumin per liter of ascites removed; however, this therapy has been found to be somewhat cumbersome and quite expensive, limiting the utility of the procedure. A recent study suggests that dextran 70, a synthetic volume expander, is as effective as albumin in preventing renal failure after large-volume paracentesis, at a considerable cost saving.[62]

If paracentesis is not possible, we often use a "Galambos cocktail," which consists of an albumin infusion followed by intravenous furosemide and mannitol to induce diuresis without compromising intravascular volume. There is a reluctance to use peritoneovenous shunting to remove ascites after gastrointestinal bleeding, as the increased intravascular volume that results may precipitate variceal bleeding. Peritoneovenous shunts may also cause severe thrombocytopenia and coagulopathy associated with DIC.[63]

If, in the presence of ascites, the urine output begins to fall and the creatinine level rises, the hepatorenal syndrome must be suspected. This is a diagnosis of exclusion and can only be made following attempts to increase intravascular volume. The prognosis for patients with hepatorenal syndrome is extremely poor unless the hepatic dysfunction is reversible, and liver transplantation may be the only chance for survival. There is no contraindication to temporary dialysis for hepatorenal syndrome if there is suspected reversibility of the underlying liver disease or if liver transplantation is planned.

Surgical Intervention for Gastrointestinal Bleeding in Liver Disease

Since the advent of fiberoptic endoscopy over two decades ago, a variety of nonsurgical hemostatic techniques have emerged for both variceal and nonvariceal bleeding. Despite these advances, surgical intervention to control acute or chronic bleeding is still often required. Careful evaluation of hepatic function is required to make the most appropriate decisions regarding the type and timing of surgery in patients with liver disease.

Unfortunately, the presence of hepatic dysfunction greatly increases the risks during the operative and postoperative periods. Patients with liver disease may suffer severe decompensation or overt hepatic failure after surgery, resulting in profound coagulopathy, encephalopathy, and renal failure. The etiology of this condition is probably hepatic ischemia, as inhalational, spinal, and epidural anesthetics all reduce hepatic blood flow by 30–50% during induction.[64] Increased sympathetic tone secondary to surgical stress elevates splanchnic vascular resistance and further reduces hepatic blood flow. Hypotension, anemia, and hepatic congestion secondary to mechanical ventilation may also contribute to decreased oxygen delivery to the liver.

Other factors contribute to the poor surgical outcome as well. Altered drug metabolism and sensitivity to sedative-narcotic agents, already discussed, are even more problematic in the postoperative state, when pain relief and anxiety reduction are necessary. Aminoglycosides may be required to treat postoperative infection and are more nephrotoxic in patients with underlying liver disease. Sepsis is also a problem in up to one-third of patients with postoperative hepatic failure because of underlying immune defects.[65] Finally, the problems of coagulopathy, ascites, and renal failure, discussed earlier in reference to gastrointestinal bleeding, exist in the perioperative state as well.

For the purposes of this section, we must stratify the surgical risk in specific patients with liver disease. In general, acute icteric viral hepatitis and severe alcoholic hepatitis both pose extremely high risks for any surgical intervention. In an older series where patients were operated on for presumed biliary obstruction on clinical grounds, every patient with acute alcoholic or viral hepatitis died perioperatively.[66] Conversely, patients with chronic viral hepatitis without cirrhosis appear to be at little increased risk for surgical procedures, although one must be careful not to underestimate the degree of underlying hepatic dysfunction based on admission transaminase values, as noted previously.[67]

Of greatest importance is the assessment of the cirrhotic patient, in whom surgery for gastrointestinal bleeding is most often required. The outcome following surgery for these patients is best predicted by the preoperative functional hepatic reserve, as determined by clinical or laboratory parameters or the modified Child's classification. Garrison et al. reviewed a series of 100 cirrhotic patients who underwent elective and emergent nonshunt laparotomy and found that the mortality was 10%, 31%, and 76% in Child's A, B, and C patients, respectively.[68] The overall mortality for the 12 patients with nonvariceal bleeding in this study was 33%. Aranha et al. similarly found 67% mortality in 51 patients with Child's B and C cirrhosis undergoing nonshunt laparotomy with mortality increasing to 83% in the presence of ascites and to 91% when the prothrombin time was elevated above 2.5 seconds.[69] In an older series from Boston City Hospital dealing specifically with surgery for nonvariceal gastrointestinal hemorrhage, there was a 57% overall mortality, with more than 90% mortality when the preoperative bilirubin level was above 4 mg/dl.[70]

Increasing mortality predicted by Child's classification has been demonstrated for selective and nonselective portosystemic shunts for acute or recurrent variceal bleeding. However, probably the most important factor influencing survival in these patients appears to be the avoidance of emergency intervention. Procedures undertaken prior to the cessation of hemorrhage and clinical stabilization have up to 50% mortality in patients with Child's C cirrhosis, almost 10 times that of an elective procedure.[71] This discrepancy between elective and emergent procedures may be due to operative factors, improvement in Child's classification during stabilization, or, more likely, elimination of doomed patients by death prior to elective surgery.

Recently, another factor has emerged in assessing a cirrhotic patient who requires surgery for gastrointestinal bleeding. Unfortunately, although portosystemic shunt surgery prevents recurrent gastrointestinal bleeding in many, survival is not prolonged because the patient is left with a diseased liver compromised by diversion of the portal nutrient blood flow. Subsequently, liver function will deteriorate and hepatocellular carcinoma may develop. These factors make liver transplantation an attractive option now that long-term survival is possible because of advances in both surgical experience and immunosuppressive therapy. Iwatsuki et al. compared the survival of patients with a history of variceal bleeding undergoing liver transplantation with that reported in the literature following portosystemic shunt surgery and found superior survival in the transplanted group.[72] This was in spite of the fact that most transplant patients were in the Child's C category, with advanced liver disease. Wood et al. similarly found that when Child's C patients alone were considered, the five-year survival of transplantation vs. selective shunt surgery was increased from 40% to 65%.[73] One must realize that any intra-abdominal surgery, particularly if it involves the portal venous system, may make subsequent hepatic transplantation more difficult, if not impossible. A thorough evaluation by a liver disease specialist and a transplant surgeon after variceal bleeding is indicated in the patient with Child's B or C liver disease to determine eligibility for present or future liver transplantation.

Clearly, a decision to operate on a patient with liver disease must be individualized, but the recommendations are as follows. In nonvariceal bleeding, surgery must be undertaken only after endoscopic attempts to stop bleeding have been exhausted, particularly if the patient has ascites or falls into the Child's C category. Arbitrary decisions to intervene operatively after a certain number of units or red cells have been transfused have to be abandoned given the poor postoperative outcome in these patients. Likewise, elective surgery to prevent the recurrence of nonvariceal bleeding, particularly from peptic ulcer disease, carries a high risk and may make subsequent transplantation more difficult. In variceal bleeding, surgery again must be reserved for patients who have had bleeding arrested, if possible, by a combination of sclerotherapy, balloon tamponade, and medical treatment, regardless of Child's classification. As noted above, the possibility of future hepatic transplantation in these patients must be considered prior to any abdominal surgical procedure.

REFERENCES

1. Banti G: Dell anemia splenica. *Arch Scuola Anat Pato (Firenze)* 2:53–122, 1833.
2. Schlichting P, Christensen E, Fauerholdt L, et al: Main causes of death in cirrhosis. *Scand J Gastroenterol* 18:881–888, 1983.
3. Everhart JE, Di Bisceglie AM, Murray LM, et al: Risk for non-A, non-B (type C) hepatitis through sexual or household contact with chronic carriers. *Ann Intern Med* 112:544–545, 1990.
4. Conn HO: Trailmaking and number-connection tests in the assessment of mental state in portal systemic encephalopathy. *Am J Dig Dis* 22:541–550, 1977.
5. Reichling JJ, Kaplan MM: Clinical use of serum enzymes in liver disease. *Dig Dis Sci* 33:1601–1614, 1988.
6. Raby N, Karani J, Powell-Jackson P, et al: Assessment of portal vein patency: Comparison of arterial portography and ultrasound scanning. *Clin Radiol* 39:381–385, 1988.
7. Polio J, Groszmann RJ: Hemodynamic factors involved in the development and rupture of esophageal varices: A pathophysiologic approach to treatment. *Semin Liv Dis* 6:318–331, 1986.
8. Dagradi AE, Mehler R, Tan DTD, et al: Sources of upper gastrointestinal bleeding in patients with liver cirrhosis and large esophagogastric varices. *Am J Gastroenterol* 54:458–502, 1970.
9. Waldram R, Davis M, Nunnerley H, et al: Emergency endoscopy after gastrointestinal hemorrhage in 50 patients with portal hypertension. *Br Med J* 4:94–96, 1974.
10. Thomas E, Rosenthal WS, Rymer W, et al: Upper gastrointestinal hemorrhage in patients with alcoholic liver disease and esophageal varices. *Am J Gastroenterol* 72:623–629, 1979.
11. Mitchell KJ, Madougall BRD, Silk DBA, et al: A prospective reappraisal of emergency endoscopy in patients with portal hypertension. *Scand J Gastroenterol* 17:965–968, 1982.
12. Tabiban N, Graham DY: Source of upper gastrointestinal bleeding in patients with esophageal varices seen at endoscopy. *J Clin Gastroenterol* 9:279–282, 1987.
13. The North Italian Endoscopic Club for Study and Treatment of Esophageal Varices: Prediction of the first variceal hemorrhage in patients with cirrhosis of the liver and esophageal varices: A prospective multicenter study. *N Engl J Med* 319:983–989, 1988.
14. Muringhini A, Cuttone M, Sciarrino E, et al: Ultrasonography and alpha-fetoprotein in diagnosis of hepatocellular carcinoma in cirrhosis. *Dig Dis Sci* 33:47–51, 1988.
15. Sherlock S: Esophageal varices. *Am J Surg* 160:9–13, 1990.

16. Christensen E, Schlichting P, Fauerholdt L, et al: Prognostic value of Child-Turcotte criteria in medically treated cirrhosis. *Hepatology* 4:430–435, 1984.
17. Cales P, Zabotto B, Mesken SC, et al: Gastroesophageal endoscopic features in cirrhosis. Observer variability, interassociations, and relationship to hepatic dysfunction. *Gastroenterology* 98:156–162, 1990.
18. Gines P, Quintero E, Arroyo V, et al: Compensated cirrhosis: Natural history and prognosis factors. *Hepatology* 7:122–128, 1987.
19. Graham DY, Smith JL: The course of patients after variceal hemorrhage. *Gastroenterology* 80:800–809, 1981.
20. Sarfeh IJ, Juler GL, Stemmer EA, et al: Results of surgical management of hemorrhagic gastritis in patients with gastroesophageal varices. *Surg Gynecol Obstet* 155:167–170, 1982.
21. McCormack TT, Sims J, Eyre-Brook I, et al: Gastric lesions in portal hypertension: Inflammatory gastritis or congestive gastropathy? *Gut* 26:1226–1232, 1985.
22. Papazian A, Braillon A, Dupas JL, et al: Portal hypertensive gastric mucosa: An endoscopic study. *Gut* 27:1199–1203, 1986.
23. Sarfeh IJ, Tarnawski A, Malki A, et al: Portal hypertension and gastric mucosal injury in rats. Effects of alcohol. *Gastroenterology* 84:987–993, 1983.
24. Sarin SK, Misra SP, Singal A, et al: Evaluation of the incidence and significance of the "mosaic pattern" in patients with cirrhosis, noncirrhotic portal fibrosis, and extrahepatic obstruction. *Am J Gastroenterol* 83:1235–1239, 1988.
25. Foster PN, Wyatt JI, Bullmore DW, et al: Gastric mucosa in patients with portal hypertension: Prevalence of capillary dilatation and campylobacter pylori. *J Clin Pathol* 42:919–921, 1989.
26. D'Amico G, Montalbano L, Traina M, et al: Natural history of congestive gastropathy in cirrhosis. *Gastroenterology* 99:1558–1564, 1990.
27. Cappell MS, Price JB: Characterization of the syndrome of small and large intestinal variceal bleeding. *Dig Dis Sci* 32:422–427, 1987.
28. Manzione N, Kiron MD, Walkoff AW: Unusual sites of upper gastrointestinal variceal bleeding. *J Clin Gastroenterol* 9:40–42, 1987.
29. Foutch PG, Sivak MV: Colonic hemorrhage after endoscopic injection sclerosis of esophageal varices: A report of three cases. *Am J Gastroenterol* 79:756–760, 1984.
30. Kirk AP, Dooley JS, Hunt RH: Peptic ulceration in patients with chronic liver disease. *Dig Dis Sci* 25:756–760, 1980.
31. Rabinovitz M, Young-Kul Y, Schade R, et al: Prevalence of endoscopic findings in 510 consecutive individuals with cirrhosis evaluated prospectively. *Dig Dis Sci* 35:705–710, 1990.
32. De Weert TM, Gostout CJ, Wiesner RH: Congestive gastropathy and other upper endoscopic findings in 81 consecutive patients undergoing orthotopic liver transplantation. *Am J Gastroenterol* 85:573–576, 1990.
33. Tabaqchali S, Dawson AM: Peptic ulcer and gastric secretion in patients with liver diseases. *Gut* 5:417–421, 1964.
34. Ostensen H, Gudmundsen TE, Ostensen M, et al: Smoking, alcohol, coffee, and familial factors: Any association with peptic ulcer disease? A clinically and radiologically prospective study. *Scand J Gastroenterol* 20:1227–1235, 1985.
35. Sugawa C: Endoscopic diagnosis and treatment of upper gastrointestinal bleeding. *Surg Clin North Am* 69:1167–1183, 1989.
36. Paquet KJ, Mercado-Diaz M, Kalk JF: Frequency, significance and therapy of the Mallory-Weiss syndrome in patients with portal hypertension. *Hepatology* 11:879–883, 1990.
37. Cowan DH, Hines JD: Thrombocytopenia of severe alcoholism. *Ann Intern Med* 74:37–43, 1971.

38. Ingeberg S, Jacobsen P, Foscher ER, et al: Platelet aggregation and release of ATP in patients with hepatic cirrhosis. *Scand J Gastroenterol* 20:285–288, 1985.
39. Owen JS, Hutton RA, Day RC, et al: Platelet lipid composition and platelet aggregation in human liver disease. *J Lipid Res* 22:423–430, 1981.
40. Francis JL, Armstrong DJ: Acquired dysfibrinogenemia in liver disease. *J Clin Pathol* 35:667–672, 1982.
41. Carr JM: Disseminated intravascular coagulation in cirrhosis. *Hepatology* 10:103–110, 1989.
42. Murray DJ, Olson JO, Strauss R, et al: Coagulation changes during packed red cell replacement of major blood loss. *Anesthesiology* 69:839–845, 1988.
43. Burroughs AK, Matthews K, Qadiri M, et al: Desmopressin and bleeding time in patients with cirrhosis. *Br Med J* 291:1377–1381, 1985.
44. Mannuccio PM, Viceantre V, Vianello L, et al: Controlled trial of desmopressin in liver cirrhosis and other conditions associated with a prolonged bleeding time. *Blood* 67:1148–1153, 1985.
45. Manucci PM: Desmopressin: A non-transfusional form of treatment for congenital and acquired bleeding disorders. *Blood* 72:1451–1455, 1988.
46. Munoz SJ, Ballas SK, Moritz MJ, et al: Perioperative management of fulminant and subfulminant hepatic failure with therapeutic plasmapheresis. *Transplant Proc* 21:3535–3536, 1989.
47. Christensen E, Krintel JJ, Hansen SM, et al: Prognosis after the first episode of gastrointestinal bleeding or coma in cirrhosis. Survival and prognostic factors. *Scand J Gastroenterol* 24:999–1006, 1989.
48. Lanthier PL, Morgan MY: Lactitol in the treatment of chronic hepatic encephalopathy: An open comparison with lactulose. *Gut* 26:415–420, 1985.
49. Erikkson SL, Conn HO: Branched-chain amino acids in the management of hepatic encephalopathy: An analysis of variants. *Hepatology* 10:228–246, 1989.
50. Gammal SH, Jones EA: Hepatic encephalopathy. *Med Clin North Am* 73:793–813, 1989.
51. Klotz U, Avant GR, Hoyumpa A, et al: The effects of age and liver disease on the disposition and elimination of diazepam in adult man. *J Clin Invest* 55:347–359, 1975.
52. MacGilchrist AJ, Birne GG, Cook A: Pharmacokinetics and pharmacodynamics of intravenous midazolam in patients with severe alcoholic cirrhosis. *Gut* 27:190–195, 1986.
53. Mazoit JX, Sandouk P, Zetlaoui P, et al: Pharmacokinetics of unchanged morphine in normal and cirrhotic subjects. *Anesth Analg* 66:293–298, 1987.
54. Schrier RW, Arroyo V, Bernardi M, et al: Peripheral arterial vasodilation hypothesis: A proposal for the initiation of renal sodium and water retention in cirrhosis. *Hepatology* 8:1151–1157, 1988.
55. Kravetz D, Sikuler E, Groszmann RJ: Splanchnic and systemic hemodynamics in portal hypertensive rats during hemorrhage and blood volume restitution. *Gastroenterology* 90:1232–1240, 1986.
56. Epstein M, Lifschitz M: Renal eicosanoids as determinants of renal function in liver disease. *Hepatology* 7:1359–1367, 1987.
57. Rector WG, Reynolds TB: Superiority of the serum-ascites albumin difference over the ascites total protein concentration in separation of "transudative" and "exudative ascites." *Am J Med* 77:83–85, 1984.
58. Runyon BA: Cardiac ascites: A characterization. *J Clin Gastroenterol* 10:410–412, 1988.
59. Editorial: Diuretics or paracentesis for ascites? *Lancet* 2:775, 1988.
60. Gines P, Arroyo V, Quintero E, et al: Comparison between paracentesis and diuretics in the treatment of cirrhosis with tense ascites. *Gastroenterology* 93:234–241, 1987.

61. Tito LJ, Gines P, Arroyo V, et al: Total paracentesis associated with intravenous albumin management of patients with cirrhosis and ascites. *Gastroenterology* 98:146–151, 1990.

62. Planas R, Gines P, Arroyo V, et al: Dextran-70 versus albumin as plasma expanders in cirrhotic patients with tense ascites: Results of a randomized trial. *Gastroenterology* 99:1736–1744, 1990.

63. Fulerwider JT, Smith RB, Redd SC, et al: Peritoneovenous shunts. *Arch Surg* 199:1133–1137, 1984.

64. Batchelder BM, Cooperman LH: Effects of anesthetics on splanchnic circulation and metabolism. *Surg North Am* 55:787–794, 1975.

65. Norton K, Moore G, Eisman B: Liver failure in the postoperative patient: The role of sepsis and immunologic deficiency. *Surgery* 78:6–13, 1975.

66. Powell-Jackson P, Greenway B, Williams R: Adverse effects of exploratory laparotomy in patients with unsuspected liver disease. *Br J Surg* 69:449–451, 1982.

67. Runyon BA: Surgial procedures are well tolerated by patients with asymptomatic chronic hepatitis. *J Clin Gastroenterol* 8:542–544, 1986.

68. Garrison RN, Cryer HM, Howard DA, et al: Clarification of risk factors for abdominal operations in patients with hepatic cirrhosis. *Ann Surg* 199:648–655, 1984.

69. Aranha GV, Greenlee HB: Intra-abdominal surgery in patients with advanced cirrhosis. *Arch-Surg* 121:275–277, 1986.

70. Wirthlin LR, Van Urk H, Malt RB, et al: Predictors of surgical mortality in patients with cirrhosis and nonvariceal gastroduodenal bleeding. *Surg Gynecol Obstet* 139:65–68, 1974.

71. Levine BA, Sirinek KR: The portocaval shunt: Is it still indicated? *Surg Clin North Am* 70:361–378, 1990.

72. Iwatsuki S, Starzl TE, Todo S, et al: Liver transplantation in the treatment of bleeding esophageal varices. *Surgery* 104:697–705, 1988.

73. Wood RP, Shaw BW, Rikkers LF: Liver transplantation for variceal hemorrhage. *Surg Clin North Am* 70:449–461, 1990.

7

DRUG-INDUCED GASTROINTESTINAL INJURY AND BLEEDING

Bernard M. Schuman, M.D.
Joseph W. Griffin, Jr., M.D.

INTRODUCTION

A number of drugs have been implicated as injurious to the gastrointestinal (GI) mucosa, with the resultant complication of bleeding or perforation. Pill-induced esophageal ulceration has been documented since 1970,[1] and in subsequent years many case reports have associated a variety of pharmacological agents with esophageal injury.[2] The most common drugs involved—tetracycline derivatives, potassium chloride, and quinidine—produce a spectrum of pathology ranging from mild esophagitis to deep ulceration, but the clinical manifestations are primarily pain and dysphagia, with bleeding being an infrequent complication.[3]

Ethanol-induced gastric injury in laboratory animals has been well recognized for many years,[4] and although it is often a factor in self-limited GI mucosal bleeding,[5] no direct role for alcohol has been established in the causation of gastroduodenal ulceration, with or without hemorrhage, in humans. There may be a potentiating effect of alcohol on the gastroduodenal mucosal damage by nonsteroidal anti-inflammatory drugs (NSAIDs),[6] but alcohol per se is not a clinically important aspect of GI bleeding.[7]

There is considerable controversy regarding the ulcerogenicity of corticosteroids. Studies purporting to show that corticosteroids induce ulcers and GI bleeding are often hampered by being retrospective, may be difficult to interpret because of the use of concomitant drugs such as aspirin and are sometimes unreliable because of failure to utilize endoscopy for diagnosis. A meta-analysis suggested that there was an association between corticosteroids and peptic ulcer[8] but, on clinical grounds, other than the risk of masking the signs of acute ulcer perforation that may occur with high-dose therapy, there is apparently not much concern among physicians that patients on standard doses of corticosteroids will develop peptic ulcer, because antiulcer therapy is infrequently prescribed as adjunct therapy. Piper et al.,[9] in a study of over 1,400 patients hospitalized for ulcer or GI bleeding, showed that the risk of developing peptic ulcer disease among users of oral corticosteroids was increased only in those who concurrently received NSAIDs; this risk was 15 times greater than that of nonusers of either drug.

Chemotherapeutic agents have well-known toxic effects on the GI tract but are not associated with clinically significant gastroduodenal ulceration when given by the standard dosage and route. However, in patients with hepatocellular carcinoma undergoing transcatheter arterial chemoembolization, 45% manifest GI ulceration, the ulcers being multiple in 13%.[10]

By far the most important drugs responsible for GI mucosal damage and bleeding are the NSAIDs, both salicylate and nonsalicylate in type.[11,12] NSAID consumption in the United States, the United Kingdom, and worldwide has shown remarkable growth based on both prescription and nonprescription use of this class of drugs. An aging population more subject to arthritis and chronic painful disorders, the availability of over-the-counter ibuprofen in the United States, and the general belief that NSAIDs are safer than aspirin are cited as reasons for this increased use. In this chapter, we will concentrate on the NSAID-injured gastroduodenal mucosa because this constitutes the major clinical basis for GI bleeding related to drug therapy.

NSAID GI MUCOSAL INJURY

Epidemiology of Bleeding

In a retrospective cohort study, Carson et al. found that patients taking NSAIDs had a rate of bleeding per 10,000 person-months one-third greater than that of patients not taking the drugs.[12] Somerville et al.,[13] by means of a case control analysis, established a relative risk for GI bleeding in NSAID users of 3.8 compared with that of hospital controls. Current use of NSAIDs in a Medicaid population over the age of 65 hospitalized for peptic ulcer disease or upper gastrointestinal (UGI) bleeding was associated with a risk of 2.4 for GI bleeding compared to hospital controls.[14] Aspirin alone has long been associated with major UGI bleeding[15] and recently has been shown to carry about the same risk as nonaspirin (NA) NSAIDs for UGI hemorrhage, based on an analysis of 57 patients hospitalized for melena or hematemesis compared with over 2,000 controls.[16] Kurata cites 11 case control studies and 5 cohort studies that appear to establish that both aspirin and NA-NSAIDs carry an increased risk ratio for the development of gastric and duodenal ulcers and consequent complications including death.[17]

Mucosal Injury with NSAIDs

The manifestations of mucosal injury by NSAIDs are submucosal hemorrhage, petechial eruption, erosions, and ulceration. The major site of injury is the gastric antrum, but the mucosa of the esophagus,[18] duodenum, small bowel, and colon may also be affected.[19] The small intestinal and colonic inflammation does not usually progress to ulceration but may be a source of occult bleeding. A recent report of endoscopically confirmed colonic (cecal and ascending colon) erosions and ulcerations associated with NSAID use highlights the potential for significant bleeding, as two of seven patients presented with massive hematochezia. Withdrawal of the NSAID resulted in healing of the lesions in all seven patients when studied by follow-up colonoscopy.[20]

Mucosal injury may occur because of direct topical damage or as a result of increased production of inflammatory mediators. Of all the NSAIDs, aspirin is the quintessential drug for demonstrating cell toxicity, disruption of the gastric mucosal barrier, reduction of adenosine 5′-triphosphate (ATP), and increased membrane permeability.[21] Back diffusion of hydrogen ions probably initiates epithelial cell damage, and the influx of other cations and water causes swelling and death of the cell.

Most NA-NSAIDs have no appreciable *direct* effect on the gastric mucosa and, of course, no effect on the distal intestinal mucosa. The other type of damage elicited by NA-NSAIDs and aspirin is caused by a systemic mechanism that involves the inhibition of cyclooxygenase, an enzyme essential to the production of prostaglandins from arachidonic acid. The depletion of gastric mucosal prostaglandins as a permissive factor in the development of mucosal injury is controversial because low prostaglandin levels have not been uniformly demonstrated in animal experiments,[22] although the preservation of gastric mucus and the microcirculation, both prostaglandin dependent, is obviously of mucosal defensive importance.[21] The prostaglandin E_1 analog, misoprostol, which has antisecretory and mucosal protective activity, was more effective in preventing gastric mucosal damage than an H-2 blocker in patients taking tolmetin,[23] an NSAID second only to sulindac as a cause of UGI bleeding.

The reduction in the amount and quality of gastric mucus by systemic effects on endogenous prostaglandin permits aspirin, for example, to permeate the epithelial cell layer when the intragastric pH is <3.5. As more cell disruption occurs, focal microcirculatory stasis develops, resulting in ischemia, and histamine is released from mast cells. Edema, submucosal hemorrhage, and erosions ensue. A continuing cycle of erosions, greater aspirin penetration of the cells, and ischemia bring about the formation of ulcers.[21] Many patients on NSAIDs, who develop hemorrhage and erosions early on, show mucosal healing even with continued administration of the NSAID. This ''mucosal adaptation'' to NSAID therapy is related to repair of the injury due to restitution of the surface epithelium by migration of cells from underlying layers. The failure of mucosal adaptation may partially explain why patients are as likely to have bleeding with short-term, acute therapy with NSAIDs as they are with chronic NSAID therapy.[24]

Although not directly responsible for gastric mucosal injury, the production of oxygen-free radicals and leukotrienes, by diversion of arachidonic acid through the lipoxygenase pathway (because of inhibition of cyclooxygenase), potentiates vasoconstriction. Most NSAIDs inhibit cyclooxygenase, but it has been difficult to show that gastric mucosal damage is related to the extent to which prostaglandin is reduced by this mechanism.[25]

There is a great deal of variation in the ulcerogenicity of NA-NSAIDs. The degree of anti-inflammatory effect and the level of prostaglandin depletion in gastric mucosa do not correlate with mucosal injury of the stomach.[26] A long plasma half-life of the drug, however, does appear to be important.[27,28] Thus, the high incidence of gastric ulcers noted in patients taking piroxicam may be a function of its long half-life. A prodrug that must be metabolized to an active agent usually does not significantly inhibit prostaglandin synthesis because, since it is nonacidic, there is little uptake by the epithelial cells. Nabumetone, for example, showed no more UGI blood loss, as measured by radioactive chromium, than placebo or control groups, whereas aspirin showed a statistically significant increased loss by comparison.[29] On the other hand, the prodrug sulindac, although

TABLE 7.1. NSAID: Relative Risk for GI Injury

Lower Risk	*Intermediate Risk*	*Higher Risk*
Nonacetylated salicylates	Fenoprofen	Aspirin
Magnesium choline trisalicylate	Ketoprofen	Indomethacin
Salsalate	Ketorolac (injectable)	Naproxen
Diclofenac	Tolmetin	Meclofenamate sodium
Diflunisal		Phenylbutazone
Etodolac		Piroxicam
Ibuprofen		Sulindac

producing little superficial damage of the mucosa, has a higher incidence of UGI bleeding from gastric ulcer than most other NSAIDs[28] (Table 7.1).

The relative risk of various NSAIDs for mucosal ulceration is summarized in Table 7.1. While none of the drugs are considered completely free of risk, the nonacetylated salicylates may be somewhat less injurious than either aspirin or the more potent, longer-acting NSAIDs.[30,31]

Because of the systemic pathways of prostaglandin inhibition, mucosal injury, GI ulceration, and bleeding are recognized effects of NSAIDs administered parenterally or rectally. The injectable NSAID ketorolac is used in the United States for postoperative analgesia and for other conditions requiring short-term pain control. While this agent may be somewhat less injurious than orally administered drugs, potential significant adverse effects, including bleeding, have been reported.[32]

Endoscopic Appearance of Mucosal Injury

Within one hour after the ingestion of aspirin, gastric erythema and petechiae are evident endoscopically. A few hours later, erosions may be seen, but these short-term effects do not necessarily persist or progress in patients taking aspirin for months or years. Similar findings occur with NA-NSAIDs, but to a lesser extent because these drugs have little or no topical toxicity. As Graham points out,[33] gastric erythema and petechiae represent trivial damage, and only erosions are really important. Presumably, a large number of erosions and greater size of the individual erosion (acute ulcer) correlate with the potential for gastric mucosal injury of the drug, but we have no data as to whether these early endoscopic findings predict chronic ulceration or bleeding.[34]

The endoscopic appearance of NSAID-induced gastric ulcer and duodenal ulcer in no way differs from that of ordinary peptic ulcers. When an erosion becomes an ulcer is subject to interpretation, but most endoscopists consider a diameter of 5 mm to be a reasonable lower limit of ulcer size. Some studies, however, have characterized 3-mm erosion as an ulcer. The appreciation of ulcer depth is in the eye of the beholder; thus, a required measured depth to make an erosion an ulcer has little scientific validity. Patients receiving chronic NSAID therapy have at least a 10% prevalence of gastroduodenal ulceration; some studies may approach 30%, obviously depending on the criteria used for the definition of ulcer.[35] The ulcers are usually found in elderly women, so the prevalence also depends on the patient population and the particular NSAIDs prescribed. When ulcers are identified endoscopically because of a bleeding complication, there is no way to know whether the ulcer preceded or was induced by NSAID therapy, or whether the ulcer is acute or chronic. Endoscopic biopsy does not differentiate typical peptic ulcer disease from NSAID ulcer. *Helicobacter pylori* may be found in antral tissue in about the same percentage (gastric ulcer 70%, duodenal ulcer 80%) in NSAID-induced ulcers as in peptic ulcers.[36]

The frequency of ulcers per month among NSAID users is 4% for gastric ulcers and 3% for duodenal ulcers.[33] Egan and Jensen, in 1991, reported that 60% of all ulcer patients admitted with UGI bleeding had ingested aspirin or an NSAID within two weeks of admission.[36] Thus, a history of NSAID use in a patient with UGI bleeding is highly predictive of the endoscopic finding of a gastric ulcer (less so for a duodenal ulcer), particularly if the patient is an elderly woman who has had previous ulcer disease and smokes.

Additional risk factors seen with NSAID-associated GI lesions have been studied extensively and can be summarized as follows: (1) age over 60 (in both men and women); (2) previous UGI events—including a history of ulcer disease, GI bleeding, and hospitalizations for UGI disease; (3) concomitant use of corticosteroids, apparently even in small doses; (4) severity of underlying rheumatological disorders, particularly rheumatoid arthritis, as related to the degree of functional impairment in these patients; (5) early in the course of NSAID therapy, namely within the first three months; and (6) the dose of the NSAID utilized.[14,37–39]

Unfortunately, NSAID-associated GI injury does not have a typical clinical presentation, as does classic peptic ulcer disease. There is a significant degree of dyspepsia in users of NSAIDs, but symptoms do not correlate with endoscopic findings, including the presence of deep ulcerations. In some series, over 50% of patients had as their initial manifestation a complication such as bleeding or perforation, but symptoms were otherwise clinically silent.[35,40,41] This clinical dilemma prevents a rational approach to both investigation and management of dyspeptic patients taking NSAIDs. While there is no accepted diagnostic algorithm for these patients, one must consider endoscopy in the NSAID-treated patient who experiences a significant change in symptoms or who has persistent/progressive dyspepsia. The explanation for the lack of typical peptic ulcer pain in NSAID users is unknown. The masking of symptoms may be related to the analgesic property of the NSAIDs themselves and to the underlying illness of these patients, which often results in chronic pain and a relative high tolerance of physical discomfort.

TREATMENT OF NSAID-INDUCED GASTRODUODENAL EROSIONS OR ULCER

For patients bleeding from multiple erosions of the stomach or duodenum, withdrawal of the NSAID usually results in prompt resolution of the hemorrhage. For bleeding ulcers, therapeutic measures described in Section V may be necessary as well. Obviously, there are some patients for whom alternative therapy such as analgesic drugs, nonacetylated salicylates, corticosteroids or immunosuppressive therapy are not effective or are contraindicated, and NSAIDs must be continued. No long-term studies show that any known ulcer therapy can prevent complications from NSAID-induced ulcers, although uncontrolled and controlled trials of traditional therapy indicate that acute mucosal disease can be attenuated and ulcers prevented or healed.[42-44] Ulcers of the stomach and duodenum will respond to treatment even in the face of ongoing NSAID therapy. Retrospective studies of high-dose antacids and H_2 receptor antagonists showed similar healing rates.[44] However, if the NSAID is continued, prolonged therapy with a full-dose ulcer regimen is usually required to achieve an acceptable healing rate. With continued NSAID administration, duodenal ulcer healing rates on full-dose H_2 antagonists may reach 80% only at eight weeks of therapy. In gastric ulcer, 75–80% will heal at 12–16 weeks if the NSAID is continued.[44-47] In a recent prospective randomized study, 40 μg daily of omeprazole (twice the dose usually employed in ulcer disease) healed more gastric ulcers than 150 μg of ranitidine twice daily in a subgroup of patients who continued NSAID therapy.[48] However, ranitidine has been found to be effective in reducing the frequency of duodenal ulcers in long-term NSAID users.[43]

Preventive Therapy

Numerous studies have been conducted in an attempt to define appropriate prophylactic or preventive therapy for NSAID-associated gut injury. There are great inconsistencies in the reported studies to date, including differences in study duration, in patient populations (healthy subjects vs. chronically ill patients), in the definition of endpoints of injury or protection, and in the doses of protective drugs employed. Many studies are not placebo controlled. In summary, at this time, the accumulated data indicate that full-dose H_2 antagonist therapy appears to be efficacious in preventing duodenal but not gastric ulceration. The H_2 drugs are well tolerated and appear safe on a long-term basis.[43,49,50] Moreover, the prostaglandin E_1 analog, misoprostol, and other prostaglandins are protective against NSAID-associated gastric ulceration. Misoprostol, at doses of 100 or 200 μg four times daily, has been shown to prevent the formation of gastric ulcers after one to three months of therapy with an NA-NSAID.[51] Compared to placebo-controlled populations, the incidence of duodenal ulcer is reduced only at the higher dose, 200 μg four times a day which is associated with acid antisecretory activity as well as with a mucosal protective mechanism.[52] Unfortunately, the adverse effects profile of the prostaglandin analogs includes a high incidence—up to 39%—of abdominal cramps and diarrhea. The abortifacient property of this class of drugs prohibits its use in women of childbearing potential.[47] Finally, there are recent studies suggesting that neither sucralfate nor antacids are superior to placebo in protecting against gastric or duodenal injury in NSAID users.[53-55]

Meta-analyses of the cost effectiveness of prophylactic therapy in both the United Kingdom and the United States have concluded that it is not cost beneficial to use prophylactic therapy across the board for patients taking NSAIDs.[56,57] Currently, the decision to use these expensive drugs to prevent gastroduodenal injury must be individualized. The use of preventive medication should be restricted to those patients who must be restarted on their NSAID after an ulcer hemorrhage or after the healing of a significant ulcer and to patients with multiple risk factors (see above).[58] Currently, there are no data on the long-term use of these agents in well-conducted, controlled trials. Furthermore, we are not aware of any study investigating the effectiveness of omeprazole as a preventive agent. It is clear that before any preventive therapy can be considered efficacious in the prophylaxis of ulcer complications, particularly bleeding, it will require a two- to three-year controlled evaluation, given the long latency period for the development of ulcers in many NSAID users.

REFERENCES

1. Pemberton D: Oesophageal obstruction and ulceration caused by oral potassium therapy. *Br Heart J* 323:267–268, 1970.
2. Kikendall JW, Friedman AC, Oyewole MA, et al: Pill-induced esophageal injury. Case reports and review of the medical literature. *Dig Dis Sci* 28:174–182, 1983.
3. Bott S, Prakash C, McCallum R: Medication-induced esophageal injury: Survey of the literature. *Am J Gastroenterol* 82:758–762, 1987.
4. Hollander D, Tarnawski A, Krause WJ, et al: Protective effect of sucralfate against alcohol-induced gastric mucosal injury in the rat. *Gastroenterology* 88:366–374, 1985.
5. Tarnawski A, Stachura J, Kleinczy RB, et al: Endoscopic appearance, transendoscopic potential difference, pH, histologic and ultrastructural changes in human gastric mucosa after alcohol. *Gastrointest Endosc* 28:145–149, 1982.
6. Lanza FL, Royer GL, Nelson RS, et al: A single blind randomized study of the potentiating effect of alcohol on the gastric and duodenal mucosa injury seen with aspirin and ibuprofen. *Am J Gastroenterol* 77:69–74, 1982.
7. Kevin JI, Roth JLA: Drug and chemical-induced injuries of the stomach, in Berk J (ed): *Bockus Gastroenterology*. Philadelphia, WB Saunders, 1985, pp 976–979.
8. Messer J, Reitman D, Sacks HS, et al: Association of adrenocorticosteroid therapy and peptic ulcer. *N Engl J Med* 309:21–24, 1983.
9. Piper JM, Ray WA, Daugherty JR, et al: Corticosteroid use and peptic ulcer disease: Role of nonsteroidal anti-inflammatory drugs. *Ann Intern Med* 114:735–740, 1991.
10. Hirakawa M, Iida M, Aoyagi K, et al: Gastroduodenal lesions after transcatheter arterial chemoembolization in patients with hepatocellular carcinoma. *Am J Gastroenterol* 83:837–840, 1988.
11. Silvoso GR, Ivey KJ, Brett JH: Incidence of gastric lesions in patients with rheumatic disease on chronic aspirin therapy. *Ann Intern Med* 91:517–520, 1979.
12. Carson JL, Strom BL, Soper KA, et al: The association of non-steroidal anti-inflammatory drugs with upper gastrointestinal bleeding. *Arch Intern Med* 147:85–88, 1987.
13. Somerville K, Faulkner G, Langman M: Non-steroidal anti-inflammatory drugs and bleeding peptic ulcer. *Lancet* 1:1302–1304, 1986.
14. Griffin MR, Piper JM, Daugherty JR, et al: Nonsteroidal anti-inflammatory drug use and increased risk for peptic ulcer disease in elderly persons. *Ann Intern Med* 114:257–263, 1991.
15. Levy M: Aspirin use in patients with major upper gastrointestinal bleeding and peptic-ulcer disease. A report from the Boston Collaborative Drug Surveillance Program, Boston University Medical Center. *N Engl J Med* 290:1158–1162, 1974.
16. Levy M, Miller DR, Kaufman DW, et al: Major upper gastrointestinal tract bleeding: Relation to the use of aspirin and other non-narcotic analgesics. *Arch Intern Med* 148:281–285, 1988.
17. Kurata JH: An assessment of nonsteroidal anti-inflammatory drugs as a risk factor in ulcer disease. *Ann Intern Med* 114:307–319, 1991.
18. Coates AG, Nostrant TT, Wilson JA, et al: Esophagitis caused by nonsteroidal anti-inflammatory medication: Case reports and review of the literature on pill-induced esophageal injury. *South Med J* 79:1094–1097, 1986.
19. Bjarnason I, Zanelli G, Smith T, et al: Nonsteroidal anti-inflammatory drug-induced intestinal inflammation in humans. *Gastroenterology* 93:480–489, 1987.
20. Stamm CP, Pearce WA, Larsen BA, et al: Colonic ulcerations associated with nonsteroidal anti-inflammatory ingestion (abstract). *Gastrointest Endosc* 37:260, 1991.
21. Szabo S: Mechanisms of mucosal injury in the stomach and duodenum: Time-sequence analysis

of morphologic, functional, biochemical and histochemical studies. *Scand J Gastroenterol* 22(Suppl 127):21–28, 1987.

22. Ligumsky M, Golanska EM, Hansen DG, et al: Aspirin can inhibit gastric mucosal cyclooxygenase without causing lesions in the rat. *Gastroenterology* 84:756–761, 1983.
23. Lanza FL, Aspinall RL, Swabb EA, et al: Double-blind, placebo-controlled endoscopic comparison of the mucosal protective effects of misoprostol versus cimetidine on tolmetin-induced mucosal injury to the stomach and duodenum. *Gastroenterology* 95:289–294, 1988.
24. Ivey KJ: Mucosal adaptation to NSAID therapy: Clinical relevance, in Ivey KJ, Currey H, (eds): *Arthritis and the Gastrointestinal Tract.* Royal Society of Medicine Round Table Series, No. 21. Oxford, Alden Press, 1990, pp 49–59.
25. Rainsford KD: Mechanisms of gastrointestinal toxicity of nonsteroidal anti-inflammatory drugs. *Scand J Gastroenterol* (Suppl 163)24:9–16, 1989.
26. Rainsford KD, Willis C: Relationship of gastric mucosal damage induced in pigs by anti-inflammatory drugs to their effects on prostaglandin production. *Dig Dis Sci* 27:625–635, 1982.
27. Carson JL, Strom BL: The gastrointestinal side effects of the nonsteroidal anti-inflammatory drugs. *J Clin Pharmacol* 28:554–559, 1988.
28. Carson JL, Strom BL, Morse ML, et al: The relative gastrointestinal toxicity of the nonsteroidal anti-inflammatory drugs. *Arch Intern Med* 147:1054–1059, 1987.
29. Lussier A, LeBel E: Radiochromium (chromium-51) evaluation of gastrointestinal blood loss associated with placebo, aspirin, and nabumetone. *Am J Med* 83(Suppl):15–18, 1987.
30. Paulus HE: Clinical pharmacology of the antirheumatic drugs, in Schumacher HR (ed): *Primer on the Rheumatic Diseases.* Atlanta, Ga, Arthritis Foundation, 1988, pp 282–288.
31. Bianchi Porro G, Caruso I, Petrillo M, et al: A double-blind gastroscopic evaluation of the effects of etodolac and naprosen on the gastrointestinal mucosa of rheumatic patients. *J Intern Med* 229:5–8, 1991.
32. Lanza FL, Karlin DA, Yee JP: A double-blind placebo controlled endoscopic study comparing the mucosal injury seen with orally and parenterally administered nonsteroidal analgesic ketorolac tromethamine at therapeutic and supratherapeutic doses (abstract). *Am J Gastroenterol* 82:939, 1987.
33. Graham DY: The relationship between nonsteroidal anti-inflammatory drug use and peptic ulcer disease. *Gastroenterol Clin North Am* 19:171–182, 1990.
34. Graham DY: Prevention of gastroduodenal injury induced by chronic nonsteroidal anti-inflammatory drug therapy. *Gastroenterology* 96(Suppl):675–681, 1989.
35. Larkai EN, Smith JL, Lidsky MD, et al: Gastroduodenal mucosa and dyspeptic symptoms in arthritic patients during chronic nonsteroidal anti-inflammatory drug use. *Am J Gastroenterol* 82:1153–1158, 1987.
36. Egan JV, Jensen DM: Long-term management of patients with bleeding ulcers. *Gastrointest Endosc Clin North Am* 1:367–385, 1991.
37. Fries JF, Williams CA, Bloch DA, et al: Nonsteroidal anti-inflammatory drug-associated gastropathy: Incidence and risk factor models. *Am J Med* 91:213–222, 1991.
38. Pincus T, Griffin M: Gastrointestinal disease associated with nonsteroidal anti-inflammatory drugs: New insights from observational studies and functional status questionnaires (editorial). *Am J Med* 91:209–212, 1991.
39. Gabriel SE, Jaakkimainen L, Bombadier C: Risk for serious gastrointestinal complications related to use of nonsteroidal anti-inflammatory drugs: A meta-analysis. *Ann Intern Med* 115:787–796, 1991.
40. Pounder R: Silent peptic ulceration: Deadly silence or golden silence? *Gastroenterology* 96:626–631, 1989.

41. Mellem H, Stave R, Myren J, et al: Symptoms in patients with peptic ulcer and hematemesis and/or melena related to the use of nonsteroidal anti-inflammatory drugs. *Scand J Gastroenterol* 20:1246–1248, 1985.

42. LoIudice TA, Saleem T, Lang JA: Cimetidine in the treatment of gastric ulcer induced by steroidal and nonsteroidal anti-inflammatory agents. *Am J Gastroenterol* 75:104–110, 1981.

43. Robinson MG, Griffin JW Jr, Bowers J, et al: Effect of ranitidine on gastroduodenal mucosal damage induced by nonsteroidal anti-inflammatory drugs. *Dig Dis Sci* 34:424–428, 1989.

44. McCarthy DM: Nonsteroidal anti-inflammatory drug-induced ulcers: Management by traditional therapies. *Gastroenterology* 96:662–674, 1989.

45. Bijlsma JW: Treatment of NSAID-induced gastrointestinal lesions with cimetidine: An international multicentre collaborative study. *Aliment Pharmacol Therap* 2S:85–96, 1988.

46. Manniche C, Malchow-Møller A, Andersen JR, et al: Randomised study of the influence of nonsteroidal anti-inflammatory drugs on the treatment of peptic ulcer in patients with rheumatic disease. *Gut* 28:226–229, 1987.

47. McCarthy DM: NSAID-induced gastrointestinal damage. A critical review of prophylaxis and therapy. *J Clin Gastroenterol* 12(Suppl 2):S13–S20, 1990.

48. Walan A, Bader JP, Classen M, et al: Effect of omeprazole and ranitidine on ulcer healing and relapse rates in patients with benign gastric ulcer. *N Engl J Med* 320:69–75, 1989.

49. Berkowitz JM, Rogenes PR, Sharp JT, et al: Ranitidine protects against gastroduodenal mucosal damage associated with chronic aspirin therapy. *Arch Intern Med* 147:2137–2139, 1987.

50. Ehsanullah RSB, Page MC, Tildesley G, et al: Nonsteroidal anti-inflammatory drug-induced gastroduodenal damage: Prophylactic effect of inhibition of gastric acid secretion. *Br Med J* 297:1017–1021, 1988.

51. Graham DY, Agrawal NM, Roth SH: Prevention of NSAID-induced gastric ulcer with misoprostol: Multicenter, double-blind, placebo-controlled trial. *Lancet* 2:1277–1280, 1988.

52. Graham DY, Stromatt SC, Jaszewski R, et al: Prevention of duodenal ulcer in arthritics who are chronic NSAID users: A multicenter trial of the role of misoprostol (abstract). *Gastroenterology* 100:A75, 1991.

53. Lanza FL, Graham DY, Davis RE, et al: Endoscopic comparison of cimetidine and sucralfate for prevention of naproxen-induced acute gastroduodenal injury: Effect of scoring system. *Dig Dis Sci* 35:1494–1499, 1990.

54. Agrawal NM, Roth S, Graham DY, et al: Misoprostol compared with sucralfate in the prevention of nonsteroidal anti-inflammatory drug-induced gastric ulcers. A randomized, controlled trial. *Ann Intern Med* 115:195–200, 1991.

55. Sievert W, Stern AI, Lambert JR, et al: Low-dose antacids and nonsteroidal anti-inflammatory drug-induced gastropathy in humans. *J Clin Gastroenterol* 13(Suppl):S145–S148, 1991.

56. Knill-Jones R, Drummond M, Harpreet K, et al: Economic evaluation of gastric ulcer prophylaxis in patients with arthritis receiving nonsteroidal anti-inflammatory drugs. *Postgrad Med J* 66:639–646, 1990.

57. Hillman AL, Bloom B: Economic effects of prophylactic use of misoprostol to prevent gastric ulcer in patients taking nonsteroidal anti-inflammatory drugs. *Arch Intern Med* 149:2061–2065, 1989.

58. Curtis WD, Griffin JW: Nonsteroidal anti-inflammatory drug-induced gastroduodenal injury: Therapeutic recommendations. *Aliment Pharmacol Ther* 5(Suppl 1):99–109, 1991.

8

HEMATOLOGIC PROBLEMS IN GASTROINTESTINAL BLEEDING

C. Lawrence Lutcher, M.D.

Bleeding diatheses due to liver disease, chemotherapy-induced thrombocytopenia, acquired platelet dysfunction, and excessive anticoagulation constitute the major problems encountered by the hematologist who is asked to see the patient with gastrointestinal bleeding. One must recognize, however, that even less frequent causes of bleeding such as untreated hematologic malignancies, congenital coagulopathies, circulating anticoagulants, and hereditary vascular or collagen disorders are also associated with gastrointestinal bleeding. Bleeding due to liver disease is discussed elsewhere in this text. The spectrum of hematologic disorders that may be associated with gastrointestinal bleeding is summarized in Table 8.1. This chapter presents important diagnostic and management aspects of hematologic disorders that may be encountered by the clinician who is caring for the patient with gastrointestinal bleeding.

HEMATOLOGIC ASPECTS OF ACUTE AND CHRONIC BLOOD LOSS

Acute blood loss is frequently associated with sufficient hemodynamic stress to result in mild elevation of the white cell and platelet counts. The hemoglobin will be normal until the intravascular volume is reconstituted (usually within 24 to 72 hours), but nucleated red cells are frequently present when acute blood loss is severe. The mean corpuscular volume (MCV) is normal immediately following acute blood loss, and will remain so if the hemoglobin is replaced promptly and bleeding does not recur. Subacute blood loss that is not totally replenished is associated with a reticulocytosis and a mild increase in the MCV that peaks within 7 to 10 days and is sustained until the hemoglobin level approaches normal. Moderate to severe thrombocytopenia occurs when stored whole

TABLE 8.1. Spectrum of Hematologic Disorders Associated with Gastrointestinal Bleeding

Platelet disorders	Combined platelet and factor disorders
Thrombocytopenia	Liver disease
Platelet dysfunction	Disseminated intravascular clotting
Coagulation factor disorders	Parahematologic disorders
Excessive anticoagulation	Vasculitis
Hemophilia	Hereditary vascular disorders
Von Willebrand's disease	Hereditary collagen disorders
Circulating anticoagulants	

blood or packed red blood cells (RBCs) are given without platelets. This usually occurs after a one- to two-volume replacement (the equivalent of 5 to 10 units of whole blood). Table 8.2 illustrates an estimate of the quantity of any blood component remaining in the best- and worse-case examples of blood loss and replacement.

Gastrointestinal blood loss frequently results in iron deficiency and mild to moderate thrombocytosis. In occult blood loss, there is generally a poor correlation between symptoms and the hemoglobin level until the anemia is moderate to severe. In postmenopausal females and adult males, iron deficiency is attributed to gastrointestinal blood loss until proven otherwise. It can be the first sign of an occult gastrointestinal malignancy and may be overlooked if the anemia responds to iron therapy before proper evaluation of the gastrointestinal tract is performed.

From 20% to 30% of patients with the anemia of chronic disorders, and a comparable percentage of black Americans as a group, have low or low normal RBC indices. Both entities are often and inappropriately treated with iron, further emphasizing the importance of precisely defining the cause of apparent iron deficiency. The anemia of chronic disorders is seldom severe (hemoglobin, 9–11 g/dl) and is associated with increased iron stores (abundant marrow iron and increased serum ferritin) in the face of low serum iron and low or low normal iron-binding capacity. The high incidence of thalassemia trait (alpha 28%, beta 1.0%) in black Americans can usually be resolved by family studies, hemoglobin electrophoresis, and quantitation of minor hemoglobins (A_2 and F). A normal to increased RBC count is a practical and cost-effective first clue to recognition of a thalassemic disorder, in comparison with iron deficiency, where there is a parallel decrement of the RBC count, hemoglobin, and indices. Like the anemia of chronic disorders, the thalassemias have normal or increased iron stores.

In the vast majority of patients, the diagnosis of iron deficiency is straightforward,

TABLE 8.2. Examples of the Percentage Blood Volume Remaining: 5-Liter Blood Volume Transfused (with 500-ml Units)

	Magnitude of Hemorrhage and Transfusion		
Situation	*1 Vol. (10 Units)*	*2 Vols. (20 Units)*	*3 Vols. (30 Units)*
Best*	37%	14%	5%
Usual	25–30%	10%	3–4%
Worst†	18%	3%	0.4%

*Best: simultaneous and equal replacement during hemorrhage.
†Worst: initial loss of one-half of blood volume, which is not replaced until hemorrhage stops.
Source: Modified with permission from Collins JA: Massive blood transfusion. *Clin Hematol* 5(1):201–219, 1976.

particularly when an adequate history and a thorough physical examination are available. An uncomplicated patient with anemia and microcytic indices, whose history indicates the cause of iron deficiency, requires only a serum ferritin or serum iron study (now widely available on biochemical screening profiles) in addition to an appropriate response to iron therapy. Patients with microcytic indices who have normal RBC counts, or evidence of normal RBC indices in the past, need not be evaluated for thalassemia. Vigorous diagnostic evaluation for the cause need not be pursued as aggressively in children and menstruating females, due to their increased requirement for iron, as in adult males and postmenopausal females.

The Hemostatic Profile

The clinician must vigorously resist the temptation to substitute laboratory tests for a history that probes for a possible bleeding disorder. This is particularly true for mild bleeding disorders, where screening tests of hemostasis are usually normal. The medical history, particularly the medication history and the patient's response to surgery or trauma, is more important than the screening tests. Moreover, certain abnormalities that are detected in screening tests (e.g., the prolonged partial thromboplastin times associated with Hageman factor deficiency and the lupus anticoagulant) are not associated with bleeding manifestations. A history of recurrent mucosal bleeding suggests a platelet disorder or von Willebrand's disease, while delayed or deep tissue hemorrhage indicates a likely factor deficiency. Mucosal petechiae or significant telangiectasias must be explained.

The essential elements of the hemostatic process, emphasizing both the primary platelet thrombus and its reinforcement by fibrin as the result of coagulation protein interactions, are shown in Figure 8.1. Recent investigations have revealed that platelet glycoproteins (GPs) Ib and IIb/IIIa are critical sites for platelet interaction with the vessel wall (adhesion) and with each other (aggregation), respectively. These sites are the targets of new antithrombotic strategems in the laboratory and are known to be deficient in certain rare platelet function disorders (e.g., the absence of GP Ib in the Bernard Soulier syndrome and of GP IIb/IIIa in Glanzman's thrombasthenia). Endothelial cells secrete von Willebrand factor (vWF), which is present in subendothelial sites and, in high molecular weight forms (vWF multimers), provides a critical ligand between the subendothelium and GP Ib on the platelet membrane. Fibrinogen provides an equally important ligand between GP IIb/IIIa sites on platelets. Infusion of desmopressin (DDAVP) causes release of vWF and factor VIII from endothelial cells, resulting in a rise of both factors that persists for several hours.

The prothrombin time (PT), activated partial thromboplastin time (aPTT), and platelet count constitute the traditional preoperative screening profile. The causes of a prolonged PT and aPTT are generally well understood and reflect the extrinsic and intrinsic systems of coagulation respectively. Other screening tests that are occasionally helpful are the bleeding time and the thrombin time.

The template bleeding time (tBT) remains the most practical way of assessing platelet function and is particularly helpful in assessing systemic factors (e.g., renal failure and medications) that can cause or contribute to platelet dysfunction. There is, however, no good correlation between prolongation of the bleeding time and clinical bleeding in most acquired platelet function disorders.[1,2] A prolonged thrombin time may be the first indication of hypofibrinogenemia, dysfibrinogenemia, or dysproteinemia.

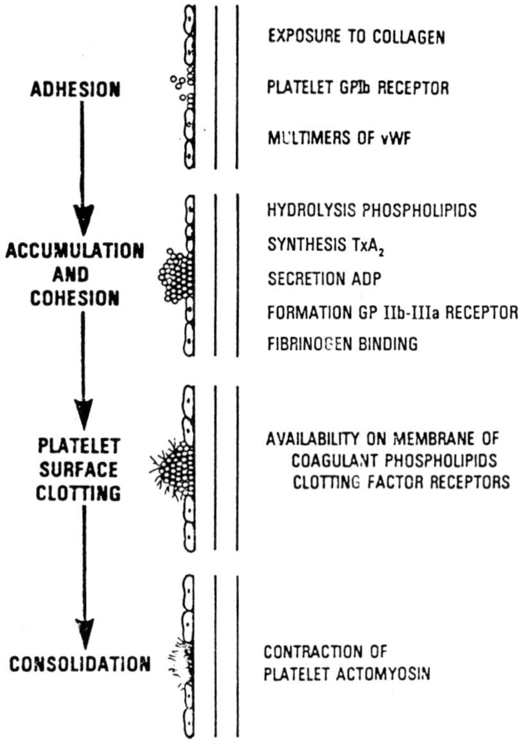

Figure 8.1. Primary and secondary components of the hemostatic plug. (Reprinted with permission and modified from Rapaport SI: Hemostasis in West JB (ed): *Best and Taylor's Physiologic Basis of Medical Practice,* ed 11. Baltimore, Williams & Wilkins, 1984, pp 409–436.)

BLEEDING DISORDERS AND GASTROINTESTINAL BLEEDING

Selected features of platelet, coagulation factor, and parahematological vascular bleeding disorders are summarized in Table 8.3. Some forms of vasculitis and primary vascular or collagen disorders are arbitrarily designated parahematologic disorders because they are frequently first seen by the hematologist due to their hemorrhagic manifestations.

PLATELET DISORDERS

Thrombocytopenia

There is a relatively good inverse correlation between the tBT and platelet counts, ranging from 10,000 to 100,000/μl (Figure 8.2). Spontaneous bleeding is quite rare when the platelet count is above 10,000/μl.

Chemotherapy-induced thrombocytopenia is by far the most common cause of

TABLE 8.3. Clinical Observations in Bleeding Disorders

Observations	*Platelet*	*Factor*	*Vascular*
Family history	Rarely	Frequently	Rarely†
Site(s) of bleeding	Mucocutaneous	Joints, muscles, viscera, mucosal*	Mucocutaneous
Signs of bleeding	Petechiae, purpura	Hematomas, pain	Rash, echymoses (Local)
Chronology	Spontaneous Parallels injury	Follows trauma Frequently delayed	Follows trauma

*Von Willebrand's disease.
†Can be positive in rare vascular and collagen disorders.

thrombocytopenia seen today and is the result of aggressive treatment regimens for many neoplasms. It is critically important that platelets be maintained at a minimal level, usually 10,000–20,000/μl, during aggressive induction chemotherapy. Skin and mucocutaneous bleeding are apparent when platelets are insufficient during intense chemotherapy. The acute leukemias and myelodysplastic syndromes frequently present with bleeding due to thrombocytopenia.

Idiopathic thrombocytopenic purpura is characterized by a relatively short bleeding time for the degree of thrombocytopenia (Figure 8.2). These patients, and those with human immunodeficiency virus–related thrombocytopenia, have far less bleeding than amegakaryocytic or chemotherapy-induced thrombocytopenic states.

Alloimmune neonatal thrombocytopenia is frequently associated with gastrointesti-

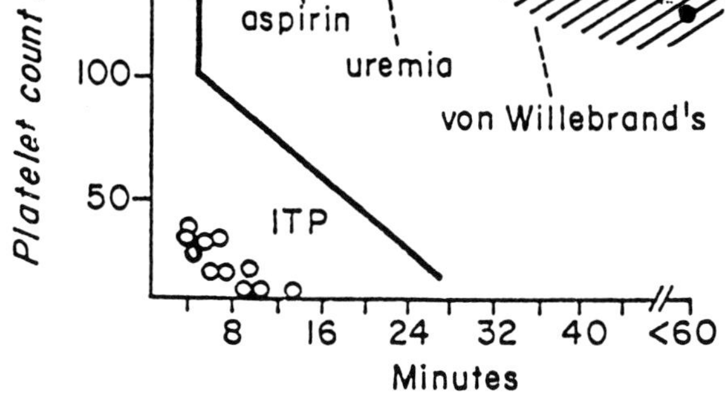

Figure 8.2. Relationships Between Bleeding Time, Platelet Count and Selected Examples of Platelet Dysfunction. (Reprinted with permission from Thompson AR, Harker LA: Approach to Bleeding Disorders in Manual of Hemostasis and Thrombosis, Philadelphia, FA Davis Co., 1974, pp 57–64.)

nal bleeding in the infant. As many as 25% of patients who ingest thiazide diuretics develop mild to moderate thrombocytopenia due to suppression of megakaryocyte production. Mucosal bleeding and ecchymosis are uncommon, but neonatal thrombocytopenia in the offspring of mothers taking these agents has presented with purpura and gastrointestinal bleeding.[3]

Drug-Induced Platelet Dysfunction

Aspirin

Aspirin increases the bleeding time in approximately 50% of recipients taking 600–975 mg/day. Thromboxane synthesis in the platelet is inhibited 100% by a single 80-mg dose or by 10 mg taken for seven days.[4] It is not known whether the antiplatelet effect is related to the ability of aspirin to produce mucosal erythema, petechiae, and erosions. It is known that rheumatoid arthritis patients who take aspirin have no undue bleeding when biopsied at endoscopy.[2] The most impressive effect of aspirin on hemostasis is noted when it is used in the setting of another hemorrhagic influence (e.g., in hemophilia; in uremia; in the presence of ethanol or anticoagulants; and in the pregnant patient before delivery). In all of these settings, an increase in bleeding tendency is readily apparent. In the pregnant patient, as a case in point, a single aspirin tablet taken within five days of delivery has resulted in increased vaginal bleeding and in systemic bleeding in the infant.[5]

A small but definite increase in surgical bleeding is recognized and mandates a judicious three- to five-day wait, without aspirin, before elective surgery is performed. Alternatively, DDAVP can be tried or platelet transfusions can be given. The overall risk of surgical bleeding in any patient is thought to be negligible, but where the minimum risk must be obtained (e.g., in cosmetic, neurological, or ophthalmological surgery), a conservative approach is justified.

Other Antiplatelet Agents

The newer nonsteroidal analgesic agents have the same mechanism of action as aspirin, but this mechanism is weaker and more transient, allowing surgery within one day of discontinuation of these agents. These agents have no untoward hemorrhagic effects in the joints of hemophiliacs and rarely produce an increase in the tBT.

β-Lactam antibiotics have a side chain that blocks a platelet receptor for aggregation, occasionally resulting in an increase in the tBT. The tBT, however, does not predict clinical bleeding.

Ethanol, anticoagulants, and fibrinolytic agents clearly enhance bleeding in the presence of aspirin. Dextran, nitrates, dipyridamole, and calcium channel blockers are not associated with clinical bleeding.

Renal Failure

Chronic renal failure is a common cause of severe platelet dysfunction. Diminished platelet aggregation and liberation of platelet phospholipid (platelet factor III) are found in the majority of patients with severe (creatinine clearance <5 cc/min) renal failure. A prolonged tBT is usually the only abnormality detected by the hemostasis profile. Platelet dysfunction is attributed to the accumulation of products (e.g., urea, guanidinosuccinic acid, and phenol derivatives) of renal failure and is not corrected by platelet transfusion.

Gastrointestinal and intracranial bleeding were common accompaniments of chronic renal failure in the predialysis era. Recurrent gastrointestinal bleeding remains a problem in some patients with chronic renal failure and has recently been associated with angiodysplastic lesions of the stomach and duodenum.[6]

Although the tBT may be shortened by a number of treatment maneuvers, e.g., frequent dialysis, infusion of cryoprecipitate or DDAVP, administration of estrogens, and by increasing the hematocrit with RBC transfusion or administration of erythropoietin, the absolute tBT value is not clearly related to hemorrhagic events. Among the treatments tested, only estrogen and erythropoietin therapy offer sustained improvement in the bleeding time, and clinical trials to date are insufficient to evaluate their efficacy in treating or changing the natural history of gastrointestinal bleeding due to renal failure.

Myeloproliferative Disorders

Approximately one-third of patients with myeloproliferative disorders (polycythemia vera, chronic granulocytic leukemia, essential thrombocytosis, and agnogenic myeloid metaplasia) have hemorrhagic manifestations.[7] In 10%, hemorrhage is a major contributor to mortality, usually from bleeding esophageal varices or peptic ulceration. Approximately one-third of these patients have mild abnormalities of platelet aggregation, and 10–20% have an increase in their bleeding times. Neither is predictive of clinical bleeding, nor is the frequently elevated platelet count. Hyperviscosity, however, as seen in polycythemia vera, is associated with postoperative bleeding. The use of aspirin and other nonsteroidal analgesics in myeloproliferative disorders is associated with bleeding episodes in as many as 30% of patients.

From 2% to 5% of patients with essential thrombocytosis present with gastrointestinal bleeding, and many are iron deficient when first seen. This frequently prompts administration of iron therapy to evaluate the possibility of polycythemia vera masked by iron deficiency.

The myeloproliferative disorders are clonal and, for the most part, slowly evolving neoplasms characterized by excessive proliferation in the marrow, an increase in one or more cell lines in the blood, and splenomegaly. Karyotypic analyses may be helpful in specifying the type of myeloproliferative disorder. With the exception of phlebotomy for polycythemia vera, no therapy is known to ameliorate the bleeding tendency in these patients.

Dysproteinemias

The amount of monoclonal (M) protein produced is roughly correlated with the incidence of platelet dysfunction in multiple myeloma. Bleeding is usually mild and is far more frequently associated with thrombocytopenia. A unique IgG(k) myeloma patient, who died of a bleeding gastric ulcer, demonstrated binding of his M protein to GP IIIa, thus inhibiting fibrinogen binding and platelet aggregation.[8] The M protein can also interfere with fibrin polymerization, causing a marked increase in the thrombin time, without resulting in bleeding.

Amyloid deposition of the primary type, as occurs in myeloma, causes fragility of vessels, resulting in purpura in areas of trauma. It is also frequently associated with acquired factor X deficiency, which may be ameliorated by splenectomy.[9]

An acquired type of von Willebrand's disease has also been seen in association with M protein disorders and has successfully been treated with plasmapheresis and chemotherapy.

Congenital Platelet Disorders

Glanzman's thrombasthenia and the Bernard Soulier syndrome are characterized by deficiencies of GPs IIb/IIIa and Ib, respectively. Most patients have consistently prolonged bleeding times, but there is considerable variation in hemorrhagic manifestations.[10] Bleeding can be very severe, particularly in patients who have become refractory to platelet transfusions. DDAVP infusion has shown some promise in dealing with acute hemorrhagic episodes in patients with the Bernard Soulier syndrome.

COAGULATION FACTOR DISORDERS

Excessive Anticoagulation

Warfarin

Warfarin, the prototypic coumarin agent, has a half-life of 48 hours. About twice that time is required to induce the anticoagulated state when conventional doses are used, and a comparable period is required for the PT to return to normal when warfarin is discontinued. The anticoagulant effect is, therefore, not subject to prompt modulation by varying the dose. Excessive anticoagulation with warfarin is associated with major hemorrhagic events (1–7%), including intramural hemorrhage of the bowel. Peptic ulceration and intracranial bleeding are the most common fatal hemorrhagic entities.

It has recently become apparent that the traditional therapeutic range for oral anticoagulation in the United States has been excessive due to the lesser sensitivity of U.S. thromboplastin reagents compared with their European counterparts. Current recommendations are that the patient's PT should be 1.3–1.5$\times$ the control versus the higher traditional range (1.5–2.0) now reserved for patients with the greatest risk of thromboembolism (e.g., those with a mechanical heart valve prosthesis and those with a history of recurrent emboli).[11]

Properly anticoagulated patients should not hemorrhage from the bowel, particularly when the recently recommended lower doses are used. The search for an underlying organic lesion should be vigorously pursued in all such patients when other possible interacting hemorrhagic effects (e.g., antiplatelet agents, uremia) are not known to be present.[12]

Major bleeding associated with excessive warfarin anticoagulation should be treated with vitamin K analogs or, in the acute setting, with fresh frozen plasma. Only modest doses of vitamin K_1 (5–10 mg) should be given, in most cases, to permit prompt resumption of anticoagulation when appropriate.

Heparin

The risk of major hemorrhage from heparin anticoagulation, based on pooled analysis of randomized trials, varies with the type of administration: 6.8% with continuous infusion vs. 14.2% with intermittent intravenous injections.[13] Recent investigations indicate that new low molecular weight formulations of heparin are associated with less bleeding while proving to be equally effective in preventing thromboembolism.[14]

Congenital Factor Deficiencies

Hemophilia

About 17,000 people in the United States have clinically detectable sex-linked hemophilia, 80% due to factor VIII deficiency (hemophilia A) and approximately 15% due to factor IX deficiency (hemophilia B). Hemophilia may be classified based on the amount of normal factor present (severe, $<1\%$; moderate, 1–5%; mild, $>5\%$). Factor XI deficiency is rare, has autosomal inheritance, and has variable clinical expression.

Historically, peptic ulcer disease and its complications accounted for one-third of deaths from hemophilia. Modern replacement therapy and the advent of H_2 blockers have changed the natural history to the point where only 10–25% of hemophiliacs now demonstrate evidence of gastrointestinal bleeding at any time. Intramural hemorrhage of the bowel may be difficult to diagnose but must be considered, because early and frequent factor replacement may be the only way to avoid obstruction. Symptoms due to gastrointestinal bleeding are uniformly responsive to the appropriate replacement therapy. Gastrointestinal bleeding seldom occurs in hemophiliacs who are only moderately or mildly affected.

Modern factor replacement has markedly decreased the morbidity of hemophilia. The majority of patients are now able to lead productive lives. The new monoclonal and recombinant DNA-derived factor concentrates are essentially free of viral contamination. Mildly affected hemophiliacs may respond to DDAVP, thus avoiding plasma products for most minor bleeds.[15]

Von Willebrand's Disease

Von Willebrand's disease may be more common than hemophilia. Most cases demonstrate autosomal dominant inheritance and many variants have been described, although classic (type I) von Willebrand's disease continues to represent approximately 70% of all cases. Most agree that variations in vWF, factor VIII clotting activity, and bleeding time occur occasionally in the same patient.[16] Thus multiple basal determinations of these parameters are frequently necessary before a diagnosis is established. Mild cases of von Willebrand's disease may not be detected until surgery or major trauma occurs. Gastrointestinal bleeding occurs in approximately 10% of patients and is the most common cause of death in these patients.[17,18] Cryoprecipitate is rich in vWF and is the traditional replacement factor for von Willebrand's disease. Certain pasteurized or solute detergent products (e.g., Humate-P, Humate-HS) now appear to be superior to cryoprecipitate because of superior vWF content and reduced viral contamination. As with hemophilia, mildly affected type I cases may require only DDAVP infusions for minor bleeds or surgery.

Acquired Factor Deficiencies

Most antibodies that attack clotting factors are directed against factor VIII; the majority occur in hemophilia as a response to replacement infusions. Others usually arise spontaneously in the elderly, in settings of altered immunity (e.g., lymphoproliferative or collagen vascular disorders), after pregnancy, after transfusions, and after taking certain drugs. Gastrointestinal bleeding is common and management often proves difficult, involving the use of heterologous plasma, immunosuppressive therapy, and extracorporeal antibody absorption. Immune tolerance has been induced in hemophiliacs with a factor VIII antibody, but at great cost and inconvenience. In the spontaneously occurring idiopathic types, particularly in older patients, as many as one-third have a spontaneous remission.

COMBINED PLATELET AND CLOTTING DISORDERS

Liver Disease

The multifactorial bleeding aspects of liver disease are presented elsewhere in this text and will not be discussed here, except to elaborate on the significance of liver biopsy in the patient with hemophilia and to briefly discuss hemorrhagic disease of the newborn.

The plasma products used by adult hemophiliacs place 15–25% of them at risk for significant liver disease. Liver biopsy based on sustained enzyme elevations was performed in 155 patients who received appropriate factor replacement.[19] The histopathological exam revealed chronic persistent hepatitis in 68%, chronic active hepatitis in 7%, and frank cirrhosis in 15%. Thirteen percent had significant bleeding, and two died as a result of the procedure. Given the recently recognized efficacy of interferon treatment in chronic active hepatitis, the morbidity and mortality of liver biopsy in this population deserve very careful attention by both gastroenterologists and hematologists.

Hemorrhagic Disease of the Newborn

Immaturity of hepatic synthetic mechanisms produces a self-limited deficiency of vitamin K–dependent procoagulants in as many as 2% of infants not receiving vitamin K at birth.[20] This entity, known as *hemorrhagic disease of the newborn (HDNB),* presents on the second or third day of life, frequently as gastrointestinal bleeding, and may cause severe anemia. HDNB is preventable by administration of vitamin K_1, preferably menadione or hykinone (0.5–1.0 mg parenterally) at birth. Synkavite is avoided due to its tendency to induce hemolysis in the newborn. Infants of mothers taking anticonvulsants such as phenytoin and phenobarbital are particularly susceptible to HDNB and require larger doses of vitamin K.[21]

Disseminated Intravascular Coagulation (DIC)

Acute promyelocytic leukemia (APL) is the prototypic example of cancer-related DIC. All patients with APL have DIC, and heparin improves the laboratory parameters without changing the mortality.[22] Patients frequently present with undue bleeding at bone marrow puncture and vascular access sites. Thromboembolism is rare. Other malignancies frequently associated with DIC are adenocarcinomas of the prostate and bowel. Gastrointestinal bleeding is not unusual in chronic DIC, though it is less frequent than in acute fulminating DIC. Peritoneovenous shunting is also invariably associated with diffuse intravascular clotting and may be an additive contribution to gastrointestinal bleeding.[23]

Blood product support is more effective in decreasing bleeding than heparin. While treating the underlying disorder, the major management issues are (1) gauging the pace of the process (with serial determinations of platelets, fibrin degradation products, and fibrinogen) and (2) providing adequate blood product replacement.

VASCULAR DISORDERS

While not strictly hematological problems, some vascular disorders are often first seen by the hematologist because of the appearance of the lesions or associated bleeding. Many such disorders cause purpura, but relatively few are associated with gastrointestinal bleeding.

Dengue infection and Henoch-Schönlein purpura are associated with fever and sterile nonthrombocytopenic vasculitis.[24,25] Both of these entities have a significant incidence of gastrointestinal bleeding in addition to cutaneous manifestations that clear within a short time. Leukocytoclastic vasculitis, as occurs in rheumatoid vasculitis, is seldom recognized as the sole cause of gastrointestinal bleeding.

Angiodysplastic lesions of the cecum and proximal colon have recently been recognized as a common cause of lower gastrointestinal bleeding in the elderly and frequently present as recurrent melena or iron deficiency.[26,27] These degenerative lesions are often multiple; may involve arteries, capillaries, and veins; and are a variant of those described in patients with aortic stenosis, radiation injury, and hereditary hemorrhagic telangiectasia.

Hereditary vascular and hereditary collagen disorders can be associated with gastrointestinal bleeding. The most common of these is hereditary hemorrhagic telangiectasia, an autosomal dominant disorder with an estimated incidence of 1/50,000.[28] Patients usually present with either epistaxis or gastrointestinal bleeding, and many are chronically iron deficient. Lesions may be present throughout the body but are most apparent on the face, lips, tongue, nail beds, and palms. The size of the lesions tends to increase with age and multiple lesions are usually apparent, although the diagnosis is occasionally first suspected when endoscopy or mesenteric angiography reveals a previously undetected bleeding site.

Among the hereditary collagen disorders, both pseudoxanthoma elasticum and the Ehlers-Danlos syndrome can present with gastrointestinal bleeding.[28] Gastroscopy frequently reveals discrete yellowish, linear or nodular densities that are caused by submucosal microaneurysms in pseudoxanthoma elasticum. The Ehlers-Danlos syndrome has also been associated with platelet dysfunction and multiple gastrointestinal abnormalities, such as spontaneous perforation, retroperitoneal hemorrhage, rectal prolapse, gastric atony, and megacolon. The treatment of vascular causes of bleeding is difficult when a single major bleeding site cannot be identified and definitively managed.

HEMATOLOGIC CONSIDERATIONS IN THE MANAGEMENT OF GASTROINTESTINAL BLEEDING

The majority of patients with iron deficiency due to gastrointestinal bleeding respond to iron therapy when it is properly administered. If iron absorption is optimal and blood loss has ceased, the marrow produces 0.2–0.3 g hemoglobin per day after 7–10 days,

TABLE 8.4. Minimal Required Hemostatic vs. Stored Blood Levels of Clotting Factors

Clotting Factors	*Hemostatic Level (% of Normal)*	*Storage (4°C × 7 Days) (% of Normal)*
XI	10%	20%
V	15%	10%
IX	20%	50–100%
II	>30%	50–100%
VII	>30%	50–100%
X	>30%	50–100%
VIII	30%	10%
Fibrinogen (I)	100 mg %*	100%
Platelets	20–50 × $10^3/\mu l$*	0%

*Absolute values

TABLE 8.5. Treatment Considerations in Gastrointestinal Bleeding Due to Hematological Disorders

Condition	*Therapy*
Thrombocytopenia	
Nonimmune	Platelet transfusions
Immune	Corticosteroids, splenectomy, immune modulation
Platelet dysfunction	
Acquired	Remove offending agent, DDAVP
Congenital	Platelet transfusion, DDAVP
Hemophilia A	
Mild	DDAVP
Moderate-severe	Factor VIII replacement
Hemophilia B	
Mild	Fresh frozen plasma
Moderate-severe	Factor IX replacement
Von Willebrand's Disease	
Mild	DDAVP
Moderate-severe	Intermediate purity factor VIII Cryoprecipitate
Excessive warfarin effect	
Major	Fresh frozen plasma, vitamin K_1 5–10 mg IV
Minor	Interrupt or modify dose, vitamin K_1 1–5 mg IV
Vascular defects	
Vasculitis	Treat basic process
Vascular defects	Consider surgery Consider trial of steroids, estrogens, or antifibrinolytics

and even severe degrees of anemia are fully corrected within two months. Iron therapy is then continued for four to six months to replenish body stores, as indicated by achieving a serum ferritin of 50–100 μg/liter. Poor compliance is the most common cause of treatment failure and is often first apparent when the patient relates a vague or ambivalent history about change in the color of the stool. Reinforcement of the goals of therapy and the physician's ability to reduce the gastrointestinal side effects will usually improve compliance.

Minimal hemostatic levels of coagulation factors and platelets are given, and compared with levels obtained from stored blood (Table 8.4). Five platelet packs per day are usually sufficient to control bleeding in patients with nonimmune forms of severe thrombocytopenia. Fresh frozen plasma (2 units/m^2) for warfarin excess and cryoprecipitate (10 bags/day) for von Willebrand's disease are recommended initiating regimens for acute bleeding episodes. For severe bleeds, hemophilia patients are given sufficient factor concentrate to raise levels to 100% initially, followed by a maintenance level of 50% for 5–10 days.

Studies of the efficacy of DDAVP therapy are sufficient to recommend its use in many hemorrhagic disorders. Intravenous (0.3 μg/kg over 30 minutes) and nasal spray (150 μg to each nostril) administration appear equally effective in mild cases of hemophilia A and type I von Willebrand's disease. A second administration may be helpful after two or three days when endothelial cell factor VIII has been restored.[29] The role of low-dose corticosteroids, estrogens, and antifibrinolytic agents remains somewhat ill defined due to a paucity of controlled clinical trials. This should not, however, discourage the judicious use of one or more of these agents in refractory bleeding disorders. Treatment considerations for hematological therapy of gastrointestinal bleeding disorders are summarized in Table 8.5.

REFERENCES

1. Rodgers RPC, Levin J: A critical reappraisal of the bleeding time. *Semin Thromb Hemost* 16:1–20, 1990.
2. O'Laughlin JC, Hoftiezer JW, Mahoney JP, et al: Does aspirin prolong bleeding from gastric biopsies in man? *Gastrointest Endosc* 27:1–5, 1981.
3. Rodriguez SU, Leikin SL, Hiller MC: Neonatal thrombocytopenia associated with antepartum administration of drugs. *N Engl J Med* 270:881–884, 1964.
4. George JN, Shattil S: The clinical importance of acquired abnormalities of platelet function. *N Engl J Med* 324:27–39, 1991.
5. Bleyer WA, Breckenridge RT: Studies in the detection of adverse drug reactions in the newborn. II. The effects of prenatal aspirin on newborn hemostasis. *JAMA* 213:2049–2053, 1970.
6. Zuckerman GR, Cornette GL, Clouse RE, et al: Upper gastrointestinal bleeding in patients with chronic renal failure. *Ann Intern Med* 102:588–592, 1985.
7. Shafter HI: Bleeding and thrombosis in the myeloproliferative disorders. *Blood* 64:1–12, 1984.
8. DiMinno G, Coraggio F, Cerbone AM, et al. A myeloma paraprotein with specificity for platelet glycoprotein IIIa in a patient with a fatal bleeding disorder. *J Clin Invest* 77:157–164, 1986.
9. Rosenstein ED, Itykowitz SH, Penziner AS, et al: Resolution of factor X deficiency in primary amyloidosis following splenectomy. *Arch Intern Med* 143:597–598, 1983.

10. Bennett JS, Hoffman R, Benz L, et al: Hereditary disorders of platelet function, in Hoffman R. *Hematology: Basic Principles and Practice*. New York, Churchill Livingstone, 1991, pp 1514–1528.
11. Hull R, Hirsh J, Jay R, et al: Different intensities of oral anticoagulant therapy in the treatment of proximal vein thrombosis. *N Engl J Med* 307:1676–1681, 1982.
12. Jaffin BW, Bliss CM, LaMont JT: Significance of occult gastrointestinal bleeding during anticoagulation therapy. *Am J Med* 83:269–272, 1987.
13. Hirsh J: Heparin. *N Engl J Med* 324:1565–1574, 1991.
14. Levine MN, Hirsh J, Gent M, et al: Prevention of deep vein thrombosis after elective hip surgery. *Ann Intern Med* 114:545–551, 1991.
15. Mannuci PM: A nontransfusional form of treatment for congenital and acquired bleeding disorders. *Blood* 72:1449–1455, 1988.
16. Gralnick HR: Von Willebrand's disease, in Ratnoff OD, and Forbes CD (eds): *Disorders of Hemostasis,* ed 2.). Philadelphia, WB Saunders, 1991, pp 203–244.
17. Larrieu MJ, Caen JP, Meyer DO, et al: Congenital bleeding disorders with long bleeding time and normal platelet count. II. Von Willebrand's disease (report of thirty-seven patients). *Am J Med* 45:354–372, 1968.
18. Ratnoff O: Personal communication, in Gralnick HR, von Willebrand's disease, in Ratnoff O, Forbes CD (eds): *Disorders of Hemostasis,* ed 2. Philadelphia, WB Saunders, 1991, pp 203–241.2
19. Aledort LM, Levine PM, Hilgartner M, et al: A study of liver biopsies and liver disease among hemophiliacs. *Blood* 66:367–372, 1985.
20. Donaldson VH: Hemorrhagic disorders of neonates, in Ratnoff O, Forbes CD (eds): *Disorders of Hemostasis,* ed 2. Philadelphia, WB Saunders, 1991, pp 318–423.
21. Serp M: Effects of antiepileptic drugs in pregnancy on the fetus and newborn infant. *Ann Clin Res* 5:205–207, 1973.
22. Kantarjian H, Keating M, Walters R, et al: Acute promyelocytic leukemia. M.D. Anderson hospital experience. *Am J Med* 80:789–797, 1986.
23. Strin SF, Fulenuider JT, Ansley JD, et al: Accelerated fibrinogen and platelet destruction after peritoneovenous shunting. *Arch Intern Med* 141:1149–1151, 1979.
24. Cream JJ, Grumpel JM, Peachey RDG: Schönlein-Henoch purpura in the adult. *Q J Med* 39:461–484, 1970.
25. Halstead SB: Dengue: Hematologic aspects. *Semin Hematol* 19:116–131, 1982.
26. Richter JM, Hedberg SE, Athanasoulis CA, et al: Angiodysplasia—clinical presentation and colonoscopic diagnosis. *Dig Dis Sci* 29:481–485, 1984.
27. Ahr DJ, Rickles FR, Hoyer LW, et al: Von Willebrand's disease and hemorrhagic telangiectasia: Association of two complex disorders resulting in life-threatening hemorrhage. *Am J Med* 62:452–458, 1977.
28. Lowe GDO: Vascular disease and vasculitis, in Ratnoff O, Forbes CD (eds): in *Disorders of Hemostasis,* ed 2. Philadelphia, WB Saunders, 1991, pp. 532–544.
29. Rose EH, Aledort LM: Nasal spray desmopressin (DDAVP) for mild hemophilia A and von Willebrand's disease. *Ann Intern Med* 114:563–568, 1991.

9

GASTROINTESTINAL BLEEDING IN THE CRITICAL CARE UNIT

Frederick H. Weber, Jr., M.D.
David A. Peura, M.D.

INTRODUCTION

Two distinct groups of patients with gastrointestinal bleeding can be distinguished in the critical care unit. First, there are those who present with upper or lower gastrointestinal bleeding as the principal reason for admission to the unit. The clinical features, diagnosis, and therapy of individuals in this first category are well outlined in other chapters of this text. The second group consists of physiologically stressed patients presenting with diverse medical or surgical illnesses who develop a characteristic pattern of upper gastrointestinal tract mucosal damage. This stress-related mucosal damage (SRMD) may lead to gastrointestinal bleeding ranging from trivial mucosal oozing to massive, life-threatening hemorrhage. These physiologically stressed patients will be the focus of this chapter.

SRMD of the upper gastrointestinal tract is now a well-recognized cause of significant morbidity in the critical care unit and an occasional cause of mortality. One of the first descriptions of SRMD was given in 1842 by Curling, who noted a relationship between acute duodenal ulceration and thermal injury.[1] Ninety-five years later, Cushing observed a similar association between brain tumors and perforated gastric ulcers.[2] Despite these early reports, the magnitude of the problem remained unappreciated because mucosal lesions were clinically recognized only when severe bleeding or perforation resulted in surgery or when autopsy revealed incidental mucosal injury.

The widespread use of fiberoptic gastrointestinal endoscopy during the past several decades has led to the recognition that the vast majority of critically ill patients will develop SRMD. In addition, advances in critical care medicine and life support technology have improved the immediate survival of critically ill patients. This has created more opportunity to manage late complications of multisystem organ failure, one of which is SRMD. Despite these facts, it appears that the incidence of clinically significant stress-related bleeding in intensive care units is declining.[3,4] The reason for this remains unclear.

Perhaps technological advances in the management of critical illness, as well as the widespread use of prophylactic therapy with antacids, H_2-receptor antagonists, and sucralfate have influenced the natural history of SRMD. Alternatively, this perception of declining incidence may be partly artifactual. The larger number of intensive care unit beds available now compared to the 1960s may have resulted in the occupancy of such beds by patients who, on average, are less sick and at lower risk for stress-related bleeding.

INCIDENCE

SRMD develops in nearly all patients subjected to the intense physiological stress of a critical illness, although certain patients seem particularly susceptible. These include patients with severe central nervous system injury (Cushing's ulcer), burns over more than 35% of the body surface area (Curling's ulcer), respiratory failure, renal failure, hepatic failure, sepsis, major trauma, uncorrectable coagulopathy, shock, acidosis, high volumes of gastric acid, and prolonged stay in the intensive care unit.[5] In such individuals, lesions can occur within hours of the initial insult. Endoscopy performed within 24 hours of admission to an intensive care unit demonstrates a 74–100% incidence of mucosal damage in patients with a variety of medical and surgical conditions (Table 9.1). One can also identify patients who do not seem to be at increased risk for SRMD. Such individuals include those with burns involving less than 35% of the body surface area, intracranial lesions without coma, dialyzed renal failure, soft tissue injury (trauma, infections), and uncomplicated cardiac disease (myocardial infarction, arrhythmias, congestive heart failure).

The overall severity of the illness appears to correlate with the incidence of SRMD and the risk of bleeding. Without prophylactic therapy, some degree of gastrointestinal bleeding is observed in 10–20% (Figure 9.1) of critically ill patients, although the exact incidence varies greatly, depending on the precise definition of bleeding. Nevertheless, clinically significant blood loss occurs in 2–7% of such patients and has an associated mortality of 50–77% with or without surgical intervention.[3,6] While not all mortality is related to bleeding, upper gastrointestinal hemorrhage can account for up to one-third of these deaths. In contrast, the overall mortality in comparable nonbleeding intensive care unit patients is 9–22% (Figure 9.2).

TABLE 9.1. Incidence of SRMD Within 18 to 24 Hours of Admission to the Intensive Care Unit

Reference	*Population*	*Endoscopic Abnormalities (%)*
Lucas (1971)	Trauma	100
Czaja (1974)	Burns	74
Peura (1985)	Medical ICU	74
Brown (1988)	Head injury	91
Munakata (1987)	Cardiac surgery	88

Source: Adapted from Peura DA, Johnson LR: Gastroduodenal mucosal damage: Techniques to prevent bleeding. Infusions of H_2-receptor antagonists inhibit acid secretion. *J Crit Illness* 3(Suppl 9):S49–S54, 1988.

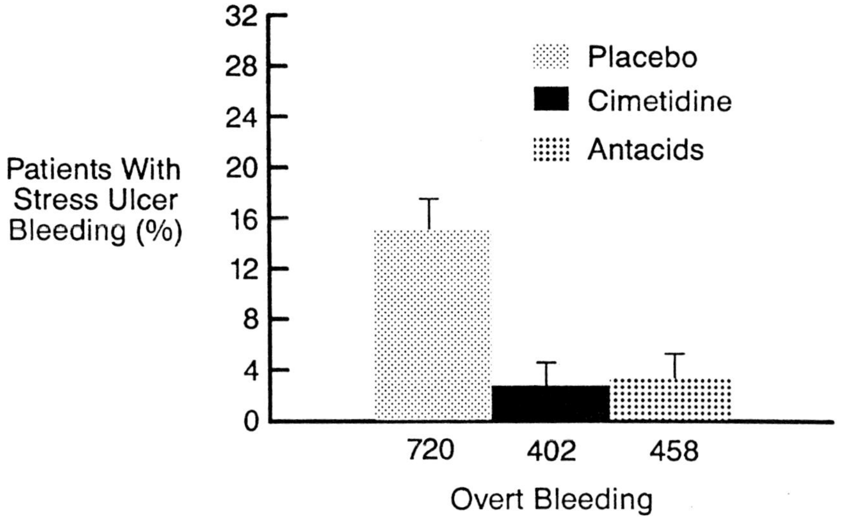

Figure 9.1. Percentage of critically ill patients with stress-related bleeding among patients receiving placebo, cimetidine, or antacids. (Adapted from Shuman RB, Schuster DP, Zuckerman GR: Prophylactic therapy for stress ulcer bleeding: A reappraisal. *Ann Intern Med* 106:562–567, 1987.)

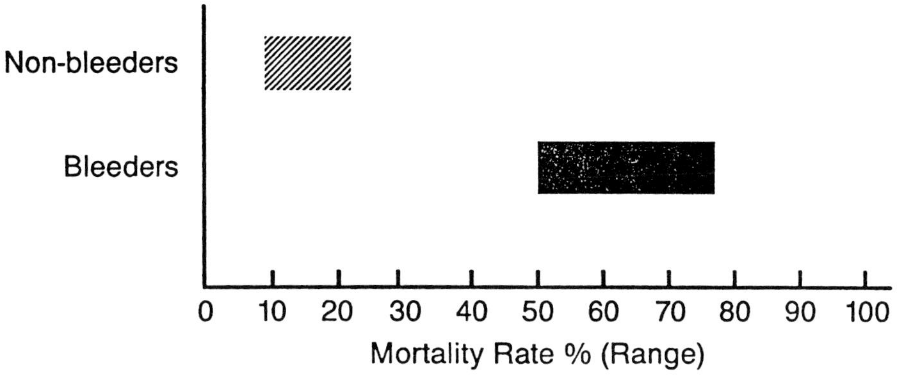

Figure 9.2. Mortality associated with SRMD. (Adapted from Zuckerman G, Shuman R: Therapeutic goals and treatment options for prevention of stress ulcer syndrome. *Am J Med* 83(Suppl 6A):29–35, 1987.)

DIAGNOSIS AND METHODS OF MONITORING

Endoscopy is clearly the most sensitive and specific method for monitoring SRMD and has provided valuable information regarding the natural history of mucosal injury. Clinical studies utilizing early endoscopy reveal that identifiable lesions are present within hours of the stressful event and, if left untreated, can progress over several days, leading occasionally to significant hemorrhage or perforation. Macroscopic lesions are initially confined to the acid-producing areas (gastric fundus and body), though on occasion they can be more extensive, involving the antrum, the duodenum, and even the distal esophagus. Serial endoscopic observations suggest that submucosal petechiae and hemorrhages occur first, followed by erosions and superficial ulcers. Lesions due to SRMD appear quite different from peptic ulcers, and due to their superficial nature, the lesions tend to ooze blood rather than bleed briskly. An exception to this pattern, however, seems to occur in patients with sepsis or central nervous system (CNS) disease. In this setting, the lesions tend to be deeper, perforation can be seen, and bleeding may more often be massive. Although endoscopy is impractical to use routinely to monitor all intensive care unit patients, it should remain the gold standard for monitoring the gastric mucosa during therapeutic trials.

Due to the impracticalities of endoscopy, the clinician must use other techniques to diagnose SRMD. Unfortunately, most of these have major shortcomings. Barium radiographs are both unreliable and impractical to perform in critically ill patients. Macroscopic upper gastrointestinal bleeding is a reliable clinical indicator of mucosal damage, but it greatly underestimates the true prevalence, since nonbleeding lesions are not recognized. Occult blood testing of the nasogastric aspirate is used frequently to infer the presence or absence of mucosal damage. However, it is a nonspecific test which suffers from both false-positive[7] and false-negative[8] results. Monitoring the hematocrit (or transfusion requirement) may prove unreliable, not only because nonbleeding lesions will be missed, but also because critically ill patients may have hematocrit changes (or require transfusions) for reasons unrelated to gastrointestinal hemorrhage. Although gastric acidity seems to be a necessary factor in the development of SRMD, intragastric pH monitoring cannot be used as a diagnostic tool. Low intragastric pH does not always equate with mucosal damage, nor does high pH guarantee its absence.

PATHOGENESIS

The precise pathogenesis of SRMD remains unknown, although the injury is best thought of as arising from an imbalance between aggressive (acid, pepsin, bile salts) and defensive (mucus, bicarbonate, mucosal blood flow, prostaglandins, epithelial cell renewal) mucosal factors. The weight of evidence to date suggests that the mucosal defense is primarily defective. This allows a normally acidic and proteolytic gastric environment to induce mucosal damage. Much of our understanding of the mechanisms underlying SRMD comes from animal models of stress-induced injury. We must await reproducible techniques to study mucosal defensive properties in humans to validate our basic knowledge in the clinical setting.

Aggressive Mucosal Factors

Intraluminal gastric acid is a prerequisite for the development of SRMD in a wide variety of experimental animal models as well as humans. Despite this, acid hypersecretion is unusual in critically ill patients, except for those with either sepsis or CNS injury. The efficiency of the various mucosal defensive factors which affect the degree of hydrogen ion back diffusion appears to be more important than the absolute quantity of acid. Experimentally, a drop in lamina propria pH below 6.7 to 6.5 results in mucosal ulceration.[9]

Pepsin also seems to be important for the development of SRMD.[10] Its activity is acid dependent, having an optimal pH of 1.8 and being inactivated at pH above 4.5. Although not responsible for the initial mucosal lesion, pepsin contributes secondarily through proteolysis of damaged tissue, as well as through its mucolytic action on gastric mucus.

The potential role of bile acids and lysolecithin as aggressive factors has been investigated in several animal models. Both in dogs[11] and in Yorkshire piglets,[12] occlusion of the pylorus during a period of sustained shock prevents the typical mucosal lesions associated with this insult. The protection afforded by pyloric occlusion is no longer apparent if taurocholic acid in high concentration is added to the gastric contents.[13] In mongrel dogs, bile acids have been shown to enhance the mucosal damage caused by acid and mucosal ischemia, although bile salts are incapable of inducing such damage by themselves.[14] They may produce damage by increasing gastric epithelial permeability to hydrogen ion, or by altering mucosal cell tolerance to back-diffusion by inhibiting various active transport processes.[15] Disturbed gastrointestinal motility in critically ill patients may contribute to increased bile reflux.

Defensive Factors

An array of defensive mechanisms allows gastric epithelial cells to exist within a hostile environment containing gastric acid and pepsin without sustaining cell injury. The interplay of these mechanisms permits a large hydrogen ion gradient to exist between the lumen and the gastric mucosa without causing tissue injury. In SRMD, this gastric mucosal barrier integrity is violated by stress-related changes in mucosal blood flow, mucus production, bicarbonate secretion, prostaglandin synthesis, and epithelial cell renewal. Back-diffusion of hydrogen ions occurs, resulting in mucosal capillary breakdown, interstitial hemorrhage, and ultimately bleeding into the gastric lumen.

Normally, gastric mucosal blood flow serves the critical functions of oxygen and bicarbonate transport to the surface of the mucosa, as well as hydrogen ion removal from the mucosa. Gastric mucosal blood flow decreases in critically ill patients,[16] and many investigators consider ischemia the most important pathogenic factor in the development of SRMD.[10,17] In experimental models, methods to maintain mucosal blood flow afford mucosal protection.[18] The mechanisms of ischemia-related epithelial cell damage may include development of an energy deficit due to diminished synthesis of high-energy phosphates,[19] reduced mucosal acid-buffering ability, and the formation of oxygen-derived free radicals or superoxides.[20] Interestingly, in experimental animals, the energy deficit appears to be more pronounced in the gastric fundus than in the antrum, which may explain the distribution of macroscopic damage described clinically.[21]

Another important defensive factor is the gastric mucus/bicarbonate layer that overlies the gastric epithelium. This thin mucus gel consists of a matrix of glycoprotein molecules joined together by physical noncovalent interactions. This mucus provides mechanical protection to the surface mucosa, maintains a pH gradient between the epithelial and luminal interfaces, and traps secreted bicarbonate for more effective buffering of back-diffusing hydrogen ion. The synthetic rate, composition, and restoration of the mucus/bicarbonate layer is altered by physiological stress.

Prostaglandins, derived from 20 C chain fatty acids, are present in high concentrations in gastric mucosa. Exogenous administration of prostaglandin analogs prevents gastric injury induced in animals by pyloric ligation, restraint, hypothermia, glucocorticoid administration, and water immersion through mechanisms independent of their antisecretory effect. They seem to enhance mucosal defense mechanisms by increasing mucosal blood flow, as well as stimulating mucus production, bicarbonate secretion, and epithelial cell growth and repair. Stress capable of causing mucosal damage reduces the synthesis and tissue activity of prostaglandins.[22]

Renewal of gastric epithelial cells is a continuous process, with cells from the mucosal proliferative zone migrating to replace senescent or damaged cells at the epithelial surface. During experimental physiological stress this process is altered, resulting in diminished cellular proliferation and DNA synthesis, along with an overall loss of RNA.[23] Such alterations also occur during fasting, a common necessity in patients with critical illness. Agents that increase protein synthesis, DNA synthesis, and cell division (e.g., pentagastrin, growth hormone, and epidermal growth factor) can prevent experimental stress ulcers in animals.[23,24] How these observations may apply to human critical illness remains unclear.

CLINICAL FEATURES

SRMD typically occurs in patients who are critically ill and have no history of upper gastrointestinal disease. Lesions are generally asymptomatic. Untreated mucosal injury can progress and result in bleeding. This bleeding commonly arises from superficial capillaries and is seldom massive. It tends to occur within 4–14 days after the initial event, and its likelihood relates to the severity of the clinical illness. The prognosis depends upon the underlying disease, although the initial severity of the endoscopic mucosal appearance and the subsequent mortality have been shown to correlate.[25]

Acid secretion tends to be normal or reduced, except for occasional patients with sepsis or CNS disease, in whom acid hypersecretion can be seen. Hence, the clinician should diligently exclude occult sepsis in critically ill patients with apparent acid hypersecretion or those in whom an acidic gastric pH persists despite therapy.

TREATMENT

The risk of bleeding from SRMD correlates with the severity and duration of the underlying disease.[26] Most of the mortality in clinical studies relates to the progression of the primary disease rather than to mucosal damage. Improvement in mucosal appearance seems to parallel clinical improvement. Therefore, therapy for SRMD should focus on the underlying cause of the physiological stress. Aggressive, prompt treatment of hypovolemia, sepsis, acid-base or electrolyte disturbances, respiratory failure, and malnutrition are at least as important as pharmacological intervention specifically directed at the gastric mucosa.[26]

Specific prophylactic pharmacotherapy of SRMD is a subject of some controversy. True prophylaxis (i.e., prevention of lesions) is not clinically practical in most cases, since SRMD is often already present when the patient first comes to medical attention. The goal of therapy is to limit the progression of early lesions and prevent clinically significant gastrointestinal bleeding. Preventing lesion progression and morbidity from bleeding are goals that are clinically obtainable using reasonably safe and effective therapies. Given that up to 20% of total intensive care unit expenditures relate to transfusion of blood products,[27] therapy of SRMD may be quite cost effective.

Antacids

Since the presence of some gastric acid is required for the development of SRMD, acid neutralization has been extensively evaluated as a mode of therapy. In addition to buffering gastric acid, antacids have several other possible mechanisms of action, which include binding bile salts, pepsin, and lysolecithin, as well as stimulating prostaglandin synthesis.

An intensive antacid regimen is known to reduce stress ulcer bleeding significantly in critically ill patients.[28,29] The optimal degree of acid neutralization required remains unclear, although achieving an intraluminal pH greater than 3.5 seems necessary. Fiddian-Green et al. have suggested that the gastric intramural pH (calculated from the gastric juice pCO_2 and arterial blood bicarbonate using the Henderson-Hasselbach equation) is a more accurate predictor of mucosal bleeding than a specific luminal pH.[30] Though attractive in theory, total elimination of gastric acid appears to be no more efficacious in preventing bleeding than a pH control greater than 3.5.

Though antacids remain a therapeutic gold standard, their effectiveness depends upon frequent dosing (every two hours in most cases) and periodic intragastric pH monitoring. Such regimens are time-consuming for the nursing staff and side-effect inducing for the patient. Frequent antacid administration may cause diarrhea, metabolic abnormalities such as the phosphate depletion syndrome, aluminum toxicity (especially in patients with renal failure), impaired drug absorption, and possibly aspiration pneumonia.[3,31] These liabilities have led to an extensive search for alternative agents.

H_2-Receptor Antagonists

H_2-receptor antagonists have been used effectively since 1977 to treat SRMD. In addition to their antisecretory effect, these agents may enhance mucosal defense mechanisms. Although the clinical significance of these enhancing properties remains unproven, it is notable that efficacy has been demonstrated with dosing regimens that do not maintain a gastric pH above 3.5.[25] Unlike antacids, H_2-receptor antagonists can be administered parenterally as well as orally.

At least 18 controlled trials have compared H_2-receptor antagonists (mainly cimetidine) to a placebo or to no treatment[3,25,32] using gastrointestinal bleeding or endoscopic changes as measures of efficacy. In 10 studies, the H_2-receptor antagonist was proven superior. In none were placebo or no treatment superior. In eight studies, there was no statistical difference between the regimens, though this may have resulted from the small number of subjects studied or the insensitivity of the endpoint determinations. Comparison of H_2-receptor antagonists with antacids has revealed the two therapies to be virtually equivalent in efficacy, as borne out by at least 15 trials.[3,32] Eleven trials revealed no statistical difference in efficacy. Antacids proved superior in two studies and H_2-receptor antagonists in two.

Most studies have utilized intermittent dosing of the H_2-receptor antagonist. More recently, continuous infusion has been proposed as a more efficient and cost-effective method of parenteral H_2-receptor antagonist administration. This technique effectively maintains therapeutic blood levels and uniform pH control with less total drug dose than bolus administration. Fluid conservation, fewer intravenous line violations, possible reduction in side effects and potential drug interactions, as well as considerable time and cost savings accompany continuous infusion therapy. For these reasons, continuous infusion is now considered the preferred method of H_2-receptor antagonist dosing in most patients, despite the lack of clinical proof of greater efficacy or safety than bolus administration. Cimetidine, ranitidine, and famotidine all seem to be equally effective when administered by intermittent or continuous infusion at the recommended doses.

Endoscopic observation suggests that as a patient's overall clinical condition improves, so does the gastroduodenal mucosal injury. Therefore, when clinical improvement occurs and oral intake is resumed, it would seem reasonable to change from costly parenteral to less costly oral therapy. Generally, patients require therapy for SRMD throughout their intensive care unit stay, and in some cases beyond their stay until they regain their previous functional status.

Sucralfate

Sucralfate, a basic aluminum salt of sucrose octasulfate, has been shown to protect the gastric mucosa in animal models and clinical trials. It is thought to act by binding to damaged mucosa, thereby forming a protective coating. It may also act as a weak buffer of acid, a binder of pepsin, and a stimulator of endogenous prostaglandins.[33] Clinical trials have not shown sucralfate to be superior to antacids or H_2-receptor antagonists. One potential advantage of sucralfate (and other drugs whose mode of action is unrelated to acid inhibition) stems from the observation that acid suppression permits bacterial overgrowth in the stomach, thereby potentially increasing the risk of nosocomial pneumonia. When looked at critically, however, the incidence of nosocomial pneumonia in patients treated with H_2-receptor antagonists alone is actually less than the incidence in sucralfate- or placebo-treated patients. This observation suggests that factors other than acid suppression and gastric bacterial colonization, such as gastric volume, may be important determinants of nosocomial pneumonia.

Clinically Unproven Therapeutic Measures

Like sucralfate, exogenously administered prostaglandins have been shown to protect the gastric mucosa in animal stress models.[34] In addition to enhancing the effects of endogenous prostanoids, they are potent acid antisecretory agents. Despite early anecdotal reports of possible efficacy,[35,36] the clinical results with prostaglandins as treatment for SRMD have been conflicting.[37-40]

Retrospective analyses suggest that clinically relevant stress bleeding rarely occurs in individuals receiving enteral alimentation.[41] However, no prospective trials have examined the effects of enteral feeding, and even if it is effective, the optimal dietary content and site of delivery (gastric vs. jejunal) remains to be elucidated.

Therapeutic doses of the H+/K+ ATPase inhibitor, omeprazole, can achieve a 1,200-fold reduction in gastric acid secretion compared to a 2- to 10-fold decrease with conventional dose H_2-receptor antagonists.[42] Although omeprazole has found a role in therapy of Zollinger-Ellison syndrome and gastroesophageal reflux, no clinical trial has examined its efficacy in preventing SRMD-related bleeding. One study observed improved bleeding cessation with 80 mg/day of intravenous omeprazole compared with 400 mg of continuous infusion of ranitidine in critically ill patients with bleeding peptic ulcers.[43] Unfortunately, a parenteral omeprazole preparation is not readily available, and the acid sensitivity of the available oral formulation precludes administration via nasogastric tube.

Somatostatin has acid antisecretory activity, as well as the ability to diminish splanchnic blood flow.[44] This latter effect could be detrimental to the gastric mucosa when used prophylactically, although it might prove beneficial in treating mucosal bleeding once the presence of SRMD is established. Despite some success in treating SRMD in rats,[45] only a marginal benefit over placebo has been shown in human studies of gastrointestinal hemorrhage.[46] It seems unlikely that somatostatin will play a major therapeutic role in SRMD.

Tranexamic acid, an agent with antifibrinolytic activity, has been evaluated in several European double-blind, randomized trials involving patients with upper gastrointestinal bleeding.[47,48] Looking specifically at patients with gastroduodenal erosions (although not necessarily critically ill or with SRMD), no clear benefit over placebo with regard to rebleeding, need for surgery, or mortality has been observed.

Pirenzepine is an anticholinergic agent with a high specificity for the M-1 muscarinic receptor located on the gastric mucosa. Not only does it have an antisecretory effect, but it seems to improve stress-induced microcirculatory disturbances and stimulate mucous secretion.[49,50] Limited clinical studies have suggested pirenzepine (30 to 60 mg intravenously per day) to be superior to placebo and at least equivalent to H_2-receptor antagonists in preventing clinically significant stress bleeding.[51]

Animal investigations have identified several agents that may warrant further clinical study. Glucagon administered subcutaneously to rats subjected to restraint and cold-immersion stress caused a fivefold decrease in acid secretion and a marked decrease in gastric ulcer size.[52] Epidermal growth factor has an antisecretory effect, stimulates epithelial proliferation, and decreases the mean ulcer area in rats subjected to aspirin-induced mucosal damage.[53] Lithium chloride is superior to placebo in rats subjected to ethanol-induced hemorrhagic gastritis.[54] Reactive oxygen metabolites, generated by mucosal xanthine oxidase after reperfusion of ischemic mucosa, have been implicated as possible factors in the production of SRMD,[55] administration of free oxygen radical scavengers and inhibitors of xanthine oxidase, such as allopurinol, have reduced mucosal injury in experimental animals.[56]

Nonpharmacological Management of SRMD

Prevention of bleeding is clearly more successful than treatment once it occurs. Although many bleeding patients respond to conservative treatment directed at improving both the underlying disease and the gastric mucosal damage, occasional patients require endoscopic therapy for persistent or massive bleeding. If endoscopic measures fail, arteriography with embolization or intraarterial vasopressin infusion should be considered.

Surgical therapy is indicated for patients with perforation or for those in whom other measures have failed to stop bleeding. No prospective studies have been performed which clearly establish the optimal surgical procedure for such patients. Rebleeding seems to be highest following vagotomy and pyloroplasty, while the mortality rate seems to be highest following vagotomy and large gastric resection. Severe underlying disease in these critically ill patients accounts for surgical mortality in more than 70%.

SPECIAL CIRCUMSTANCES

The presence of the human immunodeficiency virus merits special consideration, since such patients often undergo significant physiological stress. Upper gastrointestinal hemorrhage is an uncommon sequela of the acquired immunodeficiency syndrome (AIDS) but may occur during a phase of severe decompensation. When it occurs, an aggressive diagnostic approach is warranted in all but the terminally ill, since potentially treatable lesions may be identified. In a series of 13 patients evaluated by endoscopy at San Francisco General Hospital for upper gastrointestinal tract bleeding, 8 (62%) were bleeding from lesions associated with AIDS such as gastroduodenal Kaposi's sarcoma, gastric lymphoma, or cytomegalovirus esophagitis/duodenitis.[57] Kaposi's sarcoma accounted for one-half of the AIDS-related bleeding lesions. No patients had lesions typical of stress-related mucosal damage.

CONCLUSION

SRMD is a common problem in critically ill patients and can lead to significant morbidity and mortality. The specific features of a patient's clinical condition can be used to identify those individuals at greatest risk. The pathogenesis of SRMD involves an imbalance between aggressive and defensive mucosal factors. In addition to therapy directed at the underlying cause of physiological stress, safe and effective therapies are available which improve mucosal factor balance. Their use in the appropriate clinical setting is warranted to prevent lesion progression and morbidity from bleeding.

REFERENCES

1. Curling TB: On acute ulceration of the duodenum in cases of burns. *Med Chir Trans (Lond)* 25:123–128, 1842.
2. Cushing H: Peptic ulcers and the interbrain. *Surg Gynecol Obstet* 55:1–34, 1932.
3. Schuster DP, Rowley H, Feinstein S, et al: Prospective evaluation of the risks of upper gastrointestinal bleeding after admission to a medical intensive care unit. *Am J Med* 76:623–630, 1984.
4. Schiessel R, Feil W, Wenzl E: Mechanisms of stress ulceration and implications for treatment. *Gastroenterol Clin North Am* 19:101–120, 1990.
5. Peura DA, Johnson LF: Gastroduodenal mucosal damage: Techniques to prevent bleeding. *J Crit Illness* 3(Suppl 9):S49–S54, 1988.

6. Zuckerman G, Shuman R: Therapeutic goals and treatment options for prevention of stress ulcer syndrome. *Am J Med* 83(Suppl 6A):29–35, 1987.
7. Norfleet RG, Rhodes RA, Saviage K: False-positive "hemoccult" reaction with cimetidine (letter). *N Engl J Med* 302:467, 1980.
8. Layne EA, Mellow MH, Lipman TO: Insensitivity of guaiac slide tests for detection of blood in gastric juice. *Ann Intern Med* 94:774–776, 1981.
9. Kivilaakso E, Barzilai A, Schiessel R, et al: Experimental ulceration in rabbit antral mucosa. *Gastroenterology* 80:77–83, 1981.
10. Silen W, Merkav A, Simpson JNL: The pathophysiology of stress ulcer disease. *World J Surg* 5:165–174, 1981.
11. Guilbert J, Bounous G, Gurd FN: Role of intestinal chyme in the pathogenesis of gastric ulceration following hemorrhagic shock. *J Trauma* 9:723–742, 1969.
12. Kivilaakso E, Kalima TV: Gastric ulceration in the pig subjected to hemorrhagic shock. *Scand J Gastroenterol* 9:685–690, 1974.
13. Hamza KN, DenBesten L: Bile salts producing stress ulcers during experimental shock. *Surgery* 71:161–167, 1972.
14. Ritchie WP: Role of bile acid reflux in acute hemorrhagic gastritis. *World J Surg* 5:189–196, 1981.
15. Silen W, Forte JG: Effects of bile salts on amphibian gastric mucosa. *Am J Physiol* 228:637–644, 1975.
16. Ritchie WP: Pathogenesis of acute gastric mucosal injury. *Viewpoints Dig Dis* 5:17–20, 1983.
17. Marrone GC, Silen W: Pathogenesis, diagnosis and treatment of acute gastric mucosal lesions. *Clin Gastroenterol* 13:635–650, 1984.
18. Ritchie WP, Shearburn EW: Influence of isoproterenol and cholestyramine on acute gastric mucosal ulcerogenesis. *Gastroenterology* 73:62–65, 1977.
19. Menguy R: Role of gastric mucosal energy metabolism in the etiology of stress ulceration. *World J Surg* 5:175–180, 1981.
20. Perry MA, Wadwha S, Parks DA, et al: Role of oxygen radicals in ischemia induced lesions in the cat stomach. *Gastroenterology* 90:362–367, 1986.
21. Menguy R, Masters YF: Mechanism of stress ulcer: Differences between the antrum, corpus, and fundus with respect to the effects of complete ischemia and gastric mucosal energy metabolism. *Gastroenterology* 66:509–516, 1974.
22. Hawkey CJ, Rampton DS: Prostaglandins and the gastrointestinal mucosa: Are they important in its function, disease or treatment? *Gastroenterology* 89:1162–1188, 1985.
23. Takeuchi K, Johnson LR: Pentagastrin protects against stress ulceration in rats. *Gastroenterology* 76:327–334, 1979.
24. Robert A, Kauffman GL Jr: Stress ulcers, in Sleisenger MJ, Fordtran JS (eds): *Gastrointestinal Disease,* ed 3. Philadelphia, WB Saunders, 1984, pp 612–625.
25. Peura DA, Johnson LF: Cimetidine for prevention and treatment of gastroduodenal mucosal lesions in patients in an intensive care unit. *Ann Intern Med* 103:173–177, 1985.
26. Chamberlain CE, Peura DA: Stress ulceration and prevention. *Prob Crit Care* 3:371–384, 1989.
27. Masur H: ICU patients at risk for stress ulcers and GI bleeding. *J Crit Illness* 3:(Suppl 9):S22–S25, 1988.
28. McAlhany JC, Czaja AJ, Pruitt BA: Antacid control of complications from acute gastroduodenal disease after burns. *J Trauma* 16:645–649, 1976.
29. Hastings PR, Skillmann JJ, Bushnell LS, et al: Antacid titration in the prevention of acute gastrointestinal bleeding. A controlled randomized trial in 100 critically ill patients. *N Engl J Med* 298:1041–1045, 1978.

30. Fiddian-Green RG, McGough E, Pittenger G, et al: Predictive value of intramural pH and other risk factors for massive bleeding from stress ulceration. *Gastroenterology* 85:613–620, 1983.

31. Driks MR, Craven DE, Celli BR, et al: Nosocomial pneumonia in intubated patients given sucralfate as compared with antacids or histamine type 2 blockers. *N Engl J Med* 317:1376–1382, 1987.

32. Peura DA: Recognizing, setting up therapeutic goals, and selecting therapy for the prevention and treatment of stress-related mucosal disease. *Pharmacotherapy* 7(6 Pt 2):95S–103S, 1987.

33. Samloff IM, Odell C: Inhibition of peptic activity by sucralfate. *Am J Med* 79(Suppl 2C):15–18, 1985.

34. Gaskill HV, Sirinek KR, Levine B: 16, 16-Dimethyl PGE_2 reverses focal mucosal ischemia associated with stress ulcers. *J Surg Res* 37:83–88, 1984.

35. Groeger JS, Dazza SJ, Carlon GC, et al: Prostaglandin therapy in a case of refractory stress ulcer bleeding. *Crit Care Med* 10:46–47, 1982.

36. Weiss JB, Peskin GW, Isenberg JI: Treatment of hemorrhagic gastritis with 15 (R)-15 methyl PGE_2: A report of a case. *Gastroenterology* 82:558–560, 1982.

37. Van Essen HA, Van Blankenstein M, Wilson JH, et al: Intragastric PGE_2 and the prevention of gastrointestinal hemorrhage in intensive care unit patients. *Crit Care Med* 13:957–960, 1985.

38. Levine BA, Sirinek KR, Gaskill HV: Topical PGE_2 in the treatment of acute upper gastrointestinal tract hemorrhage. *Arch Surg* 120:600–604, 1985.

39. Skillman JJ, Lisbon A, Long PC, et al: 15(R)-15-Methyl PGE_2 does not prevent gastrointestinal bleeding in seriously ill patients. *Am J Surg* 147:451–455, 1984.

40. Zinner MJ, Rypins E, Martin LF, et al: Misoprostol versus antacid in the prevention of stress bleeding and lesions in intensive care unit patients: A multicenter prospective double-blind trial (abstract). *Gastroenterology* 92:1711, 1987.

41. Pingleton SK, Hadzima SK: Enteral alimentation and gastrointestinal bleeding in mechanically ventilated patients. *Crit Care Med* 11:13–16, 1983.

42. Pritchard PJ, Yeomans ND, Mihaly GW, et al: Omeprazole: A study of its inhibition of gastric pH and oral pharmacokinetics after morning or evening dosage. *Gastroenterology* 88:64–69, 1984.

43. Brunner G, Chang J: Intravenous therapy with high doses of ranitidine and omeprazole in critically ill patients with bleeding peptic ulcerations of the upper intestinal tract: An open randomized controlled trial. *Digestion* 45:217–225, 1990.

44. Sonnenberg GE, Keller U, Perruchaud A, et al: Affect of somatostatin on splanchnic hemodynamics in patients with cirrhosis of the liver and in normal subjects. *Gastroenterology* 80:526–532, 1981.

45. Vara-Tholbeck R, Garcia-Blanque C, Villen A: Prevention of stress ulcer by cimetidine and somatostatin in rats. *Langenbeck's Arch Chir* 351:215–218, 1980.

46. Magnusson I, Ihre T, Johansson C, et al: Randomized double-blind trial of somatostatin in the treatment of massive upper gastrointestinal hemorrhage. *Gut* 26:221–226, 1985.

47. Biggs JC, Hugh TB, Dodds AJ: Tranexamic acid and upper gastrointestinal hemorrhage—a double blind study. *Gut* 17:729–734, 1976.

48. Barer D, Oglivie A, Henry D: Cimetidine and tranexamic acid in the treatment of acute upper gastrointestinal tract bleeding. *N Engl J Med* 308:1571–1575, 1983.

49. Sato N, Hu Quan L, Kawano S, et al: Effect of H2-receptor and muscarinic receptor antagonists and PGE_1 analog on the gastric hemodynamics and oxygen sufficiency, in Braley D, Bicker HI, Reneau D (eds): *Oxygen Transport to Tissue,* Vol IV. New York, Plenum Press, 1984, pp 763–771.

50. Watanabe Y, Kobayashi R, Yoshigoe F, et al: Effect of pirenzepine on gastric mucous secretion, in *Pirenzepine: New Aspects in Research and Therapy*. Amsterdam, Excerpta Medica, 1985, p 24.

51. Tryba M: Pirenzepine as single medication for the prevention of stress bleeding—results of prospective trials, New York, *Prevention of Stress Bleeding in Critically Ill Patients—A New Concept*. Thieme Medical, 1987, pp 37–41.

52. Guth PH, Meeroff JC, Paulsen G, et al: Prevention by glucagon of experimental stress induced hemorrhagic gastritis. *Gastroenterology* 69:1048–1050, 1975.

53. Konturek SJ, Radecki T, Brzozowski T: Gastric cytoprotection by epidermal growth factor. *Gastroenterology* 81:1238–1243, 1981.

54. Wong RKH, Boedeker B, Hickey TM, et al: Lithium chloride: Protective and antisecretory properties in rats. *Gastroenterology* 87:362–371, 1984.

55. Nakamura K, Aoike A, Rokutan K: The role of oxygen radicals in the pathogenesis of gastric mucosal lesions induced in mice by feeding—restriction stress. *Scand J Gastroenterol—Supplement* 162:47–50, 1989.

56. Hirota M, Inoue M, Ando Y, et al: Inhibition of stress induced gastric mucosal injury by a long-acting superoxide dismutase that circulates bound to albumin. *Arch Biochem Biophys* 280:769–773, 1990.

57. Cello JP, Wilcox CM: Evaluation and treatment of gastrointestinal tract hemorrhage in patients with AIDS. *Gastroenterol Clin North Am* 17:639–648, 1988.

II

SITES OF BLEEDING

10

BLEEDING FROM THE ESOPHAGUS

Ross M. Bremner, Jr., M.D.
Tom R. DeMeester, M.D.

INTRODUCTION

The importance of the esophagus as a site of nonvariceal upper gastrointestinal bleeding has been underestimated. Prior reports note that such bleeding is responsible for more than 10% of acute upper gastrointestinal hemorrhage, and the mortality in these patients may be as high as 10%.[1,2] In fact, the incidence of acute hemorrhage from the esophagus or cardia from nonvariceal causes is as common as variceal bleeding (Table 10.1). Acute upper gastrointestinal hemorrhage often complicates such conditions as gastroesophageal reflux, hiatus hernia, caustic or pill-induced injury, and tumors. The esophagus may also be the site of chronic blood loss and should be considered in patients with occult anemia. Table 10.2 summarizes the disease processes that have been reported to cause bleeding from the esophagus.[3-14]

BLOOD SUPPLY OF THE ESOPHAGUS

Some insight into the different presentations of esophageal bleeding can be gained from a consideration of its arterial supply and venous drainage. The cervical and upper thoracic esophagus receives its blood supply from the inferior thyroid arteries plus smaller accessory branches from the common carotid, subclavian, and superficial cervical arteries (Figure 10.1). There is great variation in the arterial anatomy of the thoracic region, as can be appreciated by the classical work of Shapiro and Robillard in 1950.[15] This region is supplied by branches of the bronchial arteries, by two or three esophageal branches of the descending aorta, and occasionally by one or two intercostal arteries.[16] The abdominal portion of the esophagus and the lower thoracic esophagus are fed by ascending branches of the left gastric artery and inferior phrenic arteries. There is an extensive anastomotic network between these systems, which explains why the esophagus can be mobilized from the cardia to the level of the aortic arch without fear of ischemic necrosis. Recent resin-casting techniques on postmortem esophagi have shown the striking feature that all

TABLE 10.1. Benign Cardioesophageal Causes of Acute Upper Gastrointestinal Hemorrhage: Final Diagnoses

			Nonvariceal				
Reference	*Year*	*Number of Pts.*	*Esophagitis*	*Esophageal Ulcer*	*Mallory-Weiss*	*Total*	*Variceal*
Palmer et al.[3]	1971	1,500	7.2%	—	5.1%	12.3%	19.7%
Silverstein et al.[2]	1981	2,097	6.3%	1.7%	7.2%	15.2%	10.3%
Sugawa[4]	1989	3,549	5.2%	—	10.2%	15.4%	12.6%

TABLE 10.2. Causes of Esophageal Bleeding

Congenital
- Weber-Osler-Rendu disease[3,4]
- Blue rubber bleb nevus syndrome[5]
- Epidermolysis bullosa[6]
- Esophageal duplication[7]

Acquired

Inflammatory
- Reflux esophagitis
- Barrett's esophagus
- Infection
- Corrosives/pill-induced injury
- Radiation therapy
- Chemotherapy
- Crohn's disease[8]
- Behcet's syndrome[9]
- Pemphigoid[10]

Traumatic/Mechanical
- Hiatal hernia
- Mallory-Weiss syndrome
- Boerhaave syndrome
- Spontaneous intramural hemorrhage[11]
- Foreign body[12,13]
- Endoscopy

Neoplastic
- Benign
- Malignant

Vascular
- Varices
- Aortic aneurysm[14]
- Cardiac surgery

Hematological
- Anticoagulants
- Bleeding disorders

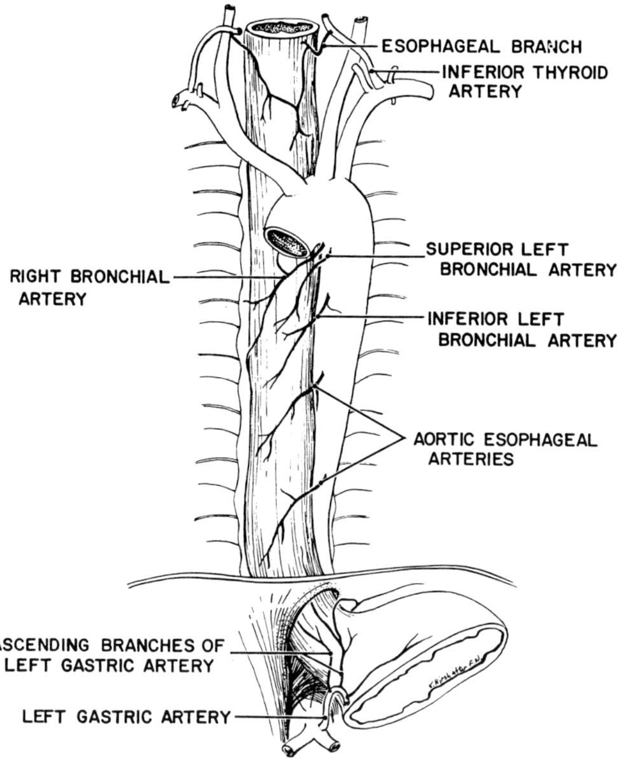

Figure 10.1. Arterial supply of the esophagus. (From Rothberg M, DeMeester TR: Surgical anatomy of the esophagus, in Shields TW (ed): *General Thoracic Surgery,* ed 3. Philadelphia, Lea & Febiger, 1989, p 76, with permission.)

arteries supplying the esophagus branch extensively before penetrating the wall.[17] Those entering the wall are less than 1 mm in diameter, and only small arterioles and capillaries are found in the mucosa and submucosa.

In 1966 De Carvalho described the patterns of venous drainage of the esophagus in the region of the cardia and lower esophagus.[18] He noted a detour of the main venous plexus of the submucosa to a more superficial level in the region of the gastroesophageal junction (Figure 10.2). Teleologically, this would make sense to avoid the obstructive effects of the tonic contractions of the lower esophageal sphincter. Using resin-casting techniques, Kitano and colleagues have described the esophageal venous system as consisting of four layers (Figure 10.3).[19] Minute intraepithelial channels drain the papillae to form a superficial venous plexus just below the muscularis mucosa. Blood from these channels drains into the deep intrinsic veins of the submucosa, which in turn drain via perforating veins into the larger adventitial veins. The relative paucity of veins in the muscularis propria allows esophageal myotomy with minimal bleeding. The adventitial veins from the cervical region drain into the inferior thyroid vein; veins from the thoracic region drain into the bronchial, azygos, or hemiazygos veins; veins from the abdominal region drain into the coronary vein.

Thus, there is a very rich arterial and venous network at the level of the mucosa and submucosa, especially near the gastroesophageal junction. The superficial venules

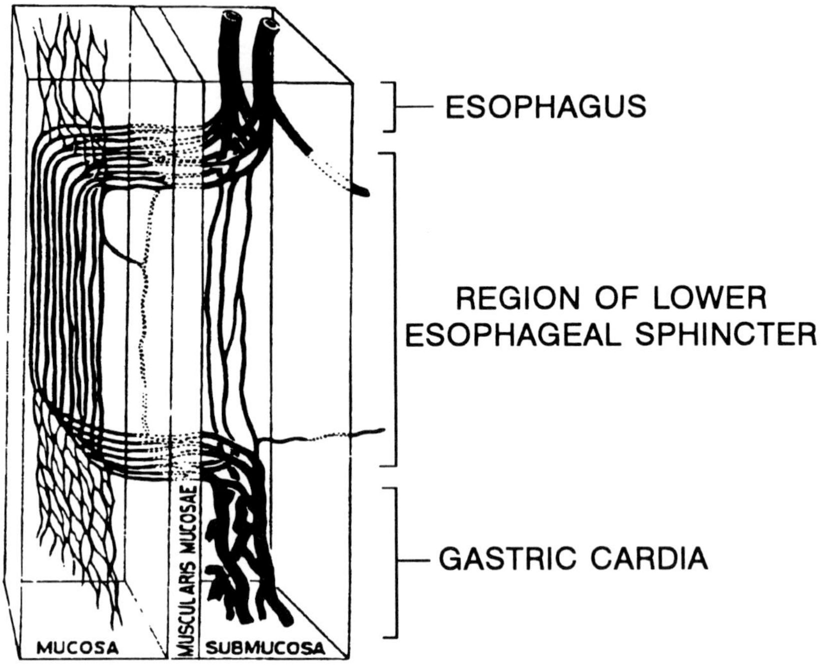

Figure 10.2. Venous drainage of the gastroesophageal junction. Note the superficial venous plexus at the region of the lower esophageal sphincter. (Adapted from De Carvalho CAF: Sur L'Angioarchitecture veineuse de la zone de transition oesophagogastrique et son interpretation fonctionelle. *Acta Anat* (Basel) 64:125–162, 1966.)

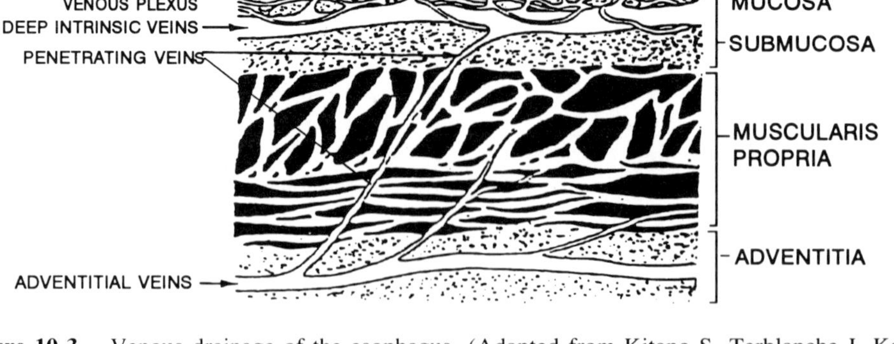

Figure 10.3. Venous drainage of the esophagus. (Adapted from Kitano S, Terblanche J, Kahn D, et al: Venous anatomy of the lower oesophagus in portal hypertension: Practical implications. *Br J Surg* 73:525–531, 1986.)

are of minute diameter but soon form significant-sized veins in the deep submucosa. The arterioles superficial to the muscularis propria are all very small in caliber. Most mucosal and submucosal bleeding is venous in origin, as the small arterial counterparts at this level have potent hemostatic contractile properties. Disruption of the venules from mucosal injury results in a slow ooze, provided that the venous pressure is normal and the veins are not dilated. This explains why most nonvariceal bleeding can be treated conservatively. Perforation of the esophageal wall or erosion of an ulcer into the wall rarely results in massive bleeding unless the process involves adjacent periesophageal vascular structures such as the aorta or the azygos vein. In this way, esophageal bleeding differs from gastric bleeding. This explains why patients with Mallory-Weiss syndrome present with bleeding, while those with Boerhaave's syndrome present with sepsis and, rarely, with hematemesis.

INFLAMMATORY CAUSES OF BLEEDING

Reflux Esophagitis

A large proportion of the population suffers from gastroesophageal reflux disease at some stage of their lives. Wienbeck and Barnett have recently estimated that the prevalence of reflux esophagitis in the Western world is approximately 2%.[20] Hemorrhage is not an uncommon complication of this disease. Palmer, in a 20-year prospective study noted that 26.6% of patients with what he termed the *hiatus hernia-esophagitis-esophageal stricture complex* were observed to have significant bleeding.[21] In a series of 3,549 endoscopies, Sugawa found esophagitis to be the primary cause of bleeding in 5.2% of patients presenting with acute upper gastrointestinal hemorrhage.[4] A large survey performed by the American Society for Gastrointestinal Endoscopy (ASGE) found the incidence to be 6.3%.[2]

This bleeding is usually a slow ooze, with pulsatile bleeding seen endoscopically in less than 1% of patients.[22] The irritant effects of refluxed gastric contents on the esophageal mucosa result in inflammation, with migration of inflammatory cells and neovascularization of the lamina propria and submucosa. These changes are especially evident in the vascular papillae or rete pegs, which are extensions of the lamina propria into the stratified squamous epithelium (Figure 10.4). Esophagitis is characterized by an increase in the number and height of rete pegs and by loss of superficial epithelial cells over them.[23,24] Consequently the congested and neovascularized lamina propria is more liable to injury, as the tips of the pegs are closer to the mucosal surface. Continuous injury to the epithelium from reflux of gastric juice results in pinpoint weeping hemorrhage from vessels in the rete pegs. The presence of refluxed gastric juice aggravates the problem by hindering coagulation and healing.

Although the bleeding is usually slow, clinically significant bleeding has been well documented. In Palmer's series, the average number of blood units administered to those patients who required transfusion for hemorrhagic esophagitis was six.[21,25] In the ASGE series, 17% of patients with hemorrhagic esophagitis required more than five units of blood.[1,2]

Rarely is surgical intervention indicated. Three of Palmer's 269 patients with hemorrhagic esophagitis underwent emergency thoracotomy and segmental esophagectomy.[21] In our experience, such surgery has never been necessary when bleeding was caused by

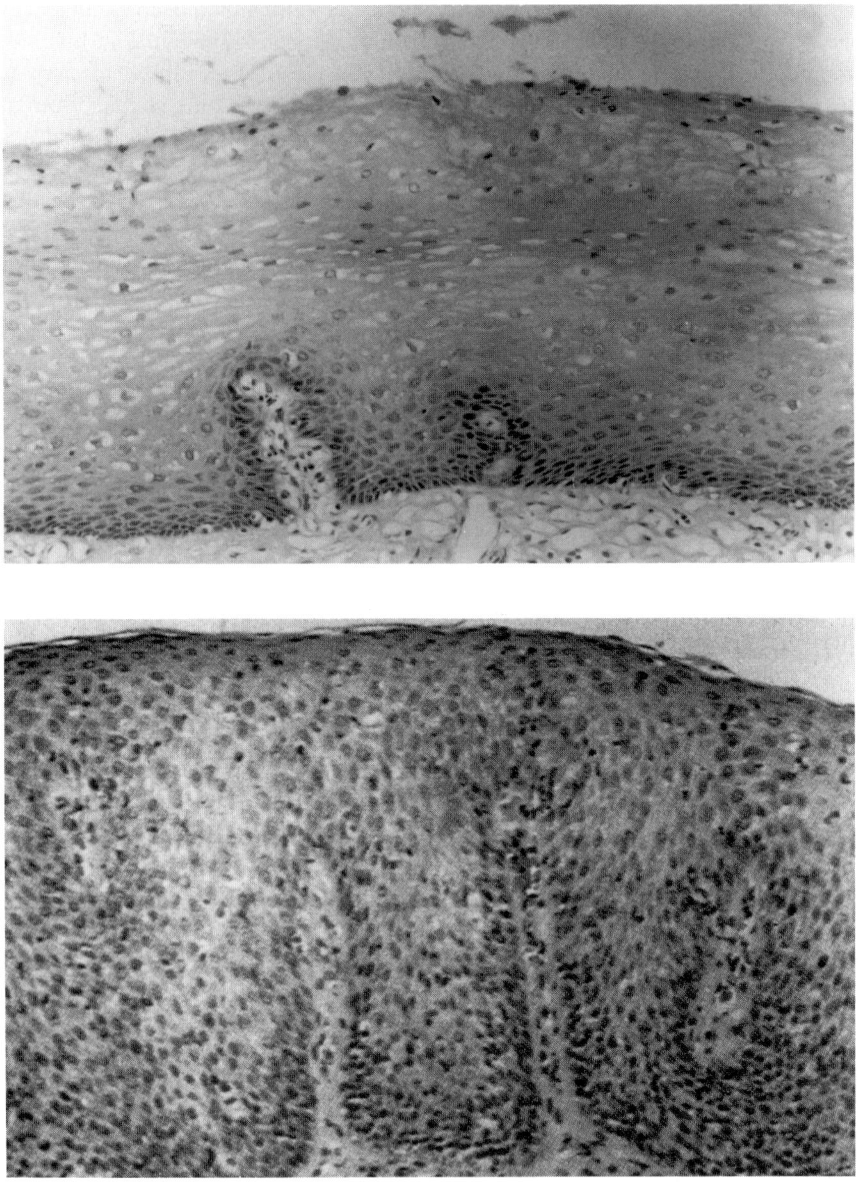

Figure 10.4. Histology of the esophageal mucosa. Normal (above) and with esophagitis (below). Note the relative increase in the height of the vascular papillae. Further loss of superficial epithelium results in erosion of the papillae and subsequent hemorrhage.

esophagitis alone. Almost all patients stop bleeding when milk or an antacid solution is dripped through a nasogastric tube placed in the upper esophagus.

Once the acute episode is over, the patient's underlying problem should be addressed. Patients with esophagitis sufficiently severe to cause hemorrhage usually have severe gastroesophageal reflux, which is difficult to control with medication.[26,27] Brossard et al. recently reported that 26% of patients with erosive esophagitis developed a complication when followed endoscopically for a mean period of 6.5 years.[28] There are a number of reasons for the continuous exposure of the esophagus to gastric juice and its resultant damage. First, the lower esophageal sphincter may be mechanically defective. This has been defined by Zaninotto et al. as a sphincter with a resting pressure less than 6 mm Hg, a total sphincter length less than 2 cm, and an intra-abdominal sphincter length less than 1 cm.[29] Documentation of a mechanically defective sphincter is important, as this is the defect that surgical antireflux procedures are designed to correct. Second, there may be inadequate clearance of physiological reflux because of abnormal esophageal body function. This may be a primary motility disorder, or associated with diseases such as diabetes and scleroderma, or secondary to severe gastroesophageal reflux.[30] Third, gastric abnormalities, such as delayed gastric emptying, increased intragastric pressure, gastric distention, and gastric hypersecretion may cause regurgitation of gastric juice into the esophagus.[30]

Since the underlying pathogenesis of reflux esophagitis is often complex and bleeding is a hallmark of severe disease, it is important that these patients undergo esophageal function studies to document and quantify the presence of gastroesophageal reflux and to determine its cause. We recommend that patients who have had a significant hemorrhage from esophagitis or who have refractory anemia secondary to esophagitis and are found to have an incompetent lower esophageal sphincter should be offered an antireflux procedure, especially since these patients are often resistant to medical therapy. Healing of the esophagitis occurs rapidly following an antireflux procedure, and previously refractory anemias are thereby corrected.

Barrett's Esophagus

The columnar lining of the esophagus, or Barrett's esophagus, is the end stage of long-standing reflux disease and is present in up to 12% of patients with persistent reflux symptoms.[31] Bleeding is a well-recognized complication of Barrett's esophagus. Bremner reported significant bleeding as a complication in 11 of 77 patients with Barrett's esophagus.[32] Others have reported an incidence of up to 30%.[33] Occult bleeding is also common; Borrie and Goldwater noted that one-third of all patients have iron deficiency anemia.[34] Significant bleeding is most commonly associated with ulceration in the columnar segment and is often more severe than the bleeding associated with reflux esophagitis. The so-called Barrett's ulcer, as described by Allison[35] and Barrett,[36] has been said to behave more like a typical gastric ulcer and to bleed in a similar way.[37] The eroding nature of such an ulcer may cause bleeding from larger vessels in the esophageal adventitia or by penetrating the aorta or atrium of the heart.[38]

In the acute situation, surgery is indicated if medical measures are unable to control the bleeding. This usually indicates a bleed from a large or deeply penetrating Barrett's ulcer, but an unsuspected concomitant peptic ulcer elsewhere in the foregut should also be considered since over 40% of patients with Barrett's esophagus have hypersecretion.[39]

Pearson et al. noted that 4 of 11 patients with Barrett's ulcers presented with massive upper gastrointestinal bleeding.[37] Those patients who need surgery to control hemorrhage nearly always require an esophagectomy, as the ulcer usually destroys the esophageal wall. However, if the bleeding can be controlled by conservative measures, the prognosis is good, as all of these ulcers will heal after subsequent antireflux surgery. We defer antireflux surgery until a full evaluation of foregut function has been obtained. Patients with Barrett's esophagus should undergo esophageal function tests, including manometry and ambulatory pH studies. Repeat endoscopy should be performed to exclude malignancy.

All six of our patients with giant Barrett's ulcers healed following antireflux surgery, and none have had a recurrence.[39] The 1968 Palmer series noted that none of 11 patients with Barrett's ulcers healed with a trial of medical therapy, whereas all of them healed following an antireflux procedure.[21] Omeprazole has been reported to heal these ulcers but is limited to short-term therapy at present.[40] Discontinuance of the drug is associated with ulcer recurrence. Gillen and Hennessy state that severe, life-threatening hemorrhage and the possibility of perforation into the mediastinum should prompt surgical intervention if medical therapy does not result in rapid healing.[41]

Infective Esophagitis

Esophagitis in as many as 10% of patients is not related to gastroesophageal reflux but rather to infection or exogenous chemical injury. Bacterial, fungal, and viral infections of the esophagus occur more commonly in the immunocompromised individual. With the widespread use of immunosuppressive agents in transplantation and the epidemic of human immunodeficiency virus (HIV) infection, the incidence of esophageal infections has dramatically increased. Candida, blastomycosis, histoplasmosis, actinomycosis, mucormycosis, tuberculosis, cytomegalovirus, and herpes virus have all been reported to cause significant bleeding.[42-50] Treatment with specific antimicrobial therapy is usually successful. Surgery is reserved for the rare patient with massive, uncontrollable bleeding and usually consists of emergency esophageal resection, cervical esophagostomy, and feeding jejunostomy; gastrointestinal reconstruction is planned for a later date.

Caustic and Pill-Induced Injury

The injury resulting from the ingestion of caustic agents depends on the nature of the ingested material and the length of exposure time to the esophageal mucosa. Whereas acidic substances are noted to cause more severe gastric injury, highly basic substances have a more destructive effect on the esophagus. Caustic soda, or lye, is a common causative agent of esophageal injury; it is present in many household cleaning preparations that are sold over the counter. Concentrated caustic soda may produce total esophageal necrosis but rarely causes acute bleeding, as thrombosis of vessels accompanies the esophageal mucosal injury.[51] Sugawa noted that when extensive ulceration and hemorrhage are seen endoscopically, the injury has extended at least to the muscle layer and may have penetrated through the entire wall.[52] Massive hemorrhage may result from caustic erosion of a major periesophageal vessel and is an indication for emergency surgery. During the healing phase of less severe burns, bleeding can result from mechanical injury to the neovascularized granulation tissue during bougienage.

There is an increasing awareness of pill-induced esophageal injury.[53] In 1983, an extensive review of the literature noted that 26 different types of pills have been implicated in causing esophageal mucosal injury.[54] The most common of these are doxycycline, potassium chloride, and emepronium bromide. Hemorrhage results from ulceration caused by prolonged contact of the pill with esophageal mucosa. Delayed transit of tablets is more likely in patients with hiatus hernias or with defects in esophageal peristalsis.[55-58] As both hernias and abnormal esophageal body function are commonly associated with gastroesophageal reflux disease, these patients are more prone to pill-induced injury, which, in turn, is often complicated by stricturing and hemorrhage. Analgesics used to alleviate heartburn may consequently aggravate esophagitis resulting from reflux disease. Recently, Lanas and Hirshowitz found that 62% of patients with active esophagitis had evidence of current aspirin use vs. only 26% of normal controls.[59] While pill-induced injury commonly results in stricture formation, hemorrhage is less common.[60] In a recent review of the literature, it was noted that only 7 of 142 patients with documented pill-induced injury experienced hematemesis. In three of these patients, however, the hemorrhage was fatal.[61]

Radiation- and Chemotherapy-Induced Bleeding

Injury to the esophagus usually accompanies irradiation for bronchogenic or esophageal carcinoma and is dose related. Yang et al. reported a series of 27 patients who developed a nonmalignant ulcer of the esophagus following radiation treatment for esophageal carcinoma.[62] Injury that occurs after a dose of 25–45 Gy is usually self-limiting and heals without sequelae.[63] Ulceration, stricture, and abnormal motility have been described as late sequelae with higher doses.[64]

Esophagitis commonly occurs in patients receiving adriamycin or actinomycin D and recurs with repetitive administration. When chemotherapy is combined with radiation therapy, injury has been described even after low doses (less than 20 Gy).[65]

MECHANICAL AND TRAUMATIC CAUSES OF ESOPHAGEAL BLEEDING

Hiatus Hernia

Hiatus hernias were associated with chronic anemia as early as 1931.[66] Windsor and Collis, in a study of 400 patients with hiatus hernias, noted an overall incidence of hemorrhage in these patients of 15%.[67] Cameron showed that anemia in 259 patients with large hiatus hernias was 18 times more common than in control subjects.[68] Since the recognition of this association, there have been many attempts to understand the cause of the bleeding. Hemorrhage has been attributed to blood loss from associated esophagitis, from stasis and erosion in the herniated pouch, from congestion of blood vessels in the pouch, and from mechanical trauma of the hernia as it rides over the crus of the diaphragm.

Understanding the pathogenesis of blood loss requires a knowledge of the various types of hernia that may occur and the incidence of blood loss associated with them. Hiatus hernias were classified by Akerlund in 1926 according to the position of the

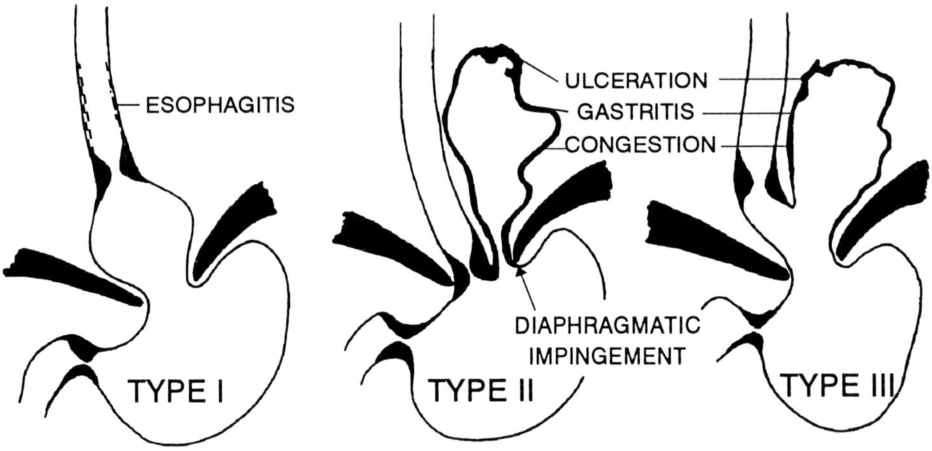

Figure 10.5. Causes of bleeding in hiatus hernias. Small sliding (type I) hernias are related to bleeding by the association of hernias with gastroesophageal reflux and the resultant esophagitis. Bleeding in type II or III hernias originates in the stomach and is a result of stasis of irritant gastric juices within the herniated pouch, as well as mechanical trauma and vascular compromise resulting from diaphragmatic impingement on the neck of the hernia.

gastroesophageal junction in relation to the diaphragmatic hiatus[69]—a concept still used today (Figure 10.5). The type I or common sliding hernia accounts for 90–95% of hiatus hernias and is associated with herniation of the gastroesophageal junction and proximal stomach into the thorax. This is often associated with a mechanically defective sphincter and gastroesophageal reflux. In these patients, bleeding is rarely from the herniated stomach. The prevalence of bleeding in patients with reducible type I hernias is small. When bleeding does occur, it is usually related to esophagitis, gastritis, or duodenal ulcer.

In type II or paraesophageal hernias, the gastroesophageal junction remains fixed in the correct anatomical position due to the attachments of the cardia to the preaortic fascia,[70] the fundus of the stomach herniates through the hiatus into the mediastinum, alongside the esophagus. Type III hernias are a combination of type I and II hernias. Types II and III both cause bleeding more commonly than type I. Windsor and Collis found that 30% of patients with types II and III hernias had anemia as opposed to only 11% of patients with type I hernias.[67] In the former patients, bleeding was from the herniated stomach and not the esophagus. Gardner in 1933 attributed the cause of bleeding in type II hernias to obstruction of venous drainage of the herniated pouch by compression of the edge of the diaphragm.[71] Truesdale and, later, Mendelsohn thought that vascular disturbance was the cause of hemorrhage.[72,73] Belsey in 1954 introduced the concept that hyperacidity was responsible for mucosal ulceration and bleeding.[74] Aylwyn analyzed the esophageal refluxate during sleep in patients with hiatus hernias and found a high concentration of acid and pepsin with a low concentration of protective mucus.[75] By instilling contrast medium into the stomach, he demonstrated that only hernial contents were refluxed into the esophagus during sleep. From these results, Marchand suggested that stasis of gastric contents within the hernial pouch can result in "auto-digestion" of the mucosa, with consequent ulceration and hemorrhage.[76] Endoscopy has revealed large gastric ulcers in the herniated pouch, riding ulcers at the neck of the pouch

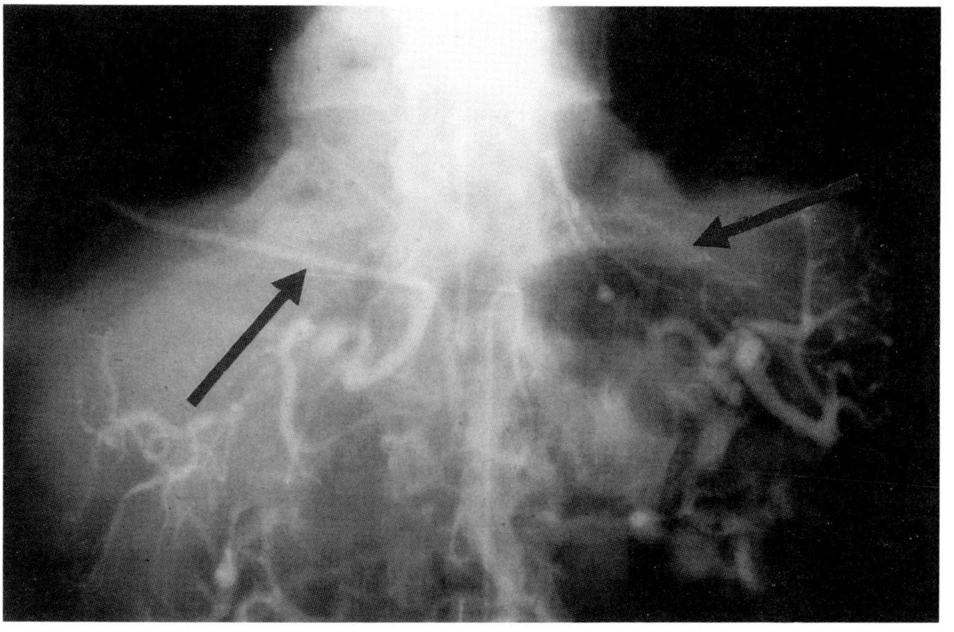

Figure 10.6. Angiogram showing the blood supply to a large type II hernia. Note the stretching of the right gastroepiploic artery (left arrow) and short gastric arteries (right arrow). (From DeMeester TR, Bonavina L: Paraesophageal hiatal hernia, in Nyhus LM, Condon RE (ed): *Hernia,* ed 3. Philadelphia, JB Lippincott Co, 1989, p 684, with permission.)

overlying the impression of the crus of the diaphragm, diffuse erosive gastritis in the hernial sac, and congestion with erythema and edema of the mucosa.[67,77] The riding ulcer was thought to have a mechanical component to its etiology.[67] Congestion, erythema, and edema of the mucosa are thought to occur from impingement of the diaphragm on the neck of the pouch and from vascular engorgement due to venous outflow obstruction. Stretching of the vascular structures has been documented in large paraesophageal hernias and can result in venous or arterial compression (Figure 10.6). Ulcers and gastritis in the herniated pouch are likely to be the result of mucosal injury from gastric juice retained within the compromised incarcerated gastric pouch.

An incompetent cardia with gastroesophageal reflux is more commonly seen in patients with paraesophageal hernias than was previously thought. Sixty percent of 18 patients treated by us for paraesophageal hernias had abnormal acid exposure of the esophagus and an incompetent cardia.[78] Esophagitis may be a contributory cause of blood loss in these patients.

Patients with paraesophageal hernias or incarcerated type III hernias require timely surgical intervention.[79] Besides the complications of bleeding, which may be life-threatening, there is the risk of strangulation, ischemic necrosis, and perforation.[80] Skinner and Belsey in 1967 reported on 21 patients with paraesophageal type II hernias that were treated conservatively because of minimal symptoms.[81] Six of these patients subsequently died from acute complications of the hernia; this experience prompted the authors to repair the hernia in the other 15 patients and to encourage surgeons elsewhere to do the same for their patients. The surgical correction of the hernia should be accompa-

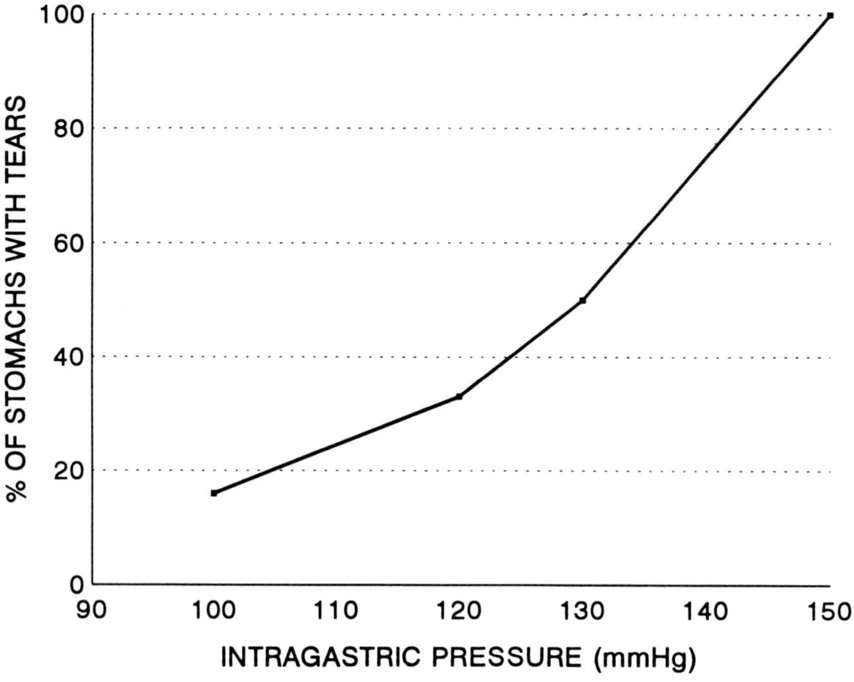

A

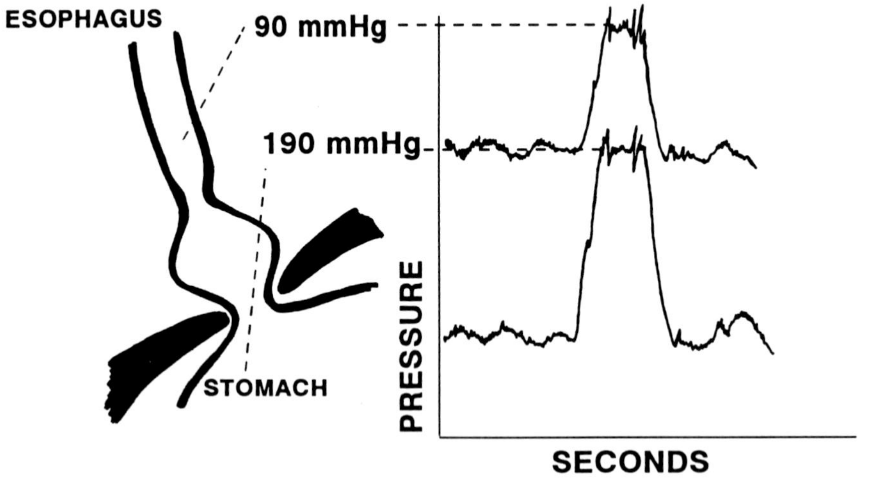

B

Figure 10.7. (A) Intragastric pressures required to produce Mallory-Weiss tears in cadaver stomachs. (B) Pressure changes in the esophagus and stomach recorded during retching. The rapid increase in intragastric pressure relative to the intraesophageal pressure results in dilatation of the lower esophagus or hernial pouch, with resultant mucosal tears. (Adapted from Atkinson M, Mitchell WM: The mechanism whereby Mallory-Weiss mucosal tears at the cardia are produced, in Smith AN (ed): *Surgical Physiology of the Gastrointestinal Tract*. Proceedings of a Symposium held in the Royal College of Surgeons of Edinburgh, 1962, pp 35–39.)

nied by an antireflux procedure, as many of these patients have coexistent incompetent sphincters and surgery at the hiatus further weakens the antireflux mechanism.[82] Skinner and Belsey found that bleeding ceases within two or three days after surgical reduction of the hernia, and ulcers heal rapidly.[83]

Mallory-Weiss Syndrome

In 1929 Mallory and Weiss reported massive hematemesis in 15 patients following an "intense alcoholic debauch" and consequent vomiting.[84] Four patients succumbed to the hemorrhage and were found at autopsy to have linear lacerations at the gastric cardia. Vomiting was purported to play a more important role than the alcohol. Before the advent of routine endoscopy, this disorder was considered a rarity, but it is now diagnosed in up to 15% of patients with acute upper gastrointestinal bleeds.[85]

There are several causes of this syndrome besides violent vomiting. Maneuvers that cause a sudden increase in abdominal pressure such as retching, hiccuping, physical straining, intense coughing, cardiopulmonary resuscitation, and childbirth have been reported to cause these mucosal tears.[86,87] Mallory-Weiss tears are often associated with radiologically demonstrable hiatus hernias, but this is not a consistent finding. Transient hernias that occur only during rapid intra-abdominal pressure changes may be the etiological factor in patients with no demonstrable hernia. A sudden distention of the lower esophagus and cardia occurs during vomiting owing to the rapid increase in the pressure gradient across the higher-pressure region of the lower esophagus and cardia of the stomach and the lower-pressure region of the thorax. The linear tears seen on endoscopy are thought to result from the sudden distention that occurs with the pressure change. Atkinson and Mitchell in 1962 found that 100% of cadaver stomachs submitted to intragastric pressures of 150 torr developed mucosal tears in the region of the cardia (Figure 10.7A).[88] In vivo studies show that intragastric pressures may reach 200 torr during retching (Figure 10.7B). Failure to vent this pressure change through the cricopharyngeal sphincter increases the probability of a tear or rupture of the cardioesophageal area. Nonrelaxation of the upper esophageal sphincter may be due to incoordination secondary to inebriation. The tears seen in Mallory-Weiss syndrome are usually limited to the mucosa because of the lesser distensibility of the mucosa compared to the underlying muscularis mucosae. Associated alcohol and aspirin ingestion may play a role in injury to the mucosal lining.[89]

Levine has noted that patients with a hernia tend to have tears in the cardia of the stomach; those with a transient hernia or no demonstrable hernia usually develop tears across the gastroesophageal junction or in the lower esophagus.[90] Sugawa et al. found that 83% of tears seen endoscopically in 224 patients with Mallory-Weiss syndrome were located on the lesser curve just below the gastroesophageal junction, only 8.7% of tears extended into the esophagus.[91]

The bleeding that results from Mallory-Weiss tears is usually self-limiting. Sugawa et al. found that only 25% of patients had active bleeding at endoscopy and 90% of these patients stopped bleeding spontaneously.[85] Surgery is rarely necessary to stop bleeding and should be considered only after more conservative measures have failed. A gastrotomy through an upper abdominal midline incision is performed, and oversewing of the tear is usually successful in stopping the hemorrhage. Intraoperative endoscopy may be useful in locating a tear that is difficult to find at the time of laparotomy and can be used to monitor the closure of a high esophageal mucosal tear through an open gastrotomy. In this setting, the surgeon can place the sutures accurately while watching the video screen. Currently, in our laboratory, we have modified percutaneous gastrostomy tubes to accept laparoscopic instruments. Endoscopic intragastric surgery for the surgical treatment of acute upper gastrointestinal hemorrhage from a variety of causes may avoid the need for laparotomy.

Endoscopy

Endoscopy, with or without biopsy, is a recognized cause of upper gastrointestinal bleeding. Besides precipitating bleeding from lesions such as esophagitis, varices, or cancers, insufflation during endoscopy may cause retching and a Mallory-Weiss-type mucosal tear. Sugawa et al. have described a mushrooming of the gastric mucosa into the esophagus during retching and have noted that this may result in mucosal tears and bleeding.[91] Kolts and colleagues have recently noted that endoscopic Mallory-Weiss tears occur in 1 in 200 endoscopies. These lesions rarely require transfusions and heal without incident.[92]

Surgery

Rarely, hypothermia and low perfusion states during cardiac surgery can result in esophageal necrosis and massive hemorrhage 7–10 days later. We operated on such a patient with massive hematemesis 10 days after aortic valve surgery. At operation there was profuse bleeding from the whole esophagus, and esophagectomy was required. Histological examination showed complete necrosis of the esophageal epithelium. The patient was subsequently reconstructed with a colon interposition, and complete restoration of gastrointestinal function.

BLEEDING FROM ESOPHAGEAL NEOPLASMS

All of the primary and secondary tumors that involve the esophagus have the potential to bleed.[93-98] These tumors rarely present with bleeding. Occult bleeding is more common and contributes to the anemia which is often present in these patients. Occasionally, acute bleeding occurs, especially in the ulcerative-type tumors which comprise 25% of squamous cell cancers.[99,100] Invasion by tumor into periesophageal vascular structures such as the aorta or the azygos vein has been described, and the consequent hemorrhage is usually lethal.[101,102]

ACKNOWLEDGMENTS

We are indebted to the expert assistance of Suzanne Talbot in the preparation of the manuscript.

REFERENCES

1. Silverstein FE, Gilbert DA, Tedesco FJ, et al: The national ASGE survey on upper gastrointestinal bleeding. I. Study design and baseline data. *Gastrointest Endosc* 27:73–79, 1981.
2. Silverstein FE, Gilbert DA, Tedesco FJ, et al: The national ASGE survey on upper gastrointestinal bleeding. II. Clinical prognostic factors. *Gastrointest Endosc* 27:80–93, 1981.
3. Palmer ED, Beck IT, Conn HO, et al: Hemorrhage at the esophagogastric junction (including bleeding esophageal varices), in Katz D, Hoffman F (eds): *The Esophagogastric Junction.* Amsterdam, Excerpta Medica, 1971, pp 57–86.
4. Sugawa C: Endoscopic diagnosis and treatment of upper gastrointestinal bleeding. *Surg Clin North Am* 69:1167–1181, 1989.
5. Kisu T, Yamaoka K, Uchida Y, et al: A case of blue rubber bleb nevus syndrome with familial onset. *Gastroenterol Jpn* 21:262–266, 1986.
6. Orlando RL, Bozymski EM, Briggaman RA, et al: Epidermolysis bullosa: Gastrointestinal manifestations. *Ann Intern Med* 81:203–206, 1974.
7. Vitale GC: Diagnostic techniques and tests of oesophageal function, in Hennessy TPJ, Cushieri A (eds): *Surgery of the Oesophagus.* London, Balliere Tindall, 1986, pp 17–47.
8. Geboes K, Janssens J, Rutgeerts P, et al: Crohn's disease of the esophagus. *J Clin Gastroenterol* 8:31–37, 1986.
9. Levack R: Behcet's disease of the oesophagus. *J Laryngol Otol* 93:99–101, 1979.
10. Foroozan P, Enta T, Winship D, et al: Loss and regeneration of the esophageal mucosa in pemphigoid. *Gastroenterology* 52:548–558, 1967.
11. Ackert JJ, Sherman A, Lustbader IJ, et al: Spontaneous intramural hematoma of the esophagus. *Am J Gastroenterol* 84:1325–1328, 1989.
12. Henderson CT, Engel J, Schlesinger P: Foreign body ingestion: Review and suggested guidelines for management. *Endoscopy* 19:68–71, 1987.
13. Beinert T, Boehm G, Pfretzschner C, et al: Esophageal injuries caused by a swallowed foreign body: A life-threatening condition. *Laryngol Rhinol Otol Stuttg* 65:518–520, 1986.
14. Brullet E, Colomer O, Riera R: Upper digestive hemorrhage caused by rupture of an aortic aneurysm into the esophagus. *Rev Esp Enferm Dig* 78:47, 1990.
15. Shapiro AL, Robillard GL: The esophageal arteries: Their configurational anatomy and variations in relation to surgery. *Ann Surg* 131:171–183, 1950.
16. Rothberg M, DeMeester TR: Surgical anatomy of the esophagus, in Shields TW (ed): *General Thoracic Surgery,* ed 3. Philadelphia, Lea & Febiger, 1989, p 76.
17. Liebermann-Meffert DMI, Luescher U, Neff U, et al: Esophagectomy without thoracotomy: Is there a risk of intramediastinal bleeding? *Ann Surg* 206:184–192, 1987.
18. De Carvalho CAF: Sur L'Angio-architecture veineuse de la zone de transition oesophagogastrique et son interpretation fonctionelle. *Acta Anat (Basel)* 64:125–162, 1966.
19. Kitano S, Terblanche J, Kahn D, et al: Venous anatomy of the lower oesophagus in portal hypertension: Practical implications. *Br J Surg* 73:525–531, 1986.
20. Wienbeck M, Barnert J: Epidemiology of reflux disease and reflux esophagitis. *Scand J Gastrtoenterol* 24(Suppl 156):7–13, 1989.
21. Palmer ED: The hiatus hernia-esophagitis-esophageal stricture complex: Twenty year prospective study. *Am J Med* 44:566–579, 1968.
22. Gilbert DA, Silverstein FE, Tedesco FJ, et al: The national ASGE survey on upper gastrointestinal bleeding. III. Endoscopy in upper gastrointestinal bleeding. *Gastrointest Endosc* 27:94–102, 1981.
23. DeNardi FG, Riddell RH: The normal esophagus. *Am J Surg Path* 15:296–309, 1991.

24. Bremner CG: Reflux oesophagitis in the baboon: The significance of the number of vascular papillae. *Gastroenterology* 73:1463, 1977.

25. Palmer ED: Subacute erosive esophagitis: Clinical impressions. *Military Med* 130:39–43, 1965.

26. Spechler SJ, Williford WO, VA Cooperative Study Group #277: Medical vs. surgical therapy for gastroesophageal reflux disease (GERD): Final results of VA Cooperative Study #277. *Gastroenterology* 100(5):A19, 1991.

27. Lanspa SJ, Spechler SJ, DeMeester TR, et al: Incidence of esophageal stricture formation in patients with complicated gastroesophageal reflux disease (GERD). *Gastroenterology* 100(5):A107, 1991.

28. Brossard E, Mannier P, Ollyo JB, et al: Serious complications—stenosis, ulcer and Barrett's epithelium—developed in 21.5% of adults with erosive reflux esophagitis. *Gastroenterology* 100(5):A36, 1991.

29. Zaninotto G, DeMeester TR, Schwizer W, et al: The lower esophageal sphincter in health and disease. *Am J Surg* 155:104–111, 1988.

30. DeMeester TR, Stein HJ: Gastroesophageal reflux disease, in Moody FG, Carey LC, Jones RS, et al: (eds): *Surgical Treatment of Digestive Disease,* ed 2. Chicago, Year Book Medical Publishers, 1989, p 65.

31. Winters C Jr, Spurling TJ, Chobanian SJ, et al: Barrett's esophagus: A prevalent, occult complication of gastroesophageal reflux disease. *Gastroenterology* 92:118–124, 1987.

32. Bremner CG: The management of columnar-lined oesophagus, in Jamieson GG (ed): *Surgery of the Oesophagus.* New York, Churchill Livingston, 1988, p 223–231.

33. Cooper BT, Barbezat GO: Barrett's oesophagus: A clinical study of 52 patients. *Q J Med* 62:97–108, 1987.

34. Borrie J, Goldwater L: Columnar cell-lined esophagus: Assessment of etiology and treatment. A 22-year experience. *J Thorac Cardiovasc Surg* 71:825–834, 1976.

35. Allison PR: Peptic ulcer of the oesophagus. *Thorax* 3:20–42, 1948.

36. Barrett NR: Chronic peptic ulcer of the esophagus and esophagitis. *Br J Surg* 38:175–182, 1990.

37. Pearson FG, Cooper JD, Patterson GA, et al: Peptic ulcer in acquired columnar-lined esophagus: Results of surgical treatment. *Ann Thorac Surg* 43:241–244, 1987.

38. Lambert DR, Llaneza PP, Gaglani RD, et al: Esophageal-atrial fistula. *J Clin Gastroenterol* 9:345–349, 1987.

39. DeMeester TR, Attwood SEA, Smyrk TC, et al: Surgical therapy in Barrett's esophagus. *Ann Surg* 212:528–542, 1990.

40. Hameeteman W, Tytgat GN: Healing of chronic Barrett ulcers with omeprazole. *Am J Gastroenterol* 81:764–766, 1986.

41. Gillen P, Hennessy TPJ: Barrett's oesophagus, in Hennessy TPJ, Cushieri A, Bennett JR (eds): *Reflux Oesophagitis.* London, Butterworths, 1989, pp 87–111.

42. Kaplan D, Warren J: Massive gastrointestinal hemorrhage due to *Candida* esophagitis. *Am J Gastroenterol* 83:463–464, 1988.

43. Maitra I, Mukherjee A, Bhattacherjee D: Oesophageal candidiasis. *J Assoc Physicians India* 37:800–801, 1989.

44. McKenzie R, Khakoo R: Blastomycosis of the esophagus presenting with gastrointestinal bleeding. *Gastroenterology* 88:1271–1273, 1985.

45. Forsmark CE, Wilcox CM, Darragh TM, et al: Disseminated histoplasmosis in AIDS: An unusual case of esophageal involvement and gastrointestinal bleeding. *Gastrointest Endosc* 36:604–605, 1990.

46. Chase RA, Haber MH, Pottage JC Jr, et al: Tuberculous esophagitis with erosion into aortic aneurysm. *Arch Pathol Lab Med* 110:965–966, 1986.
47. Mayeux GP, Smith JW: Massive esophageal bleeding from cytomegalovirus esophagitis. *Am J Gastroenterol* 85:626, 1990.
48. Iwasaki T: Alimentary tract lesions in cytomegalovirus infection. *Acta Pathol Jpn* 37:549–565, 1987.
49. Rattner HM, Cooper DJ, Zaman MB: Severe bleeding from herpes esophagitis. *Am J Gastroenterol* 80:523–525, 1985.
50. Agha FP, Lee HH, Nostrant TT: Herpetic esophagitis: A diagnostic challenge in immunocompromised patients. *Am J Gastroenterol* 81:246–253, 1986.
51. Estrera A, Taylor W, Mills LJ, et al: Corrosive burns of the esophagus and stomach: A recommendation for an aggressive surgical approach. *Ann Thorac Surg* 41:276–283, 1986.
52. Sugawa C, Lucas CE: Caustic injury of the upper gastrointestinal tract in adults: A clinical and endoscopic study. *Surgery* 106:802–807, 1989.
53. Pemberton J: Oesophageal obstruction and ulceration caused by oral potassium therapy. *Br Heart J* 32:267–268, 1970.
54. Kikendall JW, Friedman AC, Oyewole MA, et al: Pill-induced esophageal injury: Case reports and review of the medical literature. *Dig Dis Sci* 28:174–181, 1983.
55. Evans KT, Roberts GM: Where do all the tablets go? *Lancet* 1237–1239, 1976.
56. Kaul BK, DeMeester TR, Oka M, et al: The cause of dysphagia in uncomplicated sliding hiatal hernia and its relief by hiatal herniorrhaphy: A roentgenographic, manometric, and clinical study. *Ann Surg* 211:406–410, 1990.
57. Sloan S, Kahrilas P: Impairment of esophageal emptying with hiatal hernia. *Gastroenterology* 100:596–605, 1991.
58. Bailey RT Jr, Bonavina L, McChesney L, et al: Factors influencing the transit of a gelatin capsule in the esophagus. *Drug Intel Clin Pharm* 21:282–285, 1987.
59. Lanas A, Hirshowitz B: Significant role of aspirin use in esophagitis. *Gastroenterology* 100:A106, 1991.
60. Bonavina L, DeMeester TR, McChesney L, et al: Drug-induced esophageal strictures. *Ann Surg* 206:173–183, 1987.
61. Oakes DD, Sherck JP: Drug-induced esophagitis, in DeMeester TR, Skinner DB (eds): *Esophageal Disorders: Pathophysiology and Therapy*. New York, Raven Press, 1985, p 241.
62. Yang ZY, Hu YH, Gu XZ: Non-cancerous ulcer in the esophagus after radiotherapy for esophageal carcinoma: a report of 27 patients. *Radiother Oncol* 19:121–129, 1990.
63. Bremner CG: Corrosive and non-reflux oesophagitis, in Hennessy TPJ, Cushieri A (eds): *Surgery of the Esophagus*. London, Bailliere Tindall, 1986, p 262.
64. Goldstein HM, Rogers LF, Fletcher GH, et al: Radiological manifestations of radiation-induced injury to the normal upper gastrointestinal tracts. *Radiology* 117:135–140, 1975.
65. Boal DKB, Newburger PE, Teele RL: Esophagitis induced by combined radiation and adriamycin. *Am J Radiol* 132:567–570, 1979.
66. Segal HL: Secondary anemia associated with diaphragmatic hernia. *NY State J Med* 31:692–695, 1931.
67. Windsor CWO, Collis JL: Anaemia and hiatus hernia: Experience in 450 patients. *Thorax* 22:73–78, 1967.
68. Cameron AJ: Incidence of iron deficiency anemia in patients with large diaphragmatic hernia: A controlled study. *Mayo Clin Proc* 51:767–769, 1976.
69. Akerlund A: Hernia diaphragmatica hiatus oesophagei vom anatamischen und rontgenologischen gisichtspunkt. *Acta Radiol* 6:3–24, 1926.

70. Ozdemir IA, Burke WA, Ikins PM: Paraesophageal hernia: A life-threatening disease. *Ann Thorac Surg* 16:547–554, 1973.
71. Gardner KD: Diaphragmatic hernia associated with secondary anemia. *Am J Med Sci* 185: 561–568, 1933.
72. Truesdale PE: Gastric ulcer associated with diaphragmatic hernia. *N Engl J Med* 207:385–392, 1932.
73. Mendelsohn EA: Hiatus hernia of the stomach as a source of gastrointestinal bleeding. *Radiology* 46:502–506, 1946.
74. Belsey RHR: Peptic ulcer of the oesophagus. *Ann R Coll Surg Eng* 14:303–316, 1954.
75. Aylwyn JA: The physiological basis of reflux esophagitis in sliding hiatal diaphragmatic hernia. *Thorax* 8:38–43, 1953.
76. Marchand P: Hiatus hernia: A cause of gastrointestinal haemorrhage. *Br J Surg* 47:515–526, 1960.
77. Pearson FG, Cooper JD, Ilves R, et al: Massive hiatal hernia with incarceration: A report of 53 cases. *Ann Thorac Surg* 35:45–51, 1983.
78. Walther BS, DeMeester TR, Lafontaine E, et al: Effect of paraesophageal hernia on sphincter function and its implication on surgical therapy. *Am J Surg* 147:111–116, 1984.
79. Dunn DB, Quick G: Incarcerated paraesophageal hernia. *Am J Emerg Med* 8:36–39, 1990.
80. Palmer ED: Hiatus hernia and hemorrhage. *Am J Med Sci* 246:417–418, 1963.
81. Skinner D, Belsey RHR: Surgical management of esophageal reflux and hiatal hernia: Long-term results with 1,030 patients. *J Thorac Cardiovasc Surg* 53:33–54, 1967.
82. Cathcart RS III, Gregorie HB Jr, Holmes SL: Non-reflux complications of hiatal hernia. *Am Surg* 53:320–324, 1987.
83. Skinner DB, Belsey RHR: *Management of Esophageal Disease*. Philadelphia, WB Saunders, 1988, pp 631–639.
84. Mallory GK, Weiss S: Hemorrhages from lacerations of the cardiac orifice of the stomach due to vomiting. *Am J Med Sci* 178:506–515, 1929.
85. Sugawa C, Werner MH, Hayes DF: Early endoscopy: A guide to therapy for acute hemorrhage in the upper gastrointestinal tract. *Arch Surg* 107:133–137, 1973.
86. Michel L: Post-emetic laceration and rupture of the gastroesophageal junction. *Acta Chir Belg* 82:13–24, 1982.
87. Norfleet RG, Smith GH: Mallory-Weiss syndrome after cardiopulmonary resuscitation. *J Clin Gastroenterol* 12:569–572, 1990.
88. Atkinson M, Mitchell WM: The mechanism whereby Mallory-Weiss mucosal tears at the cardia are produced, in Smith AN (ed): *Surgical Physiology of the Gastrointestinal Tract.* Proceedings of a Symposium held in the Royal College of Surgeons of Edinburgh, 1962, pp 35–39.
89. MacMath TL: Alcohol and gastrointestinal bleeding. *Emerg Med Clin North Am* 8:859–871, 1990.
90. Levine GM: Upper gastrointestinal hemorrhage, in Cohen S (ed): *Clinical Gastroenterology: A Problem-Oriented Approach.* New York, Wiley, 1983, p 55.
91. Sugawa C, Benishek D, Walt AJ: Mallory-Weiss syndrome: A study of 224 patients. *Am J Surg* 145:30–33, 1983.
92. Kolts B, Achem S, Marteiro C, et al: Frequency and outcome of Mallory-Weiss tears during upper endoscopies. *Gastroenterology* 100:A10, 1991.
93. Hoevels J, Raute-Kreinsen U, Reiter J, et al: Vascular neoplasm of the esophagus with life-threatening hemorrhage. Report of a case. *Acta Radiol Diagn Stockh* 27:29–32, 1986.

94. Stadler J, Orda R, Baratz M, et al: Giant leiomyoma of the esophagus as a cause for gastrointestinal bleeding. *J Clin Gastroenterol* 9:613–615, 1987.

95. Li TD, Yang WX: Smooth muscle tumors of the alimentary tract: A review of 397 cases. *Chung Hua Chung Liu Tsa Chih* 8:287–290, 1986.

96. DiCostanzo DP, Urmacher C: Primary malignant melanoma of the esophagus. *Am J Surg Pathol* 11:46–52, 1987.

97. Chibowski D, Siezieniewska Z, Czarnecki J, et al: Hemorrhage from the digestive tract as the first clinical symptom of lymphoma of the esophagus, stomach, duodenum and the small and large intestines. *Patol Pol* 38:103–112, 1987.

98. McGrath PC, Neifeld JP, Lawrence W Jr, et al: Gastrointestinal sarcomas. Analysis of prognostic factors. *Ann Surg* 206:706–710, 1987.

99. Mannell A: Carcinoma of the esophagus, in Pantanowitz D (ed): *Modern Surgery in Africa: The Baragwanath Experience*. Johannesburg, Southern Book Publishers, 1988, pp 165–188.

100. Ming SC: Tumors of the esophagus and stomach, in *Atlas of Tumor Pathology*, Series 2, Fascicle 7. Armed Forces Institute of Pathology, pp 27–79, 1973.

101. Gable DS, Stoddard LD: Acute bacterial aortitis resulting in an aortoesophageal fistula. A fatal complication of untreated esophageal carcinoma. *Pathol Res Pract* 184:318–324, 1989.

102. Shimizu M, Itoh H, Matsuzaki T, et al: Lower-third esophageal cancer penetrating the aorta: Sudden death after emergency admission in a nontreated patient. *Am J Gastroenterol* 84: 1129–1130, 1989.

11

BLEEDING FROM THE STOMACH

W. David Curtis, M.D.
Joseph W. Griffin, Jr., M.D.

INTRODUCTION

The stomach is the most common location of bleeding lesions of the upper gastrointestinal system. Of 2,097 patients who underwent endoscopy for hemorrhage from the upper gastrointestinal tract in the American Society for Gastrointestinal Endoscopy (ASGE) Survey on Upper Gastrointestinal Bleeding, nearly two-thirds were found to be bleeding from a lesion located at or between the esophagogastric junction and the pylorus.[1] Erosions and ulcers of the gastric mucosa account for most gastric bleeding, but many other lesions can also cause this condition (Table 11.1). Discrepancy exists among different studies with regard to the frequency with which certain lesions are observed (Table 11.2). The variation can be explained by differences in the population studied, in the study design, and in the definitions of the lesions themselves.

CLINICAL PRESENTATION

The clinical presentation of patients with bleeding from the stomach can be quite diverse. Bleeding may be occult, with blood loss detected only by a positive fecal occult blood test and/or iron deficiency anemia. Acute bleeding may produce findings ranging from orthostatic syncope to hypovolemic shock. Pain may be present, particularly in patients with peptic ulcer disease. Interestingly, the pain of peptic ulcer disease is often diminished when bleeding begins. Nausea and vomiting may be present in many patients. If emesis occurs, fresh blood indicates ongoing active hemorrhage. "Coffee ground" vomitus indicates prior but not active hemorrhage. The appearance of the stool often gives an indication of the severity of bleeding. Melena is most frequent in active bleeding from the stomach, with the characteristic black, tarry, malodorous stool resulting from the conversion of hemoglobin to hematin and other pigments by hydrochloric acid and intestinal secretions. The appearance of maroon or bright red stools in a patient bleeding from a gastric lesion usually indicates rapid hemorrhage and/or rapid intestinal transit

TABLE 11.1. Causes of Bleeding from the Stomach

Gastric Mucosal Injury
Peptic ulcer disease
Acute erosive gastritis
Drug-induced mucosal injury
Alcohol-induced mucosal injury
Stress-induced mucosal injury
Mallory-Weiss tear
Vascular Anomalies
Arteriovenous malformation
Nonhereditary
Hereditary hemorrhagic telangiectasia
Gastropathy of portal hypertension
Gastric varices
Gastric antral vascular ectasia
Dieulafoy's lesion
Mesenteric vascular insufficiency
Hiatus hernia with ischemia secondary to torsion
Arterial-enteric fistula/gastric aneurysms
Tumors
Malignant
Benign
Trauma/Instrumentation
Miscellaneous
Pseudoxanthoma elasticum
Ehlers-Danlos syndrome

and is frequently accompanied by hypovolemic shock. Placement of a nasogastric tube can ascertain whether the patient is experiencing active bleeding. Of course, this maneuver does not determine the site of bleeding within the upper gastrointestinal tract and may be negative if the site of bleeding is beyond the pylorus.

GASTRIC MUCOSAL INJURY

By far the most common underlying etiology of gastric hemorrhage is alteration in the integrity of the gastric mucosa. Erosions (superficial ulcerations of the gastric mucosa that do not extend to the muscularis mucosa), erosive gastritis (multiple erosions with a variety of accompanying findings such as diffuse inflammation, erythema, friability, and/or petechiae), and ulcers (disruption of the gastric mucosa penetrating through the muscularis mucosa) are all manifestations of mucosal injury. Bleeding results when the ulcerative process invades any underlying blood vessel.

Mucosal damage results from an imbalance between the aggressive factors that promote mucosal injury (hydrochloric acid, pepsin, stress, smoking, ethanol, aspirin, and other nonsteroidal anti-inflammatory drugs, NSAIDs) and defensive factors that protect the mucosa from damage (the mucus-bicarbonate gel layer, mucosal blood flow, an

TABLE 11.2. Relative Frequency of Bleeding Gastric Lesions in Different Populations Studied for Upper Gastrointestinal Bleeding

Reference	N	*Erosive Gastritis*	*Gastric Ulcer*	*Mallory-Weiss Tear*	*Neo-plasia*	*AVMs*	*Stomal Ulcer*
Silverstein et al.[1]	2,097	29.6%	21.9%	8.0%	3.7%	0.5%	1.9%
Webb et al.[2]	117	0.8%	35.8%	9.8%	0.8%	1.6%	1.6%
Tabibian and Sutton[3]							
County	535	4.6%	23.5%	6.0%	0.4%	0.2%	—
Community	70	2.8%	21.8%	5.7%	2.8%	1.4%	—
Peterson et al.[4]	100	6.0%	18%	16%	2.%	—	—

intact gastric epithelium with epithelial renewal, and stimulation of these defensive factors by prostaglandins and epidermal growth factor.)

Peptic Ulcer Disease (PUD)

Ulceration of the gastric mucosa can occur in the absence of exogenous injurious factors such as alcohol or NSAIDs. Since gastric ulcers are known to be associated with either normal or subnormal acid secretion, the major factor in their pathogenesis is probably an alteration in gastric mucosal defenses. Gastric ulcers are typically 1–2 cm in diameter and occur most frequently in the distal body, along the lesser curvature near the angularis.[5] Massive, life-threatening hemorrhage can sometimes occur when ulcers on the lesser curvature of the stomach erode into the left gastric artery or one of its main branches. Less severe bleeding can occur when ulcers erode into arterioles.

A special category of stomach ulcer occurring in the postoperative stomach is the so-called anastomotic or stomal ulcer. From 40% to 60% of patients with postoperative recurrent PUD have bleeding as the presenting symptom.[6] The bleeding is most often chronic and occult but may be rapid and life-threatening. Several factors predispose to ulcer recurrence following surgery. Ulceration tends to recur more commonly when (1) the original surgery was done for duodenal ulcer, (2) the operation was performed by an inexperienced surgeon, (3) a hypersecretory state is present, and (4) the patient does not modify ulcerogenic factors such as NSAID use, smoking, or alcohol intake. The type of surgery performed also influences the rate of ulcer recurrence, with the highest rate of recurrence seen in patients who have undergone gastrojejunostomy without vagotomy, 30–35% of whom experience recurrent ulcer.[7]

Acute Erosive Gastritis

Acute erosive gastritis is an entity defining erosions of the gastric mucosa which occur in response to certain exogenous and endogenous stimuli. Other equally descriptive synonymous terms include *acute hemorrhagic gastritis* and *stress mucosal bleeding.* When large series of patients evaluated for upper gastrointestinal bleeding have been studied and endoscopic or surgical diagnoses reviewed, as many as 29.6% of patients have bled from acute erosive gastritis.[1,3,4] Mortality from acute erosive gastritis with hemorrhage is similar to that for hemorrhage from PUD (approximately 10%). With massive bleeding, the mortality from acute gastritis can be as high as 50%. Acute erosive gastritis can result from exogenous factors such as the ingestion of certain medications and alcohol or may be associated with a serious underlying illness or injury.

Drug-Induced Mucosal Injury

Medications can result in injury to the gastric mucosa, with resultant hemorrhage. The most commonly encountered group of offending medications is aspirin and the other NSAIDs. Roth suggested the term *NSAID gastropathy* to describe the gastric lesions associated with NSAID use.[8] When studied, as many as 31% of patients taking NSAIDs have been found to develop endoscopic evidence of gastric lesions within one year.[9] Acutely, petechiae have been noted to develop within one hour of aspirin ingestion. With further ingestion, erosions evolve in arcas containing numerous petechiae, and ultimately larger erosions or frank ulcerations may result.[10] The incidence of gastric ulcers is increased 10-fold in patients taking NSAIDs compared to patients not taking these medications.[11] Gastrointestinal hemorrhage, both minor and major, have been noted as a result of NSAID-induced gastric mucosal damage. The elderly seem to be at increased risk for hemodynamically significant bleeding.[12] Unfortunately, the typical clinical symptom complex (i.e., pain) of PUD is not usually present in patients with NSAID-related gastric mucosal injury, including those with deep ulcerations.

The role of adrenocorticosteroids in gastrointestinal bleeding is controversial. Some investigators believe that there is an association between steroid use and mucosal damage.[13] Others believe that no such association exists,[14] and still others state that corticosteroids may promote gastric mucosal injury initiated by other factors, such as NSAIDs, but do not cause injury per se.[15]

Other medications have also been associated with gastric mucosal injury and bleeding, albeit on a more anecdotal basis in most cases. Implicated drugs include ferrous sulfate,[16] potassium chloride,[17] and methotrexate. Tumor necrosis factor[18] has been found to induce hemorrhagic gastritis as well.

Alcohol-Induced Mucosal Injury

The deleterious effects of ethanol on the gastric mucosa have been known since the observations of William Beaumont in 1833. Beaumont, describing the gastric mucosa of Alexis St. Martin—a patient with a traumatically created gastric fistula—noted that when St. Martin had "been drinking ardent spirits pretty freely for eight or ten days past," the gastric mucosa was "not healthy—some erythema and aphthous patches in the mucous surface." After four or five days of abstinence, the gastric mucosa regained its normal appearance.[19] Palmer noted mucosal changes in 30 of 34 patients undergoing endoscopy within six hours of their last drink. The changes noted included patchy mucosal hyperemia, erosions, petechiae, and a purulent exudate. Follow-up endoscopy was normal in all patients after 7–20 days of abstinence.[20] Alcoholic gastritis must be considered as a potential cause of hemorrhage in the actively inbibing alcoholic patient. One group noted that gastrointestinal hemorrhage in chronic alcoholics who were actively drinking was caused by acute gastric mucosal lesions in 42.9% compared to a 12.9% incidence of bleeding from esophageal varices.[21]

Stress-Induced Mucosal Injury

Significant acute erosive gastritis has been noted to develop in patients with serious underlying illnesses. This syndrome has been known as *stress ulcerations* or *stress gastritis*.[22] These lesions have been seen in association with trauma, especially severe burns,[23] intracranial injury,[24,25] and major operations. Bleeding from stress-induced gastric lesions has also been seen in patients with serious medical illnesses. Zinner and colleagues performed a prospective study of patients in an intensive care unit and formulated an "illness severity score" to identify those patients most at risk for bleeding from stress-induced mucosal injury[26] (Table 11.3). Of the many causes of stress-induced gastric mucosal injury, only sepsis and intracranial injury have been associated with hypersecretion of acid.[27] Nonetheless, the reduction of gastric acidity with H-2 antagonists or antacids has been shown to have a protective role in patients who are susceptible to stress-induced lesions.[28,29] The goal of prophylaxis in high-risk patients is to keep the gastric pH above 5, and continuous intravenous infusion of an H-2 receptor antagonist appears to be the therapy of choice.

Mallory-Weiss Tear

Laceration of the gastroesophageal mucosa as a cause of gastrointestinal hemorrhage was described in 1929 by Mallory and Weiss.[30] The characteristic lesion is a vertically oriented mucosal laceration believed to occur as a result of violent, forceful prolapse of the upper gastric mucosa into the distal esophagus during vomiting, violent coughing, or sneezing. In patients with hiatus hernias, the laceration may be confined to the gastric mucosa.[31] The lesion tends to be especially prominent among those who abuse alcohol. Bleeding from a Mallory-Weiss tear is usually self-limited and does not recur. In one group of patients studied, 37% required no blood transfusions. The average transfusion

TABLE 11.3. Risk Factors Associated with Stress Mucosal Bleeding in the Intensive Care Unit

Ventilatory assistance >24 hours' duration
Shock (systolic BP <90 mm Hg)
Sepsis
Myocardial infarction or congestive heart failure
Acute renal failure (creatinine >3 mm/dl or BUN >50 mm/dl)
CNS injury
Steroid administration
Coagulopathy (platelet count <50 K or PT <30% of control value)
Bilirubin >5 mm/dl

No. of Risk factors	*Incidence of Bleeding*
0–2	11%
3–6	34%
>7	50%

Abbreviations: BUN, blood urea nitrogen; PT, prothrombin time.
Source: Zinner et al.[26]

requirement for all patients was 3.3 units.[32] Occasional patients have bleeding severe enough to require intervention with thermal coagulation devices via endoscopy, arteriographic embolization, balloon tamponade, and, in rare instances, surgical oversewing.

VASCULAR ANOMALIES

Vascular Malformations

Nonhereditary Malformations

Vascular malformations of the gastrointestinal tract have been identified by a multitude of different names, including *arteriovenous malformations (AVMs), angiodysplasia, telangiectasia, vascular ectasia, hemangiomata,* and others. While common in other parts of the gastrointestinal tract, these lesions are identified less frequently in the stomach. Vascular malformations of the stomach have a strong male predominance, with 87.5% of patients in one study being male.[33] Hematemesis without antecedent symptoms is the typical clinical presentation. The lesions may not be recognized on initial endoscopic evaluation, owing to their small size (typically 2–5 mm), the intermittent nature of the bleeding, their submucosal location, and their close resemblance to suction artifacts. In one series, vascular malformations were ultimately found to be the etiology of bleeding in 23.6% of the episodes of upper gastrointestinal hemorrhage initially described as being of unknown origin.[34] Patients with upper gastrointestinal bleeding caused by vascular malformations have an increased incidence of renal insufficiency, with 60% of patients in one series having a persistently elevated creatinine level above 1.5 g/dl.[35] In addition to fiberoptic endoscopy, angiography has proven beneficial in the diagnosis and sometimes the treatment of bleeding caused by vascular malformations.[36] Electrocautery is usually a successful method of treatment and prophylaxis. Surgical removal of the involved portion of the stomach may be required in some cases.

Hereditary Hemorrhagic Telangiectasia (Osler-Rendu-Weber Disease)

Gastrointestinal bleeding is second only to epistaxis as a manifestation of hereditary hemorrhagic telangiectasia (HHT). Occurring in 13–30% of HHT patients,[37] the onset of gastrointestinal bleeding is much later in life than that of epistaxis (55.5 and 11 years, respectively).[38] The gastrointestinal bleeding can at times be quite severe.[39] The stomach is a common site for telangiectasias, gastric lesions being present in 90% of one group of HHT patients studied endoscopically.[38]

Gastropathy of Portal Hypertension

In addition to esophageal varices, Mallory-Weiss tears, and acute erosive gastritis, which are the common causes of bleeding from the upper gastrointestinal tract in the alcoholic patient, a relatively new entity has been described in patients with portal hypertension. The term *congestive gastropathy* was selected by McCormack and colleagues to describe endoscopic features that included a beefy red appearance of the mucosa, petechial hemorrhages, red spots, and a red and white reticular pattern of the mucosa.[40] Of the 127 patients in their study, 28 had severe gastritis that resulted in 80 episodes of clinically significant bleeding. A controlled endoscopic study of 100 nonbleeding patients with cirrhosis revealed the presence of a mosaic pattern of multiple small, erythematous areas located primarily in the proximal stomach in 94 patients.[41] This pattern is believed to result from submucosal edema and vascular engorgement created by portal hypertension. Quintero et al. confirmed that bleeding from gastric red spots in patients with portal hypertension correlated histologically with vascular ectasia of the mucosa.[42] Acid-lowering drugs and cytoprotective agents have a limited role in stopping hemorrhage from the gastropathy of portal hypertension, but there is evidence that propranolol will reduce the risk of bleeding from congestive gastropathy.[43] Bleeding, which can be quite massive, can be controlled only by portal decompressive surgery in some patients.

Gastric Varices

Gastric varices occur less commonly than esophageal varices and have less propensity for bleeding.[44] Mathur and colleagues examined 104 patients with portal hypertension and bleeding from esophageal varices[45]; they noted gastric varices in 50 patients (48%) at the initial endoscopy. Of the 54 patients without gastric varices at initial endoscopy, 34 subsequently developed secondary gastric varices after sclerotherapy was begun. Ten percent of patients with primary gastric varices had subsequent bleeding compared to 13% of those with secondary gastric varices. Fundal varices were seen to bleed more commonly than lesser curvature varices.[45] The management of gastric variceal hemorrhage is largely dependent on the nature of the varices. Hosking and Johnson identified three types of gastric varices and emphasized the importance of each type to management.[46] Type I varices are those that appear as extensions of esophageal varices across the esophago-gastric junction. They are best managed by injection sclerotherapy. Type II gastric varices are located in the fundus and converge toward the cardia. Bleeding in this group of varices should be treated by devascularization or shunt surgery should they bleed. Type III varices are located in the fundus or body in the absence of esophageal varices and have no apparent connection to the cardia. These varices occur most commonly as a result of splenic vein thrombosis; splenectomy is curative in 90% of patients.

Gastric Antral Vascular Ectasia (Watermelon Stomach)

A vascular anomaly of the gastric antrum that is responsible for gastrointestinal blood loss (usually chronic and occult) has been described[47,48] predominantly in middle-aged females who typically present with iron deficiency anemia. At endoscopy, the gastric antrum of these patients has a very striking appearance, similar to the stripes of a watermelon, with broad, erythematous folds. Microscopically, the submucosa shows tortuous, ectatic blood vessels that appear as dilated, thrombosed capillaries with concomitant fibromuscular hyperplasia in the lamina propria. Achlorhydria or hypochlorhydria is a frequent finding. Antrectomy with Billroth I anastomosis is curative in these patients. Repeated treatments with laser and heater probe electro-coagulation have also been reported to improve this condition.[49,50]

Dieulafoy's Lesion

An entity that may appear endoscopically similar to an arteriovenous malformation was first described by Dieulafoy in 1898.[51] This lesion results from pressure erosion of the mucosa by an ectatic submucosal artery. The lesion generally occurs proximally, with a predilection for the lesser curvature of the stomach, and may produce recurrent massive hemorrhage, requiring endoscopic thermal coagulation or surgical intervention for control.[52] If not actively bleeding at the time of endoscopy, Dieulafoy's lesion is easily overlooked because of the small size of the mucosal defect. The endoscopist must have a high index of suspicion in examining a patient with massive gastrointestinal hemorrhage and no apparent lesion at endoscopy. Several endoscopic examinations may be required to establish the diagnosis. If Dieulafoy's lesion is not recognized and treated appropriately, the mortality is high.

Mesenteric Vascular Insufficiency

Compromise of the blood supply to the stomach, either secondary to atheromatous embolism or chronic mesenteric insufficiency, can lead to gastric mucosal damage and resulting hemorrhage. Patients with mesenteric ischemia typically present with postprandial pain that leads to food avoidance and subsequent weight loss.[53] Atheromatous embolization has been shown to cause multiple acute and chronic gastric ulcerations.[54] Vascular insufficiency due to atherosclerotic narrowing of the mesenteric vessels without evidence of embolization has also been shown to produce characteristic gastric mucosal changes.[55] In this group of patients, Cherry et al. observed multiple irregularly shaped shallow ulcers with sloping edges usually in the antrum. These lesions respond poorly to the usual antiulcer drugs but are uniformly healed by revascularization surgery.[56] Ischemic changes may also be seen as a result of iatrogenically induced compromise of the mesenteric circulation during surgery.

Linear Gastric Erosions in Patients with Large Hiatal Hernias

Patients with large diaphragmatic hernias have been found to have an increased incidence of chronic iron deficiency anemia.[57] An endoscopic study revealed that anemic patients with a large (more than one-third of the stomach) diaphragmatic hernia had a greater incidence of linear erosions on mucosal folds near the level of the diaphragm than did patients with similar-sized hernias but no anemia.[58] The location of the lesions suggests that they are caused by the mechanical trauma of folds abrading one another during respiration. Surgical correction of the hernia prevents recurrences of the anemia, substantiating the belief that the linear erosions are the source of blood loss.

TUMORS

Malignant and benign neoplasms of the stomach can be a source of gastrointestinal bleeding. Bleeding from adenocarcinoma of the stomach is usually occult, resulting in chronic iron deficiency anemia. More significant bleeding can occur, occasionally, resulting in hematemesis or melena. Kaposi's sarcoma of the stomach may cause significant hemorrhage in the patient with acquired immunodeficiency syndrome. Benign tumors can be responsible for bleeding as well. Leiomyomas and other submucosal tumors may on occasion erode through the mucosa, become ulcerated, and bleed significantly. Leiomyomas are often found in the fundus and can usually be identified by their characteristic appearance of an intramural mass with a central excavation.

SUMMARY

The stomach can be the site of a wide variety of bleeding lesions. After appropriate stabilization of the patient, endoscopic evaluation of the upper gastrointestinal tract by a trained observer can identify the bleeding lesion in most cases. The endoscopist, first and foremost, needs to be able to recognize the endoscopic abnormality and then be prepared to treat the bleeding lesion with endoscopic therapy if appropriate. The attending physician must also recognize the limitations of endoscopic therapy in certain patients and know when to make the necessary referral for alternative methods of treatment such as angiographic embolization or surgery.

REFERENCES

1. Silverstein FE, Gilbert DA, Tedesco FJ, et al: The national ASGE survey on upper gastrointestinal bleeding. *Gastrointest Endosc* 27:73–79, 1981.
2. Webb WA, McDaniel L, Johnson RC, et al: Endoscopic evaluation of 125 cases of upper gastrointestinal bleeding. *Ann Surg* 193:624–627, 1981.
3. Tabibian N, Sutton FM: Gastritis: A common source of acute bleeding in the upper gastrointestinal tract? *South Med J* 83:769–770, 1990.
4. Peterson WL, Barnett CC, Smith HJ, et al: Routine early endoscopy in upper-gastrointestinal-tract bleeding: A randomized, controlled trial. *N Engl J Med* 304:925–929, 1981.
5. Gelfand DW, Dale WJ, Ott DJ: The location and size of gastric ulcers: Radiologic and endoscopic evaluation. *Am J Roentgenol* 143:755–758, 1984.
6. Sharaiha ZK, Smith JL, Cain GD, et al: Recurrent ulcers after gastric surgery: Endoscopic localization to the gastric mucosa. *Am J Gastroenterol* 78:269–271, 1983.
7. Stabile BE, Passaro E Jr: Recurrent peptic ulcer. *Gastroenterology* 70:124–135, 1976.
8. Roth SH: Nonsteroidal anti-inflammatory drug gastropathy. *Arch Intern Med* 146:1075–1076, 1986.
9. Caruso I, Bianchi-Porro G: Gastroscopic evaluation of anti-inflammatory agents. *Br Med J* 1:75–78, 1980.
10. O'Laughlin JC, Hoftiezer JW, Ivey KJ: Effect of aspirin in the human stomach in normals: Endoscopic comparison of damage produced 1 hour, 24 hours and 2 weeks after administration. *Scand J Gastroenterol* 67(Suppl):211–214, 1981.
11. Graham DY, Smith JL: Gastroduodenal complications of chronic NSAID therapy. *Am J Gastroenterol* 83:1081–1084, 1983.
12. Griffin MR, Piper JM, Daugherty JR, et al: Nonsteroidal anti-inflammatory drug use and increased risk for peptic ulcer disease in elderly persons. *Ann Intern Med* 114:257–263, 1991.
13. Meltzer LE, Bockmann AA, Kanerson W, et al: The incidence of peptic ulcer among patients on long term prednisone therapy. *Gastroenterology* 35:351–356, 1958.
14. Conn HO, Blitzer BL: Non-association of adrenocorticosteroid therapy and peptic ulcer. *N Engl J Med* 194:473–479, 1976.
15. Chung RSK, Field M, Silen W: Gastric permeability to H^+: Effects of prednisolone and acetylsalicylic acid in the coefficient of H^+ diffusion (abstract). *Gastroenterology* 58:1038, 1970.
16. Laine L, Bentley E, Chandrasoma P: The effect of oral iron therapy on the upper gastrointestinal tract: A prospective evaluation. *Dig Dis Sci* 33:176–177, 1988.

17. McMahon FG, Ryan JR, Akdamar K, et al: Upper gastrointestinal lesions after potassium chloride supplements: A controlled clinical trial. *Lancet* 2:1059–1060, 1982.

18. Krigal RL, Padavic-Shaller KA, Rudolph AA, et al: Hemorrhagic gastritis as a new dose limiting toxicity of recombinant tumor necrosis factor. *J Natl Cancer Inst* 83:129–131, 1991.

19. Beaumont W: *Experiments and Observations in the Gastric Juice and the Physiology of Digestion* (facsimile of the original edition of 1833). Cambridge, Mass, Harvard University Press, 1929.

20. Palmer E: Gastritis: A re-evaluation. *Medicine* 33:199–290, 1954.

21. Valencia-Parracen J: Alcoholic gastritis. *Clin Gastroenterol* 10:389–399, 1981.

22. Lucas CE, Sugawa C, Riddle J, et al: Natural history and surgical dilemma of "stress" gastric bleeding. *Arch Surg* 102:266–273, 1971.

23. Czaja AJ, McAlhany JC, Pruitt BA: Acute gastroduodenal disease after thermal injury: An endoscopic evaluation of incidence and natural history. *N Engl J Med* 291:925–929, 1974.

24. Cushing H: Peptic ulcers and the interbrain. *Surg Gynecol Obstet* 55:1–34, 1932.

25. Kamada T, Rusamoto II, Kawano S, et al: Gastrointestinal bleeding following head injury: A clinical study of 433 cases. *J Trauma* 17:44–47, 1977.

26. Zinner MJ, Zuidema GD, Smith PL, et al: The prevention of upper gastrointestinal tract bleeding in patients in an intensive care unit. *Surg Gynecol Obstet* 153:214–220, 1981.

27. Idjadi F, Robbins R, Stahl W, et al: Prospective study of gastric secretion in stressed patients with intracranial injury. *J Trauma* 11:681–688, 1971.

28. Hastings PR, Skillman JJ, Bushnell LS, et al: Antacid titration in the prevention of acute gastrointestinal bleeding. A controlled randomized trial in 100 critically ill patients. *N Engl J Med* 298:1041–1045, 1978.

29. Priebe HJ, Skillman JJ, Bushnell LS, et al: Antacid vs. cimetidine in preventing acute gastrointestinal bleeding. *N Engl J Med* 302:426–430, 1980.

30. Mallory GK, Weiss S: Hemorrhages from lacerations of the cardiac orifice of the stomach due to vomiting. *Am J Med Sci* 178:506–515, 1929.

31. Watts HD: Lesions brought on by vomiting: The effect of hiatus hernia on the site of injury. *Gastroenterology* 71:683–688, 1976.

32. Graham DY, Schwartz JT: The spectrum of the Mallory-Weiss tear. Medicine 57:307–318, 1977.

33. Goldman RL: Submucosal arterial malformation ("aneurysm") of the stomach with fatal hemorrhage. *Gastroenterology* 46:589–594, 1964.

34. Quintero E, Pique JM, Bomsi JA, et al: Upper gastrointestinal bleeding caused by gastroduodenal vascular malformations: Incidence, diagnosis and treatment. *Dig Dis Sci* 31:897–905, 1986.

35. Clouse RE, Costigan DJ, Mills BA, et al: Angiodysplasia as a cause of upper gastrointestinal bleeding. *Arch Intern Med* 145:458–461, 1985.

36. Sherman L, Shenoy SS, Satchidanand SK, et al: Arteriovenous malformations of the stomach *Am J Gastroenterol* 72:160–164, 1979.

37. Smith CR, Bartholomew LG, Cain JC: Hereditary hemorrhagic telangiectasia and gastrointestinal hemorrhage. *Gastroenterology* 44:1–6, 1963.

38. Vase P, Grove O: Gastrointestinal lesions in hereditary hemorrhagic telangiectasia. *Gastroenterology* 91:1079–1083, 1986.

39. Amerson JR, McGarity WC: Massive gastrointestinal hemorrhage due to hereditary hemorrhagic telangectasia. *Am Surg* 26:707–712, 1960.

40. McCormack TT, Sims J, Eyre-Brook I, et al: Gastric lesions in portal hypertension: Inflammatory gastritis or congestive gastropathy? *Gut* 26:1226–1232, 1985.

41. Papazian A, Braillon A, Dupas JL, et al: Portal hypertensive gastric mucosa: An endoscopic study. *Gut* 27:1199–1203, 1986.
42. Quintero E, Pique JM, Bombi JA, et al: Gastric mucosal vascular ectasias causing bleeding in cirrhosis. *Gastroenterology* 93:1054–1061, 1987.
43. Hosking SW, Kennedy HJ, Seddon L, et al: The role of propranolol in congestive gastropathy of portal hypertension. *Hepatology* 3:337–341, 1987.
44. Karr S, Wohl GT: Clinical importance of gastric varices. *N Engl J Med* 263:665–669, 1960.
45. Mathur SK, Dalvi AN, Someshwar V: Endoscopic and radiological appraisal of gastric varices. *Br J Surg* 77:432–435, 1990.
46. Hosking SW, Johnson AG: Gastric varices: A proposal for classification leading to management. *Br J Surg* 75:195–196, 1988.
47. Jabbari M, Cherry R, Loush JO, et al: Gastric antral vascular ectasia: The watermelon stomach. *Gastroenterology* 87:1165–1170, 1984.
48. Wheeler MH, Smith PM, Cotton PB, et al: Abnormal blood vessels in the gastric antrum: A cause of upper gastrointestinal bleeding. *Dig Dis Sci* 24:155–158, 1979.
49. Petrini LJ, Johnson JH: Heater probe therapy for vascular ectasia of the antrum (abstract). *Gastrointest Endosc* 32:174–175, 1986.
50. Frager JD, Brandt LJ, Frank MS, et al: Treatment of a patient with watermelon stomach using transendoscopic laser photocoagulation. *Gastrointest Endosc* 34:34–37, 1988.
51. Dieulafoy G: Exulceratio simplex. Bull Acad Med 39–40:49–82, 1898.
52. Hoffman J, Beck H, Jensen HE: Dieulafoy's lesion. *Surg Gynecol Oncol* 159:537–540, 1984.
53. Allende HD, Ona FV: Celiac artery and superior mesenteric artery insufficiency. *Gastroenterology* 82:763–766, 1982.
54. Taylor NS, Gueft B, Lebowich R: Atheromatous embolization: A cause of gastric ulcers and small bowel necrosis. *Gastroenterology* 47:97–103, 1964.
55. Cherry RD, Jabbari M, Gorescky CA, et al: Chronic mesenteric vascular insufficiency with gastric ulceration. *Gastroenterology* 91:1548–1552, 1986.
56. Hojgaard L, Krag E: Chronic ischemic gastritis reversed after revascularization operation. *Gastroenterology* 92:226–228, 1987.
57. Cameron AJ, Higgins JA: Linear gastric erosion: A lesion associated with large diaphragmatic hernia and chronic blood loss anemia. *Gastroenterology* 91:338–342, 1986.
58. Cameron AJ: Incidence of iron-deficiency anemia in patients with large diaphragmatic hernia: A controlled study. *Mayo Clin Proc* 51:767–769, 1976.

12

BLEEDING FROM THE DUODENUM

Karl T. Esrason, M.D.
William S. Haubrich, M.D.

While the duodenum amounts to hardly 5% of the linear extent of the alimentary tract, and its mucosal surface even less, bleeding from the duodenum accounts for approximately 20% of all loss of blood from the entire tract. The intent of this chapter is to highlight the anatomy of the duodenum, with particular reference to its blood supply; to describe how bleeding from the duodenum can be manifested; to mention how the duodenum lends itself to the diagnosis of bleeding; and to enumerate, in some detail, those lesions of the duodenum that can be a source of blood loss. A more comprehensive discussion of diagnosis will be found in Section III, and the management of bleeding from the duodenum is covered in Section V.

ANATOMY

The duodenum takes its name as a Latin derivation of the Greek *dodekadaktulon,* literally "12 fingers." The explanation lies in its length, approximately equivalent to the breadth of 12 fingers. In German, the duodenum is called *der Zwölffingerdarm,* "the 12-finger intestine." The duodenum is the shortest, widest, and most fixed segment of the small intestine. Its length ranges between 20 and 30 cm, and its width varies from 3 to 5 cm. The duodenum is shaped like a horseshoe. It is adherent to the posterior abdominal wall, with the open end directed up and to the left, and the closed end adherent to the posterior parietes overlying and adjacent to the inferior vena cava. This horseshoe is conveniently subdivided into four portions (Figure 12.1). The first, most proximal, and superior portion often is called the duodenal *bulb* or *cap;* the second portion descends vertically and nestles the head of the pancreas; the third portion extends almost horizontally to the left; and the fourth portion curves upward to be anchored by the ligament of Treitz, at which point the duodenum is in continuity with the jejunum. All of the duodenum except its first portion is retroperitoneal.

The blood supply to the duodenum is exceptionally generous (Figure 12.2), being derived from major branches of both the celiac axis and the superior mesenteric artery,

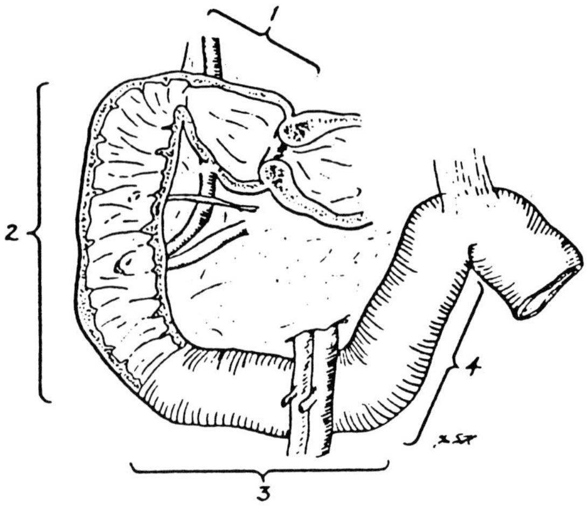

Figure 12.1. Drawing of the duodenum delineating the four portions described in the text and illustrating the relation of the duodenum to the common bile duct and to the superior mesenteric artery and vein.

which join in an anastomotic arcade. Thus, ischemia and infarction of the duodenum are virtually unknown. This arterial configuration explains, too, why bleeding from the duodenum cannot be stopped simply by ligation of a vessel leading to a bleeding site.

The superior aspect of the first portion of the duodenum is served by a supraduodenal branch of the gastroduodenal artery; the inferior aspect is served by a branch of the right gastroepiploic artery. Both of these vessels also supply adjacent areas of the gastric antrum. The second portion of the duodenum shares with the head of the pancreas an abundant blood supply from paired anterior and posterior arcades formed by anastomoses of branches from the superior pancreatoduodenal artery (derived from the celiac axis) and from the inferior pancreatoduodenal artery (derived from the superior mesenteric artery). Proximal intestinal branches of the superior mesenteric artery serve the third and fourth portions of the duodenum. Nutrient arteries of substantial caliber course within the muscular wall and submucosa of the duodenal wall; most of these run parallel to the lumen. Terminal arterial extensions permeate the wall of the duodenum to form a rich network of nourishing channels.

All arterial branches and arcades supplying the duodenum are accompanied by corresponding veins which drain into the splenic and superior mesenteric venous channels.

HOW BLEEDING CAN ORIGINATE IN THE DUODENUM

Blood can be lost from the duodenum in minute amounts with no visible evidence, i.e., *occult* or hidden in the stool, or bleeding can be of an amount and at a rate sufficient to be *overt* and readily evident as melena, hematochezia, or hematemesis.

The actual frequency of occult duodenal bleeding is unknown, as would be expected

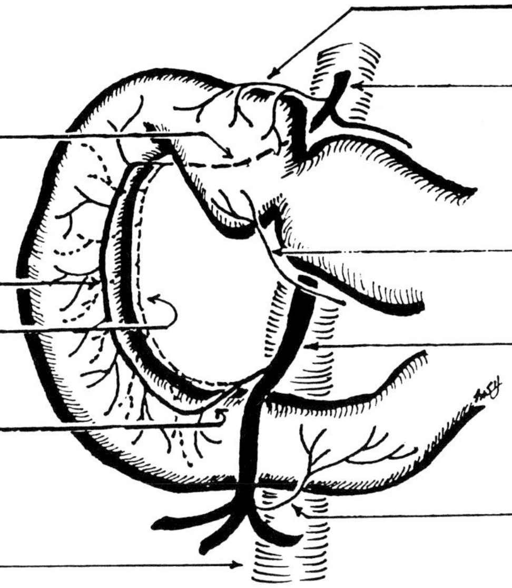

Figure 12.2. Scheme of the arterial blood supply to the duodenum. Note its close relation to the aorta, the celiac axis, and the superior mesenteric artery.

from the definition of *occult*. Doubtless, diapedesis of red blood cells can and does occur through intact duodenal epithelium, but this is insufficient in volume or rate to be registered by currently available tests for occult blood in stools; nor is diapedesis sufficient to account for iron deficiency anemia. Occult bleeding that can be detected by testing of stools commonly occurs as a result of superficial erosion of the single-layer columnar epithelium that lines the lumen of the duodenum. Such bleeding typically issues from the rich network of capillaries in the lamina propria.

Within the lamina propria of each duodenal villus are arterioles and venules that can bleed from slightly deeper and more extensive erosion. Such bleeding can be either occult or overt, depending on its volume and rate. As an example, subjects given acetylsalicylic acid (aspirin) by mouth show on electron microscopy of mucosal biopsy specimens sloughing of the protective mucus layer and the underlying surface epithelium.[1] Focal cellular degeneration can increase in depth and extent to penetrate superficial blood vessels underlying the eroded epithelium.

Still deeper ulceration can breach branches and trunks of terminal arteries and veins that course in the submucosa and muscular wall of the duodenum. The larger trunks from which terminal branches emerge often run horizontally with reference to the lumen; hence erosion from deep ulceration tends to produce bleeding from the sidewalls rather than from terminal twigs.

The duodenum is in close proximity to a number of large extramural arteries and their accompanying veins (Figure 12.2). In certain pathological states, fistulas between these vessels and the duodenum can occur, either as a result of penetration of the vascular wall by a lesion extending from the duodenum or consequent to extension of a vascular lesion to and through the duodenal wall. Hemorrhage from vascular fistulas is typically massive and life-threatening.

HOW BLEEDING FROM THE DUODENUM IS MANIFESTED

Melena most often signifies bleeding from a peptic ulcer that is usually situated in the first, most proximal portion (the bulb or cap) of the duodenum. When hemorrhage from a duodenal ulcer is copious, it can also be manifested as hematemesis, inasmuch as duodenal contents readily reflux into the stomach. Hematemesis from a bleeding ulcer rarely occurs in the absence of melena, although hematemesis may appear prior to melena. Melena also can result from lesser erosions in the duodenal mucosa, though superficial duodenitis is seldom a plausible cause of melena or iron deficiency anemia. An unusual cause of melena, peculiarly associated with intermittent, obstructive jaundice, is neoplasia at the papilla of Vater; the tumor obstructs the ampulla and then becomes necrotic, ulcerates, and bleeds.

Red blood, expressed either as *hematemesis* or visible in *maroon stools,* can originate in the duodenum and, as such, signifies massive hemorrhage. The color of exuded blood reflects not the distance it travels through the gut but rather its volume, its exposure to acid, and the length of time it lies in the gut lumen. Dark red or black blood has been degraded by acid or bacterial action; fresher, brighter red blood has been expelled so rapidly as to escape these changes. Copious hemorrhage in the duodenum is typical of hematobilia (a rare complication of intrahepatic lesions), erosion of a relatively large blood vessel in the duodenal mucosa or wall, and bleeding from an aortic fistula.

TABLE 12.1. Bleeding from the Duodenum: Causes to be Considered

- Erosive Inflammatory Lesions
  - Nonspecific duodenitis
  - Infectious duodenitis
  - Erosions and ulcerations
    - Acid—peptic
    - Idiopathic
    - Drug-related (iatrogenic)
    - Stress-related
    - Induced by foreign bodies
- Vascular Lesions
  - Intrinsic
    - Angiodysplasia
    - Hereditary hemorrhagic telangiectasia
    - Dieulafoy's lesion
    - Duodenal varices
  - Extrinsic
    - Aortoenteric fistulas
    - Arterioenteric fistulas
    - Venoenteric fistulas
    - Pancreatobiliary fistulas
- Mass Lesions (Neoplasms)
  - Benign
    - Leiomyoma
    - Lipoma
    - Adenomatous polyps
    - Neuroendocrine tumors
  - Malignant
    - Adenocarcinoma
    - Leiomyosarcoma
    - Carcinoid tumor
    - Lymphoma
    - Ampullary carcinoma
    - Metastatic lesions
- Developmental Lesions
  - Diverticula
  - Duplication cysts
- Special Circumstances
  - Postoperative bleeding
  - Bleeding incident to organ transplantation
  - Systemic conditions
    - Renal disease
    - Hemophilia
    - Hepatic disease

TABLE 12.2. Relative Frequencies of Upper Gastrointestinal Bleeding Sites

Unknown or unspecified site		~10%	(3.2–13%)
Esophagus		~25%	(22–33%)
Stomach		~35%	(28–51%)
Duodenum		~30%	(17.5–31.4%)
Duodenal ulcer	~25%		
Angiodysplasia	~4–7%		
Duodenitis	~1–1.4%		
Other	~<2%		

Source: Based on Sugawa,[2] Zuckermann et al.,[3] and Palmer.[9]

DUODENAL LESIONS LIABLE TO BLEED

Lesions responsible for bleeding from the duodenum are legion. A list of the more common ones is found in Table 12.1; the relative frequency of bleeding is noted in Table 12.2. Bleeding lesions can be conveniently classified into the broad categories of *erosive inflammations, vascular defects,* and *neoplasms,* as well as *degenerative* and *developmental lesions.* A further, clinically important category is bleeding that occurs in *special circumstances,* affecting particular patient populations.

EROSIVE AND ULCERATIVE INFLAMMATORY LESIONS

Nonspecific Erosive Duodenitis

This is a relatively rare cause of significant blood loss from the duodenum, being reported in little more than 1% of patients with upper gastrointestinal bleeding.[2,3] Duodenitis is observed endoscopically as areas of mucosal erythema and edema with scattered erosions, some of which may show pinpoint bleeding. Mere erythema of duodenal mucosa is sometimes described by endoscopists as *duodenitis.* Aside from the arguable issue of whether this is truly an inflammatory lesion, mucosal erythema alone is an unlikely setting for significant blood loss.

Acute duodenitis with macrohemorrhagic lesions has been described in patients with generalized septicemia. The histological finding of epithelial cell atypia, necrosis, and infiltration by neutrophils is characteristic.[4] Chronic duodenitis is marked by abnormally heavy round-cell infiltration of the lamina propria, often extending into and through the muscularis mucosae, along with interstitial lesions such as reticular hyperplasia.

Infectious Duodenitis

Viral, bacterial, fungal, and parasitic organisms can all inflame the duodenal mucosa, but their propensity to induce overt bleeding is low.

Duodenitis caused by viruses is an unusual source of bleeding; however, *cytomega-*

lovirus infection can be marked by mucosal erosions and aphthous lesions, notably in immunocompromised hosts.

Helicobacter pylori commonly resides in gastric mucosa and is associated with gastritis and duodenal ulcer, although a pathogenetic relation is currently debated. *H. pylori* also has been found to inhabit the mucus overlying metaplastic gastric epithelium in the duodenal cap.[5] The organism is thought to disrupt the functional, if not the structural, integrity of the protective mucosal barrier, causing subsequent acid-peptic injury and inflammation, with erosion and ulceration which can bleed. *Mycobacterium tuberculosis* rarely infects the duodenal mucosa (and almost never in the absence of pulmonary infection); bleeding from tuberculous ulcers is usually slight, although erosion into a major blood vessel can result in massive hemorrhage.[6] Gummas of *syphilis* can be found in the duodenum, but clinically significant bleeding is rare.[7]

Fungal infections can cause duodenitis, but this seldom is encountered in persons with intact immune mechanisms. *Candida albicans* can produce severe inflammation by mucosal invasion in immunocompromised patients, although clinically significant bleeding is unusual.

Parasitic infection of the duodenum, on the other hand, can cause significant hemorrhage. *Strongyloides stercoralis* has been implicated in life-threatening upper gastrointestinal bleeding.[8] *Schistosoma mansoni,* as well as *ancylostomiasis,* can produce severe duodenitis which, on rare occasions, can lead to substantial blood loss. Other offending organisms include *Giardia lamblia, Trichinella spiralis, Capillaria philippiensis, Necator americanus, Entamoeba histolytica, Isospora belli,* and *Cryptosporidium.*[7]

Acid-Peptic Erosions and Ulceration

Duodenal peptic ulcer is the most common source of bleeding from the duodenum and, indeed, is among the most frequent causes of upper gastrointestinal bleeding, accounting for 14 to 68% of all cases.[2,3,9,10] In a recent series of 445 patients with upper gastrointestinal hemorrhage observed at the University of Southern California, duodenal ulcer was responsible for 120 cases, or 27%.[11]

Peptic ulcers commonly occur in the first portion of the duodenum (the bulb or cap). The minority that occur distally as *postbulbar ulcers* are situated typically on the posterior wall, proximal to the papilla of Vater, and are especially prone to bleed.[12]

Historically, there have been remarkable and largely unexplained shifts in the incidence of peptic ulcer disease and its complications. The early 1900s saw a rapid rise in the frequency of duodenal ulcers, far surpassing that of gastric ulcers. The rise peaked at midcentury and is now declining. There has been a substantial decline in the frequency of surgical intervention in the management of peptic ulcer disease and an even more striking change in the relative indications for operation[13] (Figure 12.3). The absolute percentage of patients requiring operation for ''intractability'' has declined, but the number of patients requiring surgery for bleeding has increased (Figure 12.3). From 1970 to 1985, hospitalization for peptic ulcer hemorrhage in Britain did not change, but the age distribution of patients shifted toward a preponderance of the elderly.[14]

Bleeding from peptic ulcers is frequently self-limited and ceases spontaneously. From the Washington, D.C., Veterans Administration Medical Center, Fleischer[15] reported a series of 196 episodes of upper gastrointestinal bleeding in 175 patients; hemorrhage was severe and persistent in 20.6% (with a 44% mortality in this subgroup).

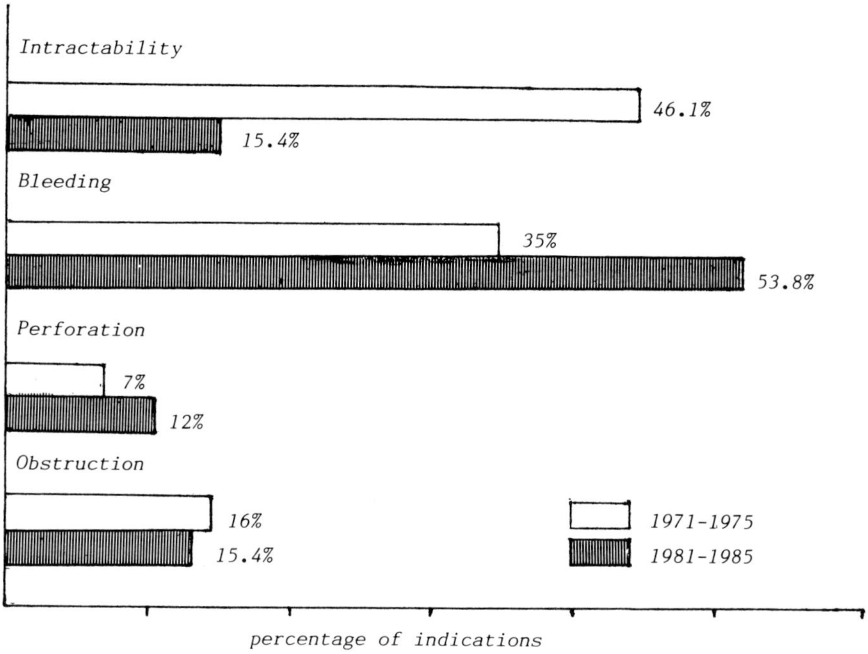

Figure 12.3. Shifting trends in indications for surgical intervention in the management of duodenal peptic ulcer disease. Bleeding is now a far more frequent indication for operation than is intractability. Data taken from Walker.[13] Reproduced with permission of Haubrich WS: Gross anatomy of small intestine in Bockus gastroenterology. 4th ed; J. Berk (ed) Philadelphia. WB Saunders Co, 1985.

Granulomatous Ulceration

Crohn's disease, while predominant in the ileum and colon, can affect the duodenum, where ulcerated granulomatous lesions may be the source of bleeding that ranges from occult to massive.[16] In sarcoidosis, eosinophilic granulomas can develop in the stomach and extend into the duodenal bulb. The overlying mucosa has been known to erode and result in bleeding.[9]

Drug-related Erosions and Ulcerations

Gastrointestinal bleeding due to drug-induced epithelial damage is a well-recognized iatrogenic complication and most often is related to the use of nonsteroidal anti-inflammatory drugs (NSAIDs). The prototype drug is acetylsalicylic acid (ASA, aspirin), which has been shown capable of inducing multiple, patchy, mucosal erosions and bleeding, mainly in the stomach, but in one-half of the cases also in the duodenum.[1] Sloughing of the mucus layer and surface epithelium leads to minute superficial erosions and capillary bleeding. Such bleeding is typically occult but in some cases can be overt.

More serious is the aggravation by NSAIDs of existing dormant or active peptic ulcers. In a series of 235 patients with grave complications of peptic ulcer disease, nearly 80% of all ulcer-related deaths occurred in patients using NSAIDs.[17]

Stress-related Erosions and Ulcerations

Gastroduodenal bleeding is observed in patients who have been stressed by serious trauma, sepsis, or grave illness. The condition may be related more to impaired mucosal blood supply than to gastric hypersecretion. Stress-induced bleeding is mainly from the stomach, though it can also occur in the duodenal mucosa; this area is thoroughly covered in the preceding chapter.

Two particular conditions affecting the duodenum need to be cited. Thomas Curling, a British physician, in 1842 described acute duodenal ulceration in 10 patients with extensive burns, a lesion that has come to be known as *Curling's ulcer*.[9] Patients with burns covering more than 35% of the body surface are especially liable to these lesions, and bleeding is a common presenting sign. Harvey Cushing in 1932 described acute mucosal ulceration in the esophagus, stomach, and duodenum of patients with severe injury to the central nervous system. Such ulcers tend to be deeply penetrating, with a propensity to bleed and perforate.[18]

Since the recognition of the benefit of prophylactic therapy against bleeding in critically ill patients, a significant reduction in bleeding from gastroduodenal stress ulceration has been achieved.

VASCULAR LESIONS

While it can be argued that all duodenal bleeding is vascular in origin, there are lesions primarily vascular, both intrinsic and extrinsic to the duodenum, that can result in hemorrhage.

Intrinsic Lesions

A variety of intrinsic vascular malformations can lead to blood loss. Various names have been given to these lesions, such as *telangiectasia, arteriovenous ectasia, vascular dysplasia,* and *angiodysplasia*. In most cases, their pathogenesis is unclear. Gilmore, in a comprehensive recent review,[19] prefers the term *angiodysplasia* and describes the general manifestation as sharply delineated, red, mucosal lesions with flat or slightly raised surfaces, of round or stellate shape, and with circumscribed, often fern-like margins.

The diagnosis of angiodysplasia is often delayed because the condition is relatively unusual and because minute lesions are easily overlooked.[20] Clouse et al.[21] found gastroduodenal angiodysplasia to be responsible for 4% of upper gastrointestinal bleeding in 676 patients referred for endoscopic examination. Lesions of gastroduodenal angiodysplasia typically are multiple, often numerous. When angiodysplasia is evident at endoscopy of the stomach, similar lesions likely will be found in the duodenum as well. The frequent occurrence of angiodysplasia in elderly persons suggests a degenerative process. However, there is a subset of patients in whom the condition becomes evident early in life, thus suggesting a developmental defect.[22] Bleeding from angiodysplasia is usually relatively benign and manageable. However, severe and protracted hemorrhage can occur.[23]

Duodenal varices are a rare cause of upper gastrointestinal bleeding.[24] Most cases are associated with esophageal varices, though isolated duodenal varices have been reported and appear to be more often associated with extrahepatic causes of portal hypertension than with cirrhosis. The observation of duodenal varices following injection sclerotherapy of esophageal varices[25] raises the possibility that duodenal varices may become more frequently encountered, and that their presence must be suspected and looked for in patients in whom bleeding recurs after apparently successful esophageal sclerotherapy.

Extrinsic Lesions

Vascular structures extrinsic to the duodenum can be the source of gastrointestinal bleeding by various mechanisms. A lesion developing within the duodenum, such as a peptic ulcer, may penetrate an adjacent vascular channel, causing an angioenteric fistula and massive hemorrhage. Moreover, extrinsic vessels may undergo degenerative changes and, by pulsatile action, erode the duodenal wall from without, resulting in a similar bleeding fistula. Expanding lesions in adjacent organs, such as the pancreas, liver, and biliary tree, can also erode into vascular structures and bleed into the duodenum through the papilla of Vater.

Massive upper gastrointestinal hemorrhage from aortoenteric fistulas is not rare. Fistulas can be *primary,* i.e., spontaneous, or *secondary,* i.e., consequent to prior operative intervention. Most primary aortoduodenal fistulas develop as a complication of atherosclerotic aneurysms; syphilitic, tuberculous, and mycotic aneurysms are rare. Of 673 patients with massive gastrointestinal bleeding reported by Mollerup and Strand,[26] 3% were found at necropsy to have aortoenteric fistulas. The third part of the duodenum, being in close retroperitoneal contact with the abdominal aorta, was the site of fistula in 62% of cases.

Aneurysms of medium-sized vessels, such as the gastroduodenal, left gastric, hepatic, and splenic arteries, can cause substantial duodenal hemorrhage by eroding into the biliary tree or into a pancreatic cyst.[27] Abdominal ultrasonography may be useful in delineating an expansile, pulsating mass. Pseudoaneurysm of the hepatic artery, with fistulization and massive upper gastrointestinal hemorrhage, has been reported as a complication of selective angiography.[28] Continuous selective intra-arterial infusion of chemotherapeutic agents has been implicated as another iatrogenic cause of arterioduodenal fistula.[29]

NEOPLASMS

Tumors of the duodenum are unusual and seldom cause exsanguinating hemorrhage. However, they may produce intermittent, self-limited episodes of acute bleeding or chronic occult blood loss.

Benign Neoplasms

Leiomyoma is a benign smooth muscle neoplasm which is relatively common in the stomach but less so in the duodenum. Leiomyomas account for about 22% of all benign small bowel tumors; one-fifth occur in the duodenum.[30] The typical presentation is bleeding, as evidenced by melena or iron deficiency anemia. *Lipomas* occur in all segments of the gastrointestinal tract but most often in the jejunum, ileum, and colon. In a series of 115,251 necropsies, 26 lipomas of the duodenum were found.[31] Most lipomas of the gastrointestinal tract are asymptomatic and discovered only incidentally; acute bleeding is a potential but rare complication of duodenal lipomas.

Adenomatous polyps are the third most frequent benign neoplasm of the small bowel. In a series of 7,346 endoscopic procedures reported by Ghazi et al.,[32] 443 gastroduodenal polyps were excised from 257 patients. Of these, 44 polypoid lesions were found in the duodenums of 19 patients; just over half were adenomas.

Malignant Neoplasms

Primary cancers of the duodenum are rare, but presentation by blood loss is typical. In a review of 29 published series of small bowel tumors, Johnson et al.[33] collected 1,397 cases. Duodenal lesions included 330 adenocarcinomas, 62 malignant carcinoid tumors, and 48 leiomyosarcomas. Approximately two-thirds of the patients had guaiac-positive stools. Ouriel and Adams[34] reported a series of 66 cases of small bowel adenocarcinomas; 34 were in the duodenum, 21 in the jejunum, and 11 in the ileum. Melena or hematochezia occurred in just five cases, whereas half of the patients were anemic.

Carcinoma of the papilla of Vater, in its growth as a fungating mass, obstructs the common bile duct and erodes easily. The combination of bleeding and acholia gives the stool a peculiar silver color.[9]

Cancer metastatic to the duodenum is infrequent but often attended by blood loss. Duodenal metastases from renal cell carcinoma have been the source of massive hemorrhage.[35] A more frequent cause of severe hemorrhage is adenocarcinoma invading the duodenal wall by direct extension from the pancreas or stomach.

DEVELOPMENTAL LESIONS

Simple, presumably congenital, diverticula of the duodenum are frequently encountered incidentally; they rarely bleed. The possibility of bleeding is increased if there are associated developmental abnormalities, such as heterotopic gastric mucosa or pancreatic rests. Occult gastrointestinal bleeding or iron deficiency anemia should never be attributed to the incidental finding of a duodenal diverticulum unless blood has actually been seen to emerge from the diverticular orifice. Knight et al.[36] reported massive hemorrhage from a duplication cyst of the duodenum.

SPECIAL CIRCUMSTANCES

The frequency and pathogenesis of gastrointestinal bleeding in certain patient groups differ from those in the general population, and recognition of these differences is important in the approach to the problem of bleeding in these patients.

Postoperative Bleeding

The nature of bleeding from the duodenum in patients following abdominal surgery depends, to a certain extent, on the primary reason for the antecedent operation, as well as on the specific procedure performed. For example, inadequate resection or incomplete vagotomy in the treatment of peptic ulcer disease can result in recurrent peptic ulcer. Also, postoperative bleeding is more likely to occur when bleeding was the indication for the initial surgical intervention.

Early postoperative bleeding can result from inadequate vascular ligation ("slipped suture"), anastomotic dehiscence, or sepsis. Later postoperative bleeding may derive from overlooked or recurrent mucosal erosions or ulcerations.[37]

The antecedent operation need not have been below the diaphragm. In patients having undergone cardiac surgery, Krasna et al.[38] reported gastrointestinal complications in 2%, among whom the mortality was 44%. While acute pancreatitis was the most frequent abdominal complication, upper gastrointestinal hemorrhage occurred in 5 of 25 patients.

Bleeding Incident to Organ Transplantation

Patients who have undergone organ transplantation can bleed from any of the causes cited above, but there are conditions peculiar to impaired immunity that can result in duodenal bleeding in patients surviving transplantation. Therapy invoked to prevent or treat rejection of transplanted organs increases the liability to opportunistic infection that can lead to mucosal disintegration. An example is the sometimes extensive ulceration caused by cytomegalovirus.[39] Even more devastating is hemorrhage throughout the alimentary tract, including the duodenum, that can occur with extensive mucosal sloughing associated with acute or chronic graft-versus-host disease.[40]

Bleeding in AIDS

Duodenal lesions are not often the cause of bleeding in patients with the acquired immunodeficiency syndrome (AIDS), but can include infectious ulceration, such as that caused by the cytomegalovirus, salmonellosis, and shigellosis, as well as the neoplastic complications of Kaposi's sarcoma and lymphoma.[41]

Systemic Conditions

Impaired hemostasis due to any cause can provoke and intensify bleeding from any of the duodenal lesions that have been cited. While it is prudent to assess the hemostatic capacity of every bleeding patient, deficient hemostasis alone does not result in bleeding from an intact duodenum.

Hemophiliacs bear the burden of an increased risk of upper gastrointestinal bleeding, which, in patients with severe afflictions, remains considerable even with the availability of factor VIII replacement therapy. Mittal et al.[42] cited gastrointestinal bleeding in 7.9% of hemophiliacs; one-fifth of the bleeding episodes was attributed to duodenal ulcer.

Patients with portal hypertension and esophageal varices can, at times, also develop duodenal varices, as noted earlier. However, cirrhosis is associated with other conditions that predispose to bleeding. In a prospective endoscopic study of 510 cirrhotic patients, duodenitis was found in 12.7% and duodenal ulcer in 5%.[43]

REFERENCES

1. Domschke S, Domschke W: Gastroduodenal damage due to drugs, alcohol, and smoking. *Clin Gastroenterol* 13:405–436, 1984.
2. Sugawa C: Endoscopic diagnosis and treatment of upper gastrointestinal bleeding. *Surg Clin North Am* 69:1167–1183, 1989.
3. Zuckermann GR, Cornette GL, Clouse RE, et al: Upper gastrointestinal bleeding in patients with chronic renal failure. *Ann Intern Med* 102:588–592, 1985.
4. Cheli R, Aste H: *Duodenitis.* Stuttgart, Thieme, 1976, p 44.
5. Chamberlain CE, Peura DA: What is new about duodenitis? *Scand Gastroenterol* 14 (Suppl 54):28–30, 1979.
6. Misra D, Rai RR, Nundy S, et al: Duodenal tuberculosis presenting as bleeding peptic ulcer (letter). *Am J Gastroenterol* 83:203–204, 1988.
7. Beck IT: Duodenitis, in Berk JE (ed): *Bockus Gastroenterology,* ed 4. Philadelphia, WB Saunders Co, 1985, p 1403.
8. Bhatt BD, Cappell MS, Smilow PC, et al: Recurrent massive upper gastrointestinal hemorrhage due to *Strongyloides stercoralis* infection. *Am J Gastroenterol* 85:1034–1036, 1990.
9. Palmer E: *Upper Gastrointestinal Hemorrhage.* Springfield, Ill, Charles C Thomas, 1970.
10. Tulassey Z, Gupta R, Papp J, et al: Somatostatin versus cimetidine in the treatment of actively bleeding duodenal ulcer; a prospective, randomized, controlled trial. *Am J Gastroenterol* 84:6–9, 1989.
11. Laine L: Upper gastrointestinal tract hemorrhage. *Western Med J* 155:274–279, 1991.
12. Goldschmiedt M, Peterson WL, Vuitch F, et al: Postbulbar duodenal ulcer in a patient with pentagastrin-fast achlorhydria. *Gastroenterology* 97:771–774, 1989.
13. Walker LC: Trends in the surgical management of duodenal ulcer; a 15-year study. *Am J Surg* 155:436–438, 1988.
14. Bloom BS, Fendrick AM, Ramsey SD: Changes in peptic ulcer and gastritis/duodenitis in Great Britain, 1970–1985. *J Clin Gastroenterol* 12:100–108, 1990.
15. Fleischer D: Etiology and prevalence of severe persistent upper gastrointestinal bleeding. *Gastroenterology* 84:538–543, 1983.
16. Wolff BG: Crohn's disease; the role of surgical treatment. *Mayo Clin Proc* 61:292–295, 1986.
17. Armstrong CP, Blower AL: Non-steroidal anti-inflammatory drugs and life-threatening complications of peptic ulceration. *Gut* 28:527–532, 1987.
18. Kamada T, Fusamoto H, Kawano S, et al: Gastrointestinal bleeding following head injury; a clinical study of 433 cases. *J Trauma* 17:44–47, 1977.
19. Gilmore PR: Angiodysplasia of the upper gastrointestinal tract. *J Clin Gastroenterol* 10:386–394, 1988.
20. Tai DI, Chou FF, Lee TY, et al: Vascular ectasia of the duodenum detected by duodenoscopy. *Am J Gastroenterol* 82:1071–1073, 1987.
21. Clouse RE, Costigan DJ, Mills BA, et al: Incidence of perforated and bleeding ulcers before and after the introduction of H2-receptor antagonists. *Ann Surg* 207:4–6, 1988.
22. Gunnlaugsson O: Angiodysplasia of the stomach and duodenum. *Gastrointest Endosc* 31:251–254, 1985.
23. Woodlock TJ, Francis CW, Rowe JM, et al: Prolonged remission after life-threatening gastrointestinal hemorrhage from coexistent angiodysplasia and acquired bleeding diathesis. *Am J Hematol* 22:125–131, 1988.
24. Manzione NC, Das KM, Wolkoff AW, et al: Unusual sites of upper gastrointestinal variceal bleeding. *J Clin Gastroenterol* 9:40–42, 1987.

25. Eleftheriadis E: Duodenal varices after sclerotherapy for esophageal varices. *Am J Gastroenterol* 83:439–441, 1988.
26. Mollerup CL, Strand L: Gastrointestinal hemorrhage due to fistula from aortic aneurysm; case report. *Acta Chir Scand* 153:631–632, 1987.
27. Hugel HE, Oser W, Bodner E: Aneurysm of the proper hepatic artery as a rare source of upper gastrointestinal bleeding. *Gastrointest Radiol* 11:158–160, 1986.
28. Aggarwal S, Berry M: Duodenal fistula: Complication of a pseudoaneurysm of the common hepatic artery. *Gastrointest Radiol* 13:230–232, 1988.
29. Kernstine NH, Kryjeski SR, Hall LJ, et al: Gastroduodenal artery—duodenal fistula: A complication of continuous floxuridine (FUDR) infusion into the gastroduodenal artery. *J Surg Oncol* 45:59–62, 1990.
30. Aagaard J: Isolated hematemesis in duodenal leiomyoma; case report. *Can J Surg* 26:552–553, 1983.
31. Michel LA, Ballet T, Collard JM, et al: Severe bleeding from submucosal lipoma of the duodenum. *J Clin Gastroenterol* 10:541–545, 1988.
32. Ghazi A, Ferstenberg H, Shinya H: Endoscopic gastroduodenal polypectomy. *Ann Surg* 200:175–180, 1984.
33. Johnson AM, Harman PK, Hanks JB: Primary small bowel malignancies. *Am Surgeon* 51:31–36, 1985.
34. Ouriel K, Adams JT: Adenocarcinoma of the small intestine. *Am J Surg* 147:66–71, 1984.
35. Lynch-Nyhan A, Fishman EK, Kadir S: Diagnosis and management of massive gastrointestinal bleeding owing to duodenal metastasis from renal cell carcinoma. *J Urol* 138:611–613, 1987.
36. Knight CD Jr, Allen MJ, Nagorney DM, et al: Duodenal duplication cyst causing massive bleeding in an adult; an unusual complication of a duplication cyst of the digestive tract. *Mayo Clin Proc* 60:772–775, 1985.
37. Rypins EP, Sarfeh IJ, Collins-Irby D, et al: Asymptomatic peptic disease in patients undergoing major elective operations: A prospective endoscopic study. *Am J Gastroenterol* 83:927–929, 1988.
38. Krasna MJ, Flanebaum L, Trooskin SW, et al: Gastrointestinal complications after cardiac surgery. *Surgery* 104:773–780, 1988.
39. Johnson R, Peitzman AB, Webster MW, et al: Upper gastrointestinal endoscopy after cardiac transplantation. *Surgery* 103:300–304, 1988.
40. McDonald GB, Shuliman HM, Sullivan KM, et al: Intestinal and hepatic complications of human bone marrow transplantation. (Part I). *Gastroenterology* 90:460–477, 1986.
41. Friedman SL, Owen RL: Gastrointestinal manifestations of AIDS and other sexually transmitted diseases, in Sleissinger MH, Fordtran JF (eds): *Gastrointestinal Disease,* ed 4. Philadelphia, WB Saunders Co, 1989, p 1242.
42. Mittal R, Spero JA, Lewis JH, et al: Patterns of gastrointestinal hemorrhage in hemophilia. *Gastroenterology* 88:515–522, 1985.
43. Rabinovitz M, Voo VK, Schade RR, et al: Prevalence of endoscopic findings in 510 consecutive individuals with cirrhosis evaluated prospectively. *Dig Dis Sci* 35:705–710, 1990.

13

BLEEDING FROM THE SMALL INTESTINE

Blair S. Lewis, M.D.
Jerome D. Waye, M.D.

Bleeding lesions in the small intestine are uncommon and often difficult to diagnose. In 3–5% of patients with gastrointestinal (GI) bleeding, the site is located between the second portion of the duodenum and the ileocecal valve.[1] Because of the inability to localize a bleeding site in the small bowel, these patients may present with prolonged occult blood loss or with recurrent melena or maroon hematochezia of undetermined origin. Often multiple transfusions are required to support these patients, in whom repeated examinations of colonoscopy, upper intestinal endoscopy, barium enema, upper GI series, and bleeding scan are negative. An early diagnosis of the bleeding site in these patients is rarely made.[1-5] Several factors influence the failure to find the source of blood loss. Besides being an unusual site of bleeding not routinely considered, the small bowel is relatively inaccessible compared to the stomach and colon. The usual diagnostic techniques are confounded by the length of the small intestine and by its free intraperitoneal location, vigorous contractility, and overlying loops. These attributes limit the diagnostic capability of barium studies, endoscopic intubation, and the special imaging techniques of nuclear medicine scans and angiography. In addition to these technical problems of access, the bleeding rate may be slow or intermittent, thereby precluding identification by either angiography or bleeding scan. The yield of a small bowel series for diagnosing tumors of the small intestine is quite low; even enteroclysis double-contrast studies cannot diagnose angiodysplasias, which are the most common cause of small bowel bleeding. Until recently, the small intestine has been considered relatively unapproachable by endoscopic evaluation.

Various causes of small bowel bleeding may be encountered, but vascular ectasias account for 70–80% of bleeding episodes (Table 13.1). Angiodysplasias can present with either brisk or occult bleeding. These submucosal collections of dilated capillaries and veins develop secondary to prolonged intermittent obstruction of venous outflow.[6] The chronic obstruction leads to increased back-pressure in the capillary bed, resulting in incompetence of the prearteriolar sphincters and development of small arteriovenous shunts. The mucosa overlying these small shunts may receive an inadequate blood supply, resulting in localized ischemia with ulceration and subsequent bleeding. Diagnosis is

TABLE 13.1. Causes of Small Intestinal Bleeding

Angiodysplasia
Small bowel tumors
Leiomyoma
Hemangioma
Carcinoid
Leiomyosarcoma
Adenocarcinoma
Lymphoma
Aortoenteric fistula
Jejunal diverticula
Meckel's diverticulum
Duplication cyst
Ulcerating diseases of the small bowel

usually made endoscopically, though there are several characteristic angiographic signs such as early filling vein, vascular blushes, and delayed emptying of veins[7] (Plate 17).

Although tumors of the small bowel account for only 6% of all GI tract tumors, they are the second most common cause of obscure bleeding and comprise 5–10% of all cases of small intestinal hemorrhage.[8,9] More than half of these tumors are benign. These patients are generally younger than those with angiodysplasia of the small bowel. The patient with a small bowel tumor has an average age of 51 compared to 69 for the patient with angiodysplasia.[10] Bleeding is the presenting complaint in 25–50% of patients with small bowel tumors. Since bleeding is often the sole symptom, the diagnosis is often delayed, thus contributing to the poor prognosis in patients with malignant tumors. Leiomyomas and leiomyosarcomas, distributed throughout the small bowel, are the most common tumors that bleed (Plate 18). Bleeding, which may be brisk, occurs from these submucosal smooth muscle tumors when there is necrosis and ulceration of the overlying mucosa. Due to their vascularity, 99m-Tc pertechnetate scanning may be positive in leiomyomas; angiography has been reported to show a tumor blush in 86% of lesions.[9] There is no sex predilection, and these lesions occur most frequently in the fifth to seventh decades. Gradual but more chronic blood loss is usually associated with other small bowel tumors, including carcinoids, adenocarcinomas, and lymphomas. Adenomatous polyps and adenocarcinomas are most frequently found within the proximal bowel, with 90% of lesions located within the duodenum and the first 20 cm of the jejunum. Lymphomas, on the other hand, tend to involve the distal jejunum or ileum. Melanoma and breast tumors are the most common tumors that metastasize to the small bowel. Colonic cancer can also involve the small intestine by metastasis. Pancreatic cancer can directly invade the duodenum and present with bleeding. Small bowel tumors are often not identified on routine small bowel series, but the addition of enteroclysis may increase the yield.

Ulcerative diseases within the small intestine also cause small bowel bleeding. Crohn's disease is the most common ulcerative disease. Gross bleeding is unusual in Crohn's disease, occurring in 4–10% of patients with ileitis.[11-13] Transmural inflammation, the pathological hallmark of the disease, can extend into large submucosal vessels, causing massive bleeding. These episodes are usually self-limited and not recurring.[13]

Bleeding is not usually the sole symptom in these patients, since most also have the more common symptoms of Crohn's disease such as diarrhea and abdominal pain.[12] The diagnosis is virtually always made based on small bowel x-ray series.

Meckel's diverticulum is a remnant of the vitelline duct and is usually located within 100 cm of the ileocecal valve. This anomaly occurs in 2% of the population and is more common in men than women. This entity is diagnosed in two-thirds of men under the age of 30 presenting with small bowel bleeding.[14] The bleeding is almost always brisk, resulting from ulceration within the diverticulum or the adjoining ileum secondary to acid production from ectopic gastric mucosa lining the diverticular wall. Preoperative diagnosis is uncommon, though radionuclide scanning using 99m-Tc pertechnetate is available to label parietal cells within the gastric mucosa. An intestinal duplication cyst can also be lined with ectopic gastric mucosa, leading to ulceration and bleeding. Unlike a Meckel's diverticulum, these congenital cysts may be located anywhere in the bowel. Other causes of small bowel ulcerations include Zollinger-Ellison syndrome, certain infectious agents, medications, and various vasculitides (Table 13.2).

Jejunal diverticula can cause small bowel bleeding. These are acquired pseudodiverticula that develop on the mesenteric border of the intestine at the site of perforating blood vessels. Jejunal diverticula, found in 1–2% of individuals in autopsy studies, are usually asymptomatic. Less than 5% of all people with jejunal diverticula actually bleed from them.[1] Thus, when discovered on a small bowel series, the jejunal diverticula should be considered incidental findings, since angiographic or radionuclide scanning evidence of active bleeding is necessary to conclude that the diverticula are the site of bleeding. When bleeding does occur from jejunal diverticula, it is usually massive and is associated with a 20% mortality.

TABLE 13.2. Ulcerating Diseases of the Small Intestine

Acid-induced
Ectopic gastric mucosa (Meckel's diverticulum, duplication)
Zollinger-Ellison syndrome
Infectious
Tuberculosis
Syphilis
Typhoid
Histoplasmosis
Drug-induced
Potassium
Nonsteroidal anti-inflammatory drugs
6-Mercaptopurine
Vasculitis
Atherosclerotic ischemic disease
Radiation
Polyarteritis nodosa
Henoch-Schonlein purpura
Idiopathic
Crohn's disease
Ulcerative jejunitis

EVALUATION OF OBSCURE BLEEDING

A routine small bowel series results in a low yield of positive findings when patients present with obscure bleeding. Although Crohn's disease and large ulcerations of the small bowel can readily be diagnosed using this standard examination,[15] only about 5% of small bowel follow-through exams detect a bleeding site.[16] Enteroclysis radiographic examinations can increase that yield to 10%.[17] During this procedure, a tube is positioned radiographically in the duodenum and a mixture of barium, air, water, or methylcellulose is instilled (Figure 13.1). The x-rays obtained are comparable to the double-contrast studies of the colon. Although a tumor can be overlooked by this examination, there is a better chance of demonstrating intraluminal pathology than with the single-column barium x-ray of the small bowel (Figure 13.2). Angiodysplasias cannot be identified by means of barium radiographic modalities.

Radioisotope bleeding scans may be diagnostic when there is bleeding distal to the ligament of Treitz.[18] The ready availability, low cost, and safety of this procedure have led to its universal acceptance. It is often a prerequisite for emergency angiography. Technetium-labeled red blood cell scintigraphy has replaced the older sulfur colloid scans. These earlier scans had a short (three-minute) intravascular half-life due to rapid uptake of the colloid by reticuloendothelial cells in the liver and spleen. Active bleeding

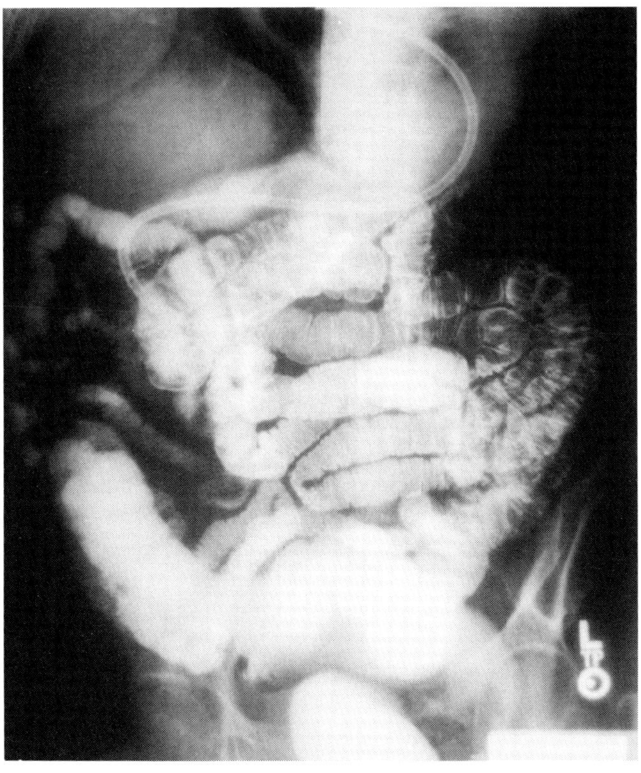

Figure 13.1. A normal enteroclysis showing a double-contrast study of the small bowel.

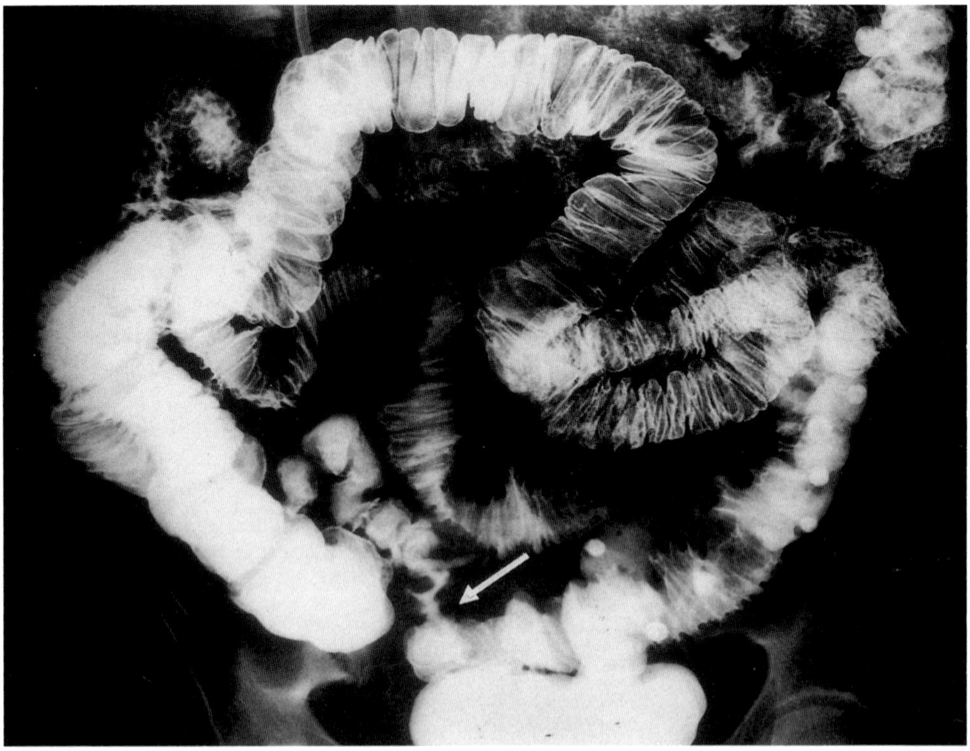

Figure 13.2. Radiograph of a jejunal lymphoma, identified by enteroclysis, not seen on a routine small bowel series. (Courtesy of S. Freedman, M.D., Medical College of Georgia.)

at the time of injection is required to make a correct diagnosis. With current bleeding scans, red blood cells are labeled either in vitro or in vivo with a radionuclide tag and, during an acquisition time of one or two hours, as little as 5 cc of intraluminal blood will give a positive scan. Another advantage to red blood cell scans is the intravascular half-life of 24 hours, permitting a longer scanning time whereby sequential scans increase the probability of identifying the bleeding site. Small bowel bleeding can be identified on nuclear scans as the tracer-labeled blood takes a serpiginous route through the gut in subsequent pictures, unlike the course of blood in colonic bleeding, which follows a more specific movement pattern. The effectiveness of the scan is somewhat dependent on the affinity between the radioactive technetium and the red cell. In vitro labeling results in a tighter bond between the tag and the red cell, whereas multiple transfusions can adversely alter the binding mechanism, limiting the effectiveness of the scan.[19]

Meckel's diverticulum may be detected by 99m-Tc pertechnetate, which binds to parietal cells. The sensitivity of this nuclear scan used in the evaluation of small bowel bleeding is reported to be 75–100%, with false-positive scans reported in 15% of instances and false-negatives reported in 25%.[14] Pentagastrin and cimetidine have been shown to increase the uptake of pertechnetate by parietal cells, and a so-called enhanced Meckel's scan using either of these pharmacological agents has been used to increase the sensitivity of this test.[20]

Angiography can detect bleeding at a rate of 0.5 ml/min. This radiographic technique can localize a site of bleeding in 50–72% of patients with massive hemorrhage, but this yield decreases to 25–50% when active bleeding has slowed.[21] In addition to the demonstration of active bleeding, angiography can diagnose nonbleeding lesions such as angiodysplasias and small bowel tumors. Unfortunately, the detection of a bleeding site in patients with chronic occult bleeding is only in the range of 10–15%.[22]

Exploratory surgery is often considered in the patient with recurrent obscure GI bleeding. At laparotomy the surgeon can inspect the small bowel in several ways, including palpation, transillumination, and creation of multiple enterotomies. However, there is a low success rate for simple exploration when unaccompanied by other simultaneous evaluations such as intraoperative endoscopy[23,24] (see Chapter 18).

Endoscopy of the small intestine can be accomplished in several ways.[15,25,26] The usual techniques of upper endoscopy and colonoscopy intubating the ileocecal valve provide visualization of the most proximal and distal ends of the gut. Routine esophagogastroduodenoscopy generally reaches the junction of the second and third portions of the duodenum. Extended upper intestinal endoscopy, also termed *push enteroscopy,* using an orally passed adult or pediatric colonoscope or a specialized instrument, can inspect up to 60 cm of jejunum beyond the ligament of Treitz[25-27] (Plates 17, 18 and Figure 13.3).

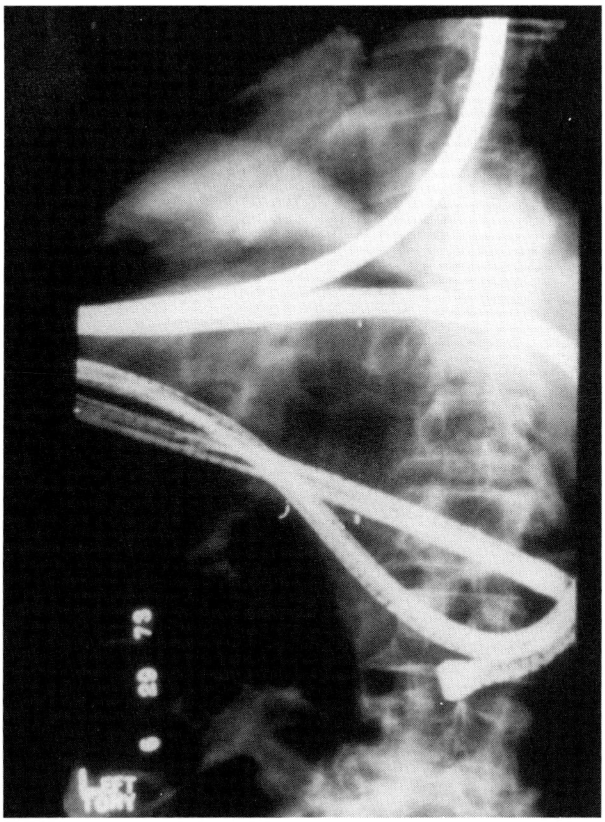

Figure 13.3. An x-ray showing push enteroscopy, with the tip of the endoscope 40 cm past the ligament of Treitz.

Gas sterilization of the 130- to 165-cm-long instrument is not necessary when performing this exam, since a clean, disinfected colonoscope may be used safely. Colonoscopes provide four-way directional tip deflection of 160–180°, unlike gastroscopes. Thus, greater tip deflection, along with increased length, allows this deep intubation.

Passage of the pylorus is readily accomplished with gentle pressure using these larger-caliber instruments, whose tip diameters vary from 11 to 14 mm. The ligament of Treitz is usually encountered 100 cm from the incisor teeth and frequently requires extreme tip deflection to locate the lumen at that juncture. When push enteroscopy has been used in patients with suspected small bowel bleeding, presumptive sites have been identified in 15–38%.[27] Angiodysplasias are the most common finding, and therapeutic cauterization is possible through these instruments. In an effort to extend the reach of this therapeutic procedure, a new push enteroscope measuring 200 cm has been developed.[28] This instrument utilizes an overtube which is initially backloaded onto the shaft of this orally passed endoscope. Once the tip of the endoscope is within the jejunum, the overtube is advanced through the esophagus until its distal tip rests within the second portion of the duodenum. This stiffening tube limits intragastric and intraduodenal looping of the push enteroscope, a hindrance to deep small bowel intubation. The push enteroscope can then be advanced 6–7 feet beyond the ligament of Treitz, effectively extending endoscopic evaluation and therapeutic intervention to the entire jejunum.

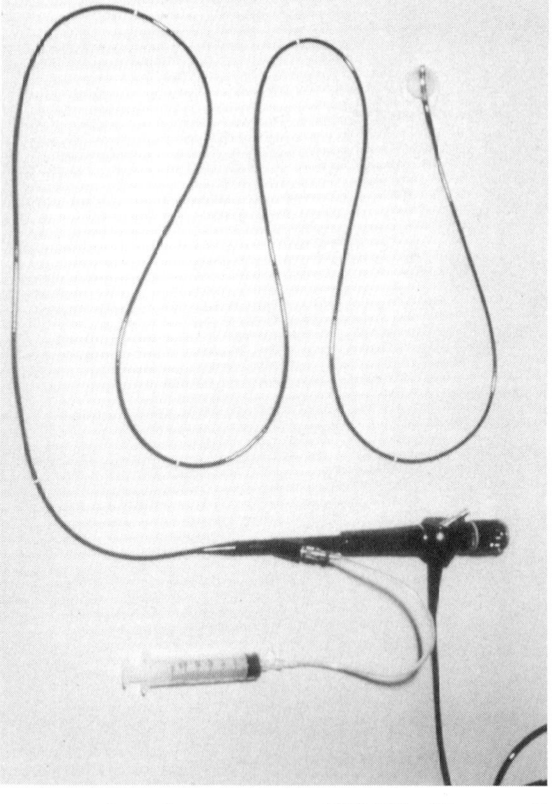

Figure 13.4. The transnasal sonde enteroscope (SIF-SW, Olympus Corporation of America, Lake Success, N.Y.)

A long, flexible fiberoptic instrument propelled through the intestine by peristalsis provides a nonsurgical alternative to viewing the remainder of the small intestine. Sonde enteroscopy, also termed *small bowel enteroscopy,* employs a small transnasal instrument with a balloon at its tip[25,26] which acts as a foreign body bolus, permitting peristalsis to pull the endoscope into the small intestine. This instrument is 2,560 mm long and has a tip diameter of 5 mm (Figure 13.4). There are two internal channels, one for inflation of the balloon and another for air insufflation of the intestinal lumen. This instrument has no therapeutic capability, nor can it mark sites of bleeding for later therapy. Because of the absence of tip deflection capability, its intraluminal view is limited to 50–75% of the mucosal surface.

Sonde and push enteroscopy are closely linked, since the sonde instrument is carried into the proximal jejunum by the push instrument. Placing the tip of the sonde enteroscope into the small bowel hastens the overall examination, since passive movement of the scope through the pylorus may require several hours. In this procedure, a push enteroscope grasps a suture affixed to the tip of the sonde instrument while both instruments lie within the stomach. They are then advanced into the small bowel. The orally passed push enteroscope is then removed, leaving the sonde enteroscope in place. During a transit time that averages seven hours, the ileum is reached in 75% of patients and the ileocecal valve or colon in 10%[29] (Figure 13.5). Previous surgery with adhesions may limit the depth of intubation. The small bowel is examined upon withdrawal of the instrument. Sonde enteroscopy of the small bowel in cases of obscure GI bleeding has a diagnostic yield of 40%.[29,30] Angiodysplasia accounts for 80% of the findings, while small bowel tumors account for 10% including patients who had a normal enteroclysis

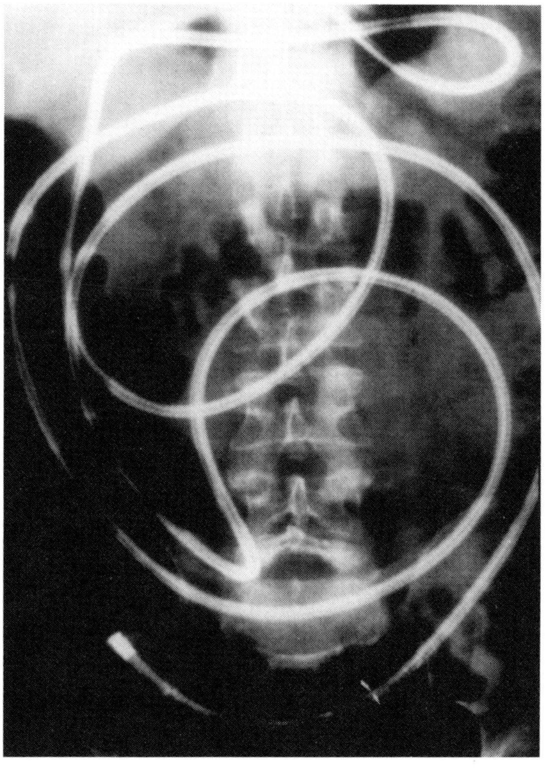

Figure 13.5. An x-ray of the sonde enteroscope with total intubation of the small bowel.

study. Though sonde enteroscopy does not provide complete inspection of the entire small bowel, when compared to intraoperative enteroscopy exact correlation of findings has been reported in 77% of cases.[31]

DIAGNOSTIC APPROACH

With massive hemorrhage from the small bowel, the source of bleeding is usually diagnosed rapidly by bleeding scan and angiography, and exploratory surgery is usually successful. If bleeding is not brisk or is intermittent, the bleeding site may not be readily apparent at surgery; then exploration must be coupled with intraoperative endoscopy, angiography, or scintigraphy.[24] Difficulty in diagnosis commonly is encountered in the patient presenting with anemia, melena, or a positive fecal occult blood test when the diagnosis has not been established by barium radiography or endoscopy. Once all the standard examinations are negative, the small bowel is assumed to be the source of blood loss. Because of the increased yield of significant pathology provided by push enteroscopy when all other diagnostic tests are unrevealing, this procedure should be considered prior to repeating any of the previous examinations. Finally, sonde enteroscopy can evaluate the remainder of the small intestine and provide the diagnosis in a significant number of patients. Bleeding scans and angiography are withheld unless the patient is actively bleeding. Depending on these results, exploratory surgery can then be carried out, coupled with intraoperative endoscopy in a select group of patients. When diffuse angiodysplasias of the small intestine are discovered by enteroscopy, the patient may not be amenable to surgical therapy. Despite lack of a preoperative diagnosis in patients with normal enteroscopic exams, exploratory surgery is advocated especially in the patient younger than 50 years when small bowel tumors and Meckel's diverticulum are most likely.

CONCLUSIONS

The small intestine is an uncommon site for gastrointestinal bleeding. However, in the patient with obscure bleeding, the small bowel is often found to be the source of blood loss. Most causes of bleeding are benign, but the diagnosis is often hindered by the small intestine's inaccessibility. Enteroscopy has permitted a new and fruitful method of evaluation in these patients. When standard diagnostic tests are negative, enteroclysis should precede enteroscopy. A red cell–labeled radioisotope scan may be appropriate before enteroscopy when persistent bleeding is suspected. Angiography is rarely of benefit in the investigation of chronic obscure bleeding. Exploratory laparotomy has a role in examination of the patient who requires multiple blood transfusions for obscure bleeding, but the surgeon should be prepared to utilize intraoperative endoscopy of the small bowel.

REFERENCES

1. Netterville R, Hardy J, Martin R: Small bowel hemorrhage. *Ann Surg* 167:949–957, 1968.
2. Thompson J, Salem R, Hemingway A: Specialist investigation of obscure gastrointestinal bleeding. *Gut* 28:7–51, 1987.

3. Spechler S, Schimmel E: Gastrointestinal tract bleeding of unknown origin. *Arch Intern Med* 142:236–240, 1982.
4. Peterson W: Obscure gastrointestinal bleeding. *Med Clin North Am* 72:1169–1176, 1988.
5. Thompson J, Hemingway A, McPherson G, et al: Obscure gastrointestinal haemorrhage of small-bowel origin. *Br Med J* 288:1663–1665, 1984.
6. Boley S, Sammartano R, Adams A, et al: On the nature and etiology of vascular ectasias of the colon. *Gastroenterology* 72:650–660, 1977.
7. Boley S, Sprayregen S, Sammartano R, et al: The pathophysiologic basis for the angiographic signs of vascular ectasias of the colon. *Radiology* 125:615–621, 1977.
8. Martin L, Max M, Richardson J, et al: Small bowel tumors: Continuing challenge. *South Med J* 73:981–985, 1980.
9. Ashley S, Wells S: Tumors of the small intestine. *Semin Oncol* 15:116–128, 1988.
10. Lewis B, Kornbluth A, Waye J: Small bowel tumours, yield of enteroscopy. *Gut* 32:763–765, 1991.
11. Farmer R, Hawk W, Turnbull R: Clinical patterns in Crohn's disease: A statistical study of 615 cases. *Gastroenterology* 68:627–635, 1975.
12. Gryboski J, Spiro H: Prognosis in children with Crohn's disease. *Gastroenterology* 74:807–817, 1978.
13. Sparberg M, Kirsner J: Recurrent hemorrhage in regional enteritis: Report of 3 cases. *Am J Dig Dis* 8:652–657, 1966.
14. Brown C, Olshaker J: Meckel's diverticulum. *Am J Emerg Med* 6:157–164, 1988.
15. Bowden T: Endoscopy of the small intestine. *Surg Clin North Am* 69:1237–1247, 1989.
16. Rabe F, Becker G, Begozzi M, et al: Efficacy study of the small-bowel examination. *Radiology* 140:47–50, 1981.
17. Rex D, Lappas J, Maglinte D: Enteroclysis in the evaluation of suspected small intestinal bleeding. *Gastroenterology* 97:58–60, 1989.
18. Markisz J, Front D, Royal H: An evaluation of 99M-Tc labeled red blood cell scintigraphy for the detection and localization of gastrointestinal bleeding sites. *Gastroenterology* 83:394–398, 1982.
19. Bunker S, Brown J, McAuley R: Detection of gastrointestinal bleeding sites: Use of in vitro Tc 99m-labelled RBC's. *JAMA* 247:789–792, 1982.
20. Khettery J, Effmann E, Grand R, et al: Effect of pentagastrin, histalog, glucagon, secretin, and perchlorate on the gastric handling of 99mTc pertechnetate in mice. *Radiology* 120:629–631, 1976.
21. Browder W, Cerise E, Litwin M: Impact of emergency angiography in massive lower gastrointestinal bleeding. *Ann Surg* 204:530–536, 1986.
22. Fiorito J, Brandt L, Kozicky O, et al: The diagnostic yield of superior mesenteric angiography: Correlation with the pattern of gastrointestinal bleeding. *Am J Gastroenterol* 84:878–881, 1989.
23. Retzlaff J, Hagedorn A, Bartholomen L: Abdominal exploration for gastrointestinal bleeding of obscure origin. *JAMA* 177:104–107, 1961.
24. Biener A, Palestro C, Lewis B, et al: Intraoperative scintigraphy for active small intestinal bleeding. *Surg Gynecol Oncol* 171:388–392, 1990.
25. Tada M, Kawai K: Small bowel endoscopy. *Scand J Gastroenterol* 19(Suppl 102):39–52, 1984.
26. Lewis B, Waye J: Small bowel enteroscopy in 1988: Pros and cons. *Am J Gastroenterol* 83:799–802, 1988.

27. Foutch P, Sawyer R, Sanowski R: Push enteroscopy for diagnosis of patients with gastrointestinal bleeding of obscure origin. *Gastrointest Endosc* 36:337–341, 1990.

28. Shimizu S, Tada M, Kawai K: Development of a new insertion technique in push-type enteroscopy. *Am J Gastroenterol* 82:884–887, 1987.

29. Lewis B, Waye J: Chronic gastrointestinal bleeding of obscure origin, the role of small bowel enteroscopy. *Gastroenterology* 94:1117–1120, 1988.

30. Lewis B: Conquering the last frontier: Is it necessary? *Gastrointest Endosc* 37:97–99, 1991.

31. Lewis B, Wenger J, Waye J: Small bowel enteroscopy and intraoperative enteroscopy for obscure gastrointestinal bleeding. *Am J Gastroenterol* 86:171–174, 1991.

14

LARGE BOWEL SOURCES OF BLEEDING

Frank J. Harford, M.D.
Jack Pickleman, M.D.

Once nasogastric suction, with or without upper endoscopy, has established that the source of blood loss is distal to the ligament of Treitz, diagnostic efforts should be directed first to the large bowel, which bleeds more frequently than the small bowel. The colon is also more accessible for investigative procedures. The assessment should begin with anoscopy and proctosigmoidoscopy performed with a proper light source. The anoscopic exam begins with manual traction on the perianal skin to evert all the anoderm up to the dentate line. This is best done with the patient in the jackknife position. When this is not possible, a left lateral position with the knees flexed is acceptable. This permits visualization of anal fissures, which are typically confined to the anoderm and do not extend above the dentate line. Fissures may easily be missed if this maneuver is neglected and one proceeds directly to anoscopy, since the folds of anoderm collapse when the anoscope is removed rapidly, obscuring the view of a fissure. After visual inspection, an anoscope is gently inserted to assess the anal canal for the presence of hemorrhoids or other bleeding sources in the anal canal or lower rectum. After anoscopy, a proctoscope is inserted. This procedure is best done with a rigid sigmoidoscope, which permits rectal irrigation and evacuation of any clot. If no bleeding source is found with proctoscopy and the bleeding is moderate or mild, one may attempt colonoscopy. Massive amounts of clot or continuous brisk bleeding make colonoscopy futile. When continuous bleeding is apparent, one should proceed to a radionuclide scan to confirm ongoing bleeding and to identify its approximate location. A positive scan should lead to contrast angiography to pinpoint the source of bleeding more precisely and possibly to intervene therapeutically. If it is obvious that there is continued brisk bleeding, the nuclear scan should be bypassed in favor of immediate arteriography. Most authorities feel that an angiogram is not indicated if the radionuclide scan is negative (Figure 14.1), but two recent studies have cast some doubt on the sensitivity of tagged red cell scan.[1,1a]

DIVERTICULAR BLEEDING

Although there are many causes of lower gastrointestinal (GI) bleeding, the most common etiology of massive lower GI bleeding is diverticulosis.[2-3] Parks, in an unse-

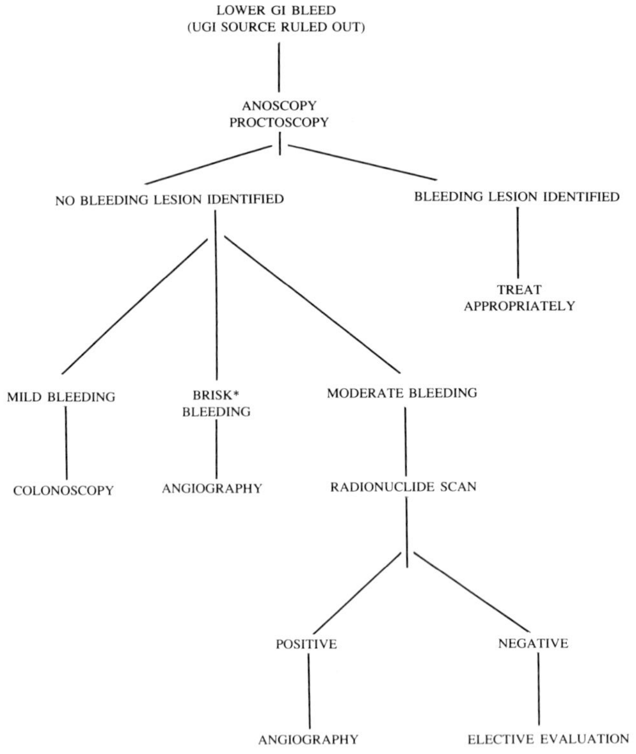

Figure 14.1. Diagnostic evaluation.

lected autopsy study done in the United Kingdom, found that 40% of the population at age 60 had diverticula and that the incidence increased with advancing age.[4] The purported incidence of bleeding in diverticular disease varies from 3 to 5%.[5] Hemorrhage from diverticulosis occurs in the absence of diverticulitis; is often massive, causing a significant change in hematocrit, if not hypotension; and usually ceases spontaneously with conservative management. Once the bleeding has stopped, the incidence of rebleeding is 25%. Surviving patients who bleed a second time will likely bleed a third time if they are not resected.[6,7] Minor bleeding from colonic diverticula is probably due to the presence of granulation tissue within a diverticulum, whereas massive hemorrhage is secondary to erosion of the vasa recta at the base of the diverticula.[8]

Browder et al. reported visualization of extravasated contrast in 36 of 50 patients (72%) who underwent emergency angiography for active lower GI bleeding. Lack of contrast extravasation in the remaining 14 patients probably reflected cessation of bleeding while waiting for the study to be performed. Hemorrhage in 19 of the 36 patients with positive arteriograms appeared to emanate from diverticulosis. Most of the remaining 17 patients bled from angiodysplastic lesions. Vasopressin infusion stopped the bleeding in 20 of 22 patients (91%), but 10 of the 20 (50%) rebled after the infusion was stopped.[2a] Both the diverticular and the angiodysplastic bleeding lesions responded equally well to vasopressin infusion, but rebleeding occurred more frequently in the patients bleeding from diverticulosis. These results are similar to those previously obtained by Athanasoulis et al., who reported cessation of bleeding in 22 of 24 patients with massive hemorrhage from diverticular bleeding and a 23% rebleeding rate while still hospitalized.[9]

Other authors have not found arteriography or vasopressin infusion to be as useful. Leitman et al. were able to identify the bleeding site clearly in patients undergoing emergency arteriography for massive lower GI hemorrhage in only 27 (40%) of 68 patients. Twelve (29%) of the patients with a negative arteriogram required emergency operative intervention.[3] Intra-arterial infusion of vasopressin or embolization (1 patient) was successful in 5 of 14 patients in whom it was attempted (36%), but 2 patients died from procedure-related complications, namely, myocardial infarction during vasopressin infusion and intestinal infarction after attempted embolization.[3]

If bleeding from a diverticulum has been identified and controlled acutely with vasopressin, the incidence of rebleeding while in the hospital varies from 22% to 50%. The remaining patients discharged without rebleeding have a 25% probability of a later bleed.[9] This incidence of rebleeding after discharge approximates the expected rebleeding rate seen in patients whose hemorrhage stopped spontaneously.[7]

When a patient is admitted with an obvious and refractory massive lower GI bleed from a lesion not seen on anorectal examination or by angiography, immediate operative exploration for possible subtotal colectomy is warranted. During surgery, a thorough evaluation of the small bowel helps rule out a more proximal cause of the bleeding. The intraoperative finding that all of the intraluminal blood is confined to the colon despite ongoing active hemorrhage reassures the surgeon that the bleeding is, in fact, from the large intestine. In contrast, the presence of blood in the terminal ileum raises the possibility that the bleeding point may be located proximal to the colon and did not reach the terminal ileum by retrograde reflux.

When a specific bleeding site is localized in the colon by angiography but bleeding does not stop with vasopressin infusion, the choice of operation is somewhat controversial. One must decide between a segmental colon resection and a subtotal (abdominal) colectomy. This dilemma is especially pertinent when the bleeding has been localized in the right colon in a patient with known diverticular disease in the left colon seen on prior studies or discovered during laparotomy. Welsh and Newhall and their colleagues recommend subtotal colectomy in this situation,[10,11] while Boley and Wright and their co-authors advocate segmental resection whenever a bleeding site has been identified.[2,12] We usually prefer a subtotal colectomy in the patient with bleeding localized to one side of the colon with disease on the opposite side as well (Figure 14.2).

ANGIODYSPLASIA

Prior to 1960, most massive lower GI bleeding was ascribed to diverticular disease.[6] This was a presumptive diagnosis based on the finding of diverticulosis on barium enema, a nondiagnostic rigid proctosigmoidoscopy, and the absence of an upper GI source of bleeding. In 1960, Margulis et al. demonstrated a bleeding arteriovenous malformation on visceral angiography.[13] Since that time, most reports of massive lower GI bleeding have included significant numbers of patients with angiodysplasia,[2-3,10,12,14] although some studies report a low incidence of bleeding angiodysplasia.[15,16] Comparison of various published series is somewhat problematical, as the patient populations are not well defined, the methods of diagnosis differ, and uniform criteria for confirming a given diagnosis are not established.

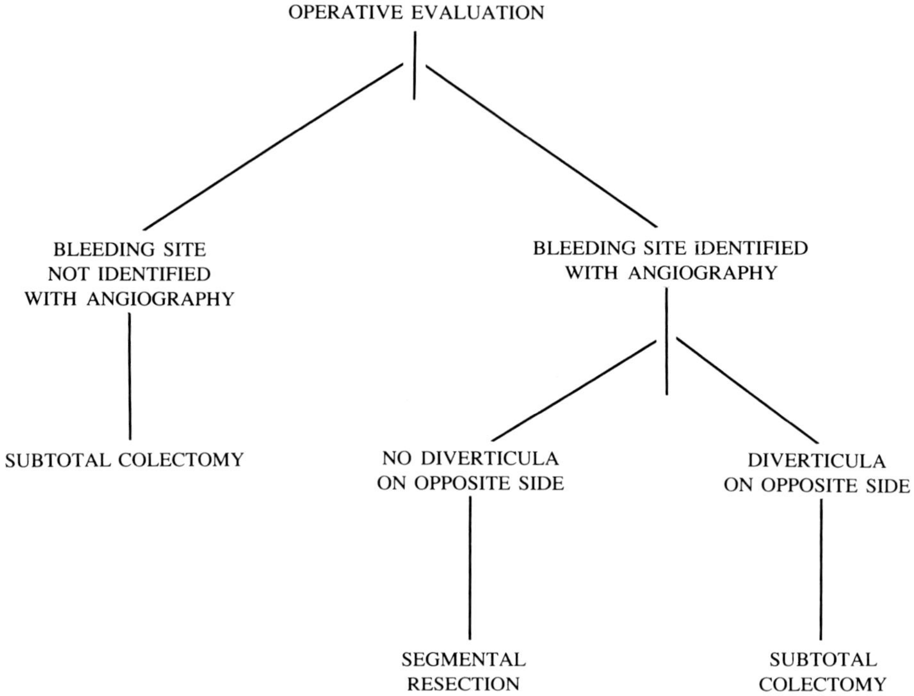

Figure 14.2. Operative evaluation.

These lesions have been referred to as *vascular ectasias, angiomas, arteriovenous malformations,* and *angiodysplasias*. They are thought to be degenerative lesions caused by the intermittent obstruction of submucosal veins by a contraction of the muscular coat of the bowel wall. The submucosal veins eventually become dilated and tortuous. With time, the small venules of the arteriolar-capillary-venular units also become dilated. Eventually, the capillary rings surrounding the crypts become dilated and the precapillary sphincters become incompetent, forming a small arteriovenous fistula.[17] These changes can be depicted angiographically. The earliest and most frequent sign is the presence of a dilated, slowly emptying intramural vein, usually seen on the antimesenteric border of the bowel. This dilation is noted in 90% of the patients with angiodysplasia. A vascular tuft, namely, dilation of the mucosal veins and capillaries, is seen in 70–80% of patients. An early filling vein, seen in 60–70% of patients, highlights the arteriovenous fistula stage. All three findings are found in over half of the patients with bleeding angiodysplastic lesions.[18]

Most angiodysplastic lesions are located in the right colon. The 20% of patients with transverse or left colon lesions often have synchronous lesions in the right colon. These lesions are multiple in 25–50% of patients.[2a,14,19] Bleeding from angiodysplasia is most often low grade and recurrent. Only about 15% of patients present with massive lower GI hemorrhage. Boley and Brandt have pointed out that the nature and degree of bleeding frequently vary in the same patient with different bleeding episodes.[18] Some patients (20–25%) have only dark-colored stools, whereas others in (10–15%) show only an iron deficiency anemia. Bleeding stops spontaneously in over 90% of patients.[18] As with diverticulosis, most patients with angiodysplasia never bleed. Boley et al. have estimated that 25% of the population over the age of 60 have angiodysplasia.[17] In contrast, Richter et al. estimated that only 1.4% of people over the age of 50 have angiodysplasia.[20] Studies of the natural history of nonbleeding angiodysplastic lesions are few, but when these lesions are visualized as incidental findings, future bleeding is infrequent.[20]

A diagnosis of angiodysplasia can be made with angiography or colonoscopy. The angiographic criteria have been described. Given the usually intermittent nature of the bleeding in angiodysplasis, it is not surprising that only 10–20% of patients have extravasation demonstrated angiographically. When extravasation is demonstrated in patients with active hemorrhage, the success rate in controlling the bleeding with vasopressin infusion is about the same as in diverticular bleeding, namely, about 70%.[2a] This procedure, however, is not risk free. Boley[18] has observed infarction of the sigmoid colon and ischemia of the leg following vasopressin infusion in the inferior mesenteric artery. Recognizing that blood flow through the inferior mesenteric artery is only a small fraction of that through the superior mesenteric artery, he advocates a reduction in the usual 0.1 to 0.4 units/min doses of vasopressin. Arterial embolization of lesions has been reported but carries certain risks. Both bowel infarction and late stricture have been observed following this treatment.[21,22] Embolization thus should be reserved for the most desperate situations.

The colonoscopic diagnosis of angiodysplasia is based on the finding of clusters of dilated submucosal arterioles 2–10 mm in diameter that are flat or slightly raised and have a prominent draining vein originating with the tuft. Several methods for the treatment of angiodysplasia with thermal energy are available. These include monopolar and bioplar electrocoagulation, heater probe, and laser.[23] Of the electrosurgical techniques available, bipolar coagulation appears to be the safest in the experimental model.[24] Rutgeerts et al. reported a decrease in bleeding episodes and transfusion requirements using the YAG laser. This, however, was associated with a 6% rate of perforation. They recommend that the total energy applied to each lesion should not exceed 200 joules. They also observed that the greater the number of lesions present, the less effective was the laser treatment. Patients with Weber-Osler-Rendu syndrome did poorly, as did those with von Willebrand's disease.[25] Theoretically, the argon laser would be a safer modality, as it causes less tissue destruction. There has been some accumulated experience with this laser in treating upper GI bleeding;[26] however, there is no large reported experience with large bowel bleeding. Richter et al. followed patients who were treated with coagulation using the hot biopsy forceps technique, as well as those who were treated surgically, for comparison to a group treated only with medical supportive measures. The bleeding rate in those patients treated medically or endoscopically was 2½ times that of the surgical group.[20] A controlled trial of the various treatment modalities has yet to be done.

Surgical treatment in the Richter et al. series was associated with rebleeding rates of 16% within one year and 24% within three years.[20] This approximates the incidence of rebleeding reported by Boley et al. after segmental resection.[27] The Hammersmith Hospital team found that 22% of patients undergoing operations for colonic angiodysplasia also had small bowel lesions which were found during celiotomy or when the patient returned later for recurrent bleeding.[28] We recommend intraoperative enteroscopy at the time of segmental colon resection in patients with angiodysplasia.

Table 14.1. Hemangiomas

Type	*Histological Characteristics*	*Gross Characteristics*
Capillary	Closely packed capillary-like vascular structures No true capsule	Red spots on mucosa Usually asymptomatic
Cavernous	Large, thin-walled vascular channels No true capsule	Discrete, diffuse, and expansile or infiltrating
Phlebectasia	Collections of multiple small, discrete cavernous lesions	Lesions less than 5 mm Usually asymptomatic

HEMANGIOMAS

The first case of hemangioma of the rectum was described by Philips in 1839.[29] Since that time, approximately 200 cases of large bowel hemangiomas have been reported.[30] The majority of these lesions are located in the rectum or rectosigmoid.

These patients usually present with a history of repeated episodes of hematochezia, often starting in childhood. Occasionally patients may have symptoms of tenesmus, urgency, or incomplete defecation. In the series of cases reported from St. Mark's Hospital, 80% of the patients had undergone at least one surgical procedure before the correct diagnosis was made.[31] Skin lesions may be seen in association with colorectal hemangiomas. Nader and Margolin found cutaneous lesions in half of their pediatric patients with large bowel hemangiomas.[32] Those patients with associated skin lesions were likely to have multiple rather than solitary intestinal lesions. A familial tendency to develop gastrointestinal hemangiomas has also been noted. Cavernous hemangiomas may be found occasionally in association with a Klippel-Trenaunay syndrome.[33]

Hemangiomas can be classified as capillary, cavernous, or mixed. The large majority of large bowel hemangiomas are cavernous. Capillary hemangiomas are composed of networks of tiny capillary-like vascular structures. These vessels are closely packed together but have no true capsule. Cavernous hemangiomas are composed of large, thin-walled vascular channels. These lesions may be discrete, diffuse and expansive, or infiltrating. There is a variety of cavernous hemangioma, called *multiple phlebectasia,* which consists of collections of multiple small, discrete, cavernous lesions. They are usually asymptomatic. A small number of hemangiomas have elements of both capillary and cavernous characteristics. The expansive, infiltrating type of lesions may extend into adjacent structures such as the bladder or uterus, but they usually retain their own vascular supply[34] (Table 14.1).

Whether these lesions are truly neoplastic or simply congenital vascular malformations remains controversial. There is, however, general agreement that they develop from embryonic sequestrations of mesodermal tissue. Capillary hemangiomas are considered to be a result of anomalous development in the first stage of mesodermal stem cell differentiation. Cavernous hemangiomas reflect aberrations in a later stage of development.[34]

The diagnosis of rectal hemangioma can usually be made without difficulty on physical and proctoscopic examinations. One should be alerted to a possible hemangioma by a history of recurrent, painless hematochezia, usually starting in childhood. Any cutaneous hemangioma found on general physical examination should enhance one's suspicions. Many of these patients are also anemic.[35] Cavernous hemangiomas also may be associated with thrombocytopenia, defibrination, and depression of factors V and VIII. This has been referred to as the *Kasabach-Merritt syndrome*.[36] On digital examination, the tumor may be felt as a soft, compressible mass that is poorly defined. The stool is often hemoccult positive. On proctoscopic examination, these lesions will be seen as wine- or plum-colored masses that collapse with insufflation of pressure from the proctoscope. A small cavernous hemangioma may present as a bluish discoloration on a polyp. Capillary hemangiomas often appear as cherry red spots on the mucosa. These are usually asymptomatic. The rectal mucosa over the lesions may show chronic inflammatory changes on both gross and microscopic examinations. This, on occasion, will result in a misdiagnosis. When a cavernous hemangioma is present on digital and endoscopic examination, biopsy is ill advised. Total colonoscopy should be done to assess the extent of the lesion and to search for multiple lesions. Fifty percent of patients with intestinal hemangiomas will have phlebolith clusters noted on plain abdominal films (Figure 14.3). Mesenteric angiography will detect these lesions in two-thirds of patients. Some authors advocate angiography in all patients with a cavernous hemangioma in order to define the vascular supply of the lesion.[37] Computed tomography (CT) scanning may help define the limits of the lesion and detect infiltration of local structures.[37] Magnetic resonance

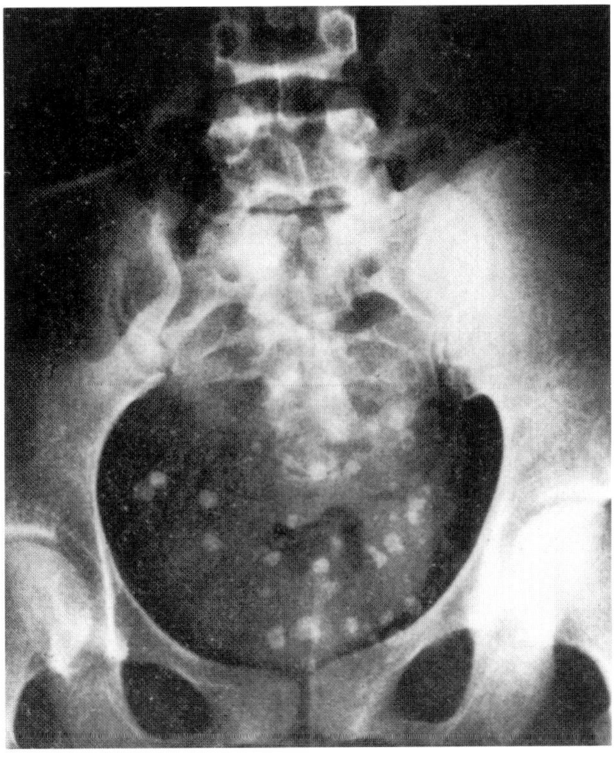

Figure 14.3. Phlebolith clusters in a patient with rectal hemangioma. Reprinted with permission from Bland RI, Abney HT, MacGregor AMC, et al: Hemangiomatosis of the colon and anorectum. *Am Surgeon* 40:626–635, 1974.

imaging (MRI) has also been used, but no clear advantage over CT has been demonstrated.[38]

Capillary hemangiomas or small cavernous hemangiomas may be treated endoscopically with electric snare cautery or with local resection. Larger cavernous hemangiomas, however, do not lend themselves to local treatment. Various reported nonoperative remedies have included injection of sclerosing agents, radiotherapy, and cryosurgery, but surgical resection is clearly the therapy of choice in the medically fit patient.[30] Although abdominoperineal resection has been recommended[39] as a treatment for rectal cavernous hemangiomas, recent successful applications of sphincter-sparing procedures are gaining in popularity.[31,39-41]

VARICES OF THE LARGE INTESTINE

Varices of the large intestine are an uncommon source of lower GI bleeding. Most colonic varices arise in patients with portal hypertension, and the remainder are probably secondary to vascular malformations. Gudjonsson et al. reviewed the literature in 1986 and found 69 cases of colonic varices.[42]

Normally, there are communications between the portal and systemic venous circulations in the esophagus, the diaphragm, the retroperitoneum, and the rectum. Portal hypertension causes enlargement of these natural shunts and can also open embryological vessels, as seen when the periumbilical veins dilate and develop into a caput medusae.[43] Other portal systemic shunts open in areas of adhesions of the bowel to the abdominal wall at incision sites or at the mucocutaneous junction of ileostomies, colostomies, or ureterostomies. Portal hypertension in most of the reported patients is secondary to alcoholic cirrhosis and is due to portal vein obstruction in the remainder. There is one case report of colon varices following vena caval ligation, an example of so-called downhill varices.[44] Britton studied 92 patients with splenoportography and found that the coronary-azygos system was the main portosystemic connection in most patients, whereas 25% of the patients had the inferior mesenteric-internal iliac communication as the major portosystemic shunt.[45] There have been several reports of bleeding from large bowel varices following obliteration of esophageal varices with sclerotherapy.[46,47]

One should make the distinction between rectal varices and hemorrhoids. Internal hemorrhoids are vascular cushions located in the anal canal. Thomson, in his careful anatomical studies, demonstrated that hemorrhoids are not varicose veins, but rather vascular tissue composed of arterioles and venules with communications between the two in a stroma of fibro-collagenous supportive tissue, without any direct connection to the branches of the portal vein.[48] These findings have been confirmed by others.[49,50] Jacobs et al. surveyed a large portal hypertensive population and found that the incidence of hemorrhoids in this group was not increased compared to the normal population.[51] They noted, however, that the hemorrhoids appeared to be under increased pressure in patients with portal hypertension. They postulated that coagulation abnormalities played an important part in hemorrhoidal bleeding in the cirrhotic.

Varices appear as bulging veins in the rectal vault which may extend all the way down to the anal canal or even the anal verge. When present at the anal verge, they may be distinguished from external hemorrhoids by their easy compressibility and prompt refilling once pressure is released. Hemorrhoids, in contrast, appear as engorged vascular cushions in the anal canal and do not decompress easily with digital pressure. Gudjonsson et al. demonstrated that colonic varices were located within the inferior mesenteric vein system in 66% of patients, within the superior mesenteric vein in 26%, and within both systems in the remainder.[42] Those patients with diffuse varices throughout the colon have associated vascular anomalies. Manzi and Samanta have reported a patient with varices with adhesions in the absence of portal hypertension or other associated conditions;[52] possibly this patient had an underlying vascular malformation, prompting the subtotal colectomy which led to the adhesions in which the varices were thought to have developed. The entity of adhesion-related colonic varices without some associated portal hypertension or vascular anomaly remains problematic.

The diagnosis of colorectal varices can be made with various methods. Anorectal varices are easily diagnosed with a rigid proctoscope or anoscope. Colonic varices may be seen with a colonoscope. One must recognize that insufflation of air may compress the varices, which may then be overlooked. Careful viewing of the luminal surface without excessive air insufflation circumvents this problem. Visceral angiography has a 95% sensitivity in collected series.[42] Barium enema is reported to be falsely negative in half of the cases, but this, again, may be technique dependent. Detection with a technetium 99m-labeled red cell scan[42] and a 99m technetium-sulfur colloid scan[53] has been reported. Transhepatic portography is very effective in outlining the varices and is more likely than arteriography to demonstrate extravasation in the presence of bleeding. Portal pressures may, of course, be measured at the same time.[54]

There have been three reports of successful local therapy of rectal varices using sclerosing agents.[53-56] In one instance, a large rectal ulcer developed. Caution is advised if the varices are injected above the peritoneal reflection. One patient who was considered too sick for a portosystemic shunt[57] had successful embolization of rectal varices with Gelfoam and coils via a transhepatic portal catheter. Several authors report successful treatment of rectal varices by ligation with running locking sutures.[58-60] Johansen et al. described inserting a gauze pack in the anal canal after suture ligation to tamponade bleeding from the needle holes.[60] Such patients require careful monitoring, since recurrent bleeding will no longer be evident as hematochezia. There is also one report describing the successful use of cryosurgery.[61]

The operative treatment of colonic varices in patients with portal hypertension should be a portosystemic shunt, as the results with resection are uniformly dismal.[42] In contrast, resection is the procedure of choice if the varices are secondary to a vascular malformation. Resection would also be indicated in those patients with segmental occlusion of portal venous outflow. Patients who have variceal bleeding from a colostomy or another enterocutaneous stoma may be treated locally with suture ligation or with reconstruction of the stoma. The latter can be accomplished with a local anesthetic by incising the mucocutaneous junction and carefully dissecting out the large veins for division and ligation. This is a temporary but extremely effective method for dealing with stomal varices.[62] A portosystemic shunt provides long-term resolution for stomal varices, but the risk of this approach precludes its application to a problem which can be controlled with a safe local procedure even if it must be repeated from time to time.

In the presence of portal hypertension, internal hemorrhoids are no more common than they are in the general population. However, when they do occur, bleeding may be more troublesome. Nichols advocates treating true hemorrhoids with rubber band ligation, either alone or accompanied by infrared coagulation.[63] Nivatvongs has advised suture ligation.[64] Jacobs et al. have advocated initial rubber band ligation and, if this fails, single-quadrant hemorrhoidectomy to control refractory bleeding; if bleeding persists from other sites, they recommend staging further quadrant excisions.[51]

INFLAMMATORY BOWEL DISEASE

Although minor GI bleeding is common in patients with inflammatory bowel disease, severe hemorrhage is considerably less frequent. Major bleeding occurs in up to 6% of patients with equal frequency in both Crohn's disease and ulcerative colitis.[65,66] Robert and co-workers reported on 21 patients with Crohn's disease and GI hemorrhage.[65] The majority of these patients had ileocolitis (66%) rather than enteritis alone (19%) or colitis alone (14%). This bleeding incidence represented 0.7% of the patients being followed for isolated small bowel disease and 1.7% of patients with colonic involvement. The bleeding stopped spontaneously in 50% of the patients, of whom 30–35% rebleed. There were three deaths among the 21 patients; two deaths occurred in patients treated nonoperatively, and one death was due to a severe hemorrhage seven years after a subtotal colectomy and ileostomy for a prior hemorrhage. These authors recommend bowel resection at the time of the first bleed, considering the 33% incidence of rebleeding with conservative management.

This same group reported on 25 patients with ulcerative colitis and severe hemorrhage.[66] Twenty-two (88%) of these patients were treated surgically. Half of the operations were done emergently, and half were semielective resections. Four of the surgical patients also had toxic megacolon, which was the prime reason that prompted the operation. Five patients underwent total proctocolectomy and 17 patients had a subtotal colectomy, usually with a mucus fistula. One patient had a one-stage ileosigmoidostomy. Two patients had postoperative bleeding from the remaining rectum. We would suggest that patients operated on for severe hemorrhage have a very low anterior resection, amputating the rectum at the levator muscles. This should eliminate any problems with postoperative bleeding while at the same time preserving the option of a subsequent ileoanal pull-through operation. If pathological interpretation of the surgical specimen favors Crohn's disease rather than ulcerative colitis, the remaining rectum and anus can be removed via a perineal approach, thus eliminating the need for a second laparotomy.

ISCHEMIC COLITIS

Although bloody diarrhea with pain is commonly the presenting symptom complex in ischemic colitis, the bleeding itself is occasionally acute or massive enough to merit emergent surgical intervention. Ischemic colitis is usually a self-limiting process, but occasionally the patient has a smoldering course with continuing significant but not massive blood loss. Surgical resection is indicated in both of these situations.[67] One must be particularly concerned that the colon remaining after resection is well perfused.

RADIATION INJURY

Severe chronic radiation injury in the form of proctosigmoiditis may be seen following pelvic radiation. This may result in stricture, fistulization, severe pain and tenesmus, and chronic bleeding.[68,69] Complete diversion of the fecal stream with colostomy is sometimes effective.[70] However, if bleeding is the only problem, laser photocoagulation using either the Argon or YAG laser has been shown to be helpful.[71-73]

ANAL CANAL LESIONS

Occasionally, hemorrhoids can cause significant lower GI bleeding. When a patient with lower GI bleeding is hemodynamically unstable, ligation is the procedure of choice. This may serve as the definitive treatment. After stabilization, additional procedures, when needed, include rubber band ligation, bipolar coagulation, infrared coagulation, and formal surgical hemorrhoidectomy.

Bleeding from anal fissure is usually a self-limiting episodic occurrence, but on occasion the bleeding may persist. When this occurs, the bleeding is almost always coming from the edges of the anoderm and can be easily controlled with cautery.

MISCELLANEOUS LESIONS

Any tumor, benign or malignant, from either the small or the large bowel, can bleed massively, but this is an uncommon presentation for these neoplasms. Massive bleeding has been reported from a Dieulafoy's ulcer (exulceratio simplex) in both the jejunum and the colon.[74-76] These lesions are minute mucosal erosions of large submucosal arteries. They are rare and are usually located in the stomach. The treatment of small bowel or colonic lesions is surgical resection.

REFERENCES

1. Bentley DE, Richardson JD: Role of tagged red blood cell imaging in the localization of gastrointestinal bleeding. *Arch Surg* 126:821–824, 1991.

1a. Voeller GR, Bunch G, Britt LG: Use of technetium-labeled red blood cell scintigraphy in the detection and management of gastrointestinal hemorrhage. *Surg* 110:799–804, 1991.

2. Boley SJ, Brandt LJ, Frank MS: Severe lower intestinal bleeding: Diagnosis and treatment. *Clin Gastroenterol* 10:65–91, 1981.

2a. Browder W, Cerise EJ, Litwin MS: Impact of emergency angiography in massive lower gastrointestinal bleeding. *Ann Surg* 209:530–536, 1986.

3. Leitman IM, Paull DE, Shires GT: Evaluation and management of massive lower gastrointestinal hemorrhage. *Ann Surg* 209:175–180, 1989.

4. Parks JG: Postmortem studies on the colon with special reference to diverticular disease. *Proc R Soc Med* 61:932–934, 1968.

5. Sleisinger MH, Fortran JS. *Gastrointestinal Disease*, ed 4. Philadelphia, WB Saunders Co, 1989.

6. Noer RJ: Hemorrhage as a complication of diverticulosis. *Am Surg* 141:674–685, 1955.

7. McGuire HH, Hayes BW: Massive hemorrhage from diverticulosis of the colon. *Ann Surg* 175:847–855, 1972.

8. Meyers MA, Alonso DR, Gray GF, et al: Pathogenesis of bleeding colonic diverticulosis. *Gastroenterology* 71:577–583, 1976.

9. Athanasoulis CA, Baum S, Rosch J, et al: Mesenteric arterial infusions of vasopressin for hemorrhage from colonic diverticulosis. *Am J Surg* 129:213–216, 1975.

10. Welch CE, Athanasoulis CA, Galdabini JJ: Hemorrrhage from the large bowel with special reference to angiodysplasia and diverticular disease. *World J Surg* 2:73–83, 1978.
11. Newhall SC, Lucas CE, Ledgerwood AM: Diagnostic and therapeutic approach to colonic bleeding. *Am J Surg* 47:136–142, 1981.
12. Wright HK, Pelliccia O, Higgins EF, et al: Controlled, semielective, segmental resection for massive colonic hemorrhage. *Am J Surg* 139:535–538, 1980.
13. Margulis AR, Heinbecker P, Bernard HR: Operative mesenteric arteriography in the search for the site of bleeding in unexplained gastrointestinal hemorrhage: A preliminary report. *Surgery* 48:534–539, 1960.
14. Emanuel RB, Weiser MM, Shenoy SS, et al: Arteriovenous malformations as a cause of gastrointestinal bleeding: The importance of triple-vessel angiographic studies in diagnosis and prevention of rebleeding. *J Clin Gastroenterol* 7:237–246, 1985.
15. Giacchino L, Geis WP, Pickleman J, et al: Changing perspectives in massive lower intestinal hemorrhage. *Surgery* 86:368–376, 1979.
16. Eaton AC: Emergency surgery for acute colonic hemorrhage—a retrospective study. *Br J Surg* 68:109–112, 1981.
17. Boley SJ, Sammartano RH, Adams A, et al: On the nature and etiology of vascular ectasias of the colon: Degenerative lesions of aging. *Gastroenterology* 72:650–660, 1977.
18. Boley SJ, Brandt LJ: Vascular ectasias of the colon—1986. *Dig Dis Sci* 31:26S–42S, 1986.
19. Tedesco FJ, Griffin JW, Khan AQ: Vascular ectasia of the colon: Clinical, colonoscopic, and radiographic features. *J Clin Gastroenterol* 2:233–238, 1980.
20. Richter JM, Christensen MR, Colditz GA, et al: Angiodysplasia. Natural history and efficacy of therapeutic interventions. *Dig Dis Sci* 34:1542–1546, 1989.
21. Matalo NM, Link DO: Selective embolization for control of gastrointestinal hemorrhage. *Am J Surg* 138:840–844, 1979.
22. Mitty HA, Efremidis S, Keller RJ: Colonic structure after transcatheter embolization for diverticular bleeding. *Am J Roentgenol* 133:519–521, 1979.
23. Schrock TR: Colonoscopic diagnosis and treatment of lower gastrointestinal bleeding. *Surg Endosc* 69:1309–1325, 1989.
24. Johnston JH, Jensen DM, Auth D: Experimental comparisons of endoscopic yttrium—aluminum garnet laser, electrosurgery, and heater probe for canine gut arterial coagulation. *Gastroenterology* 92:1101–1106, 1987.
25. Rutgeerts P, Van Gompel F, Geboes K, et al: Long term results of treatment of vascular malformations of the gastrointestinal tract by neodynium yag laser photocoagulations. *Gut* 26:586–593, 1986.
26. Swain CP: Laser photocoagulation in alimentary bleeding. *World J Surg* 7:710–718, 1983.
27. Boley SJ, Sammartano R, Brandt LJ, et al: Vascular ectasia of the colon. *Surg Gynecol Obstet* 149:353–359, 1979.
28. Steger AC, Galland RB, Hemingway A, et al: Gastrointestinal hemorrhage from a second source in patients with colonic angiodysplasia. *Br J Surg* 74:726–727, 1987.
29. Philips B: Surgical cases. *London Med Gaz* 23:514–517, 1839.
30. Lyon DT, Mantia AG: Large bowel hemangiomas. *Dis Colon Rectum* 27:404–414, 1984.
31. Jeffrey PH, Hawley PR, Parks AG: Colo-anal sleeve anastomosis in the treatment of diffuse cavernous hemangioma involving the rectum. *Br J Surg* 63:678–682, 1976.
32. Nader PR, Margolin F: Hemangioma causing gastrointestinal bleeding. *Am J Dis Child* 111:215–221, 1966.
33. Ghahremani GG, Kangarloo H, Volberg F, et al: Diffuse cavernous hemangioma of the colon in the Klippel-Trenaunay syndrome. *Radiology* 118:673–678, 1976.

34. Gentry RW, Docterty MB, Clagett OT: Vascular malformations and vascular tumors of the gastrointestinal tract. *Int Abst Surg* 88:281–323, 1949.
35. Bland RI, Abney HT, MacGregor AMC, et al: Hemangiomatosis of the colon and anorectum. *Am Surgeon* 40:626–635, 1974.
36. Rodriguez-Erdman F, Button L, Murray JE, et al: Kasabach-Merritt syndrome–coagulo-analytical observations. *Am J Sci* 261:9–15, 1971.
37. Aylward CA, Orangio GR, Lucas GW, et al: Diffuse cavernous hemangioma of the rectosigmoid—CT scan, a new diagnostic modality and surgical management using sphincter-saving procedures: Report of three cases. *Dis Colon Rectum* 31:797–802, 1988.
38. Lupetin AR: Diffuse cavernous hemangioma of the rectum: Evaluation and MRI. *Gastrointest Radiol* 15:343–345, 1990.
39. Coppa GF, Eng K, Localio SA: Surgical management of diffuse cavernous hemangioma of the colon, rectum, and anus. *Surg Gynecol Obstet* 159:17–22, 1984.
40. Cunningham JA, Garcias V, Quispe G: Diffuse cavernous rectal hemangioma—sphincter-sparing approach to therapy. *Dis Colon Rectum* 32:344–347, 1989.
41. Wang CH: Sphincter-saving procedure for treatment of diffuse cavernous hemangioma of the rectum and sigmoid colon. *Dis Colon Rectum* 28:604–607, 1985.
42. Gudjonsson H, Zeiler D, Gamelli RL, et al: Colonic varices: Report of an unusual case diagnosed by radionuclide scanning, with review of the literature. *Gastroenterology* 91:1543–1547, 1986.
43. Edwards EA: Functional anatomy of the portal-systemic communications. *Arch Intern Med* 88:137–154, 1991.
44. Bersou H, Wiringer P: Varices coliques chez une malade agant sulu une ligature de le veine cave inferieure. *J Radiol Electrol Med Nucl* 42:416–417, 1961.
45. Britton RCA: Influence of portal-systemic collateral patterns and distribution of varices on results of surgical treatment of bleeding esophageal varices. *Surgery* 53:567–574, 1963.
46. Foutch PG, Sivak MV: Colonic variceal hemorrhage after endoscopic injection sclerosis of esophageal varices: A report of three cases. *Am J Gastroenterol* 79:756–760, 1984.
47. Keane RM, Britton DC: Massive bleeding from rectal varices folowing repeated injection sclerotherapy of oesophageal varices. *Br J Surg* 73:120, 1986.
48. Thomson WHF: The nature of haemorrhoids. *Br J Surg* 62:542–552, 1975.
49. Bernstein WC: What are hemorrhoids and what is their relationship to the portal venous system? *Dis Colon Rectum* 26:829–834, 1983.
50. Haas PA, Fox TA, Haas GP: The pathogenesis of hemorrhoids. *Dis Colon Rectum* 27:442–450, 1984.
51. Jacobs DM, Bubrick MP, Onstad GR, et al: The relationship of hemorrhoids to portal hypertension. *Dis Colon Rectum* 23:567–569, 1980.
52. Manzi D, Samanta AK: Adhesion-related colonic varices. *J Clin Gastroenterol* 7:71–75, 1985.
53. Barry JW, Engle CV: Detection of hemorrhage in a patient with cecal varices using 99m Tc-sulphur colloid. *Radiology* 128:489–490, 1978.
54. Hseih JS, Huang CJ, Huang YS, et al: Demonstration of rectal varices by transhepatic inferior mesenteric venography. *Dis Colon Rectum* 29:459–461, 1986.
55. Richnon J, Berclaz R, Schneider PA, et al: Sclerotherapy of rectal varices. *Int J Colorect Dis* 3:132–134, 1988.
56. Weiserbs DB, Zfass AM, Messmer J: Control of massive hemorrhage from rectal varices with sclerotherapy. *Gastrointest Endosc* 32:419–420, 1986.
57. Weinshel E, Chen W, Falkenstein DB, et al: Hemorrhoids or rectal varices: Defining the cause of massive rectal hemorrhage in patients with portal hypertension. *Gastroenterology* 90:744–747, 1986.

58. McCormack TT, Bailey HR, Simms JM, et al: Rectal varices are not piles. *Br J Surg* 71:163, 1984.
59. Hosking SW, Johnson AG, Chir M: Bleeding anorectal varices—A misunderstood condition. *Surgery* 104:70–73, 1988.
60. Johansen K, Bardin J, Orloff MJ: Massive bleeding from hemorrhoidal varices in portal hypertension. *JAMA* 244:2084–2085, 1980.
61. Mashiah A: Massive bleeding from hemorrhoidal varices in portal hypertension. (Letter to the editor). *JAMA* 246:2323, 1981.
62. Beck DE, Fazio VW, Grundfest-Broniatowski S: Surgical management of bleeding stomal varices. *Dis Colon Rectum* 31:343–346, 1988.
63. Nichols TW: Internal hemorrhoidal bleeding in patients with portal hypertension. (Letter to the editor). *Gastrointest Endosc* 33:335, 1987.
64. Nivatvongs S: Suture of massive hemorrhoidal bleeding in portal hypertension. *Dis Colon Rectum* 28:878–879, 1985.
65. Robert JR, Sachar DB, Greenstein AJ: Severe gastrointestinal hemorrhage in Crohn's disease. *Ann Surg* 213:207–212, 1990.
66. Robert JR, Sachar DB, Aufses AH, et al: Management of severe hemorrhage in ulcerative colitis. *Am J Surg* 159:550–555, 1990.
67. Chou YH, Hsu S-C, Wang C-Y, et al: Ischemic colitis as a cause of massive lower gastrointestinal bleeding and peritonitis. *Dis Colon Rectum* 32:1065–1070, 1989.
68. Stuart M, Failes DG, Killingback MJ, DeLuch C: Irradiation injuries of the large intestine. *Dis Colon Rectum* 23:94–97, 1980.
69. Haddar GK, Grodzinsky C, Allen H: The spectrum of radiation enteritis: Surgical considerations. *Dis Colon Rectum* 26:590–594, 1983.
70. Anseline PF, Lavery IV, Fazio VW, et al: Radiation injury of the rectum. *Ann Surg* 194:716–724, 1981.
71. Buchi KN, Dixon JA: Argon laser treatment of hemorrhagic radiation proctitis. *Gastrointest Endosc* 33:27–30, 1987.
72. Ahlquist DA, Gostout CS, Viggianot R, et al: Laser therapy for severe radiation induced rectal bleeding. *Mayo Clin Proc* 61:927–931, 1986.
73. Alexander TJ, Dwyer RM: Endoscopic Nd: yag laser treatment of severe radiation injury of the lower gastrointestinal tract: Long term follow-up. *Gastrointest Endosc* 34:407–411, 1988.
74. Matuchansky C, Babin P, Abadier JC, et al: Jejunal bleeding from a solitary large mucosal artery. *Gastroenterology* 75:110–113, 1978.
75. Richards WO, Grove-Mahoney D, Williams LF: Hemorrhage from a Dieulafoy type ulcer of the colon: A new cause of lower gastrointestinal bleeding. *Am Surg* 54:121–124, 1988.
76. Ma CK, Harsant P, Pace EH, et al: Submucosal arterial malformation of the colon with massive hemorrhage: Report of a case. *Dis Colon Rectum* 32:149–152, 1989.

III

DIAGNOSIS

15

DIAGNOSTIC IMAGING IN GASTROINTESTINAL HEMORRHAGE

David W. Gelfand, M.D.
William D. Routh, M.D.
Robert J. Cowan, M.D.

Three areas of diagnostic imaging are potentially useful in a patient with significant gastrointestinal (GI) hemorrhage: barium examinations, radioisotope studies, and angiography. To a large extent, the advent of universally available endoscopy has altered the frequency and manner in which diagnostic imaging techniques are employed. In particular, the ability to examine the upper GI tract and colon rapidly with the fiberoptic endoscope has made possible the diagnosis of the cause and site of bleeding by direct endoscopic observation rather than by indirect radiological imaging.

BARIUM EXAMINATIONS IN GI HEMORRHAGE

The availability of upper GI panendoscopy in particular has greatly reduced the call for emergency upper GI barium examinations. The upper GI series is now employed almost exclusively when there is physical obstruction to the passage of the endoscope. Apart from situations of restricted access, there are few circumstances in which the site or cause of hemorrhage would more likely be visible radiologically rather than endoscopically.

The small intestine is a more fertile site for radiological investigation of the cause of hemorrhage. Although enteroscopy is now becoming available, it is time consuming, uncomfortable, and expensive compared to the radiographic examination of the small intestine. In planning the radiological investigation of the small bowel in patients with hemorrhage, it is important that studies involving barium sulfate be scheduled only after all other pertinent imaging studies of the abdomen have been performed. The presence of barium sulfate in the bowel interferes with virtually every other form of abdominal imaging, including sonography, computed tomography (CT) scanning, radionuclide scanning, and angiography.

Two general methods of radiological investigation of the small bowel are available: peroral small bowel examination with barium sulfate suspension and enteroclysis. The peroral examination can be performed in approximately one hour and imposes no discomfort on the patient. However, it is of limited accuracy for detection of small, isolated bleeding lesions, such as a small leiomyoma, adenocarcinoma, or Meckel's diverticulum. Enteroclysis is the more useful radiological method of examining the small intestine in a patient with an undiagnosed source of hemorrhage because of its more accurate delineation of structural detail.

Enteroclysis is in essence a prograde barium enema of the small intestine that is accomplished by placing one of several tubes made for this purpose into the distal duodenum or proximal jejunum under fluoroscopic control.[1] The process of placing the tube involves moderate patient discomfort, particularly for individuals with an active gag reflex. Also, there are occasional patients in whom the enteroclysis tube cannot be properly placed because of an unusual shape of the stomach or prior gastric surgery. Once the tube is in the proximal small bowel, a dilute barium suspension is injected and intermittent fluoroscopy is used to follow its progress. The barium injection may be supplemented by injection of air or methylcellulose solution to provide a double-contrast examination. To date, no advantage has been demonstrated for double-contrast enteroclysis versus the single-contrast study, and the single-contrast examination is more straightforward and rapid.

Neoplasms are somewhat uncommon in the small intestine. However, at least three types—leiomyoma, adenocarcinoma, and carcinoid tumors—are capable of causing significant GI hemorrhage.

Leiomyoma has a very specific radiological appearance, presenting as a spherical or hemispherical lesion with a smooth outline due to its mucosal covering. A bleeding ulceration on the surface of the leiomyoma usually cannot be demonstrated.

Adenocarcinoma of the small intestine occurs most frequently in the proximal small bowel. Although an occasional adenocarcinoma of the small intestine may be detected while still having a polypoid configuration, most are partially or completely circumferential at the time of detection. Adenocarcinomas are a potential source of small intestinal bleeding, but these lesions are more likely to present with symptoms of obstruction because of their tendency to rapidly become circumferential. Enteroclysis is particularly useful in detecting a partially obstructing adenocarcinoma because it emphasizes the distention seen proximal to the lesion.

Carcinoid tumors may be benign or malignant, most often the latter. They are usually singular but may be multiple. The most common location for a carcinoid tumor of the small bowel is in the distal ileum. Their wide range of aggressiveness results in tumors that may have either a typically benign radiological appearance or a frankly malignant presentation.

Ischemia of the small intestine produces a radiographic appearance that is characteristic and relatively easy to detect on both peroral studies and enteroclysis. Loss of integrity of the capillaries in the submucosa causes edema and submucosal hemorrhage that thicken the semilunar folds over a variable length of the small bowel. This relatively smooth, uniform fold thickening is easily demonstrated on radiographic studies (Figure 15.1). In more severe cases of ischemia involving loss of integrity of the mucosa, one may detect a length of bowel without a visible mucosal pattern and a relatively featureless lumen.

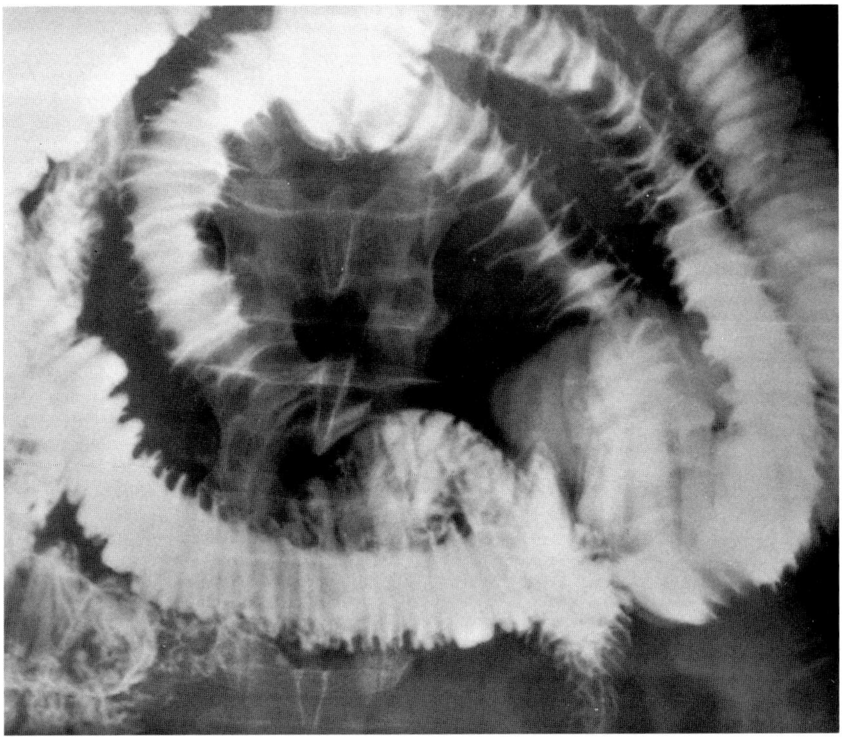

Figure 15.1. Ischemia of the small bowel as seen by enteroclysis, producing smooth, relatively uniform thickening of the valvulae conniventes.

Meckel's diverticulum can be detected with either a peroral small bowel study or enteroclysis (Figure 15.2), although the recent literature tends to suggest that enteroclysis is more sensitive.[2] This congenital abnormality is invariably located in the distal half of the small intestine.

The major causes of hemorrhage of colonic origin are diverticulosis, adenocarcinoma, and angiodysplasia, diseases mainly of the elderly. Internal hemorrhoids are an uncommon source of significant colonic bleeding. Of these potential sources of acute hemorrhage, diverticulosis and adenocarcinoma are amenable to radiological diagnosis with a very high degree of accuracy. As with the upper GI tract, the major reason for employing radiological examination of the colon rather than colonoscopy in a patient with acute GI hemorrhage is access. Colonoscopy may be impaired by fecal material or large amounts of blood. Also, in up to 25% of attempts,[3] colonoscopy does not reach the cecum, thereby leaving the proximal colon unexamined.

The radiological detection of colon carcinoma is probably as accurate as that achieved with colonoscopy when the fraction of endoscopic examinations that do not view the entire colon is taken into consideration. Also, in the presence of a radiologically demonstrated carcinoma, there is usually little doubt about the source of bleeding. The radiological appearances of polypoid and circumferential carcinomas of the colon are so well established that they need not be elucidated in this text.

Diverticulosis is similarly detected with great accuracy radiologically. However, in the presence of diverticula involving a considerable length of the colon, the radiological

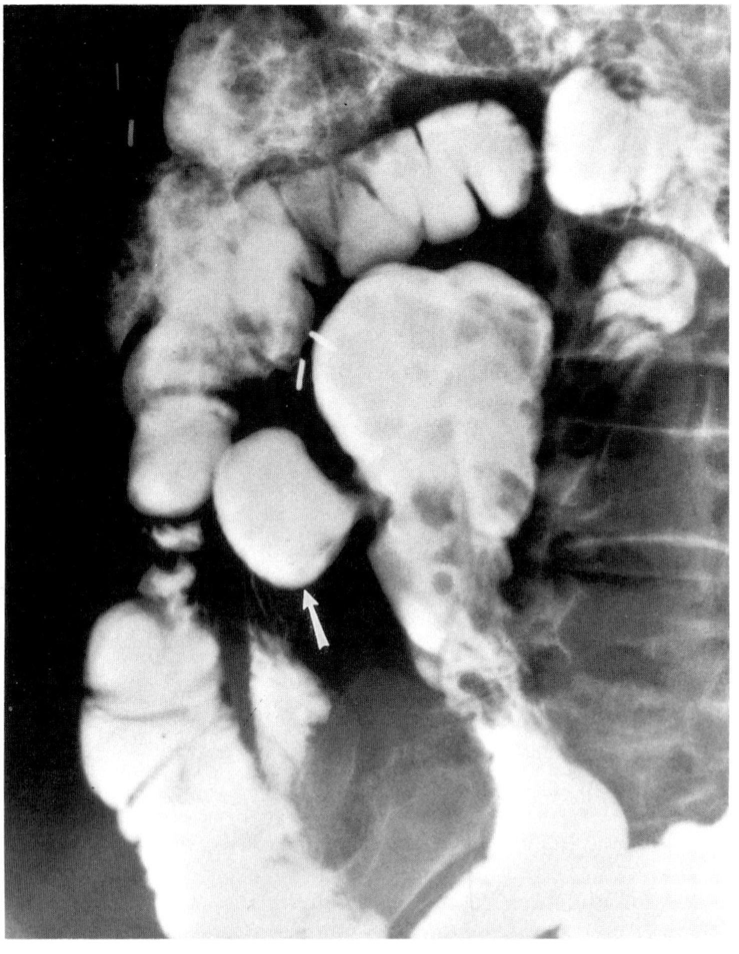

Figure 15.2. Meckel's diverticulum (*arrow*) seen on enteroclysis as a smooth outpouching from the distal small intestine.

examination cannot determine which of the diverticula is bleeding and thus may require resection. Although this does not present a problem when diverticula are confined to a limited segment of the colon, an alternative means of diagnosis, such as angiography or colonoscopy, may be required to localized the bleeding prior to surgery. This is particularly true in patients with demonstrated diverticula, but the source of bleeding is actually an angiodysplasia in a segment of colon devoid of diverticula.

SCINTIGRAPHIC EVALUATION OF GI HEMORRHAGE

Nuclear medicine imaging procedures have been widely used for the detection of GI hemorrhage since the 1970s. Current techniques are more sensitive than angiography and offer the advantage of prolonged monitoring, which is particularly useful in patients with intermittent bleeding. Scintigraphic studies can provide information on the location of the bleeding site but rarely are able to characterize the type of lesion causing the hemorrhage. These procedures do not replace angiography, but they do provide assistance in selecting the most appropriate timing of the angiogram and in directing the angiographer to areas of concern. Their greatest application at present is in the patient with intermittent melena or moderately severe acute bleeding suspected of arising from the lower GI system. The yield is low in patients with upper GI bleeding or occult bleeding. With massive acute bleeding, the patient may be referred directly to angiography.

Radiopharmaceuticals and Technique

The most commonly used agents are Tc-99m S-colloid and Tc-99m red blood cells (RBCs). Alavi introduced Tc-99m S-colloid and demonstrated experimentally in dogs that bleeding rates as low as .05–0.1 ml/min could be detected scintigraphically. Initial reports in patients[4] confirmed the ability to detect bleeding with a sensitivity significantly greater than that of angiography.

Typically, a bolus of 10 mCi (adult dose) of Tc-99m S-colloid is injected intravenously. Following an initial angiographic phase, serial 1- to 2-minute images are acquired for 30 to 45 minutes. Tc-99m S-colloid is rapidly cleared from the blood by the reticuloendothelial systems. This results in very low background activity, which facilitates detection of small amounts of extravasation. However, the rapid blood clearance is also a major disadvantage. Bleeding must be occurring at the time of injection to be detected. Since many patients bleed intermittently, their Tc-99m S-colloid study may not identify the abnormality. Although reinjection is possible, this increases the radiation burden. In addition, most of the initially injected Tc-99m S-colloid will have been deposited in the liver and spleen, and the large amount of activity in these organs will obscure the upper abdomen and interfere with evaluation of the proximal GI tract.

Use of a radiopharmaceutical with a longer resident time in the circulation improves the detection of intermittent hemorrhage. Winzelberg et al.[5] introduced the use of Tc-labeled autologous RBCs, which has become the most commonly employed radiopharmaceutical. A variety of methods are available for labeling the patient's own RBCs. The simplest in vivo technique suffers from variable labeling efficiency and frequent "free" Tc pertechnetate which is excreted by the GI tract. Better labeling efficiency is provided by the modified in vivo technique refined by Callahan et al.[6] Pure in vitro kits afford the highest labeling efficiency, but none of these have received Food and Drug Administration approval. All of these procedures depend on pretreatment of the RBCs with a reducing agent such as stannous pyrophosphate which penetrates into the cell. When Tc-99m pertechnetate is then introduced, it become reduced inside the RBCs and binds to hemoglobin, forming a stable tag.

From 20 to 25 mCi (adult dose) of tagged RBCs are usually reinjected into the patients as a bolus for an initial angiographic series of images. Longer static images (up to 5 minutes each) are then recorded for 90 to 120 minutes. If available, continuous digital recording at 30- to 60-second intervals is useful. Viewing of digital images in a cinegraphic mode may improve detection of small amounts of bleeding, help in separating vascular structures from extravasation, and assist in localizing the bleeding point. If no definite abnormality has been identified by 90–120 minutes, delayed images can be obtained for up to 24 hours. The ability to do prolonged monitoring with tagged RBCs

TABLE 15.1. Tc-99m RBC Detection of GI Bleeding

Reference	*Year*	*Sensitivity (%)*	*Specificity (%)*
Winzelberg et al.[8]	1981	91	95
Markisz et al.[10]	1982	91	
Ovecchia et al.[11]	1985	94	
Szasz et al.[12]	1985	91	76
Nicholson et al.[13]	1989	97	85

is a major advantage of this radiopharmaceutical. Indeed, many patients whose images were negative during the first hour after injection have been found to have abnormal studies.[7]

Early reports suggested that Tc-99m RBC scans would be positive in a patient with a transfusion requirement of more than 500 ml in 24 hours.[8] Additional reports estimated that a bleeding rate of only 0.1 ml/min was needed.[9] In a canine model similar to that used to evaluate Tc-99m S-colloid, imaging of Tc RBCs detected lower GI bleeding within 10 minutes at bleeding rates of 0.2–4.6 ml/min and by 55 minutes at rates down to 0.04 ml/min.[9] The authors estimated that only 2–3 ml of extravasated blood was needed for detection. These lower rates are comparable to those found with Tc S-colloid. Multiple studies with Tc RBCs have confirmed the ability of the test to demonstrate GI hemorrhage (Table 15.1).

Comparative paired studies have consistently demonstrated a higher sensitivity with Tc-RBCs.[7,14] For most patients, Tc-99m RBCs have thus become the agent of choice. However, Tc S-colloid may be preferred in the emergent patient when time is not available to label the RBCs or when prolonged imaging is not possible. Tc S-colloid may also be advantageous in cirrhotic patients with varices, since blood pool activity in these vascular structures may be misleading on the RBC images.

Interpretation

With either Tc S-colloid or Tc RBCs, initial images are helpful mainly in identifying highly vascular structures such as arteriovenous malformations or very vascular neoplasms. Actual bleeding is rarely seen during this initial sequence. On subsequent static images, the Tc S-colloid progressively accumulates in the liver and spleen and, to a lesser extent, in the bone marrow. Early images may have activity in vascular organs such as the kidneys, but blood pool activity declines rapidly. If active extravasation is detected, it is usually evident as a focus of persistent activity not corresponding to the normal reticuloendothelial distribution, and on serial images it should move consistent with progression in the GI tract. Since the radiopharmaceutical is in the blood for only a brief period, the amount actually extravasated may be relatively small.

Tc RBC images show considerable blood pool activity throughout the examination. Liver and spleen activity is less than with the colloid preparation. Vascular structures such as the aorta, inferior vena cava, portal vein, and large venous collaterals may be visible. There is often activity in the bladder, especially if the in vivo or modified in vivo techniques are used for RBC labeling. Active extravasation gradually increases and may eventually fill sufficient bowel to characterize the location accurately. Movement of the extravasated material also helps in localization. It is imperative to examine all of the images to identify the earliest bleeding site, since accumulation on delayed images may occur at some distance from the actual bleed.

Care must be taken not to mistake a vascular structure for a site of hemorrhage. Potential pitfalls include kidney, either in the normal position or ectopic; the uterus, placenta, bladder, and external genitalia; aneurysms, vascular tumors, hyperemic inflammatory lesions, hepatic hemangiomas, and varices; and poor RBC tagging and gallbladder excretion with hemolytic anemias.[15,16] The characteristics of true GI bleeding include persistence of activity on serial images, gradual increase with time, and movement which conforms to gastrointestinal anatomy and peristaltic movement (Figure 15.3).

Application

Scintigraphic detection of GI bleeding is most applicable to the lower GI tract. Although on occasion gastric and proximal small bowel bleeding may be demonstrated, the high liver/spleen activity tends to obscure the upper abdomen and limit the sensitivity of the test in this region. In patients with suspected distal small bowel and lower GI bleeding, the scintigraphic test complements the angiographic examination. Since the radionuclide study is generally more sensitive than the angiogram, a negative study can obviate the need for an emergent arteriogram and, if positive, can aid the angiographer in performing the sequence of injections. When the extravasation is clearly demonstrated

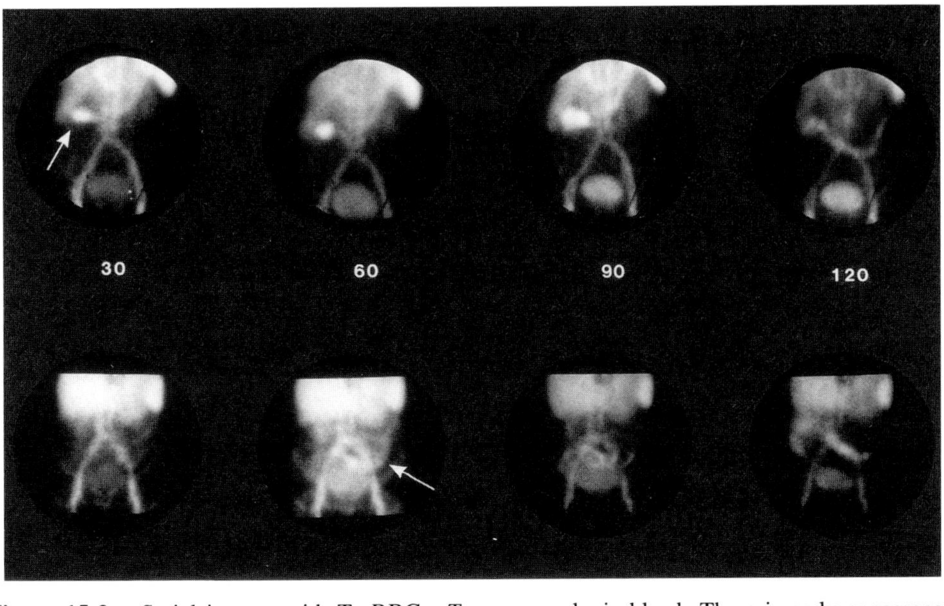

Figure 15.3. Serial images with Tc-RBCs. *Top row:* colonic bleed. There is early appearance of activity in the hepatic flexure (*arrow*), with eventual filling of the entire transverse colon. *Bottom row:* small bowel bleed. Although only colonic activity is seen on the 120-minute image, earlier frames show initial extravasation in loops of small intestine (*arrow*).

on early sequential images, accurate localization may be possible. This may provide sufficient information for clinical management by conservative therapy.

Although the radioisotopic study is sensitive for detection of small amounts of bleeding, it is rarely relied upon for localization of the abnormality if surgery is anticipated. With slow bleeding, especially when it is evident only on delayed images, exact localization of the bleeding sites may be difficult. In a recent report,[17] reliance solely on the scintigraphic study led to incorrect localization in at least 25% of patients, presumably from migration of the extravasated blood between scans.

The greatest application of the scintigraphic technique is in patients with suspected mild to moderate lower GI bleeding. The ability to image the patient over a prolonged period is extremely useful in demonstrating intermittent bleeding. The study can assist in appropriate timing of the angiographic examination and guide the angiographer in the selection of injection sequences. The angiogram may provide better localization and characterization of the lesion and permit therapeutic intervention.

SCINTIGRAPHY FOR MECKEL'S DIVERTICULUM

Meckel's diverticulum, the most common congenital anomaly of the GI tract, occurs in approximately 2% of the population. It is usually asymptomatic, although 20–30% may be complicated by diverticulitis, obstruction, perforation or bleeding. Most diverticula with bleeding contain acid-secreting ectopic gastric mucosa responsible for peptic ulceration of the diverticulum or adjacent small bowel.[18] Since Tc-99m pertechnetate is concentrated in gastric mucosa, this radiopharmaceutical can be used to localize the abnormality noninvasively. The patient need not be bleeding at the time of the study, since uptake does not depend on the presence of hemorrhage. Pertechnetate imaging is not useful in detecting those diverticula which do not contain ectopic gastric mucosa.

Technique

Ten-15 mCi (adult dose) of Tc-99m pertechnetate is injected as a bolus. A rapid-sequence flow phase of images is followed by serial static images for approximately one hour. In preparation, the patient should fast for several hours and should have had no recent barium. The bladder should be emptied immediately prior to imaging. Pharmacological approaches have been investigated to increase the concentration of pertechnetate in the gastric mucosa. Pentagastrin has been used to increase gastric mucosal secretion with and without glucagon to show intestinal transit and minimize washout from the diverticulum. Studies in an animal model have demonstrated that pretreatment with cimetidine may result in superior target:background ratios.[19] Cimetidine, 300 mg every six hours (adults), has been recommended for 24 to 48 hours prior to imaging.[20]

Interpretation

The initial flow images are more helpful in delineating other causes of bleeding, such as arteriovenous malformations or vascular tumors. On the subsequent static images, uptake is normally seen in the stomach, and variable amounts may appear in the proximal small bowel if the patient has recently eaten. Since pertechnetate is excreted by the kidneys, bladder activity is commonly present.

Accumulation in a Meckel's diverticulum is usually seen by 30 minutes. Characteristic findings include a single rounded focus of activity, usually in the right lower quadrant, which parallels the intensity of the stomach, persists throughout the hour of imaging, and can clearly be separated from structures containing urine.[21] Oblique or lateral views may aid in distinguishing renal or bladder activity. Slight movement of the focus, especially if the patient turns or is allowed to stand, does not exclude a Meckel's diverticulum, since the position of the small bowel can shift.

Results

Reviews indicate a sensitivity of approximately 85%.[22,23] Most of the studies have been in children without cimetidine pretreatment. Causes of false-negative examinations include lack of sufficient gastric mucosa, ischemia or necrosis of the diverticulum, rapid washout of the secreted pertechnetate, overlap by adjacent organs such as the bladder, and procedural error. With current techniques, sensitivity and specificity are greater than 90%. However, pertechnetate is not specific for gastric mucosa, and false-positive studies have been reported due to intussusception, duplication cysts, inflammatory bowel disease, focal urine collections, and highly vascular lesions.

Pertechnetate images provide a simple, noninvasive technique for localizing ectopic gastric mucosa and suggesting the diagnosis of Meckel's diverticulum in patients (especially children) with bleeding. Although false-positive studies occasionally occur, rectal bleeding is rarely caused by a Meckel's diverticulum when the pertechnetate study is negative. If the patient is actively bleeding at the time of the study, Tc-99m RBC or Tc-99m S-colloid may be preferable. Occasionally, a Meckel's diverticulum has been demonstrated by barium studies or angiography in patients with negative scintigraphy.

ANGIOGRAPHY IN GI HEMORRHAGE

In 1963 Baum and associates first reported the success of selective visceral angiography for the precise preoperative detection of GI bleeding sites.[24] Subsequently, numerous clinical series have confirmed the diagnostic efficacy of this modality, especially in patients with acute, severe GI hemorrhage. In spite of the increased use of endoscopy for early evaluation of such patients, angiography continues to play a valuable role in their management.

In a given patient with GI bleeding, the decision to proceed with angiography will depend on factors including the severity and time course of hemorrhage, the apparent general location of the bleeding site (upper vs. lower GI tract), and the general condition of the patient (especially the operative risk).

ACUTE UPPER GI BLEEDING

Patients with hematemesis can be assumed to have an upper GI source for their bleeding (i.e., proximal to the ligament of Treitz). Melena usually indicates an upper GI or small bowel source but, less often, can be due to colonic bleeding, depending upon the severity of hemorrhage and the degree of gut motility. Hematochezia is most often a manifestation of active colonic bleeding but is occasionally seen during brisk upper GI bleeding. In such a situation, one would anticipate clinical evidence of the acute hemodynamic effects of bleeding (tachycardia, hypotension).

Doubt regarding the location (upper vs. lower GI) of the bleeding site should be resolved prior to angiography by prompt placement of a nasogastric (NG) tube. Aspiration of blood confirms an upper GI source, while a negative NG aspirate makes active upper GI bleeding unlikely, although occasionally a duodenal ulcer can bleed briskly without reflux into the stomach. Endoscopy of the upper GI tract may be required to exclude a bleeding lesion if uncertainty still remains in regard to the upper or lower GI source of GI bleeding.

Indications for Angiography

Most episodes of upper GI hemorrhage will abate with conservative therapy. In patients with persistent bleeding, the primary role of angiography is to guide specific transcatheter hemostatic intervention by embolization and/or vasoconstrictor infusion after endoscopy has localized and characterized the bleeding lesion. Diagnostic angiography is reserved for situations where endoscopy fails to localize the bleeding site. In patients with acute GI bleeding, barium studies must be avoided, since residual barium interferes with detection of the bleeding site.

Technique

Selective celiac angiography is performed first in patients with upper GI hemorrhage. If angiographic evidence of gastric bleeding is noted or a gastric source is suspected based on endoscopic or clinical findings, a subselective left gastric angiogram is performed next (Figure 15.4). Eighty-five percent of angiographically detected acute gastric bleeding sites are supplied by branches of the left gastric artery.[25] If a gastric bleeding site is not defined on the left gastric injection, subselective splenic and/or gastroduodenal arterial studies should be performed. More selective positioning of the catheter improves the detection of active bleeding and is necessary for subsequent embolotherapy. If duodenal bleeding is clinically suspected or noted on the celiac study, a common hepatic or gastroduodenal angiogram should then be performed.

When angiographic evaluation of the celiac axis is unrevealing, selective superior mesenteric angiography should always be performed, since bleeding duodenal lesions may receive an arterial supply from the superior mesenteric artery via the inferior pancre

Figure 15.4. Angiographic localization of gastric bleeding site in a 50-year-old woman with acute hematemesis. Upper endoscopy revealed extensive blood clot in the gastric fundus, but no specific bleeding lesion was detected. (A) Selective celiac arteriogram reveals a small focus of extravasated contrast (*arrow*) projecting over the body of the stomach. (B) Superselective left gastric angiography better demonstrates extravasation with pooling of contrast in a gastric ulcer of the posterior wall (*arrowhead*). Transcatheter embolization of the left gastric artery with gelatin sponge particles acutely controlled the hemorrhage, thereby avoiding operative therapy.

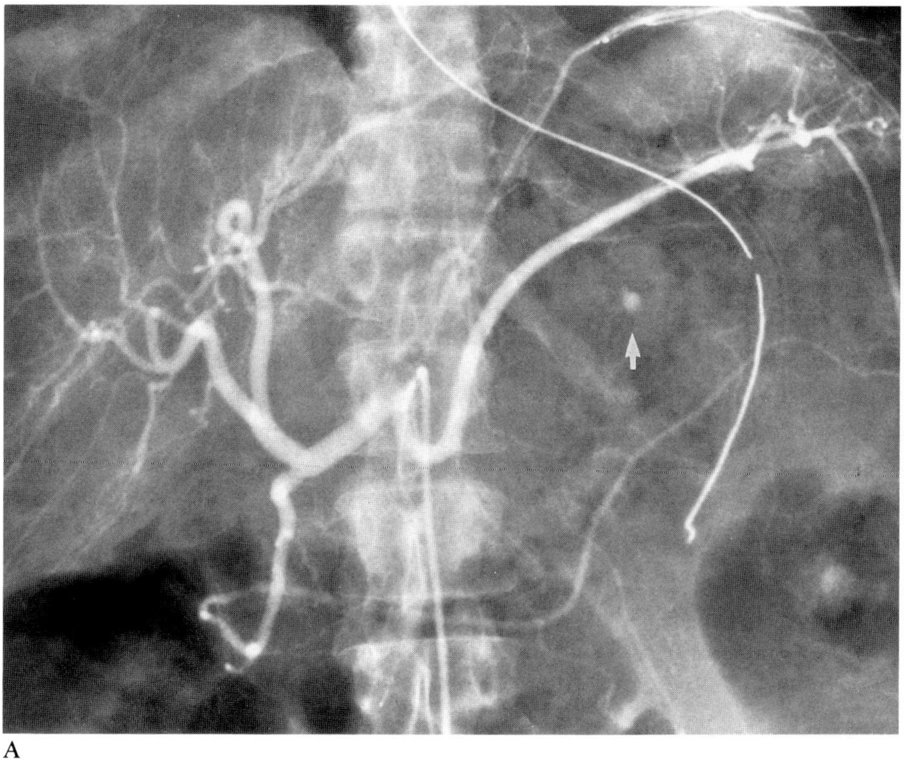

A

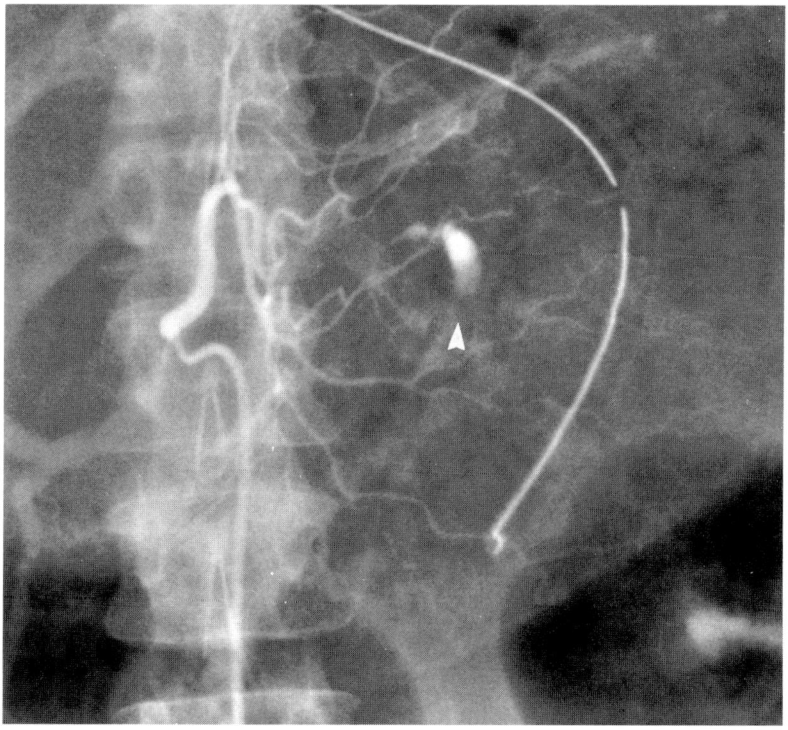

B

aticoduodenal artery. Unsuspected bleeding sites distal to the ligament of Treitz may also be detected.

ACUTE LOWER GI BLEEDING

Patients with active lower GI bleeding beyond the ligament of Treitz may present with hematochezia or melena, depending on the proximity of the bleeding site to the rectum, the bleeding rate, and gut motility. Since the clinical presentation can overlap that of a patient with upper GI bleeding, an NG tube should be inserted. A positive NG aspirate for blood or the absence of bile in the NG aspirate should prompt the performance of upper GI endoscopy.

In the patient with hematochezia but no evidence of an upper GI source, anoscopy or sigmoidoscopy may quickly define a distal colonic or rectal lesion. Although colonoscopy has been suggested in patients with acute colonic bleeding, problems with visibility in patients with severe hemorrhage may limit its applicability. In such patients, angiography should be considered.

Indications for Angiography

Patients who have persistent hematochezia, require repeated blood transfusions, and have no upper GI or distal colorectal source of bleeding identified by the above measures should undergo emergency visceral angiography. In contrast to an important therapeutic role for acute upper GI hemorrhage, angiography for lower GI bleeding is employed primarily for its diagnostic value in localization of undetermined sites of the bleeding site. In selected patients, the angiographic catheter may also provide a route for selective infusion of vasopressin, which may definitively control bleeding or allow for temporary pre-operative stabilization. To date, transcatheter embolotherapy has had a much more limited role in the treatment of small bowel and colonic bleeding than gastroduodenal bleeding.

Timing of Angiography

Studies by Nusbaum and Baum in the 1960s demonstrated that active bleeding at a rate of at least 0.5 cc/min was required for detection by selective visceral angiography.[24,26] Since lower GI bleeding is often intermittent, proper timing of angiography is imperative to maximize the diagnostic yield. Although in patients with acute upper GI bleeding NG aspiration can usually determine bleeding activity, clinical evaluation of the activity of lower GI bleeding is much more problematic. Bloody stools may be noted hours after bleeding has stopped. Also, a significant delay often exists between the onset of bleeding and a detectable decrease in hematocrit, making this test imprecise in assessing acute blood loss. Hemodynamic effects of acute lower GI bleeding, including tachycardia, hypotension, and orthostasis, are important clues to acute recurrence of bleeding and may be noted prior to the passage of bloody stools.

Radionuclide studies have been advocated to assess the activity of lower GI bleeding prior to angiography.[27] In patients with a negative scan, angiography will also likely be negative and should therefore be postponed. However, due to the much greater sensitivity of the radionuclide study and its ability to detect intermittent bleeding, a positive scan does not necessarily predict a positive angiogram. With severe active hemorrhage, angiography should be performed immediately, bypassing the nuclear medicine study.[28,29] In the time required to obtain a tagged RBC scan, the patient may temporarily stop bleeding, and an opportunity for specific angiographic documentation of the bleeding site will have been lost.

In spite of inherent problems with timing, the sensitivity of selective visceral angiography for detecting sites of acute lower GI bleeding has ranged from 58% to 86% in clinical trials.[28]

Technique

The left femoral approach should be utilized to facilitate catheterization of the inferior mesenteric artery (IMA). Unless a Foley catheter drains the urinary bladder, the IMA should be studied first to avoid obscuring distal colonic or rectal bleeding sites by bladder contrast. The superior mesenteric artery (SMA) is then examined (Figure 15.5). If no bleeding site is detected, a celiac angiogram should be performed to exclude an unsuspected upper GI source or an anomalous vascular supply from the celiac artery to the colon via the dorsal pancreatic artery.[29]

Conventional film-screen angiography is generally preferred to ensure maximum coverage and spatial resolution. Care must be taken to cover the entire vascular distribution of each of the visceral arteries studied. This may require multiple angiographic runs, especially for the SMA in large patients.

CHRONIC GI BLEEDING

Patients with chronic GI blood loss warrant initial evaluation with barium studies, endoscopy, and radionuclide scans. If these fail to detect the cause of bleeding, then elective visceral angiography is indicated. From the left femoral approach, the IMA, SMA, and celiac arteries are sequentially examined, looking for lesions manifested by abnormalities of vessels rather than contrast extravasation. Examples of such lesions include vascular malformations, neoplasms, and Meckel's diverticula. Reported angiographic detection rates of such lesions in patients with undiagnosed chronic GI bleeding average 40%.[30,31]

COMPLICATIONS OF ANGIOGRAPHY

In a survey of more than 83,000 transfemoral angiographic procedures, Hessel et al. reported an overall complication rate of 1.73%. Puncture site complications including bleeding, arterial obstruction, pseudoaneurysm, and arteriovenous fistula were noted in less than 0.5% of cases.[32] Surgical intervention for puncture site complications has been required in less than 0.2% of cases.

Catheter-guidewire complications including breakage, embolism, vessel perforation, or contrast extravasation occur in less than 1% of transfemoral angiographic cases.[32] In a series of more than 1,000 visceral artery catheterizations, subintimal contrast injection

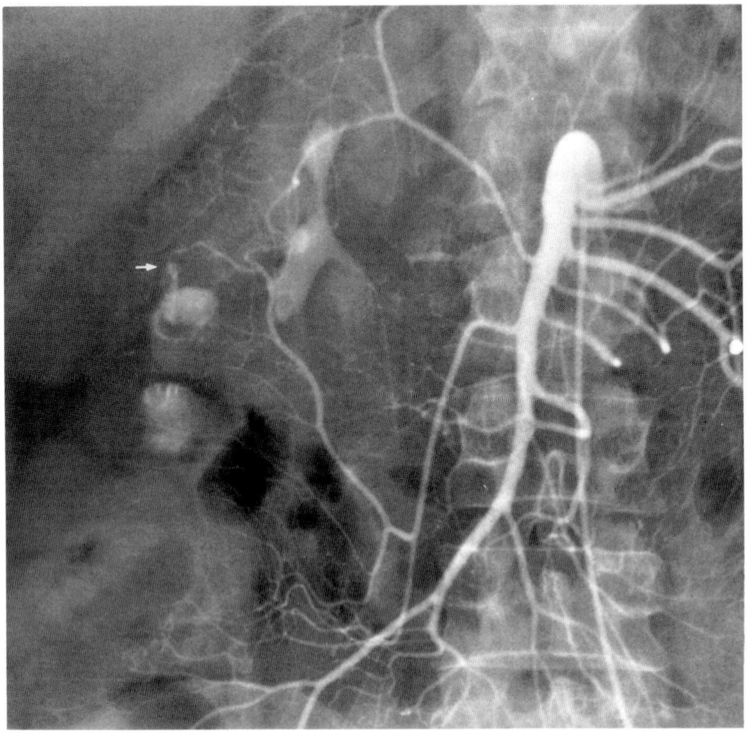

A

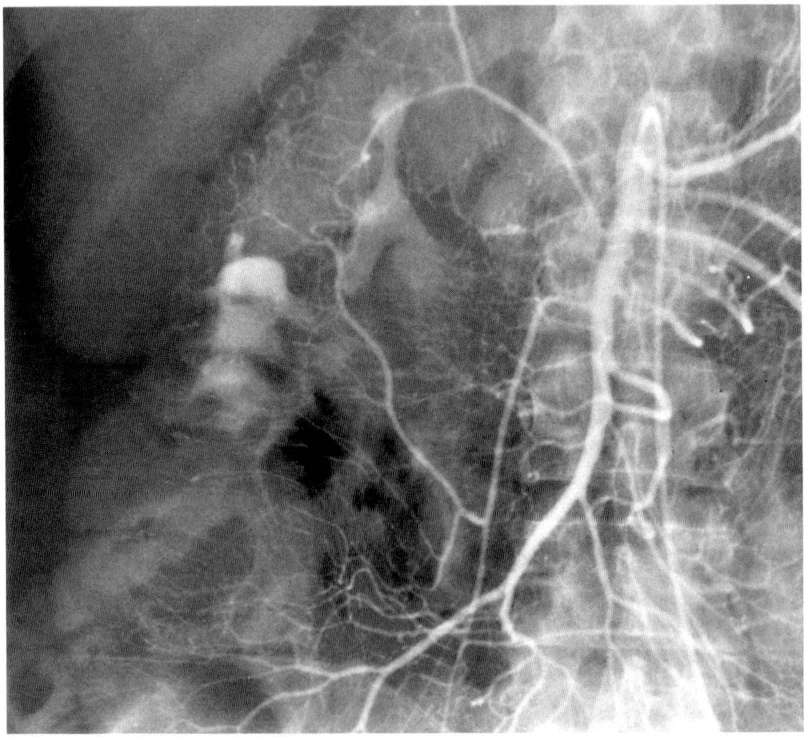

B

(reflecting vessel injury by guidewire or catheter manipulation) was noted in 2.6% of cases and considered "potentially serious" in 0.5%. Collateral circulation appeared to protect against ischemic complications in most cases, especially with injuries of the celiac axis.[33]

The most common cardiovascular complication of angiography is a vasovagal reaction, which occurs in less than 0.2% of cases. More severe cardiac complications such as angina, arrhythmias, and heart failure occur in less than 0.1%.[32]

Adverse reactions to radiographic contrast have been reported in 2.6% and 3.6% of patients in two large angiographic series.[32,33] Less than 50% of those reacting required any therapy, and less than 20% required hospitalization. Only one death was noted in more than 28,000 aortographic and nonneurological angiographic procedures.[34] These data were obtained during the era of conventional ionic contrast media use. Reduction in the incidence of contrast reactions may result from the use of newer, nonionic contrast agents.

Contrast-induced nephrotoxicity must be considered when performing angiographic procedures for acute GI bleeding in patients who are elderly and dehydrated. Renal insufficiency, diabetes mellitus, and multiple myeloma have also been suggested as risk factors for contrast-associated renal impairment.[35] Intravascular volume expansion and diuresis may afford some degree of protection. However, in situations of acute, life-threatening hemorrhage, prophylactic measures may not be possible.

REFERENCES

1. Gelfand DW: Enteroclysis in small bowel disease. *Postgrad Radiol* 6:221–234, 1986.
2. Maglinte DDT, Elmore MF, Isenberg M, et al: Meckel diverticulum: Radiologic demonstration by enteroclysis. *AJR* 134:925–932, 1980.
3. Gilbert DA, Shaneyfelt SL, Silverstein FE: The national ASGE colonoscopy survey—analysis of colonoscopic practices and yield. *Gastrointest Endosc* 30:143–147, 1984.
4. Alavi A, Ring EJ: Localization of gastrointestinal bleeding: Superiorityof ^{99m}Tc sulfur colloid compared with angiography. *AJR* 137:741–748, 1981.
5. Winzelberg GG, McKusick KA, Strauss HW, et al: Evaluation of gastrointestinal bleeding by red blood cells labelled in vivo with technetium-99m. *J Nucl Med* 20:1080–1086, 1979.
6. Callahan RJ, Froelich JW, McKusick KA, et al: A modified method for the in vivo labeling of red blood cells with Tc-99m. *J Nucl Med* 23:315–318, 1982.
7. Siddiqui AR, Schauwecker DS, Wellman HN, et al: Comparison of technetium-99m sulfur colloid and in vitro labeled technetium-99m RBCs in the detection of gastrointestinal bleeding. *Clin Nucl Med* 10:546–549, 1985.
8. Winzelberg GG, Froelich JW, McKusick KA, et al: Radionuclide localization of lower gastrointestinal hemorrhage. *Radiology* 139:465–469, 1981.

Figure 15.5. Emergency mesenteric angiography in a 53-year-old man with acute, severe hematochezia. (A) Early and (B) later arterial phases of a selective superior mesenteric arteriogram demonstrate extravasation of contrast from a peripheral right colic branch (arrow), with progressive luminal opacification of the ascending colon. There were no specific angiographic signs to help define the nature of the bleeding lesion. Hemorrhage was acutely controlled by local intra-arterial infusion of vasopressin, providing a period of clinical stabilization prior to definitive treatment by right hemicolectomy. The pathological diagnosis was bleeding from a colonic diverticulum.

9. Thorne DA, Datz FL, Remley K, et al: Bleeding rates necessary for detecting acute gastrointestinal bleeding with technetium-99m-labeled red blood cells in an experimental model. *J Nucl Med* 28:514–520, 1987.
10. Markisz JA, Front D, Royal HD, et al: An evaluation of ^{99m}Tc-labeled red cell scintigraphy for the detection and localization of gastrointestinal bleeding sites. *Gastroenterology* 83:394–398, 1982.
11. Ovecchia PM, Hensley EK, McDonald PT, et al: Localization of lower gastrointestinal hemorrhage. *Arch Surg* 120:621–624, 1985.
12. Szasz IJ, Morrison RT, Lyster DM: Technetium-99m-labeled red cell scanning to diagnose occult gastrointestinal bleeding. *Can J Surg* 28:512–514, 1985.
13. Nicholson ML, Neoptolemos JP, Sharp JF, et al: Localization of lower gastrointestinal bleeding using in vivo technetium-99m-labeled red blood cell scintigraphy. *Br J Surg* 76:358–361, 1989.
14. Bunker SR, Lull RJ, Tanasescu DE, et al: Scintigraphy of gastrointestinal hemorrhage: Superiority of ^{99m}Tc red blood cells over ^{99m}Tc sulfur colloid. *AJR* 143:543–548, 1984.
15. Dorfman GS, Cronan JJ, Staudinger KM: Scintigraphic signs and pitfalls in lower gastrointestinal hemorrhage: The continued necessity of angiography. *Radiographs* 7:543–562, 1987.
16. Boyd CM, Williamson MR: Technetium-99m RBC bleeding studies in normal subjects: Confusion with gastrointestinal bleeding sites. *Clin Nucl Med* 14:202–209, 1989.
17. Hunter JM, Pezim ME: Limited value of technetium-99m-labeled red cell scintigraphy in localization of lower gastrointestinal bleeding. *Am J Surg* 159:504–506, 1990.
18. Ghahremani GG: Radiology of Meckel's diverticulum. *CRC* 26:1–43, 1986.
19. Yeker D, Buyukunal C, Benli M, et al: Radionuclide imaging of Meckel's diverticulum: Cimetidine versus pentagastrin plus glucagon. *Eur J Nucl Med* 9:316–319, 1984.
20. Baum MD: Pertechnetate imaging following cimetidine administration in Meckel's diverticulum of the ileum. *Am J Gastroenterol* 76:464–465, 1981.
21. Sfakianakis GN, Conway JJ: Detection of ectopic gastric mucosa in Meckel's diverticulum and other aberrations by scintigraphy: II. Indications and methods—a 10-year experience. *J Nucl Med* 22:732–738, 1981.
22. Sfakianakis GN, Conway JJ: Detection of ectopic gastric mucosa in Meckel's diverticulum and other aberrations by scintigraphy: I. Pathophysiology and 10-year clinical experience. *J Nucl Med* 22:647–654, 1981.
23. Cooney DR, Duszynski DO, Camboa E, et al: The abdominal technetium scan (a decade of experience). *J Pediatr Surg* 17:611–619, 1982.
24. Nusbaum M, Baum S: Radiographic demonstration of unknown sites of gastrointestinal bleeding. *Surg Forum* 14:374–375, 1963.
25. Kelemouridis V, Athanasoulis CA, Waltman AC: Gastric bleeding: An angiographic study. *Radiology* 149:643–648, 1983.
26. Baum S, Nusbaum M, Blakemore WS, et al: The preoperative radiographic demonstration of intra-abdominal bleeding from undetermined sites by percutaneous selective celiac and superior mesenteric arteriography. *Surgery* 58:797–805, 1965.
27. McKusick KA, Froelich J, Callahan RJ, et al: ^{99m}Tc red blood cells for detection of gastrointestinal bleeding: Experiences with 80 patients. *AJR* 137:1113–1118, 1981.
28. Browder W, Cerise EJ, Litwin MS: Impact of emergency angiography in massive lower gastrointestinal bleeding. *Ann Surg* 204:530–536, 1986.
29. Tillotson CL, Geller SC, Kantrowitz L, et al: Small bowel hemorrhage: Angiographic localization and intervention. *Gastrointest Radiol* 13:207–211, 1988.

30. Best EB, Teaford AK, Rader FH: Angiography in chronic/recurrent gastrointestinal bleeding: A nine year study. *Surg Clin North Am* 59:811–828, 1979.

31. Fiorito JJ, Brandt LJ, Kozicky O, et al: The diagnostic yield of superior mesenteric angiography: Correlation with the pattern of gastrointestinal bleeding. *Am J Gastroenterol* 84:878–881, 1989.

32. Hessel SJ, Adams DF, Abrams HL: Complications of angiography. *Radiology* 138:273–281, 1981.

33. Sigstedt B, Lunderquist A: Complications of angiographic examinations. *Am J Roentgenol* 130:455–460, 1978.

34. Shehadi WH, Toniolo G: A report from the committee on safety of contrast media of the international society of radiology. *Radiology* 137:299–302, 1980.

35. Miller DL, Chang R, Wells WT, et al: Intravascular contrast media: Effect of dose on renal function. *Radiology* 167:607–611, 1988.

16

DIAGNOSTIC ENDOSCOPY OF UPPER GASTROINTESTINAL BLEEDING

Bernard M. Schuman, M.D.
Choichi Sugawa, M.D.

INTRODUCTION

We have believed for many years that the best diagnostic approach for the patient with upper gastrointestinal (GI) bleeding is endoscopic.[1-4] Barium study of the upper GI tract is fraught with problems of diagnostic interpretation because of retained blood and clot that makes for poor definition of mucosal disease and failure to identify ulcers filled with clot. The inability to determine which one of multiple lesions may be bleeding also limits the diagnostic capability of the upper GI series. Another important consideration is that barium retained in the gut will interfere with urgent angiography should it be required later. In recognition of these difficulties, most radiologists have given up evaluation of the emergent bleeding patient to the endoscopist. However, for the chronic bleeder in whom no diagnosis has been established, barium study, particularly of the small bowel, is essential. Moreover, the angiographer may have to be called on to localize the level of bleeding and, perhaps, control hemorrhage should esophagogastroduodenoscopy (EGD) show that no bleeding site is present above the ligament of Treitz.

PRESENTATION OF THE PATIENT

Assessment and Resuscitation

The course of upper GI hemorrhage is unpredictable. A patient who is seen after passage of one melenic stool and appears to be hemodynamically stable may go on to have massive hematemesis. Thus assessment and resuscitation go hand in hand. Endoscopy should not be undertaken until assessment indicates that vital signs are stable and that there are no underlying medical disorders that might compromise the patient's ability to tolerate the procedure. The patient should be restored to as good a cardiopulmonary status as possible. This usually requires an infusion of colloid solution or packed red blood cells via large-bore catheters before EGD can be undertaken. In most circumstances, the endoscopist should know the patient's blood count, urea nitrogen and electrolytes, blood sugar, platelets, and prothrombin time, and should have reviewed the electrocardiogram and chest x-ray prior to embarking on EGD. It goes without saying that at least 3 units of packed red blood cells should have been typed and cross-matched soon after venous access was obtained. This pre-EGD evaluation takes on added importance when one appreciates that the population is aging and that the morbidity and mortality in the elderly are increased not only by the GI hemorrhage per se, but probably by the stress of invasive procedures as well.

Once the patient is resuscitated, alert, and responsive, consent for EGD should be obtained. If the patient is not competent to give consent, the responsible relative should agree to the procedure. After a full explanation of the technique of EGD and its possible complications is given, the patient and family should be informed of the nature of any required endoscopic therapeutic intervention and its possible complications. We believe that EGD in the setting of upper GI bleeding should not be undertaken unless the endoscopist is qualified to proceed with the endoscopic therapy appropriate for the lesion encountered. We recognize that the diagnostic capabilities of EGD alone, although excellent, are probably not sufficient to alter patient mortality. The prospective study by Peterson et al. of 206 bleeding patients randomized to diagnostic EGD or no EGD found no statistically significant differences in deaths, blood transfusions, or length of hospital stay.[5] However, this study was not restricted to a specific bleeding lesion and therapy was not altered by the EGD diagnosis, so the effect of EGD on mortality and morbidity may or may not be salutary. Nevertheless, we believe that whatever benefit is derived from endoscopic diagnosis will be compounded by interventional endoscopic therapy, as demonstrated by Swain et al.[6] and Laine[7] in controlled trials.

It is a good idea to consider on clinical grounds the presumptive level of bleeding and the degree of bleeding because these may influence where, when, and how EGD will take place. Thus patients with hematemesis are bleeding from the esophagus, stomach, or duodenum to a moderate or greater degree, whereas those with melena and a clear nasogastric aspirate are likely but not necessarily bleeding from the distal stomach or duodenum to a lesser degree. In the former case, EGD should be preceded by thorough gastric lavage and performed on an urgent basis; in the latter, EGD can proceed without lavage and delayed for a more propitious time. Other clinical data will obviously influence judgment as well.

ENDOSCOPIC EXAMINATION

Patient Considerations

All patients undergoing EGD for upper GI bleeding are not equal. Thus the requirements for support and premedication in an otherwise healthy young man will not be the same as those in an elderly, frail woman with cardiopulmonary disease. In community hospitals with a nonalcoholic clientele, the typical patient will be over the age of 55 and, in fact, 20% will be 71 or older.[8] The elderly patient particularly requires judicious premedication and monitoring of vital signs and oxygen saturation. The bleeding patient seen in an inner-city hospital tends to be younger and to have alcohol-related disease.[9] Special attention to the complications of acute and chronic liver disease is also essential to avoid problems related to sedation and coagulopathy.

Facility

The emergency room is a less than ideal place to undertake EGD. Most patients with upper GI bleeding are admitted to the hospital via the emergency room, but resuscitation should have been sufficient to allow the patient to be transferred to the intensive care unit. Patients who do not achieve hemodynamic stabilization in the emergency room because of continuing hemorrhage belong to that small group of bleeding patients (2–3%) who must be moved to the operating room, where, under endotracheal anesthesia, EGD can be carried out while the patient is being prepared for surgery.

Most patients with active bleeding have EGD in an intensive care unit, where monitoring and resuscitative resources are at hand and nursing support is available. For those patients who never showed hemodynamic decompensation and do not have evidence of active bleeding, EGD may be delayed and performed in the endoscopy unit.

Timing

A high rate of positive diagnosis of the bleeding lesion depends on the observation of active bleeding—oozing, dripping, or spurting—or the presence of stigmata of recent bleeding—a red or black clot or a visible vessel. It has been well established by the American Society for Gastrointestinal Endoscopy's (ASGE) bleeding survey[8] that the largest percentage of actively bleeding cases (41.5%) will be seen in the first 12 hours after admission, whereas in a group of patients having endoscopy 12–24 hours after admission, the percentage drops to 29.4%. It is obvious that patients with severe bleeding, persistent moderate hemorrhage, or recurrent bleeding require urgent EGD, but stabilized patients without evidence of active bleeding can be deferred for study to an elective time without compromising the opportunity for a dependable diagnosis.

Preliminary Steps

Consultation with a medical or surgical service should be sought prior to EGD for actively bleeding patients. If a gastroenterologist is the endoscopist, the surgical service should have already been involved and then invited to observe the findings. With videoendoscopy, a tape or hard copy photos will be available for review by physicians caring for the patient. If a surgeon is the endoscopist, a medical opinion should have been sought in most cases, particularly in patients who are elderly or have underlying disease of the liver, cardiopulmonary, or renal systems.

The prudent diagnostic approach for the bleeding patient should involve thorough lavage with room-temperature water. The purpose of this procedure is to remove as much solid material, usually blood clots, as possible. This requires a large-bore tube with multiple distal openings (e.g., a 37F Edlich tube) and lavage with 2–4 liters, depending on the return. Ice water does not hasten clotting and should not be used because it may lower body temperature. Patients with a clear nasogastric tube aspirate generally will not require lavage. It is possible to view most of the stomach, even if bloody content is present, by moving the patient into a prone or semisupine position from the usual lateral decubitus position. In a few cases, insertion of an endotracheal tube can be done when it is essential to ensure that pulmonary aspiration does not occur, but this is generally considered only for a prolonged procedure that involves therapeutic maneuvers.

The patient is placed in the left lateral decubitus position, the oximeter clip is attached to the finger, and the cuff for blood pressure monitoring is applied. If the patient is in an intensive care unit, these devices as well as an electrocardiographic monitor are already in place.

At some point before the administration of premedication, usually at the time consent is obtained, the patient should be psychologically prepared for EGD. It is important to emphasize that EGD is not painful but that uncomfortable distention may occur. Testing the sensitivity of the patient's gag reflex may be a guide to how well the patient will tolerate intubation and the dosage of premedication. The patient should be assured that the gag reflex can be controlled, and anxiety and discomfort allayed, by drug therapy.

The endoscopist should make preparations for his or her own protection. A long-sleeved, long gown should be put on over clothes or a scrub suit. Latex gloves should be pulled up over the cuffs of the gown. The use of a surgical mask and goggles is imperative. EGD for a bleeding patient is a situation where contact exposure to blood and secretions and, if present, the human immunodeficiency virus is not unlikely; thus, it is foolhardy not to take all appropriate precautions.

Premedication

Although routine EGD can be done successfully without premedication,[10] particularly if a small-diameter pediatric endoscope is used, the importance of establishing a diagnosis in a bleeding patient mandates drug therapy so that the patient is as cooperative as possible. Topical pharyngeal anesthesia with a benzocaine preparation spray facilitates intubation but may increase the risk of aspiration during the procedure. Aspiration of the spray into the tracheobronchial tree can lead to high blood levels and cardiovascular or central nervous system toxicity. We prefer intravenous meperidine or midazolam, alone or in combination, for sedation. The elderly patient, the patient with obstructive lung disease, and, perhaps, the patient with established liver disease is usually given meperidine alone, primarily because the side effects—respiratory depression, hypotension, stupor—can be reversed by naloxone. Midazolam alone is used for younger, generally healthy patients, and the combination may be required for alcoholic patients who are difficult to sedate. A benzodiazepine antagonist that effectively reverses respiratory depression is now available, so we use meperidine less often. Fentanyl and diazepam are other drugs that are used effectively for sedation.

Equipment

For the diagnosis of an upper GI bleeding lesion, the standard forward-viewing instrument with an outer diameter of less than 12 mm and a biopsy channel of less than 3 mm is the workhorse. However, it is important to have available other endoscopes for special circumstances. For example, a pediatric endoscope may be useful for examining without premedication an elderly patient with respiratory compromise. On occasion, the side-viewing duodenoscope can be helpful in examining the gastric side of the cardia or the proximal wall of the descending duodenum. A double-channel or a large-diameter, single-channel endoscope may make it possible to aspirate a large puddle of blood covering gastric mucosa.

In the patient with a history of prosthetic repair of an abdominal aortic aneurysm, it is essential to examine the transverse portion of the duodenum. Excluding bleeding at that site with certainty can be done only if the tip of the endoscope is seen fluoroscopically crossing the vertebral spine. Another circumstance where a bleeding patient requires endoscopic examination under fluoroscopy is when, after a negative EGD, a pediatric colonoscope is employed in an attempt to examine the proximal jejunal mucosa, looking for neoplastic disease or telangiectasias.

As videoendoscopic systems become increasingly miniaturized and mobile, undoubtedly the fiberoptic instrumentation will be replaced and diagnosis should be enhanced by large-screen, high-resolution television monitors.[11]

Special Aspects of Technique in the Bleeding Patient

The endoscope should be passed under direct vision so that the hypopharynx can be examined and retained fluid in the esophagus suctioned. A large quantity of liquid in the stomach is best suctioned, but otherwise, the endoscope should be advanced into the duodenum as far and as speedily as it will go. On withdrawal, an inspection of the papilla of Vater is worthwhile to exclude hemobilia. A thorough survey of the duodenal bulb is essential, and it may be necessary to make multiple pyloric intubations to be satisfied that the bulb is free of ulceration. The prepyloric and antral areas usually present no impediment to complete visualization, and the angulus can be seen well with the retroflexed endoscope, which is then brought up to the gastric side of the cardia. A thorough perusal of the gastric mucosa may require rotating the patient slowly around to the right decubitus position in order to move retained clots. Sometimes abdominal compression over the distended stomach will drain bloody lacunae. In the esophagus, varices large enough to bleed are readily apparent, and no special maneuvers are necessary to demonstrate them. Only an experienced endoscopist who can readily interpret mucosal alteration and is prepared to proceed with interventional therapy should be responsible for examining a patient with upper GI hemorrhage. An inadequately trained endoscopist should not undertake EGD in these hazardous circumstances unsupervised.

Findings

In the 1981 National ASGE survey, 75% of the lesions responsible for upper GI bleeding were due to acid-peptic disease—gastric erosions and duodenal and gastric ulcers.[8] Fifteen percent of patients had bleeding varices but, interestingly, there were an additional 109 patients with varices who were bleeding from other lesions—erosions, Mallory-Weiss tears, and gastroduodenal ulcers, for the most part. One-third of the patients in the ASGE study had multiple lesions, with none or one or more bleeding at the time of EGD.[8]

Upper GI bleeding in an urban hospital shows a somewhat different distribution of causes of bleeding, with fewer patients with esophagitis and duodenal ulcer and more with varices and Mallory-Weiss tears.[9] There can be marked differences in etiology from region to region; two recent series, for example, showed a frequency of acute gastric mucosal lesions of 41% in one[12] and 7% in the other.[13]

The findings are also of value in formulating an estimate of the outcome of the bleeding lesion. Thus Foster et al. found that the presence of a visible vessel, clot, or black spot in the base of a peptic ulcer is a predictor of recurrent bleeding or the need for surgical management.[14] Moreover, active bleeding at the time of EGD by itself portends double the mortality rate of patients who do not have oozing or spurting from a lesion.[8] Active bleeding may in fact obscure the lesion and make a diagnosis impossible, but at least a level of bleeding can be ascertained so that when these patients go to surgery (and many are destined for the operating room), the surgeon knows where to find the bleeding vessel.

Specific Lesions

Varices

It is sometimes difficult to ascribe bleeding to varices, particularly if blood is absent at the time of EGD, but when no other cause is apparent and previous nasogastric suction revealed blood, the circumstantial evidence is sufficient to warrant the diagnosis of bleeding varices. If the varices have red color (cherry spots) signs, there is a good likelihood of previous variceal hemorrhage.

Gastric Ulcer

Ulcers are more frequently seen at or near the angulus on the lesser curve of the stomach. The margins are sharp and the base is clean and white except for a clot, red or black spots, or a protuberant pink visible vessel that might mar the surface.

Duodenal Ulcer

Postbulbar ulcers may be difficult to see on the medial aspect of the proximal descending limb. The best view of the bulb can be obtained by putting the tip of the endoscope just inside the pylorus. The presence of duodenitis suggests an associated ulcer, but the mucosal inflammation may, by itself, be responsible for bleeding.

Mallory-Weiss Syndrome

A gastric mucosal laceration running parallel to the long axis of the stomach and extending to and sometimes beyond the esophagogastric junction is not infrequently found in the setting of esophageal varices or erosive gastritis.[15] This is not surprising, since these tears usually occur predominantly in alcoholics and are brought about by vigorous vomiting or retching.

Erosive Gastritis

Erosions of the stomach have a variable appearance, depending on their age. Thus erosions start out as petechiae, which progress to red erosions that may develop black centers and then evolve into white lesions.[4] A large erosion may in fact be an ulcer if it extends below the muscularis mucosae. Erosions related to nonsteroidal anti-inflammatory drugs occur in the antrum and, with severe disease, extend into the duodenum. Stress or alcohol-induced erosions affect the proximal gastric mucosa but with severe disease may progress into the antrum.

COMPLICATIONS OF EGD IN BLEEDING PATIENTS

The mortality and morbidity related to urgent diagnostic EGD for bleeding patients are, as expected, higher than those for elective examination in nonbleeding patients.[16] In the ASGE survey of 2,320 endoscopies, there were five cases of perforation, four of aspiration, and three of hemorrhage, with one death in each subgroup, for a procedure-related mortality of 0.1%,[17] over 10 times that seen in routine EGD. Minor complications consist of medication reactions, hypotension, and cardiac arrhythmia. As more patients receive endoscopic therapy for bleeding lesions, procedural complications and deaths can be expected to increase somewhat, but these should be more than compensated for by a decrease in overall mortality from GI bleeding.

SUMMARY

Endoscopy is the diagnostic procedure of choice for upper GI bleeding. The cause of bleeding can be safely established by EGD in over 90% of cases, permitting rational therapy to be undertaken and facilitating surgical management should it become necessary. A natural outcome of diagnostic endoscopy is endoscopic interventional treatment, which has become the first-line therapeutic approach. Combined diagnostic and therapeutic endoscopy has already been shown to reduce transfusion requirements, hospital stays and costs, and the need for emergency operation in upper GI hemorrhage.[7] It is anticipated that, in time, additional controlled studies will support Swain et al., who showed a reduction in mortality in patients bleeding from peptic ulcer.[18]

REFERENCES

1. Allen HM, Block MA, Schuman BM: Gastroduodenal endoscopy. Management of acute upper gastrointestinal hemorrhage. *Arch Surg* 106:450–455, 1973.
2. Sugawa C, Werner MH, Hayes DF, et al: Early endoscopy: A guide to therapy for acute hemorrhage in the upper gastrointestinal tract. *Arch Surg* 107:133–137, 1973.
3. Sugawa C, Schuman BM: Upper gastrointestinal bleeding, in Sugawa C, Schuman BM (eds.): *Primer of Gastrointestinal Fiberoptic Endoscopy*. Boston, Little, Brown, 1982, pp 61–67.
4. Sugawa C: Endoscopic diagnosis and treatment of upper gastrointestinal bleeding. *Surg Clin North Am* 69:1167–1183, 1989.
5. Peterson WL, Barnett CC, Smith HJ, et al: Routine early endoscopy in upper-gastrointestinal-tract bleeding. *N Engl J Med* 304:925–929, 1981.
6. Swain CP, Storey DW, Brown SG, et al: Nature of the bleeding vessel in recurrently bleeding gastric ulcers. *Gastroenterology* 90:595–608, 1986.

7. Laine L: Multipolar electrocoagulation in the treatment of active upper gastrointestinal tract hemorrhage: A prospective controlled trial. *N Engl J Med* 316:1613–1617, 1987.
8. Gilbert DA, Silverstein FE, Tedesco FJ, et al: The National ASGE Survey on upper gastrointestinal bleeding III: Endoscopy in upper gastrointestinal bleeding. *Gastrointest Endosc* 27:94–102, 1981.
9. Sugawa C, Steffes CP, Nakamura R, et al: Upper GI bleeding in an urban hospital: Etiology, recurrence and prognosis. *Ann Surg* 212:521–527, 1990.
10. Al-Atrakchi HA: Upper gastrointestinal endoscopy without sedation: A prospective study of 2000 examinations. *Gastrointest Endosc* 35:79–81, 1989.
11. Takemoto T, Karita M, Okita K: Electronic endoscopy: Its present and future. *J Gastroenterol Hepatol* 4:75–80, 1989.
12. Larson G, Schmidt T, Gott J, et al: Upper gastrointestinal bleeding. Predictors of outcome. *Surgery* 100:765–772, 1986.
13. de Bombal FT, Clarke JR, Clamp SE, et al: Prognostic factors in upper GI bleeding. *Endoscopy* 18:6–10, 1986.
14. Foster DN, Miloszewski KJA, Losowsky MS: Stigmata of recent haemorrhage in diagnosis and prognosis of upper gastrointestinal bleeding. *Br Med J* 1:1173–1177, 1978.
15. Sugawa C, Benishek DJ, Walt AJ: Mallory-Weiss syndrome: A study of 224 patients. *Am J Surg* 145:30–33, 1983.
16. Shahmir M, Schuman BM: Complications of fiberoptic endoscopy. *Gastrointest Endosc* 26: 89–91, 1980.
17. Gilbert DA, Silverstein FE, Tedesco FJ, et al: National ASGE survey on upper gastrointestinal bleeding: Complications of endoscopy. *Dig Dis Sci* 26(Suppl):55s–59s, 1981.
18. Swain CP, Kirkham JS, Salmon PR, et al: Controlled trial of Nd-YAG laser photocoagulation in bleeding peptic ulcers. *Lancet* 1:1113–1116, 1986.

17

DIAGNOSTIC ENDOSCOPY IN LOWER INTESTINAL BLEEDING

Jerome D. Waye, M.D.

Rectal bleeding is a common complaint and always indicates a pathological process. The origin of bleeding must be investigated; the causes range from the innocuous hemorrhoid as the most frequent source to colon cancer as the most serious problem. About 20% of patients referred to the gastroenterologist with rectal bleeding will have anal disease as an etiology. In approximately 30%, no cause will be found. Examination in half of the patients will reveal clinically relevant pathology such as adenocarcinoma, adenoma, inflammatory bowel disease, angiodysplasia, or diverticular disease.[1-7]

One should look beyond the obviously visible hemorrhoids, since one-quarter of patients who present with rectal bleeding will have serious pathology combined with anal disease. In the massively bleeding patient, the physician must determine the best approach to both diagnosis and therapy. The following definitions are important for establishing the diagnostic approach to the bleeding patient.

Lower intestinal bleeding: The site is distal to the ligament of Treitz. This includes bleeding from the rectum, as well as from a small bowel source. A significant proportion of patients presenting with hematochezia may actually bleed from a site proximal to the ligament ot Treitz. The rate and volume of blood lost will determine whether the patient presents with occult bleeding found via a chemical test for blood or with a torrential flow of blood.

Massive bleeding: The patient with massive rectal bleeding requires an emergency approach considerably different from the approach to the loss of smaller amounts of blood. Massive rectal bleeding may be defined as the passage of copious quantities of bloody bowel movements requiring 2 or more units of blood transfusion to stabilize the hematocrit at 30%, or bleeding which results in clinical signs of hypovolemia, including shock, postural hypotension, tachycardia, and pallor. Immediate resuscitative efforts must be directed toward sustaining life, and decisions must be made to institute both diagnostic and/or therapeutic procedures to identify and treat the source of bleeding. Massive lower intestinal bleeding is a medical emergency.

Nonmassive bleeding: Most patients who present with rectal bleeding, even frequent bloody stools, do not fulfill the criteria for massive bleeding. The actual amount of blood lost with each bowel movement may be moderate, and when bleeding emanates from a hemorrhoid or colitis, frequent bowel movements may be associated with red-colored water in the toilet bowl, but the true amount of blood loss may be relatively small. In a prospective evaluation of mild to moderate red rectal bleeding, investigations yielded a definitive diagnosis in almost 90% of patients.[8] Pathological anal conditions such as hemorrhoids, fissures, and tears were seen in half of the patients but were the most clinically important diagnosis in only 17%, since many had other causes of bleeding.

A positive test for occult blood in the stool should be evaluated, since colorectal cancer will be found in 5–10% of patients and an adenoma in 20–40%.[9,10] Unfortunately, a negative test does not permit complacency about the absence of colorectal neoplasia. The sensitivity for neoplasia is only 21% because many tumors do not bleed continuously or because the amount of blood lost may be too small for chemical detection.[11] Adenomas less than 2 cm in diameter do not often bleed, and tumors of the right colon are less likely to bleed than those in the left colon.[12]

HISTORY AND PHYSICAL EXAMINATION

There may be events in the patient's medical history to suggest the site of lower gastrointestinal bleeding. A detailed description of the color of bleeding, its relationship to bowel movements, and its frequency are important historical events that may determine the subsequent diagnostic approach. The patient who is massively bleeding will have frequent bloody bowel movements, with passage of red blood or clots. Most massive bleeding episodes are not accompanied by brown stool. When brown stool is present along with red blood, the site of origin is usually in the left colon and will often be found in the rectosigmoid area. On the other hand, blood from a proximal source completely mixes with fecal contents, so that brown stool will not be identifiable during massive bleeding from the right colon or from a more proximal source in the small bowel. Even with massive bleeding, blood from the proximal colon will often be changed by the action of bacteria, causing a dark coloration of the rectal effluent.

The presence of abdominal pain preceding a massive bleeding episode suggests either ischemia or inflammatory bowel disease, but rarely may accompany the rupture of an aortic aneurysm into the duodenum. A history of diarrhea, aphthous stomatitis, arthritis, or systemic symptoms of anorexia and fever may indicate inflammatory bowel disease. Painless massive bleeding is common in diverticulosis, in telangiectasia, or from a Meckel's diverticulum in younger patients. Although rare, hemorrhoids may present with massive hematochezia,[13] especially in the patient with underlying portal hypertension. Whenever rectal bleeding is associated with evidence of hypovolemia, strong consideration must be given to a proximal source, and a detailed history of a potential upper gastrointestinal bleeding site must be sought.

Although drugs do not directly contribute to lower gastrointestinal bleeding, an upper gastrointestinal site may be suspected in a patient taking aspirin, nonsteroidal anti-inflammatory agents, or ethanol. Patients taking salicylates may have an increased tendency to bleed. These patients and anyone with a history compatible with a bleeding diathesis should have a coagulation workup to rule out any bleeding tendency.

A history of radiation to the rectum, prostate, or female pelvic organs may be associated with radiation colitis years after treatment was completed. Radiotherapy may induce marked neovascularization of the mucosal surface, which can bleed profusely.

The most common presentation of rectal bleeding is a history of recurrent small amounts of blood staining the toilet tissue or in the toilet bowl following defecation. Blood spurting (or dripping) into the toilet bowl following a normal evacuation is always duc to a perirectal lesion, the most common being hemorrhoids. The sudden appearance of blood is frightening to the patient and convinces him or her that it represents a major bleeding episode, but the physician must independently ascertain the severity of bleeding based on the history and physical examination.[14]

Most causes of lower gastrointestinal bleeding have no findings on physical examination, but a murmur of aortic stenosis, with or without cutaneous or retinal telangiectasias, may point to bleeding from arteriovenous malformations. Arterial bruits or a pulsatile abdominal mass may indicate ischemic colitis or an aneurysmal-duodenal leak. Blood in the small bowel acts as a peristaltic stimulant, and increased bowel sound activity associated with the passage of dark or bright blood per rectum provides a clue suggesting its origin in the upper intestinal tract. A diminished blood volume from acute blood loss causes circulatory instability with pallor, tachycardia, diaphoresis, and postural hypotension.

SIGMOIDOSCOPY

A sigmoidoscopic examination should be performed on every patient examined for rectal bleeding. In addition to identifying a bleeding site in the rectum or anus, visualization of the mucosa may determine the presence of ulcerative colitis or proctitis. When a bleeding lesion is present in the rectum and the instrument, either rigid or flexible, can be passed above the bleeding site, the distal localization of the bleeding site is highly accurate.

NONENDOSCOPIC STUDIES

The barium enema plays no role in the management of patients with acute rectal bleeding. Barium will preclude the subsequent use of either angiography or colonoscopy. Several studies have investigated the yield of the barium study along with sigmoidoscopy in the patient with nonmassive bleeding. A randomized clinical trial of patients who had positive fecal occult blood tests[15] determined that colonoscopy was the best strategy for detecting colonic neoplasms in patients over 55, but the combination of barium enema, x-ray studies, and sigmoidoscopy was more cost effective in younger people. Another report showed that colonoscopy was better for the assessment of adenomas or carcinoma, whereas the barium enema x-ray was superior for detecting diverticular disease.[8]

A radionuclide scan is valuable in the presence of significant ongoing rectal bleeding. Tc-99m sulfur colloid is an agent that is removed from the circulation rapidly after injection. It is effective in the diagnosis of bleeding sites in only 8% of patients with massive bleeding.[16] Winn et al.[17] identified only 13 sites of bleeding in 63 patients in whom Tc-99m sulfur colloid was used. The intermittent nature of gastrointestinal bleeding renders the sulfur colloid scan relatively insensitive. Labeled red blood cells which have prolonged intravascular activity provide a longer time frame during which imaging can be performed. Approximately 95% of the injected activity with tagged red cells persists in the vascular compartment beyond 30 minutes, allowing prolonged circulation of the radionuclide agent to permit diagnostic imaging for several hours. In the series by Bunker and Lull,[16] 90 minutes of continuous imaging with labeled red blood cells detected 83% of active bleeding. Other authors have found this technique less rewarding.[18-20]

Wright estimates that angiography may localize a site of bleeding in 80–85% of patients when the bleeding rate is at least 0.5 ml/min.[21] Other reports on the use of this modality have been less favorable.[18,22] Since the leading causes of lower gastrointestinal bleeding are diverticulosis and angiodysplasias, both a superior and an inferior mesenteric angiogram should be performed. In the investigation of patients with diverticulosis, intra-arterial vasopressin may be infused through the catheter; this controls bleeding in approximately 90% of patients.[23] The catheter can be left in place for continuous intra-arterial infusion, since rebleeding within the first 48 hours remains a common occurrence. In patients considered to be actively hemorrhaging, a nuclear scan immediately followed by angiography would be the sequence of choice, with the scan providing a guide that blood loss is continuing. The angiographic diagnosis of vascular ectasia is well established, but colonoscopy has probably superseded its use for both diagnosis and therapy of bleeding angiodysplasia.

COLONOSCOPY

Colonoscopy is of paramount importance in the examination of patients with chronic, unexplained rectal bleeding.[24] When colonoscopy is performed under these circumstances and a negative barium enema has already been performed, approximately 30–40% of patients will have a specific lesion discovered by endoscopy (Plate 19–24), 15% of this patient group will have a colon polyp at colonoscopy, and 10% will have an undiagnosed carcinoma.[3] A prospective study of patients with nonmassive rectal bleeding determined that colonoscopy should be the first investigation in subjects likely to require biopsy or therapeutic intervention.[8] This report stated that for the diagnosis of adenoma, carcinoma, and angiodysplasia, colonoscopy is clearly more sensitive than sigmoidoscopy and barium enema x-ray.

In the patient with massive bleeding, the endoscopic yield ranges from 10% to 60% in defining the etiology; the wide variation in positive findings reflects the input from several institutions with varying colonoscopic expertise.[22,25] Upon cessation of massive bleeding, there is an impressive yield on colonoscopic examination because adequate preparation can be provided before endoscopy.[26] A review of the data on 74 patients with recent lower gastrointestinal bleeding showed that 25% with a normal preceding barium enema had an etiology found on colonoscopy.[27] The lesions included polyps greater than 1 cm in diameter, two carcinomas, and several angiodysplasias.

ACUTE LOWER GASTROINTESTINAL BLEEDING

Eighty consecutive patients[22] with severe ongoing hematochezia who underwent emergency colonoscopy after oral purge have been reported. Seventy-four percent were found to have colonic lesions, with 30% of these being angiodysplasia, 17% diverticulosis, 11% polyps or cancer, and 9% focal colitis or ulcers. Eleven percent of the patients with massive rectal bleeding were found to have upper gastrointestinal lesions on upper endoscopy, which was performed in all patients. In comparison, 22 of these same patients also had emergency angiography, with a diagnostic yield of only 14%. The authors believe that an oral purge is an effective and safe method of cleaning the colon and that emergency upper endoscopy should be performed in any patient with lower gastrointestinal hemorrhage. Urgent colonoscopy was safe and frequently diagnostic, and in 39% of patients, therapeutic endoscopy could be performed at the time of the initial colonoscopic examination. In another report of emergency colonoscopy in 35 patients with acute hematochezia,[28] bleeding lesions were identified in 24 patients following oral purge. Therapeutic endoscopy was successful in 11 of these patients who had no complications.

Colonoscopy in an actively bleeding patient may be difficult and may carry a somewhat increased risk of perforation. Suction is difficult because of the presence of blood clots and visualization is difficult due to the dark coloration of blood in the colon. Treat and Forde[29] and Forde[30] analyzed the findings in 40 patients who underwent emergency colonoscopy for massive rectal bleeding. Seven patients had active lesions identified, and 16 had presumptive site localization because of the finding of fresh blood in an area with nonbloody contents proximally. Six of the seven patients with a documented colonoscopic lesion had the diagnosis confirmed at surgery.

A variety of surgical procedures have been performed for torrential bleeding in patients known to have diverticular disease. ''Blind'' left hemicolectomy or segmental colectomy without knowing the site of bleeding is associated with a rebleeding rate of approximately 30% and a mortality rate of 20–40%. Blind subtotal colectomy with ileoproctostomy is rarely indicated for patients too unstable for further preoperative assessment. Even in this severely ill subset of patients it is important to perform an upper endoscopic examination (done intraoperatively, if necessary), and remove most of the colon after failing intraoperative attempts to identify the source of blood which fills the colon but is not seen in the small intestine.[31] It has been suggested that emergency laparotomy after resuscitation should be performed with high-flow antegrade colonic irrigation (via a cecostomy) followed by intraoperative colonoscopy.[32] This will permit precise localization of the bleeding site to guide appropriate surgical therapy. The risk of soilage from the distended cecum is significant despite precautions.

There is clearly potential for both diagnostic and therapeutic use of colonoscopy in the setting of massive lower gastrointestinal bleeding. This procedure should be an integral part of the workup, but the requirement for an expert in the field to perform the endoscopy suggests that this investigation probably should follow the radionuclide scan.

BLEEDING ETIOLOGY

Hemorrhoids are the most common cause of lower gastrointestinal bleeding (Plate 25). Blood loss is usually minimal, but in rare cases chronic bleeding may have a cumulative effect, resulting in iron deficiency anemia.[33] Characteristically, bright red blood coats the stool or drips into the toilet bowl and frequently is noticed on the toilet tissue. Severe hemorrhage rarely occurs; however, reflux of blood into the sigmoid colon may prompt a fruitless and expensive search for a more proximal site.

Meckel's diverticulum is a significant cause of massive bleeding in the young adult. Gastric or duodenal mucosa within the diverticulum leads to peptic ulceration and bleeding. Children usually have multiple episodes of bleeding before the correct diagnosis is made by radioactive technetium picked up by the aberrant mucosa.

Beliefs about the most common cause of massive lower gastrointestinal bleeding in adults have changed over the past few decades. Diverticulosis was once considered the most common etiology,[34] but most authors now accept vascular ectasia as the leading etiology.[22] Although diverticulosis is more common in the left colon, most diverticular bleeding emanates from the right colon.[35] The high incidence of bleeding from the right colon may be related to the wider necks within the diverticulum, with the vasa rectae being more exposed to erosion/ulceration over a greater length of colon. Simultaneous bleeding from more than one diverticulum is unusual, except in the presence of uremia or a coagulopathy. The clinical presentation consists of an abrupt onset of rectal bleeding. In a series of 78 patients[36] with diverticular bleeding, 49 (63%) were admitted in shock or with a hematocrit lower than 30%. Even in these patients, spontaneous cessation of bleeding is common and, therefore, conservative management with fluid, blood transfusions, and bed rest should be considered before surgery. Most patients bleed only once, but 20–25% of patients have recurrent bleeding. It is distinctly uncommon for diverticula to present with persistent minor bleeding, such as occult blood loss.

Vascular ectasias or arteriovenous malformations (AVMs) are a cause of colonic bleeding, with some authors considering it common and others uncommon.[37-40] There is usually low-grade bleeding, with tarry stools in 20–25% of cases and iron deficiency anemia in 10–15%. Despite the common opinion that AVMs cause torrential bleeding, only 15% of patients who bleed from AVMs have massive blood loss. The majority of patients (over 90%) stop bleeding spontaneously, although bleeding frequently recurs.

Vascular ectasias are dilated blood vessels which result from degenerative vascular disease.[41,42] Most AVMs (77–89%) are found in the right colon, although they may be scattered throughout the large bowel. The diagnosis can be made by angiography, which is best performed during acute bleeding, but extravasation of contrast medium may occur in only 6% of cases. There is controversy concerning the relative roles of colonoscopy and angiography in the diagnosis of AVMs that has yet to be settled, although most endoscopists believe that AVMs can easily be seen colonoscopically.[22] The lesions are frequently associated with aortic stenosis, mitral valve prolapse, Osler-Weber-Rendu disease, and aging, but heart disease has not been definitely implicated as an independent variable.[43]

Treatment of vascular ectasias involves electrocoagulation using a hot biopsy (monopolar) forceps, with control of bleeding achieved in the majority of patients in whom this therapy is applied.[44] Endoscopic treatment can often eliminate AVMs and markedly reduce the rebleeding rate.[44] At St. Mark's Hospital in London,[45] 34 patients were found with AVMs out of a total experience of 10,000 colonoscopies, but the incidence in patients having colonoscopies for lower intestinal bleeding was 2%, and when colonoscopy was performed for anemia, AVMs were found in 9% of the cases. This group found that AVMs are present in the right colon in 76% of cases, in the transverse colon in 12%, and in the left colon in 12%.[44]

The Cleveland Clinic reported its experience[46] with the diagnosis of vascular ectasias in 71 patients utilizing colonoscopy. Forty-four percent of the patients had a history of recurrent rectal bleeding or melena, and the average number of previous bleeding episodes was six per patient. Bleeding was evident as anemia in 50% of the patients (hemoglobin less than 10 g %), fecal occult blood test positivity in 47%, melena in 25%, and tachycardia in 12%. The patients ranged in age from 9 to 88 years, with an average age of 62. Nineteen percent of the patients had AVMs in more than one colon segment, and often in both the right and left colons, with the majority (47 out of 77) occurring in the cecum. Twenty-eight patients were treated at the time of colonoscopy, and half of these had repeat bleeding. A second endoscopic coagulation was performed, which achieved control in one-third of the rebleeders. The overall endoscopic success rate was 68%, but it should be noted that 6 out of 11 patients treated with only blood transfusions did not rebleed, and therefore would also have been counted as treatment successes.

In a recent report of 30 patients with AVMs, all had lesions in the right colon and 2 had coexisting lesions in the left colon.[47] Ninety percent of the patients presented with either acute or chronic gastrointestinal bleeding, with an average hematocrit of 34%. Fifty-six percent had red rectal bleeding, 30% occult blood, and 15% melena. In this series, in 9 out of 10 patients in whom angiography was performed, a positive diagnosis was made. The remaining diagnoses were made with colonoscopy. In 13 patients, endoscopic fulguration was performed, with one perforation. Two patients required repeat endoscopic coagulation because of rebleeding and one of these had colectomy for uncontrolled bleeding. At the time of colonoscopy, 15 patients had biopsy of lesions. A definitive histological diagnosis was made in 9 of these patients (60%), while in the remaining 6 patients, the biopsy revealed ''chronic inflammation of colonic mucosa.'' The authors suggest that an endoscopic biopsy should be attempted for all patients with symptomatic vascular ectasia.

The Mayo Clinic[48] has reported on 93 consecutive patients with transfusion-dependent gastrointestinal bleeding from mucosal vascular malformations. Twenty-four patients had angiography, 12 of which were suggestive of angiodysplasia. Angiography failed to demonstrate 83% of the vascular malformations seen endoscopically because many of these malformations were small and located in the mucosa.

The colonoscopic diagnosis of AVMs is well established. The diagnosis may be made by angiography, but one cannot tell, without extravasation of dye, whether the lesion demonstrated is responsible for the bleeding. Many AVMs may be submucosal and may not be a clinical problem, although they will demonstrate a typical angiographic lesion. An excellent right colon preparation is necessary to identify these lesions colonoscopically and an electrolyte preparation seems to be a good way of achieving bowel cleansing in the patient in whom a cause for anemia or bleeding is sought. The treatment of AVMs seems to be adequately served by colonoscopy and fulguration with the hot biopsy forceps technique. Many patients rebleed and require additional electrocoagulation to control the bleeding. There is no reason to coagulate AVMs found on incidental colonoscopy in the patient who is not bleeding or anemic.

About 25% of patients with bleeding diverticulosis will have persistent bleeding or will rebleed within 48 hours.[49,50] This group of patients will require surgery, which can be limited if the site of bleeding is localized, but a subtotal colectomy with ileorectal anastomosis is required if no site is found before surgery. Every effort should be made to identify specifically the site of blood loss.[51] Fifteen percent of patients who have had a surgical hemicolectomy and in whom no site has been identified prior to surgery will have rebleeding, a figure that tends to support the performance of a subtotal colectomy in this group of patients. If angiodysplasia results in recurrent massive bleeding or if the patient becomes transfusion dependent, a decision requiring surgery should be based upon endoscopic or angiographic examinations.

In the elderly patient, an important as well as common cause of gastrointestinal hemorrhage is colonic ischemia. The left colon receives its major blood supply from the inferior mesenteric artery and a rich collateral supply from the marginal vessels. Atherosclerosis may interfere with flow through the marginal arteries, causing ischemia and subsequent necrosis, especially in the area near the splenic flexure. Ischemic colitis may present as "abdominal angina" due to transient ischemia, with a classic clinical triad of postprandial pain, weight loss, and sitophobia. The occurrence of ischemia after abdominal aortic surgery is a well-known entity and represents a serious complication of such surgery.[52,53] Bleeding results when true ischemia, of either the reversible kind[54] or the progressive type that results in colonic gangrene,[55,56] occurs. Blood loss is not usually massive, but its appearance following an episode of pain is characteristic. Patients with ischemic colitis are usually above age 65 and have a history of arteriosclerosis. Pain in the left lower quadrant may be the first symptom, with bloody diarrhea 24 to 48 hours later. Colonic ischemia may also account for bleeding in young patients taking oral contraceptives. The association with oral contraceptives is not understood but vessel wall damage, alterations in blood clotting, and immunological mechanisms have been reported.[57] In ischemia colonoscopy usually demonstrates sparing of the mucosa in the rectum, with gray to purple coloration of the sigmoid and descending colon. There may be a sharp demarcation between involved and uninvolved bowel, and biopsy of the ischemic mucosa usually produces very little bleeding.

Rarely, patients with a colonic polyp or carcinoma will present with significant rectal bleeding. The most common presentation of these lesions is with occult bleeding or minimal gross blood in the stool. Adenomas in the left colon bleed more than those in the right colon, with the amount of bleeding correlating with polyp size and the proportion of the villous component. Carcinomas tend to bleed more than adenomas, with greater blood loss when they are large, poorly differentiated, or lacking in mucin production.[58] Macrae and Johns[59] studied patients with known colonic adenomas or carcinomas and found that right-sided carcinomas bled more than 10 ml/day, whereas distal lesions had a mean blood loss of less than 6.5 ml/day. Patients with adenomas had blood loss greater than 2 ml/day only when the polyps were larger than 2 cm in diameter. The incidence of visible bleeding depends on the location of the tumor. Red blood in the stool is most frequent with rectosigmoid cancers, with a reported incidence of 75% in these patients. Left-sided lesions above the sigmoid present with gross blood on the stool in approximately 45% of patients, and right-sided lesions present with visible bleeding in approximately 10–15%.[60] Patients with polyps or carcinomas seldom present with massive blood loss.

Among other causes of lower gastrointestinal bleeding are inflammatory bowel disease and ulcers. Inflammatory bowel disease rarely presents with bleeding as an initial symptom; a good history and sigmoidoscopy should enable one to make the diagnosis. Ulcers of the colon may bleed, especially the solitary rectal ulcer syndrome wherein repetitive mucosal prolapse of the rectal mucosa results in chronic ulceration.

In the evaluation of patients with hematochezia, it is important to note that lesions proximal to the sigmoid colon may present with bright red bleeding. Shinya and Cwern[61] reported that 5% of patients who noted rectal bleeding had right-sided carcinomas, with 38% having carcinomas proximal to the splenic flexure. Colonoscopy has proven to be more sensitive than the barium enema in detecting malignancy or the presence of polyps in the colon.

DIAGNOSTIC EVALUATION

When occult blood is present in the stool, the entire colon must be evaluated. Flexible sigmoidoscopy and barium enema may be more cost effective in patients under age 55, but colonoscopy is indicated in older patients because of the probability of finding adenomas or cancer that may require polypectomy or tissue retrieval for biopsy.[15] The role of upper gastrointestinal endoscopy in occult bleeding is controversial.[51] Significant upper tract lesions are seldom found on endoscopy in patients who have occult fecal blood in the absence of upper tract symptoms. The yield from small bowel x-ray series is also quite low. Thus, if colonoscopy is negative, if there are no symptoms of upper gastrointestinal disease, and if the patient is not anemic, no further tests need to be done. However, if occult bleeding persists, further studies are indicated.

In the presence of nonmassive rectal bleeding, sigmoidoscopy with anoscopy may be diagnostic for perianal lesions. When the history includes blood entwined with the stool or presented as a stripe on the stool, a more proximal site should be considered and colonoscopy performed because of the capability for polypectomy or biopsy.

Massive bleeding must be handled as a medical emergency. If possible, an electrolyte purge should be followed by urgent colonoscopy. Emergency upper gastrointestinal endoscopy should be performed to exclude an upper bleeding site. Use of the nasogastric tube does not provide the same degree of diagnostic assurance gained from endoscopy. The efficiency of scintigraphy and visceral angiography has been reported to be rather variable, with scans being accurate in 30–90% of patients and angiography in 14–72%.[24,50,62]

The cornerstone of an accurate diagnosis is a complete history obtained from the patient.[63] Although each of the many possibilities of a bleeding site must be considered in every patient with rectal bleeding, the differential diagnosis may be markedly narrowed by an accurate history and pinpointed by the appropriate diagnostic procedure.

REFERENCES

1. Chapuis PH, Goulston KJ, Dent OF, et al: Predictive value of rectal bleeding in screening for rectal and sigmoid polyps. *Br Med J* 290:1546–1548, 1985.
2. Thoeni RF, Venbrux AG: The value of colonoscopy and double-contrast barium-enema examinations in the evaluation of patients with subacute and chronic lower intestinal bleeding. *Radiology* 603–607, 1983.
3. Tedesco FJ, Waye JD, Raskin JB, et al: Colonoscopic evaluation of rectal bleeding: A study of 304 patients. *Ann Intern Med* 89:907–909, 1978.
4. Knutson CO, Max MH: Value of colonoscopy in patients with rectal blood loss unexplained by rigid proctosigmoidoscopy and barium contrast enema examinations. *Am J Surg* 139:84–87, 1980.
5. Winawer SJ, Leidner SD, Boyle C, et al: Comparison of flexible sigmoidoscopy with other diagnostic techniques in the diagnosis of rectocolon neoplasia. *Dig Dis Sci* 24:277–281, 1979.

6. Bat L, Pines A, Rabau M, et al: Colonoscopic findings in patients with hemorrhoids, rectal bleeding and normal rectoscopy. *Isr J Med Sci* 21:139–51, 1985.
7. Rex DK, Lehman GA, Lappas JC, et al: Sensitivity of double contrast barium study for left colon polyps. *Radiology* 158:69–72, 1986.
8. Irvine EJ, O'Connor J, Frost RA, et al: Prospective comparison of double contrast barium enema plus flexible sigmoidoscopy v. colonoscopy in rectal bleeding; Barium enema v. colonoscopy in rectal bleeding. *Gut* 29:1188–1193, 1988.
9. Simon JB: Occult blood screening for colorectal carcinoma: A critical review. *Gastroenterology* 88:820–837, 1985.
10. Winawer SJ, Andrews M, Miller CH, et al: Review of screening for colorectal cancer using fecal occult blood testing, in Winawer SJ, Schottenfeld D, Sherlock P (eds): *Colorectal Cancer: Prevention, Epidemiology, and Screening*. New York, Raven Press, 1980, p. 249.
11. Rozen P, Ron E, Fireman Z, et al: The relative value of fecal occult blood tests and flexible sigmoidoscopy in screening for large bowel neoplasia. *Cancer* 60:2553–2558, 1987.
12. Schrock TR: Colon and rectum: Diagnostic techniques, in Condon RE (ed): *Surgery of the Alimentary Tract*, ed 3, Vol 4: *Colon and Anorectum*. Philadelphia, WB Saunders Co, 1991, pp 22–37.
13. Thompson WH: The nature of hemorrhoids. *Br J Surg* 62:542–552, 1975.
14. Waye JD: A diagnostic approach to colon bleeding. *Mt Sinai J Med* 51:491–500, 1984.
15. Rex DK, Weddle RA, Lehman GA, et al: Flexible sigmoidoscopy plus air contrast barium enema versus colonoscopy for suspected lower gastrointestinal bleeding. *Gastroenterology* 98:855–861, 1990.
16. Bunker SR, Lull RJ: Scintigraphy of gastrointestinal hemorrhage. *Am J Radiol* 143:543–548, 1984.
17. Winn M, Weissman HS, Sprayregen S, et al: The radionuclide detection of lower gastrointestinal bleeding sites. *Clin Nucl Med* 8:389–395, 1983.
18. Potter GD, Sellin JH: Lower gastrointestinal bleeding. *Gastroenterol Clin North Am* 17:341–356, 1988.
19. Rosen AM, Fleischer DE: Lower GI bleeding: Updated diagnosis and management. *Geriatrics* 44:49–60, 1989.
20. Kalloo AN, Collen MJ, Benjamin SB, et al: Technetium 99m-labeled red blood cell scans: Are they really useful in the diagnosis of lower gastrointestinal bleeding? (abstract). *Gastroenterology* 94:5, 1988.
21. Wright HK: Massive colonic hemorrhage. *Surg Clin North Am* 60:1297–1304, 1980.
22. Jensen DM, Machicado GA: Diagnosis and treatment of severe hematochezia. The role of urgent colonoscopy after purge. *Gastroenterology* 95:1569–1574, 1988.
23. Athanasoulis CA, Waltman AC, Phillips DA, et al: The role of arteriography in colonic hemorrhage, in Clearfield HR, Dinoso VP (Eds): *Gastrointestinal Emergencies*. New York, Grune & Stratton 1976, pp 159–165.
24. Schuman B: When should colonoscopy be the first study for active lower intestinal hemorrhage? *Gastrointest Endosc* 30:372–374, 1984.
25. Brenna E, Skreden K, Waldum HL, et al; The benefit of colonoscopy. *Scand J Gastroenterol* 25:81–88, 1990.
26. Rex DK, Weddle RA, Lehman GA, et al: Flexible sigmoidoscopy plus air contrast barium enema versus colonoscopy for suspected lower gastrointestinal bleeding. *Gastroenterology* 98:855–861, 1990.
27. Todd GJ, Forde KA: Lower gastrointestinal bleeding with negative or inconclusive radiographic studies: The role of colonoscopy. *Am J Surg* 38:627–628, 1979.

28. Caos A, Benner KG, Manier J, et al: Colonoscopy after Golytely® preparation in acute rectal bleeding. *J Clin Gastroenterol* 8:46–49, 1986.

29. Treat MR, Forde KA: Colonoscopy, technetium scanning and angiography in acute rectal bleeding. An algorithm for their combined use. *Surg Gastroenterol* 2:135–138, 1983.

30. Forde KA: Causes, diagnosis, and management of colonic bleeding. *Compr Ther* 15:45–48, 1989.

31. Newhall SC, Lucas CE, Ledgerwood AM: Diagnostic and therapeutic approach to colonic bleeding. *Am Surg* 47:125–130, 1981.

32. Berry AR, Campbell WB, Kettlewell MG: Management of major colonic haemorrhage. *Br J Surg* 75:637–640, 1988.

33. Elta GH: Approach to the patient with gross gastrointestinal bleeding, in Yamada T (ed): *Textbook of Gastroenterology*. Philadelphia, JB Lippincott Co, 1991, pp 591–616.

34. Heald RJ, Ray JE: Bleeding from diverticula of the colon. *Dis Colon Rectum* 14:420–427, 1971.

35. Cassarella WJ, Kanter IE, Seaman WB: Right-sided colonic diverticula as a cause of acute rectal hemorrhage. *N Engl J Med* 286:450–453, 1972.

36. Quinn WC: Diverticular disease of the colon with hemorrhage, a study of 78 cases. *Am Surg* 26:170–174, 1960.

37. Boley SJ, Brandt LJ: Colonic ectasias and lower intestinal bleeding. *Hosp Pract* 17:137–144, 1982.

38. Weaver GA, Alpern HD: Gastrointestinal angiodysplasia associated with aortic stenosis; Part of a spectrum of angiodysplasia of the gastrointestinal tract. *Gastroenterology* 77:1–11, 1979.

39. Welch CE, Athanasoulis CA: Hemorrhage from the large bowel with special reference to angiodysplasia and diverticular disease. *World J Surg* 2:73–83, 1978.

40. Harford WV: Gastrointestinal angiodysplasia: Clinical features. *Endoscopy* 20:144–148, 1988.

41. Boley SJ, Sammartano R, Adams A, et al: On the nature and etiology of vascular ectasias of the colon. Degenerative lesions of aging. *Gastroenterology* 72:650–660, 1977.

42. Reinus JF, Brandt LJ: Upper and lower gastrointestinal bleeding in the elderly. *Gastroenterol Clin North Am* 19:293–318, 1990.

43. Imperiale TF, Ransohoff DF: Aortic stenosis, idiopathic gastrointestinal bleeding, and angiodysplasia: Is there an association? *Gastroenterology* 95:1670, 1988.

44. Lanthier P, D'Harveng B, Vanheuverzwyn R, et al: Colonic angiodysplasia: Follow-up of patients after endoscopic treatment for bleeding lesions. *Dis Colon Rectum* 32:296–298, 1989.

45. Danesh BJZ, Spiliadis C, Williams CB, et al: Angiodysplasia—an uncommon cause of colonic bleeding: Colonoscopic evaluation of 1,050 patients with rectal bleeding and anaemia. *Int J Colorect Dis* 2:218–222, 1987.

46. Trudel JL, Fazio VW, Sivak MV: Colonoscopic diagnosis and treatment of arteriovenous malformations in chronic lower gastrointestinal bleeding. Clinical accuracy and efficacy. *Dis Colon Rectum* 31:107–110, 1988.

47. Roberts PL, Schoetz DJ Jr, Coller JA: Vascular ectasia. Diagnosis and treatment by colonoscopy. *Am Surg* 54:56–59, 1988.

48. Gostout CJ, Bowyer BA, Ahlquist DA, et al: Mucosal vascular malformations of the gastrointestinal tract: Clinical observations and results of endoscopic neodymium: Yttrium-aluminum-garnet laser therapy. *Mayo Clin Proc* 63:993–1003, 1988.

49. Farrands PA, Taylor I: Management of acute lower gastrointestinal hemorrhage in a surgical unit over a 4-year period. *J R Soc Med* 80:79–82, 1987.

50. Forde KA, Webb WA: Acute lower gastrointestinal bleeding. *Persp Colon Rectal Surg* 1:105–112, 1988.

51. Schrock TR: Colonoscopic diagnosis and treatment of lower gastrointestinal bleeding. *Surg Clin North Am* 69:1309–1325, 1989.

52. Scherpenisse J, van Hees PAM: The endoscopic spectrum of colonic mucosal injury following aortic aneurysm resection. *Endoscopy* 21:174–176, 1989.

53. Zelenock GB, Strodel WE, Knol JA, et al: A prospective study of clinically and endoscopically documented colonic ischemia in 100 patients undergoing aortic reconstructive surgery with aggressive colonic and direct pelvic revascularization, compared with historic controls. *Surgery* 106:771–780, 1989.

54. Heron HC, Khubchandani IT, Trimpi HD, et al. Evanescent colitis. *Dis Colon Rectum* 24:555–561, 1981.

55. Marston AM, Phiels MT: Ischemic colitis. *Gut* 7:1–15, 1966.

56. Marcusan RW: Ischemic colitis. *Clin Gastroenterol* 1:745–765, 1972.

57. Kilpatrick ZM, Silverman JF: Vascular occlusion of the colon and oral contraceptives. *N Engl J Med* 278:438–440, 1968.

58. Sobin LH, The histopathology of bleeding from polyps and carcinomas of the large intestine. *Cancer* 55:577–581, 1985.

59. Macrae FA, St Johns DJ: Relationship between patterns of bleeding with hemoccult sensitivity in patients with colorectal cancers or adenomas. *Gastroenterology* 82:891–898, 1982.

60. Woolley PV 3d: Clinical manifestations of cancer of the colon and rectum. *Semin Oncol* 3:373–376, 1976.

61. Shinya H, Cwern M: Colonoscopic diagnosis and management of rectal bleeding. *Surg Clin North Am* 62:897–903, 1982.

62. Leitman IM, Paull DE, Shires GT III: Evaluation and management of massive lower gastrointestinal hemorrhage. *Ann Surg* 209:175, 1989.

63. Waye JD: Diagnosis and treatment of lower intestinal bleeding, in Tytgat GNJ, Blankenstein M van (eds): *Current Topics in Gastroenterology and Hepatology*. Stuttgart and New York, Thieme, 1990, pp 23–31.

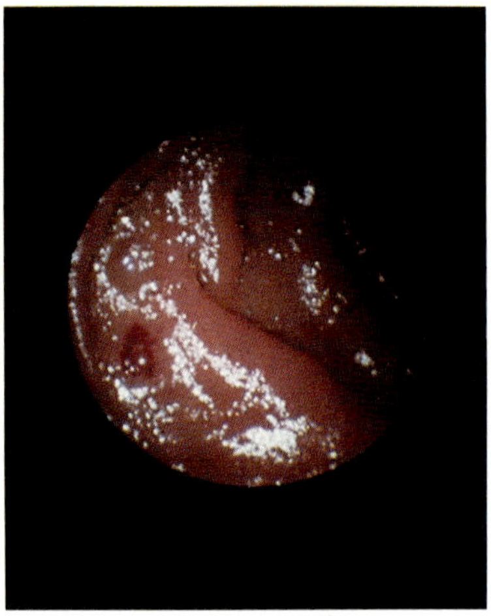

Plate 17. An angiodysplasia within the distal duodenum discovered at push enteroscopy.

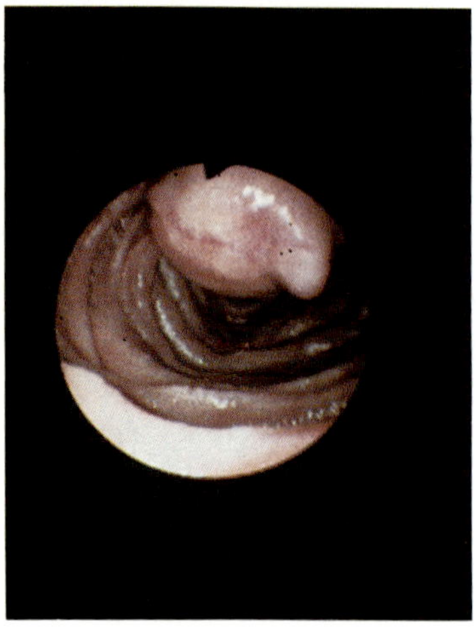

Plate 18. A leiomyoma within the jejunum.

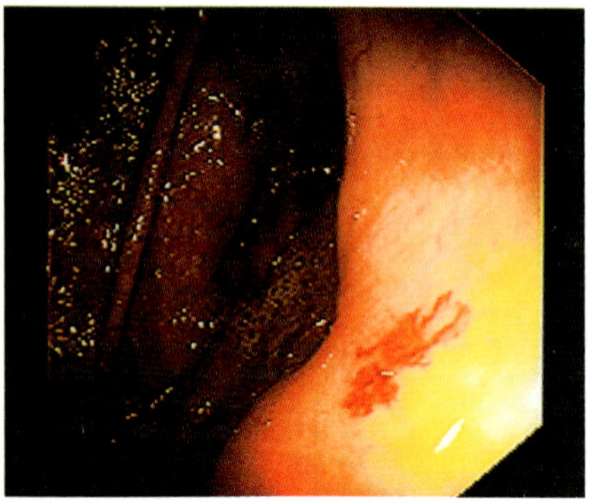

Plate 19. AVM. The typical racimose appearance of an AVM is seen on the ileocecal valve.

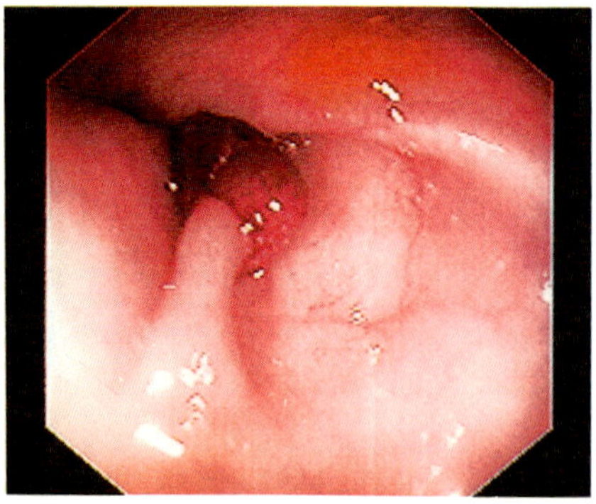

Plate 20. Pedunculated polyp. This cherry red adenoma accounted for a streak of blood on the stool. These lesions rarely cause massive bleeding.

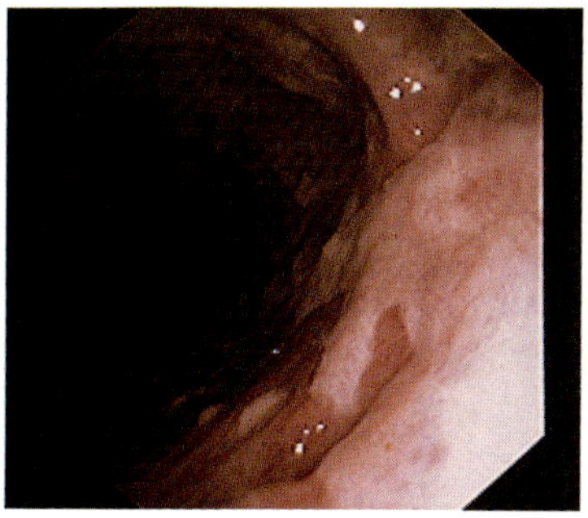

Plate 21. Ischemia. This patient's copious rectal bleeding followed shortly after the onset of abdominal cramps. Endoscopy two days later demonstrated diffuse superficial ulcerations.

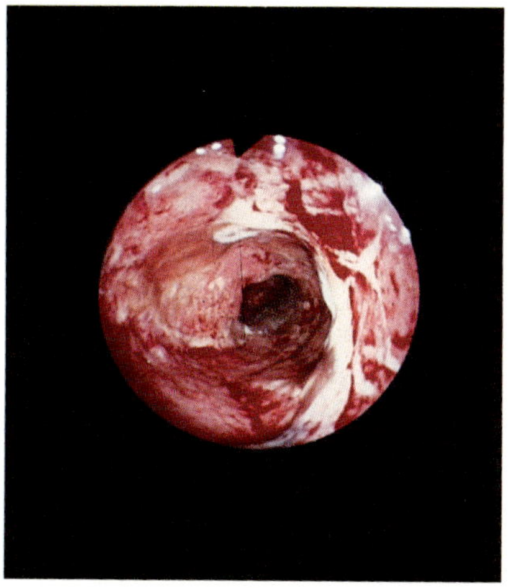

Plate 22. Inflammatory bowel disease. Extreme friability of the bowel walls leads to the symptoms of diarrhea, urgency and rectal bleeding in ulcerative colitis.

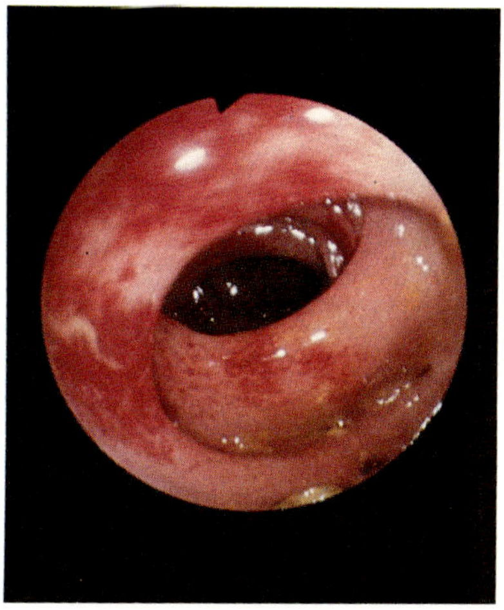

Plate 23. Diverticulosis. The trauma of stools passing an area of muscular hypertrophy may damage the mucosal surface, resulting in bleeding. This is not diverticulitis.

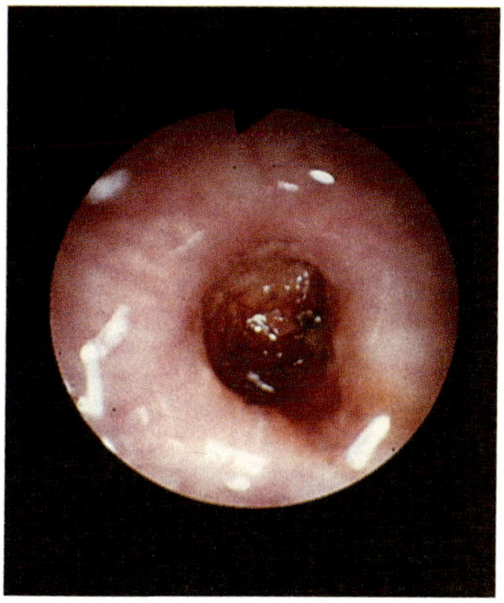

Plate 24. Diverticular bleeding. Blood is seen to emanate from a single diverticulum. This is an unusual finding that pinpoints the site of acute rectal bleeding.

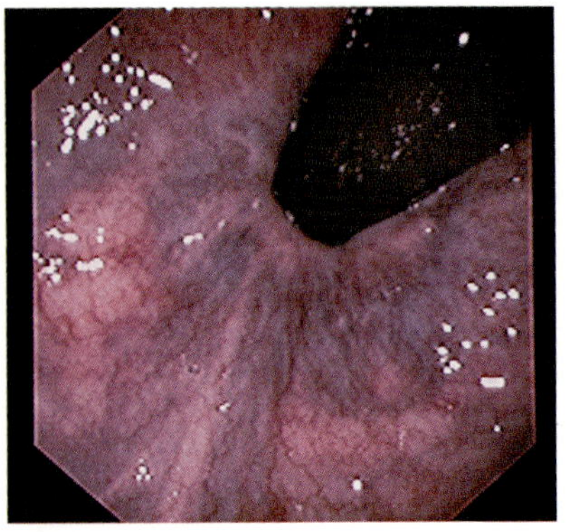

Plate 25. Hemorrhoids. A U-turn maneuver in the rectum demonstrates the presence of internal hemorrhoids, which may be a cause of copious bleeding.

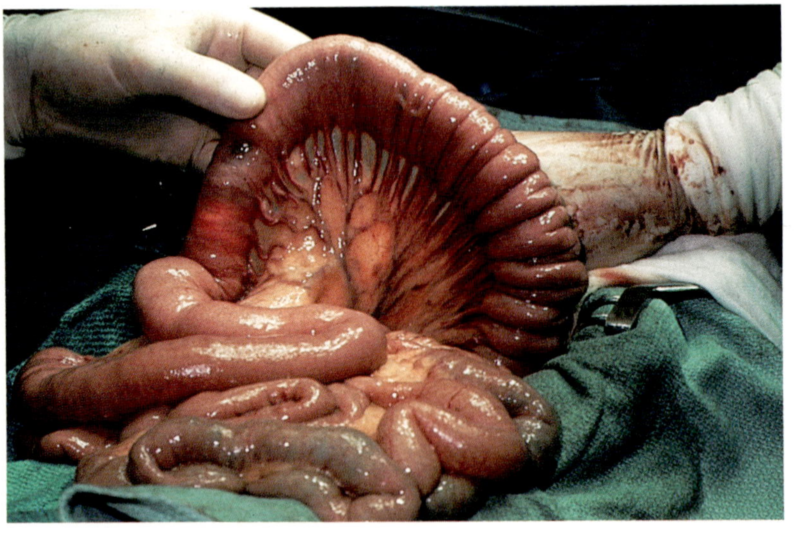

Plate 26. Corkscrew configuration forming as the bowel is pleated on the shaft of the instrument.

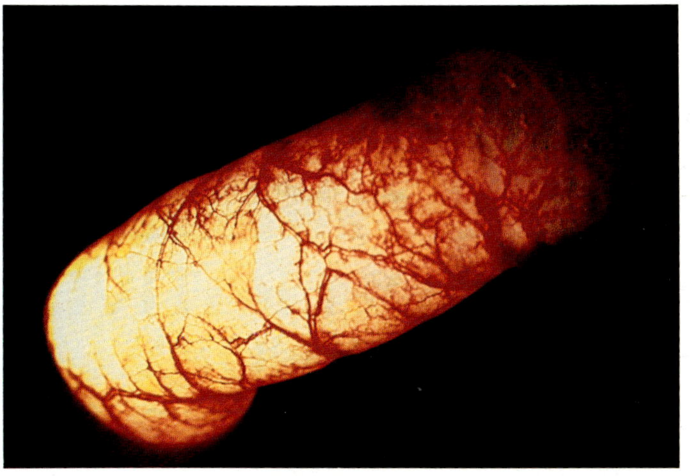

Plate 27. Transilluminated view of the normal jejunal vascular network.

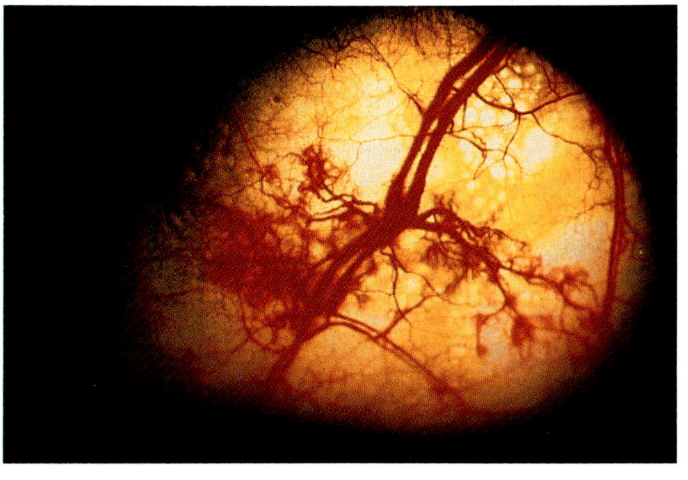

Plate 28. Transilluminated view of a cecal vascular malformation.

18

INTRAOPERATIVE ENDOSCOPY

Talmadge A. Bowden, Jr., M.D.

BACKGROUND

Approximately 95% of all cases of gastrointestinal (GI) bleeding can be accurately diagnosed with conventional flexible fiberoptic endoscopy, angiography, radioisotope scanning, and contrast barium studies. The remaining 5% are a source of frustration to all who manage these clinical problems. Formerly, exploratory laparotomy was performed as a last-ditch effort in these difficult patients, with disappointing results. In 1969 the concept of *blind* subtotal colectomy was introduced for the treatment of patients with cryptogenic lower GI bleeding.[1] Although initial experience with this technique seemed to be satisfactory, Gianfrancisco and Abcarian in 1982 pointed out in a retrospective study that there were many pitfalls in this approach.[2] These authors concluded that every effort should be made to identify the exact source of bleeding and thus proceed with targeted surgery rather than subject the patient to blind subtotal colectomy.

Before the development of the flexible endoscope, the interior of the intestinal tract could be examined during laparotomy only by introducing a rigid sigmoidoscope through an opening in the bowel. This technique was first used in 1952 by Kline and Scarboro and was termed *coloscopy*. It was popular for approximately 20 years, but the flexible colonoscope has replaced this cumbersome procedure.

The concept of performing intraoperative endoscopy without opening the GI tract was first reported in 1967 by Sugawa in a correlated study of intraoperative photography and subsequent histological diagnosis in patients undergoing gastric resection for stress-related gastric bleeding.[3] Sweeting[4] in 1968 reported enteroscopy using the flexible esophagoscope through enterotomies: he examined the entire small bowel and observed multiple vascular lesions in a patient with hereditary familial telangiectasia. In 1972 Lucas and Sugawa,[5] expanding on their original study, reported on 16 patients undergoing laparotomy for acute upper GI tract hemorrhage in whom preoperative gastroscopy could not be accomplished. In 15 patients the source of bleeding was identified without opening the GI tract. In the same year, Marcozzi and Montori[6] described the technique of intraoperative colonoscopy without colotomy. Bombeck[7] in 1975 concluded from a review of intraoperative endoscopy that the technique had a wide variety of applications but had been largely overlooked. Additional reports in the later 1970s described the experience and benefits of intraoperative endoscopy in locating the source of obscure GI tract bleeding, particularly when the hemorrhage was from the small bowel. Lipshutz et al. in 1978,[8] and Evensen et al.[9] that same year, also confirmed the usefulness of this technique in patients with small bowel hemorrhage. Bowden et al.[10] demonstrated the value of intraoperative endoscopy in patients with obscure GI tract bleeding when they defined the source of hemorrhage in six of eight patients thus examined. Bowden et al.[11] in 1982 reviewed the records of 17 patients with intestinal vascular ectasia and found that the actual distribution of lesions was not fully appreciated even though both preoperative angiography and colonoscopy gave a high diagnostic yield. Intraoperative endoscopy not only defined the exact distribution of the vascular lesions but also allowed precise localization for subsequent accurate histological examination. Intraoperative endoscopic findings also influenced the eventual surgical decision in half of these patients.

More recently, the sonde enteroscope has been used by a few investigators, who have shown that the procedure is safe and relatively effective. Available data[12] indicate that the ileum can be reached with a sonde enteroscope in 77–84% of patients. When used to define the etiology of obscure bleeding in problematic patients, this technique allows accurate diagnosis in approximately one-fourth to one-third of such patients. When sonde enteroscopy was compared to intraoperative enteroscopy performed with a colonoscope in 23 patients with bleeding, the concordance for detection of bleeding lesions between the two methods was 77%.[13] As the sonde enteroscope becomes more sophisticated and practical, it is anticipated that many patients with unexplained anemia will be examined. However, since the instrument does not presently have therapeutic potential, most of these patients will still require intraoperative enteroscopy for specific treatment of small bowel bleeding lesions. Rather than being replaced by enteroscopy, intraoperative endoscopy will continue to have a significant impact on the diagnosis and management of patients with bleeding of obscure etiology.

INDICATIONS

Over the past 25 years, the literature has been replete with case reports and small series utilizing intraoperative endoscopy for a wide variety of indications. These are summarized in Table 18.1. Most reports on intraoperative endoscopy focus on the diagnosis and management of occult intestinal bleeding. In the majority of the patients presented in these reports, the source of hemorrhage could have been localized only by intraoperative endoscopy. Intraoperative endoscopy offers a detailed view of the intestinal vascular network as a definitive aid in the localization of sources of GI bleeding. Many patients with GI bleeding of obscure etiology have intestinal vascular lesions that pose special diagnostic and therapeutic problems. These lesions may be single or multiple and may be found in areas other than the right colon. Both angiography and colonoscopy have shortcomings in detecting these lesions and defining their true extent. Occasionally, in an acute situation, an exact bleeding point may not be seen but can be "surrounded," avoiding blind resection.

Patients requiring small bowel enteroscopy are few, since only 1–5% of all patients with GI hemorrhage bleed from the small intestine. However, when a small bowel source of bleeding is suspected, based on the process of elimination or evidence generated

Table 18.1. Intraoperative Endoscopy: Uses

Localization of subtle colonic lesions
Localization of polypectomy sites
Difficult polypectomy
Synchronous lesions (proximal obstruction)
Polyposis syndromes
Mallory-Weiss tears
Congo Red mapping
Check suture lines
Intraoperative dilemmas
Aid in tube placement
Bleeding of obscure etiology

by barium contrast studies, preoperative enteroscopy, or angiography, the technique of intraoperative endoscopy offers the only consistent method of specific intraoperative localization of those lesions which are neither palpable nor identifiable from the serosal surface of the bowel. An additional fringe benefit is the opportunity to clear the entire GI tract of all other potential lesions.

TECHNIQUE

In many instances, the surgeon will possess endoscopic skills; however, if this is not the case, consultation should be sought early with an available endoscopist in order to discuss the sequential steps of management. The anesthesiologist should also be alerted that intraoperative endoscopy is planned, since it will be necessary for the anesthesia equipment and monitoring devices to be placed at the patient's right side to allow the endoscopist to work from the left side with the endoscopic instruments. If the procedure is both planned and elective, preoperative mechanical preparation of the bowel should be thorough and complete to ensure the best examination possible. Under these elective circumstances, lavage clears the small and large bowels effectively. Even when the procedure is being done in an acute situation, lavage should also be done if time is available. Occasionally, laparotomy and intraoperative endoscopy are required when the bowel is filled with blood and the source or suspected area of hemorrhage has not been identified preoperatively. Intraoperative lavage of the colon can be done through a catheter inserted into the cecum and the bowel cleared of blood. Additionally, lavage through the small intestine can be done via the endoscope during the procedure.

Since multiple sources of bleeding can be present, examination of the entire GI tract during laparotomy may be appropriate or even desirable. Unless otherwise contraindicated, the patient should be placed in stirrups in the lithotomy position. This will allow easy access to the rectum by the endoscopist, and the intestinal tract can be visualized simultaneously, both endoscopically and with transillumination. The instrument selected is usually an adult or pediatric colonoscope. The endoscope should be prepared with thorough mechanical cleaning and disinfection techniques. Intraoperative examination is enhanced for all participants if the endoscopic image can be displayed on a television monitor by means of either a videoendoscope or a clip-on television camera. If a videoendoscope is selected, a state-of-the-art color chip instrument must be used because the scintillation effects from the older instruments will not yield the continuous light beam necessary for a detailed examination.

The endoscope is inserted prior to the abdominal incision. But before the instrument is passed, a small-bore nasogastric tube should be placed into the stomach. This maneuver has a dual purpose: it acts as a guide for proper placement of the endoscope past the endotracheal tube and prevents overdistention of the stomach during the examination. During preparation of the skin, the endoscope should be passed as far into the duodenum as is easily possible. Intubation of the duodenum is always much easier if done before the abdominal incision is made and the tamponade effect of the abdominal wall is lost. One should note that as the endoscope is advanced through the duodenum and into the proximal jejunum, two loops will form—one along the greater curvature of the stomach and another at the curve of the duodenum. These loops must be prevented from becoming excessive. A member of the operating team should maintain counterpressure on the greater curvature with the right hand and on the C-loop of the duodenum with the left hand (Figure 18.1). This position of the hands will keep the endoscope as straight as possible and should be maintained until the entire small bowel has been intubated.

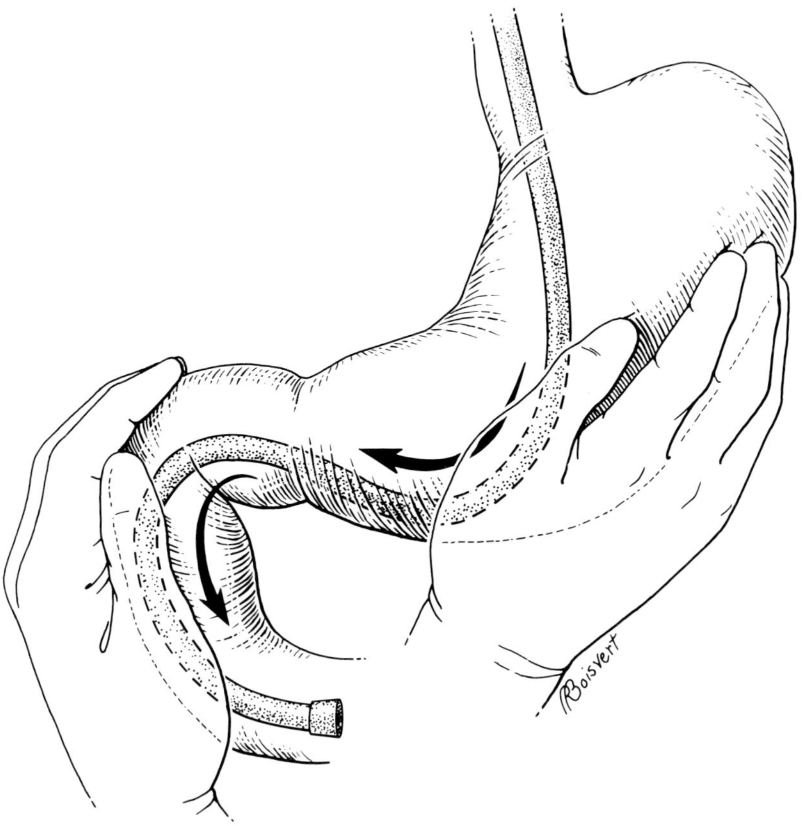

Figure 18.1. To avoid creation of loops at the greater curvature of the stomach and the descending duodenum, gentle but firm, continuous counterpressure is applied in the manner shown. Reprinted with permission of Mosby-Yearbook, Inc. Intraoperative Endoscopy of the Gastrointestinal Tract. in Surgical Endoscopy. Dent TL, Strodel WE, Turcotte JG (Eds), Chicago, 1985.

Prior to advancing the endoscope into the proximal small bowel, the surgeon should thoroughly explore the abdomen and lyse any adhesions. In some instances, obvious disease will be discovered by exploration, which may make further examination unnecessary. From this point on, the surgeon and endoscopist work together as a team, advancing the endoscope through the bowel. The utmost care is taken to avoid the creation of mucosal artifacts that can cause diagnostic dilemmas. Progress through the small bowel is made by slowly advancing the instrument and pleating the bowel over the shaft of the endoscope (Figure 18.2). The instrument tip must be advanced under *direct vision,* using minimal amounts of air. As the endoscope is passed further into the intestinal tract, a corkscrew configuration of the bowel will form (Plate 26). The mesentery should be examined frequently, and tension should not be allowed to become excessive. When the terminal ileum is reached, the operating room lights are dimmed and the instrument is gradually withdrawn. The intestines should be examined in 10-cm segments by distending the bowel with air and examining the entire circumference. As the instrument is withdrawn in 10-cm segments, the bowel is decompressed. The transilluminated intestinal vascular network is quite striking (Plate 27). Any suspicious lesions should be confirmed by both luminal and transilluminational views (Plate 28) and, if deemed significant, marked by a silk suture (Figure 18.3). The lesion will be removed at the conclusion of the examination by whatever means is deemed appropriate, including snare cautery, laser ablation, endoscopically directed suture ligation, simple elliptical excision, wedge resection, or bowel resection. The bowel should be completely decompressed in segments as the instrument is withdrawn.

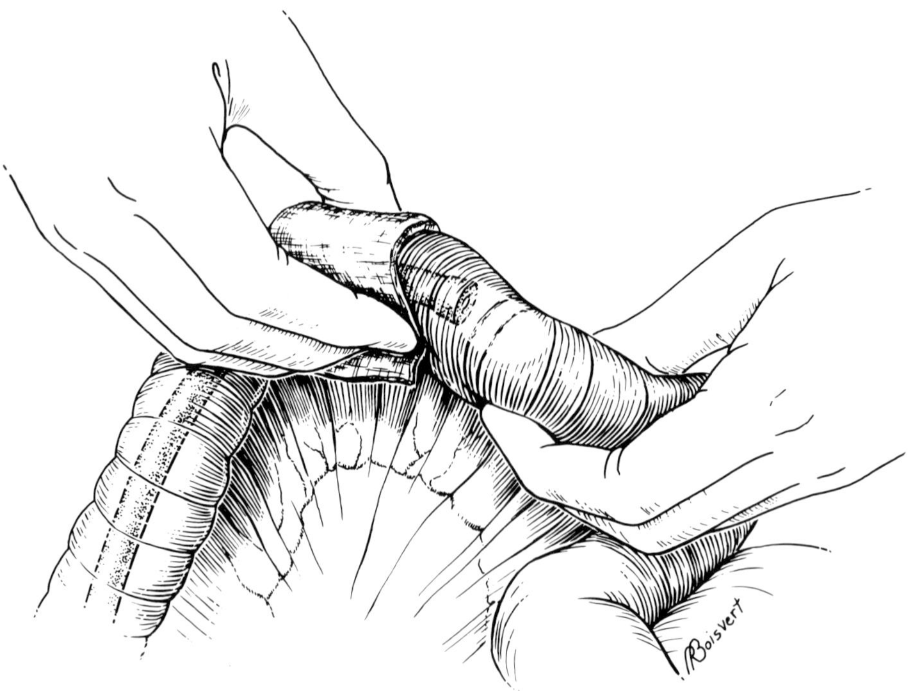

Figure 18.2. The endoscope is advanced slowly through the small bowel, and the bowel is telescoped over the shaft. The instrument is advanced under *direct vision,* using small amounts of air. Reprinted with permission of Mosby-Yearbook, Inc. Intraoperative Endoscopy of the Gastrointestinal Tract in Surgical Endoscopy. Dent TL, Strodel WE, Turcotte JG (Eds), Chicago, 1985.

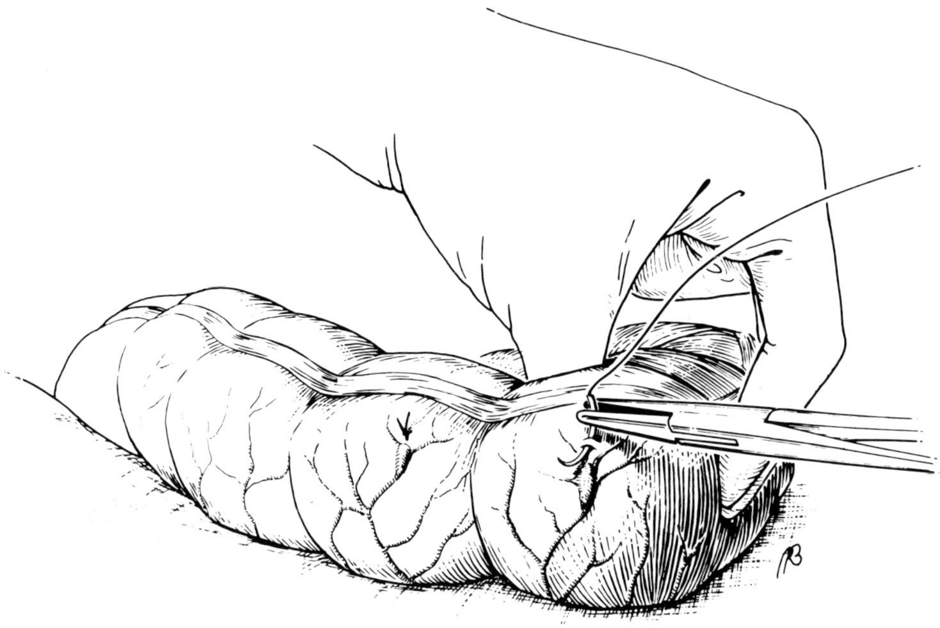

Figure 18.3. Suspicious lesions are marked with a fine silk suture placed only through the serosa. The suture is placed adjacent to but *not* through the vascular lesion. This tag will be used by the pathologist for direct histological examination. Reprinted with permission of Mosby-Yearbook, Inc. Intraoperative Endoscopy of the Gastrointestinal Tract in Surgical Endoscopy. Dent TL, Strodel WE, Turcotte JG (Eds), Chicago, 1985.

Once the small bowel examination is complete, the endoscopist can pass the endoscope per anus to examine the colon. Because the large intestine lacks the mobility of the small bowel, a complete and thorough examination may be more difficult. In some instances, flexures may occasionally need to be mobilized in order to enhance passage of the instrument to the cecum; counterpressure on the sigmoid colon is usually required (Figure 18.4). As with the small intestine, decompression of the colon is done after various segments are examined. Intraoperative endoscopy is similar to other endoscopic and surgical procedures in that it requires patience and attention to detail.

RESULTS

The literature on intraoperative endoscopy testifies to the usefulness of this technique in patients with occult GI bleeding, either massive or subtle.[14] Usually, intraoperative endoscopy is the final evaluation and therapeutic effort in these patients. Over the past 15 years at the Medical College of Georgia, 45 patients have undergone intraoperative endoscopy as part of their assessment for bleeding of obscure etiology. A real or potential source of bleeding was identified in 93% of these patients, including 25 patients who were found to have vascular ectasias (Table 18.2). Of the vascular ectasias identified, many were located in the cecum and ascending colon, but most of the patients had additional or separate vascular lesions outside the right colon, with vascular malformations discovered in the small bowel of nine patients. Intraoperative endoscopy, in 1982, was compared with colonoscopy and angiography in this patient population.[11] Both colonoscopy and angiography had a high degree of diagnostic accuracy, but angiography failed

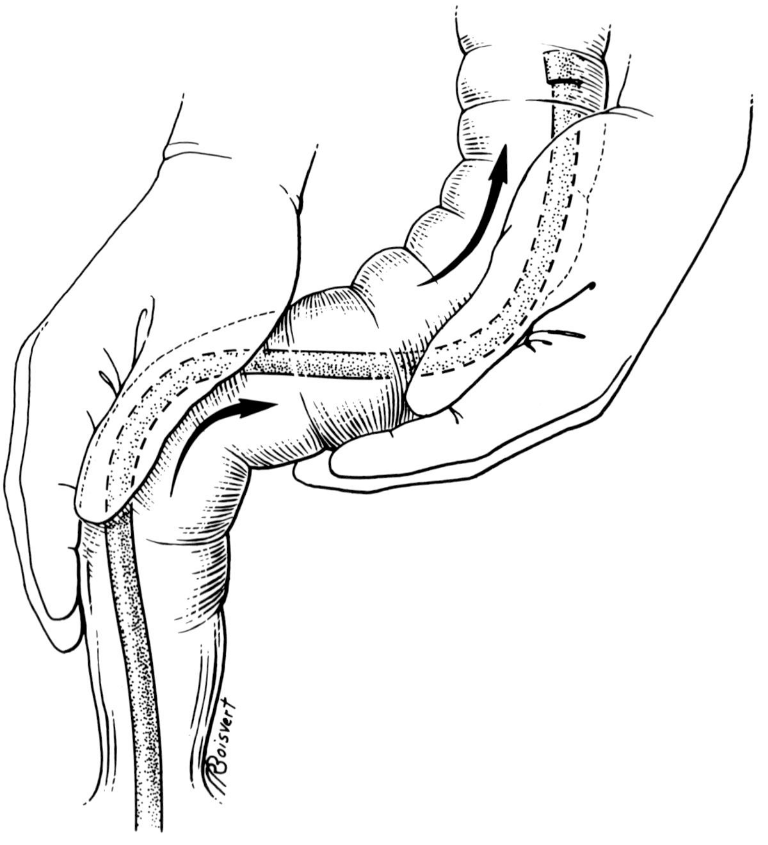

Figure 18.4. Counterpressure is applied to the sigmoid colon to avoid development of a large loop which would impede advancement of the endoscope. Reprinted with permission of Mosby-Yearbook, Inc. Intraoperative Endoscopy of the Gastrointestinal Tract. in Surgical Endoscopy. Dent TL, Strodel WE, Turcotte JG (Eds), Chicago, 1985.

to demonstrate some lesions seen by colonoscopy. Since angiography and colonoscopy, used either alone or in combination, do not always define the precise distribution of vascular malformations, intraoperative endoscopy remains the best method for defining the exact distribution of these lesions. Intraoperative endoscopy has been shown to influence the eventual surgical decision in 50% of patients with GI bleeding of obscure etiology.

When these patients rebleed, reassessment is necessary. Seven (15%) of the 45 patients in my series had rebleeding after intraoperative endoscopy. When these patients were reevaluated, the source of rebleeding was identified as gastritis, esophageal varices, radiation proctitis, hemorrhoids, and, in one patient, Osler-Weber-Rendu syndrome. Other lesions were noted to be actively bleeding at the time of reexploration and repeat intraoperative endoscopy in the patient with Osler-Weber-Render syndrome.

LIMITATIONS AND COMPLICATIONS

Few complications have been reported with intraoperative endoscopy. Review of these reports shows that most of the adverse affects could have been prevented by careful

Table 18.2. Intraoperative Endoscopy: Bleeding of Obscure Etiology

Vascular ectasias	25
Diverticulosis	4
Small bowel ulceration	3
Dieulafoy's disease	3
Osler-Weber-Rendu syndrome	2
Early Crohn's disease	2
Polyarteritis nodosum	1
Jejunal diverticula	1
Small bowel cancer	1
Failure to identify	3
Total	45

attention to detail by both the surgeon and the endoscopist. In 1981 Frank et al.[15] reported a single case of submucosal hemorrhage in a patient undergoing intraoperative small bowel endoscopy for bleeding of obscure etiology. They reported small, superficial mucosal ulcerations and elevated hemorrhagic lesions when removing the endoscope, emphasizing that the lesions were not seen on entering the bowel. These lesions were probably more commonplace when colonoscopes utilizing a hood over the tip of the instrument were used. With a modern blunt-tipped instrument, this complication should be diminished. Small suction artifacts may be created during the examination; these "lesions" can be resolved by the technique of reverse transillumination. Reverse transillumination is easily accomplished by focusing the operating room light on the area in question. The endoscope light is then turned off and, utilizing the magnification of the instrument, the fine vascular network of an angiectasia can be identified. If the lesion is a submucosal hemorrhage, this branching appearance will be absent.

Sjogren et al.[16] observed serosal laceration as a consequence of pneumatic overdistention of the colon when cross-clamping was employed to enhance the view without distending the rest of the colon. This complication can be easily prevented by not cross-clamping the ileum, by using judicious amounts of air, and by removing the air in segments as the examination progresses. Trauma to the spleen may result from overdistention of the stomach and loop formation of the endoscope along the greater curvature. Splenic injury from pressure of gastric distention can be prevented by placing a nasogastric tube prior to inserting the endoscope and using continuous nasogastric suction during the procedure. In addition, if the right hand of the assistant is placed along the greater curvature of the stomach at all times during the examination, the endoscope shaft will not impinge on the spleen. Other problems related to the procedure, such as minor wound infections and ileus, have been reported, but infrequently.

SUMMARY

The usefulness of intraoperative endoscopy as an addition to the surgical armamentarium has been supported by reports in the literature of the past 25 years. Those authors reporting their experience emphasize that the technique has been of value in almost every clinical setting in which it has been utilized. In patients with GI bleeding of obscure etiology, either an active or a potential source of hemorrhage was identified in over 90% of these highly selected patients. With that identification, the limits of resection may be extended or restricted based on the combined observations of the operating surgeon and endoscopist. Lesions not palpable through the colonic wall can be localized. Unsuspected lesions can be visualized and tissue can be obtained endoscopically for definitive diagnosis. Vascular malformations can be located and marked with a suture so that resection and subsequent accurate histological examination and definitive diagnosis can be made. The technique of total GI tract examination can be mastered, but there is a learning curve. Both patience and perseverance will be required.

REFERENCES

1. Taylor FW, Epstein LI: Treatment of massive diverticular hemorrhage. *Arch Surg* 98:505–508, 1969.
2. Gianfrancisco JA, Abcarian H: Pitfalls in the treatment of massive lower gastrointestinal bleeding with "blind" subtotal colectomy. *Dis Colon Rectum* 25:441–445, 1982.
3. Sugawa C: A study of gastrocamera findings of gastric ulcer: Precise comparison between gastrocamera photographs and pathological findings. *Gastrointest Endosc* 9:395–417, 1967.
4. Sweeting JG: Fiberoptic examination of the small intestine in a case of familial telangiectasia. *Gastrointest Endosc* 14:152–153, 1968.
5. Lucas CE, Sugawa C: Diagnostic endoscopy during laparotomy for acute hemorrhage from the upper part of the gastrointestinal tract. *Surg Gynecol Obstet* 135:285–286, 1972.
6. Marcozzi G, Montori A: Endoscopy during operation: New diagnostic possibilities. *Chir Gastroenterol* 6:23–25, 1972.
7. Bombeck CT: Intraoperative esophagoscopy, gastroscopy, colonoscopy, and endoscopy of the small bowel. *Surg Clin North Am* 55:135–142, 1975.
8. Lipshutz GR, Katon RM, Eidemiller L: Gastrointestinal bleeding due to an invaginated and intussuscepted Meckel's diverticulum diagnosed by intraoperative ileoscopy. *Gastrointest Endosc* 24:177–178, 1978.
9. Evensen SA, Blomhoff JP, Flatmark H: Peroperative endoscopic diagnosis of small intestinal bleeding. *Scand J Gastroenterol* 13:593–597, 1978.
10. Bowden TA, Hooks VH, Mansberger AR: Intraoperative gastrointestinal endoscopy in the management of occult gastrointestinal bleeding. *South Med J* 72:1532–1534, 1979.
11. Bowden TA, Hooks VH, Mansberger AR: Intestinal vascular ectasia: A new look at an old disease. *South Med J* 75:1210–1217, 1982.
12. Lewis BS, Waye JD: Chronic gastrointestinal bleeding of obscure origin: Role of small bowel enteroscopy. *Gastroenterology* 94:1117–1120, 1988.
13. Lewis BS, Wenger JS, Waye JD: Small bowel enteroscopy and intraoperative endoscopy for obscure gastrointestinal bleeding. *Am J Gastroenterol* 86:171–174, 1991.
14. Bowden TA: Endoscopy of the small bowel, in Schrock T (ed): *Surgical Clinics of North America,* Vol. 69. Philadelphia, WB Saunders Co, 1989, p 1237.
15. Frank MS, Brandt LJ, Boley SJ: Iatrogenic submucosal hemorrhage, a pitfall of intraoperative endoscopy. *Am J Gastroenterol* 75:209–210, 1981.
16. Sjogren RW, Johnson LF, Butler ML: Serosal laceration: A complication of intraoperative colonoscopy explained by transmural pressure gradients. *Gastrointest Endosc* 24:239–242, 1978.

IV

EMERGENCY MANAGEMENT

19

ACUTE MANAGEMENT AND IDENTIFICATION OF RISK FACTORS

Gregory L. Eastwood, M.D.

The principles of the acute management of virtually all patients with active gastrointestinal bleeding are the same, although specific diagnostic tests will vary, depending on the presumed site of bleeding (Table 19.1). In the presence of active gastrointestinal bleeding, the usual orderly sequence of history taking, physical examination, diagnostic evaluation, and treatment frequently is altered to meet immediate demands. The important aspects of each often commingle in the first critical moments of managing the actively bleeding patient. In patients who are hemodynamically stable, a careful history and physical examination may be appropriate, whereas in other patients who are unstable, prompt resuscitative measures are necessary.

INITIAL MANAGEMENT

History

Healthy people normally lose about 1 to 2 ml of blood from the gastrointestinal tract daily as a result of transudation of red blood cells across the mucosa and small amounts of bleeding from tiny abrasions.[1] The clinical manifestations of gastrointestinal bleeding generally require rates of blood loss that are far in excess of the normal amount.

Occult blood in the stool can be detected with as little as 15 ml of blood loss per day. Melena, or black stool, may develop with as little as 50 ml of blood loss per day.[2,3] Although melena usually signifies bleeding from the upper gastrointestinal tract, it can result from a source as low as the proximal colon. Brisker rates of bleeding may appear as red blood per rectum (hematochezia) or vomiting of blood (hematemesis). The action of gastric acid on blood quickly forms dark particles that resemble coffee grounds. Hematemesis of either frank red blood or coffee ground–appearing material usually signifies a source in the upper gastrointestinal tract, but it can result from swallowed

TABLE 19.1. Principles of Initial Management of Active Gastrointestinal Bleeding

- I. Perform in order as determined by activity of bleeding and stability of the patient
  - A. Take a history
  - B. Determine vital signs
  - C. Perform physical examination, including rectal examination
  - D. Insert large-bore intravenous catheter(s)
  - E. Draw blood for initial studies
  - F. Administer intravenous electrolyte solutions
- II. Pass NG tube
  - A. If aspirate is clear initially or clears promptly with lavage, remove tube
  - B. If aspirate is bloody, continue to lavage
- III. Transfuse blood or volume expander
- IV. Notify surgeon
- V. Survey for concomitant disease (heart, lung, renal, liver, cerebrovascular)
- VI. Make a diagnosis
  - A. If upper gastrointestinal bleeding is likely:
    - 1. Attempt endoscopy
      - a. If stigmata of recent hemorrhage* are present or esophageal varices are seen, consider therapeutic endoscopic procedure or surgery
      - b. If stigmata are not identified, treat medically as indicated by findings (e.g., treatment of peptic ulcer or gastritis)
      - c. If blood or clots obscure visibility and bleeding continues, consider radionuclide scan or selective arteriography
    - 2. If bleeding is massive and uncontrolled, consider immediate surgery; endoscopy may be attempted in operating room under anesthesia
  - B. If lower gastrointestinal bleeding is likely:
    - 1. Perform flexible or rigid sigmoidoscopy in all patients
    - 2. If bleeding stops with resuscitative efforts, perform colonoscopy 12–24 hours later after bowel preparation
    - 3. If bleeding continues despite resuscitative efforts or recurs after initial cessation, consider emergency colonoscopy after bowel lavage
      - a. If diagnosis is evident, treat accordingly
      - b. If blood or clots obscure visibility and bleeding continues, consider radionuclide scan or selective arteriography
    - 2. If bleeding is massive and uncontrolled, consider immediate surgery

*Stigmata of recent hemorrhage are a visible vessel in an ulcer crater, a fresh clot or a black eschar over a bleeding site, or active bleeding.

blood from the respiratory tract. Hematochezia is usually a sign of lower gastrointestinal tract bleeding, although profuse upper gastrointestinal bleeding, such as from esophageal varices or from an eroded artery in the base of an ulcer, may produce hematochezia. Stools may remain positive for occult blood for nearly two weeks after an acute loss of 1,000 ml or more of blood from an upper gastrointestinal source.[3]

Blood loss and peripheral vasoconstriction cause cool extremities and pale conjunctivae, mucous membranes, nail beds and palmar creases. The rectal examination provides direct access to the gastrointestinal tract and should not be omitted, even in instances of apparently obvious upper gastrointestinal bleeding. In addition to providing information that can be learned about the anus, perianal area, and rectum, this examination allows the character of the stool to be assessed. As indicated previously, red blood per rectum usually signifies lower gastrointestinal bleeding, whereas melena may indicate an upper gastrointestinal source. Vomiting of blood or coffee ground material in the presence of brown stool or stool negative for occult blood indicates that the bleeding has been of brief duration.

Volume and Blood Replacement

A large-bore intravenous catheter should be inserted promptly into a peripheral vein. In a profusely bleeding patient, a single peripheral intravenous catheter often is not sufficient to provide adequate blood or crystalloid replacement; two or more intravenous catheters may be required. When a peripheral vein is not accessible, venous access should be established via a jugular, subclavian, or femoral vein. Further, a central venous pressure catheter or Swan-Ganz catheter may be necessary to evaluate the effects of volume replacement and the need for continued infusion of blood, particularly in elderly patients or those with cardiovascular disease. Finally, monitoring of urine output will provide a reasonable indication of vital organ perfusion. In severely ill patients, a urinary catheter is essential to evaluate the adequacy of rehydration and renal perfusion.

Normal saline should be allowed to infuse rapidly until blood for transfusion is available. In patients with excess total body sodium, such as those with ascites and peripheral edema, there may be reluctance to infuse large amounts of saline, but the restoration of hemodynamic stability should take precedence over other considerations. In other words, if the patient is bleeding profusely and blood for transfusion is not yet available, saline should be infused without regard to the patient's sodium balance. When bleeding is less severe, hypotonic sodium solutions may be infused until blood for transfusion arrives.

Laboratory Studies

Blood for initial studies should be drawn promptly. Such studies should include a complete blood count, electrolytes, blood urea nitrogen (BUN), creatinine, glucose, calcium, phosphate, magnesium, blood for typing, and any other studies that seem relevant. Hemoglobin and hematocrit usually are low, with the fall in both reflecting the amount of blood loss. However, some patients bleed so rapidly that there is insufficient time for the blood volume to equilibrate, and the hemoglobin and hematocrit are normal or only slightly reduced. In acutely bleeding patients, changes in blood pressure and pulse and the direct evidence of continued bleeding from nasogastric aspiration or rectal output are better indicators than the hemoglobin and hematocrit for guiding the volume of crystalloid solutions and blood replacement.

Clotting status should be assessed by means of the platelet count, prothrombin time, and partial thromboplastin time. If a defect in clotting exists, prompt correction of the deficiency is crucial. Extensive blood transfusion will dilute platelets and clotting factors, particularly factors V and VII. This condition can be treated by infusion of platelets and fresh frozen plasma as needed. Also, a high proportion of patients who bleed while taking therapeutic anticoagulants do so from a clinically significant lesion. Thus, it is important to evaluate these patients for gastrointestinal pathology in addition to correcting their clotting status.

Elevation of the white blood cell count may be associated with acute gastrointestinal bleeding, but it is usually not in excess of $15{,}000/mm^3$. Leukocytosis should not be attributed to acute blood loss without first considering possible sources of infection.

An elevated BUN in a patient whose BUN has recently been normal or whose serum creatinine is normal suggests an upper gastrointestinal bleeding source if the site of bleeding is not initially apparent. The rise in BUN can result from digestion of blood in the small intestine and absorption of nitrogenous products. However, hypovolemia resulting from acute blood loss of either upper or lower gastrointestinal origin can also raise the BUN.

The magnitude of the nitrogen load to the intestine in an actively bleeding patient can be appreciable, since normal blood contains about 15 g of hemoglobin and 5 to 7 g of albumin and globulin per 100 ml. Thus, 1,000 ml of blood arriving in the small intestine from an upper gastrointestinal source carries a protein load of approximately 200 g. This is far in excess of the average dietary intake of 60 to 100 g of protein per day. In patients with marginal liver function, the increased protein load from blood in the gut may be sufficient to induce or aggravate hepatic encephalopathy. Thus, gastric lavage and control of bleeding are of particular importance to these patients.

Because of rapid fluid shifts during gastrointestinal bleeding and the infusion of blood, blood products, and other fluids, frequent assessment of serum electrolytes, including sodium, potassium, calcium, phosphate, and magnesium, is necessary. In severely ill patients, blood gases should be monitored to recognize impending cardiac or pulmonary difficulties. Central venous pressure monitoring may be necessary, in addition to the determination of blood pressure, pulse, and urine output.

Nasogastric Intubation

A nasogastric (NG) tube should be passed in patients with a history of melena or hematemesis. Blood from an esophageal or gastric source will pool in the stomach and, in more than 90% of bleeding duodenal ulcers, the blood will reflux back across the pyloric channel into the stomach.[4] If the aspirate is clear or clears promptly with lavage, the NG tube may be removed. If there is a large amount of blood or retained material, the stomach should be lavaged with a large-bore sump tube (20–24 French) or an Ewald tube. Removal of the gastric contents will facilitate subsequent endoscopy and will decompress the stomach. Because the NG tube is uncomfortable for the patient, predisposes to gastroesophageal reflux and pulmonary aspiration, and may irritate the esophageal and gastric mucosa, it should be removed when it no longer fulfills a useful purpose.

Antacids and Acid Inhibitory Drugs

The reduction of intragastric acid in patients with upper gastrointestinal bleeding is helpful in two ways. First, the direct harmful effects of acid and pepsin on the bleeding lesion are diminished. Second, a less acid environment promotes platelet aggregation and clotting.

After the bleeding has abated and gastric lavage is no longer necessary, an appropriate initial regimen is to administer 30 ml of antacid by NG sump tube every two hours. The tube is clamped for the first hour and suctioned for the second hour. Measurement of intragastric pH just before the next antacid dose will indicate whether the frequency and dose of antacid should be increased. The intent is to maintain the intragastric pH above 4. Whether the use of intravenous H_2 antagonists (cimetidine, ranitidine, or famotidine) is as efficacious as antacids for the control of gastric acid in acute upper gastrointestinal bleeding is controversial. After the NG tube has been removed, the patient may be treated with oral antacids and an acid-antisecretory agent.

Consultations

The management of acute gastrointestinal bleeding involves a team of health care workers. Specific diagnostic studies usually require the skills of a gastroenterologist or a radiologist. The surgeon, when consulted early, may offer valuable assistance in managing the patient and is in a better position to make a decision regarding operative intervention should the need arise later.

RISK FACTORS

Risk Factors in the Clinical Presentation

Volume of Blood Loss

In general, clinical indicators of a large initial bleed increase the morbidity and mortality.[5] These indicators include presentation with red hematemesis or black hematemesis plus melena,[6] delay or failure to clear a red nasogastric aspirate with lavage,[7] elevation of the BUN above 20 μg/dl, hemoglobin below 10 g/dl, and tachycardia. Clinical shock carries the worst prognosis.[8]

Associated Medical Conditions

The number of associated medical conditions is directly related to the increasing risk of mortality in acute gastrointestinal bleeding. In one study, mortality in patients with no accompanying medical conditions was 1.2%, whereas in those with four or more associated illnesses the mortality was 71%.[9]

Patients with liver disease are at risk to develop esophageal varices, which may bleed. However, although most patients with known esophageal varices and acute upper gastrointestinal bleeding are likely to be bleeding from the varices, other sources must be sought by appropriate endoscopic and radiographic studies.[10,11]

Ingestion of Gastric Mucosal Irritants

The recent ingestion of aspirin, other nonsteroidal anti-inflammatory drugs, or alcohol raises the possibility that erosive gastritis or other mucosal injury has developed. Aspirin not only causes direct mucosal injury but also interferes with platelet adhesion; thus, bleeding lesions in patients who take aspirin are less likely to clot.

Age

Advanced age worsens the prognosis of acutely bleeding patients.[5] The age of the patient also will make some diagnoses more or less likely, particularly with regard to lower gastrointestinal bleeding. The differential diagnosis of acute lower gastrointestinal bleeding in a person over age 60 includes ischemic colitis, carcinoma of the colon, arteriovenous malformation, and diverticulosis, whereas none of these is a serious consideration in a 25-year-old person. On the other hand, bleeding from inflammatory bowel disease or a Meckel's diverticulum is more likely in a child or young adult.

Irradiation

A history of abdominal or pelvic irradiation raises the possibility that lower gastrointestinal bleeding is due to radiation enteritis or colitis.[12] Patients may develop gastrointestinal bleeding from the acute effects of irradiation on the gut, or bleeding may occur months to years later; the latter is a form of ischemic colitis that is accelerated by the perivascular inflammation which results from the effects of irradiation.

Characteristic Clinical Presentations

Mallory-Weiss Gastroesophageal Tear. Bleeding from a Mallory-Weiss mucosal tear at the esophagogastric junction traditionally has been associated with repeated vomiting or retching before the appearance of hematemesis. However, in a large review of patients with documented Mallory-Weiss lesions, such a history was obtained in less than a third of the patients.[13] Consequently, the diagnosis of Mallory-Weiss mucosal tear must be made by endoscopic visualization of the lesion, which is usually found on the gastric side of the esophagogastric junction toward the lesser curvature.

Aortoenteric Fistula. Patients with an aortoenteric fistula typically present with massive hematemesis or hematochezia. The initial bleeding often stops abruptly—the sentinel bleed. Recurrent bleeding is usually fatal. The majority of fistulas occur in patients who have had aortic grafts.[14,15] The fistulas develop where the graft is sewn to the aorta and communicate with an adjacent portion of the gastrointestinal tract, usually the duodenum. However, a fistula may develop between unoperated aneurysms and the gastrointestinal tract, or may extend from any vascular aneurysm or replacement prosthesis to any portion of the gastrointestinal tract. When an older patient presents with massive gastrointestinal bleeding that stops abruptly, particularly if there is a history of aneurysm or surgery for aneurysm, the alert clinician should promptly arrange upper endoscopy. The fistula itself is rarely identified at endoscopy, but the absence of other causes of bleeding should prompt diagnostic studies in the stable patient. The unstable patient should be considered for emergency surgery. Computed tomography of the abdomen may show a leaking aneurysm or fistula and therefore is helpful in making the decision on whether or not to operate.[16]

Intestinal Ischemia. Risk factors in addition to advanced age also can be identified for patients with ischemic colitis or enteritis. Two types of ischemic bowel disease are recognized: occlusive and nonocclusive. Occlusion of the celiac axis, the superior mesenteric artery, the inferior mesenteric artery, or their branches can result from thrombosis or embolus. A dissecting aortic aneurysm also can produce an occlusion of one or more of these major vessels. If collateral circulation is inadequate, the bowel becomes acutely ischemic and the patient experiences severe abdominal pain. The most common risk factor for thrombosis is ordinary atherosclerotic vascular disease. Emboli may accompany acute myocardial infarction, ventricular aneurysm, atrial fibrillation, valvular heart disease, or bacterial endocarditis.

Nonocclusive ischemic vascular disease of the bowel takes two forms: abdominal angina and ischemic colitis. Abdominal angina is characterized by severe postprandial midabdominal pain that lasts for minutes to hours but typically is not associated with gastrontestinal bleeding. A minority of patients develop intestinal infarction after weeks to months of ischemic symptoms. Signs of weight loss are usually evident. Risk factors for the development of abdominal angina are coexisting arteriosclerotic disease of the heart and peripheral vessels and diabetes. The second form of nonocclusive ischemic bowel disease, ischemic colitis, typically is associated with lower gastrointestinal bleeding.[17] Mucosal ischemia is thought to result from transient low blood flow through an inadequate vascular system. Risk factors are age over 60 and a cardiovascular condition, such as congestive heart failure or an arrhythmia, that predisposes to a transient reduction in bowel perfusion. Aortic aneurysmectomy also places a patient at risk for the development of ischemic colitis because of interruption of inferior mesenteric artery blood flow in the absence of adequate collateral circulation. Ischemic colitis usually involves the region of the splenic flexure or the sigmoid colon. Patients with ischemic colitis characteristically present with an abrupt onset of moderate lower abdominal pain and bloody stool. Typically, the adomen is soft. In most patients, the course is self-limited, with spontaneous recovery in several days. A minority of patients will develop bowel infarction and peritonitis and require surgical intervention.

Risk Factors in Patient Management

NG Tube

Use of an NG tube is an important and accepted part of the routine management of patients with gastrointestinal bleeding. Removal of gastric contents has several beneficial effects: identification and characterization of the appearance of blood, monitoring of the rate of bleeding, decompression of the stomach, removal of gastric acid to lessen peptic damage, and removal of gastric contents to facilitate subsequent endoscopy. However, use of the NG tube can be associated with certain risks. Besides being uncomfortable, NG intubation predisposes to gastroesophageal reflux and pulmonary aspiration, and may irritate the esophageal and gastric mucosae, thereby aggravating existing mucosal lesions. If the initial NG aspirate is clear or clears promptly with lavage, the NG tube may be removed. It should be removed when it is no longer performing a useful function.

Stigmata of Recent Hemorrhage

Identification of the so-called stigmata of recent hemorrhage (SRH) within an ulcer crater has some prognostic and therapeutic implications. SRH include a protruding, visible vessel, an adherent clot, a black eschar, and actual oozing or spurting of blood. Patients with SRH are more likely to have uncontrolled or recurrent bleeding and to require intervention by therapeutic endoscopy or surgery.[18-20] The treatment of bleeding lesions through the endoscope has become widely available using a variety of methods, including thermal electrocoagulation, laser photocoagulation, injection of ethanol or hypertonic solutions, and injection sclerosis of esophageal varices.[21,22]

Stress Ulceration

Some patients who are severely ill, such as those in the intensive care unit or those who have suffered severe trauma or major surgery, are at high risk to develop so-called stress ulceration and bleeding. The pathogenesis of stress ulceration is unclear but probably is related to a breakdown in the normal mucosal defense mechanisms in conjunction with the injurious effects of acid and pepsin on the mucosa. The clinical setting usually is one of severe and often multisystemic illness.

Treatment of stress ulceration may place the patient at an additional risk of developing bacterial overgrowth and aspiration pneumonia, perhaps as high as 50%.[23-25] Although patients who develop stress ulcers typically do not secrete large amounts of gastric acid, acid does appear to be involved in the pathogenesis of the lesions. Thus, conventional treatment has been either to neutralize acid with antacids or inhibit its secretion with an antisecretory drug. However, maintenance of intragastric pH above 4 predisposes to bacterial colonization of the stomach and pharynx and to subsequent development of pneumonia with the same organisms. Because clinically significant bleeding from stress ulcerations usually occurs in less than 5% of patients in an intensive care unit, this raises the question of whether prophylaxis to prevent gastrointestinal bleeding is trading a high-risk condition (pneumonia) for a low-risk one. Recent evidence suggests that treatment with sucralfate is as effective as antacids or H_2 antagonists in preventing bleeding but does not predispose to pneumonia.[25] In any event, it is appropriate to restrict prophylactic treatment to patients in the intensive care unit who are at high risk for bleeding, namely, those who are on respirators and have multisystem disorders and those with a history of peptic ulcer or upper gastrointestinal bleeding.

REFERENCES

1. Leonard JR, Levy G, Niemczura R: Gastrointestinal blood loss during prolonged aspirin administration. *N Engl J Med* 289:1020–1022, 1973.
2. Daniel WA Jr, Egan S: The quantity of blood required to produce a tarry stool. *JAMA* 113:2232, 1939.
3. Schiff L, Stevens RJ, Shapiro N, et al: Observations on the oral administration of citrated blood in man. II. The effect on the stools. *Am J Med Sci* 203:409–412, 1942.
4. Luk GD, Bynum TE, Hendrix TR: Gastric aspiration in localization of gastrointestinal hemorrhage. *JAMA* 241:576–578, 1979.
5. Peterson WL: Clinical risk factors. *Gastrointest Endosc* 36:S14–S15, 1990.
6. Wara P, Stodkilde H: Bleeding pattern before admission as guideline for emergency endoscopy. *Scand J Gastroenterol* 20:72–78, 1985.
7. McLaughlin WD, Kolts BE, Achem SR: Nasogastric lavage compared with outcome in 101 patients seen in an emergency room for upper gastrointestinal hemorrhage (abstract). *Gastroenterology* 92:1529, 1987.
8. Bornman PC, Theodorou NA, Shuttleworth RD, et al: Importance of hypovolemic shock and endoscopic signs in predicting recurrent haemorrhage from peptic ulceration: A prospective evaluation. *Br Med J* 291:245–247, 1985.
9. Pimpl W, Boeckl O, Waclawiczek HW, et al: Estimation of the mortality rate of patients with severe gastroduodenal hemorrhage with the aid of a new scoring system. *Endoscopy* 19:101–106, 1987.

10. McCray RS, Martin F, Amir-Ahmadi H, et al: Erroenous diagnosis of hemorrhage from esophageal varices. *Am J Dig Dis* 14:755–760, 1969.
11. Sutton FM: Upper gastrointestinal bleeding in patients with esophageal varices. *Am J Med* 83:273–275, 1987.
12. Earnest DL, Trier JS: Radiation enteritis and colitis, in Sleisenger MH, Fordtran JS (eds): *Gastrointestinal Disease. Pathophysiology Diagnosis Management,* ed 4. Philadelphia, WB Saunders Co, 1989, pp 1369–1382.
13. Graham DY, Schwartz JT: The spectrum of the Mallory-Weiss tear. *Medicine* 57:307–318, 1978.
14. Steffes BC, O'Leary JP: Primary aortoduodenal fistula: A case report and review of the literature. *Am Surg* 46:121–129, 1980.
15. Grande JP, Ackermann DM, Edwards WD: Aortoenteric fistulas. A study of 28 autopsied cases spanning 25 years. *Arch Pathol Lab Med* 113:1271–1275, 1989.
16. Raptopoulos V, Cummings T, Smith EH: Computed tomography of life-threatening complications of abdominal aortic aneurysm. The disrupted aortic wall. *Invest Radiol* 22:372–376, 1987.
17. Wittenberg J, Athanasoulis CA, Williams LF, et al: Ischemic colitis. *Radiology and pathophysiology. Am J Roentgenol* 123:287–300, 1975.
18. Griffiths WJ, Neuman DA, Welsh JD: The visible vessel as an indicator of uncontrolled or recurrent gastrointestinal hemorrhage. *N Engl J Med* 300:1411–1413, 1979.
19. Storey DW, Bown SG, Swain CP, et al: Endoscopic prediction of recurrent bleeding in peptic ulcers. *N Engl J Med* 305:915–916, 1981.
20. Johnston JH: Endoscopic risk factors for bleeding peptic ulcer. *Gastrointest Endosc* 36:S16–S20, 1990.
21. Fleischer D: Endoscopic therapy of upper gastrointestinal bleeding in humans. *Gastroenterology* 90:217–234, 1986.
22. Fleischer D: Endoscopic control of upper gastrointestinal bleeding. *J Clin Gastroenterol* 12(Suppl 2):S41–S47, 1990.
23. DuMoulin GC, Paterson DG, Hedley-Whyte J, et al: Aspiration of gastric bacteria in antacid-treated patients: A frequent cause of postoperative colonisation of the airway. *Lancet* 1:242–245, 1982.
24. Craven DE, Kunches LM, Kilinsky V, et al: Risk factors for pneumonia and fatality in patients receiving continuous mechanical ventilation. *Am Rev Respir Dis* 133:792–796, 1986.
25. Driks MR, Craven DE, Celli BR, et al: Nosocomial pneumonia in intubated patients given sucralfate as compared with antacids or histamine type 2 blockers. *N Engl J Med* 317:1376–1382, 1987.

20

TREATMENT OF HEMORRHAGIC SHOCK INSULT

Charles E. Lucas, M.D.
Anna M. Ledgerwood, M.D.

INTRODUCTION

Factors contributing most to serious morbidity and mortality in association with gastrointestinal bleeding include the age of the patient, associated diseases, Laennec's cirrhosis, the inability to stop bleeding without emergent surgery, and rebleeding in the hospital after temporary cessation.[1,2] The last two factors are additive in that they both lead to hemorrhagic shock and the inevitable physiological and pathological sequelae of inadequate tissue perfusion, especially in the aged.[3] Our objectives are to define these responses and outline a plan of therapeutic intervention. Since the extent of the metabolic change varies directly with the severity of the hemorrhagic shock insult, the therapeutic challenges addressed apply primarily to those patients with major blood loss and the need for multiple transfusions to maintain vital signs.[4,5]

NORMAL PHYSIOLOGY

An appreciation of normal physiology provides a basis upon which the responses of hemorrhagic shock may be compared.[6] The typical 70-kg person is composed of 60% water, with 28 liters distributed in the intracellular fluid space (ICF) and 14 liters in the extracellular fluid space (ECF). The ICF contains the red blood cell volume (RBCV) of 2 liters and the muscle-organ mass of 26 liters. The ECF contains the plasma volume (PV) of 3 liters and the interstitial fluid space (IFS) of 11 liters. The PV and RBCV give a total blood volume (BV) of 5 liters, which circulates each minute. The heart and lungs work in concert to deliver oxygen and other nutrients to the capillaries, where a complex

Supported by the Interstitial Fluid Fund, Account 4-44966.

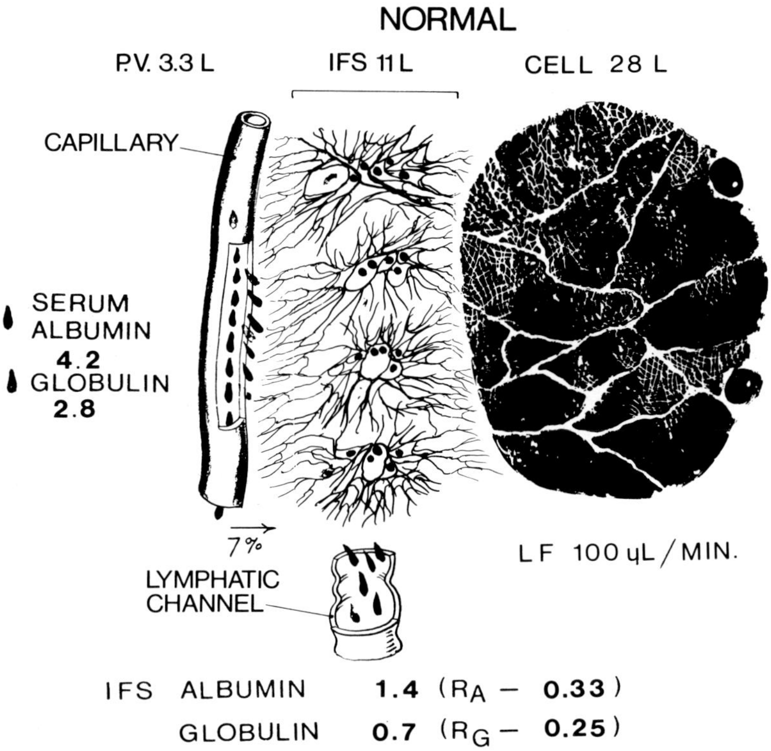

Figure 20.1. A 70-kg person has 42 liters of water; 28 liters is within cells (ICF) and 14 liters is outside cells (ECF). Salt and water exit plasma by hydrostatic forces; proteins exit by convective forces into the ICF. Salt and water reenter plasma by osmotic and oncotic forces; proteins reenter plasma via lymphatics. PV = plasma volume, LF = lymphatic flow, R_A = lymph to plasma albumin ratio, R_G = lymph to plasma globulin ratio. (Reprinted from: Resuscitation Through the Three Phases of Hemorrhagic Shock After Trauma, with permission of the Canadian Medical Association, *CJS*, 33(6), 1990.)

series of exchanges occur between the PV and the IFS and, thence, between the IFS and the ICF.[7] Fluid flux through capillaries is controlled by hydrostatic, osmotic, and oncotic forces. Salt, water, and other nutrients enter the IFS under the predominant influence of hydrostatic forces as the plasma proteins are carried into the IFS by convective forces (Figure 20.1). Since the capillary wall contains many small pores and a few large pores, protein flux into the IFS is selective, causing the IFS/PV ratio of albumin to exceed the IFS/PV ratio of larger globulins.[8] Nutrients carried with proteins reach the ICF and maintain cellular homeostasis. The IFS salt and water reenter the PV at the venular end of the capillary due to oncotic and osmotic forces. In contrast, IFS proteins leave the IFS through the lymphatic system for PV reentry at a remote site. While in the IFS, proteins exist in equilibrium between the collagenous IFS matrix or gel and the free fluid or sol. Factors regulating IFS protein include size, shape, pH, and charge.

When the matrix expands, ultrafine proteoglycans in the gel bind or trap proteins; this process is called *reduced albumin exclusion.* When the matrix contracts, proteoglycans release proteins to the sol for transport through the lymphatics to the PV; this process is called *increased albumin exclusion.*[8]

TABLE 20.1. Three Phases of Hemorrhagic Shock

Phase I:	Active bleeding period extending from the onset of hemorrhage to spontaneous or procedure-induced cessation
Phase II:	Obligatory sequestration period extending from cessation of bleeding to maximal weight gain or fluid retention within the ICF and IFS
Phase III:	Mobilization and diuretic period extending from the time of maximal weight gain to that of lowest new weight

PHYSIOLOGICAL RESPONSE OF BLEEDING

The hemorrhagic shock insult may be divided into three physiological phases reflecting sequential but different responses to severe bleeding[4,5] (Table 20.1). Phase I is the period of active hemorrhage and extends from the onset of bleeding until its cessation, either spontaneously or by therapeutic intervention. Phase II is the period of obligatory extravascular fluid sequestration which occurs in response to inadequate tissue perfusion. Patients requiring 10 or more blood transfusions in phase I typically sequester 5–10 liters over the ensuing 18–30 hours. The amount and duration of fluid sequestration correlate with the severity and duration of shock. Once phase III begins, mobilization with diuresis of previously sequestered fluid is usually complete by four days. Patients with Laennec's cirrhosis have prolonged phase II and phase III responses. Patients with a lethal shock insult never enter phase III.

ORGAN RESPONSE TO ACUTE HEMORRHAGIC SHOCK

Macrocirculation

The immediate response to acute hemorrhage includes a peripheral release of catecholamines which induce vasoconstriction in the periphery and in selected capillary beds.[9-11] This reduces blood flow to the limbs, kidneys, mesentery, spleen, and skin. Resultant clinical manifestations include pale, cold, clammy skin with later mottling. Contraction of capillary beds protects perfusion pressures temporarily. Further blood loss leads to sequential reductions in systolic pressure, pulse pressure, diastolic pressure, and mean arterial pressure (MAP). During this insult, flow is preferentially maintained to the heart and brain.

Microcirculation

Within the capillary unit, precapillary vasoconstriction reduces hydrostatic pressure, which slows the egress of water, electrolytes, and proteins from the PV to the IFS.[12] Concomitantly, contraction of the IFS matrix augments protein movement from the IFS through the lymphatics into the PV at a remote site.[13,14] At the venular end of the capillary unit, the oncotic and osmotic pressures rise, facilitating water and electrolyte flux from the IFS into the PV.

Cardiac Response

The decrease in PV lowers venous return, which reduces stroke volume and thus cardiac output.[10] Simultaneously, the catecholamine release produces a chronotropic response; the increased pulse rate partially compensates for the reduction in stroke volume.[15] Vasodilation to the coronary arteries helps maintain cardiac perfusion until the hypovolemic shock insult becomes extreme.[16] This accommodates a demand for increased cardiac work and oxygen consumption. The decreased venous return reduces the central filling pressures until late in the hemorrhagic shock insult, when cardiac decompensation occurs and the central filling pressures rise.[16,17] Although reduced tissue perfusion compromises oxygen delivery—which, to some degree, is compensated for by increased unloading of oxygen—this compensatory response is limited, so that a significant fall in cardiac output and oxygen delivery causes reduced oxygen consumption, resulting in metabolic acidosis.

Pulmonary Response

The shock-induced fall in PV is associated with a rise in pulmonary vascular resistance due to postcapillary vasoconstriction.[18,19] The resultant increase in capillary hydrostatic pressures favors the egress of fluid and protein from the capillaries into the pulmonary IFS. With a severe shock insult, the release of cytokines may enhance capillary leakage and worsen the oxygenation problems typically seen after fluid resuscitation. Impaired oxygenation is confirmed by the increase in the percentage of physiological shunting in the lung and by the reduced ratio of arterial oxygen tension (pAO_2) to percentage of inspired oxygen (FiO_2). Compensatory tachypnea enhances oxygen uptake and also causes hypocapnia with respiratory alkalosis. This tendency toward respiratory alkalosis partially compensates for the metabolic acidosis from inadequate tissue perfusion. The rise in pulmonary vascular resistance also slows the passage of red cells through the capillary unit, thereby permitting more efficient oxygen uptake.

Renal Response

The peripheral release of catecholamines causes renal vasoconstriction. The combination of renal catecholamine perfusion, decreased perfusion pressure across the juxtaglomerular apparatus, and decreased sodium delivery to the distal tubule promotes the release of renin, which enters the systemic circuit and converts angiotensin 1 to angiotensin 2.[20-22] The latter hormone enhances vasoconstriction and initiates the release of aldosterone from the adrenal gland.

A mild to moderate hypovolemic insult causes selective postcapillary or postglomerular vasoconstriction, which leads to a reduction in renal plasma flow while glomerular filtration is maintained.[23] As the hypovolemic shock becomes severe, a reduction in glomerular filtration parallels the further fall in renal plasma flow. The combination of reduced renal plasma flow and reduced filtration rate with increased release of aldosterone and antidiuretic hormone (ADH) results in a fall in urine output, osmolar clearance, and sodium clearance. Once this occurs, aggressive resuscitation is essential to circumvent the onset of renal failure.

Endocrine Response

In addition to the peripheral release of norepinephrine, shock causes a central release of epinephrine from the adrenal glands.[9,10] The norepinephrine causes marked peripheral vasoconstriction, whereas the epinephrine causes increased inotropic force of the heart. Both lead to gluconeogenesis and hyperglycemia.[11,20] Consequent to the increased serum glucose is hyperinsulinemia; the tissues, however, develop insulin resistance, so that the hyperglycemia persists.[24,25] The hemorrhagic insult is also associated with an increase in serum osmolality.[24] The combination of hyperosmolemia and reduced systolic pressure leads to ADH release from the pituitary gland.

Concomitantly, there is an adrenal cortical steroid release, so that the circulating steroid levels remain elevated until resuscitation is complete and the patient is stabilized. In randomized control trials the addition of exogenous steroids does not appear to augment the body's response to shock.[26] The pituitary-parathyroid axis is also part of the response to hemorrhagic shock.[27] Patients with an intact thyroid axis have an enhanced response to the circulating catecholamines. The increased triiodothyronine (T_3) levels may facilitate an increased thyroid response to resuscitation by influencing the release of thyroid-releasing hormone and thyroid-stimulation hormone.[28] The parathyroid glands also respond to hemorrhagic shock. The reduction in ionized calcium seen with hypoparathyroidism impairs the response to resuscitation, whereas the circulating parathyroid hormone levels rise in response to hemorrhagic shock.[29]

Cerebral Response

During severe hemorrhagic shock, cerebral blood flow, particularly outer cortical flow, falls precipitously; this is associated acutely with confusion.[30] The brain, however, is one of the last organs to exhibit deprivation from hemorrhagic shock, as flow to the brain is preferentially maintained. Possibly the hyperventilation with hypocarbia typically seen in such patients serves to protect cerebral perfusion. Changes in the intracellular calcium metabolism may also affect cerebral function, as evidenced by the marked rise in intracellular calcium in animals dying of hemorrhagic shock. These changes, however, probably reflect the process of death and should not preclude calcium supplementation, which is beneficial for cardiac inotropism in hypotensive, hypocalcemic patients.[28] Cerebral edema and increased intracerebral pressure may also be seen in the postresuscitation period when maximal extravascular fluid sequestration has occurred.[5] These changes usually abate as the patient recovers fully from the hemorrhagic shock insult and mobilizes the excess fluid stores.

Gut Alterations

The hemorrhagic shock causes mesenteric vasoconstriction. This is manifested in the stomach by areas of pallor which can be seen endoscopically during surgery for control of bleeding elsewhere.[31] The pallor is most prominent in the proximal stomach or parietal cell mass, which is the site of the later development of acute gastric mucosal lesions. These lesions may become problematic despite prophylaxis if the hemorrhagic shock is followed by a severe septic insult. Otherwise, they heal within 7 to 10 days.[32]

The hemorrhagic shock–induced small bowel vasoconstriction probably releases humeral factors which cause fluid sequestration within the bowel wall. The degree of intramural edema, or swelling, parallels the duration and severity of the shock insult; extensive swelling precludes surgical closure of the abdominal incision in patients requiring emergency surgery for massive hemorrhage. Such patients must be packed open until the edema from the bowel wall and other areas has subsided.[33] The presence of blood within the small bowel lumen increases the difficulty of mobilization, handling, and intraluminal aspiration of contents from the small intestine. Hemorrhagic shock does not usually cause marked intramural edema of the colon. The dilated colon in patients with severe bleeding is caused instead by air passing through the small bowel and may lead to massive distention. Presumably, the increased intestinal gas results from the instinctive increase in air swallowing seen in any patient with severe gastrointestinal bleeding. In contrast to the transit time for food, that for swallowed air is very short.

Hepatic Response

The mesenteric vasoconstriction of hemorrhagic shock affects the liver, which shows an injury pattern that can be directly related to the severity of the shock insult.[34,35] There is an acute rise of the hepatocellular liver enzymes, which, in some patients, is associated with clinical jaundice; the bilirubin levels frequently reach 2–5 mg/dl. The direct bilirubin fraction seldom exceeds 60% of the total bilirubin. Light microscopic examination of liver biopsy specimens from such patients shows little abnormality, whereas electron microscopic exam suggests hepatocyte injury with reduced intracellular transferase; this intracellular insult impedes the movement of conjugated bilirubin from the cell to the canaliculi bile.[34] Protein synthesis in this setting remains normal; the reduction in serum albumin concentration typically seen in these patients reflects protein relocation in the extravascular space rather than reduced synthesis.[36] When these insults occur in a patient who has had a prior liver insult such as Laennec's cirrhosis, the outcome is often fatal.

CLINICAL STAGING OF HEMORRHAGIC SHOCK

The severity of acute hemorrhagic shock may be graded by the extent of hypovolemia (Table 20.2).[6] A mild hemorrhagic insult is seen in patients with an acute 5–10% reduction of the circulating BV. This insult causes little or no change in blood pressure, minimal tachycardia, and no measurable change in cardiac output. Orthostatic changes include mild tachycardia and narrowed pulse pressure. The renal blood flow or renal perfusion is marginally decreased, whereas glomerular filtration and the renal excretion of salt, water, and osmoles are maintained.[23]

A grade II hemorrhagic insult results from an acute 15–20% reduction in circulating BV. This produces a modest fall in blood pressure and pulse pressure plus tachycardia. A small catecholamine release increases peripheral vascular resistance, leading to a fall in cardiac output and cool extremities. The added decrease in renal perfusion due to postglomerular vasoconstriction causes some decrease in filtration and in the excretion of water, osmoles, and sodium.

A grade III hemorrhagic insult due to an acute 25–30% reduction in circulating BV

TABLE 20.2. Severity of Hemorrhagic Shock Insult

	Blood Pressure (torr)	*Blood Volume (ml)*	*IFS (L)*	*RBF (ml/min)*	*GFR (ml/min)*	*Urine (ml/min)*
Normal	120/80	5000	11	1300	125	60
Grade I	120/80	4500	10	800	120	50
Grade II	115/80	3700	9	500	80	20
Grade III	85/65	3100	7.5	250	20	10
Grade IV	60/—	2100	5.5	50	—	—

IFS = interstitial fluid space, RBF = renal blood flow, GFR = glomerular filtration rate.

causes hypotension with a systolic blood pressure below 90 torr and tachycardia to more than 120/minute. Peripheral vasoconstriction causes cold, clammy extremities and a fall in cardiac output below 3 liters/min. Renal blood flow and filtration fall below 50% of normal as the patient becomes oliguric, with less than 0.3 ml/min urine output.

A patient with grade IV hemorrhagic shock insult has more than a 35% acute reduction in BV, is in severe shock with a systolic pressure below 70 torr, and likely has a pulse rate greater than 140/min. The cardiac output falls below 2.5 liters/min; the concomitant release of catecholamines, ADH, renin, and aldosterone causes profound vasoconstriction with compromised renal and peripheral perfusion, cold extremities, and anuria.[16]

PHASE I—THERAPEUTIC CHALLENGES

The early resuscitation of the bleeding patient must be directed not only to restoring the RBCV but also to replacing the huge fluid and electrolyte deficits in both the PV and the IFS[15,37] (Figure 20.2). The volume requirements of crystalloid replacement exceed those of blood replacement for two reasons: (1) the excessive IFS losses which occurred in response to the acute hemorrhage and (2) the subsequent extravascular fluid sequestration into both the IFS and the ICF during phase II. One may predict that the ratio of crystalloid infusion to the estimated acute whole blood loss will exceed 2/1 in patients resuscitated with whole blood and may reach 3/1 in patients resuscitated with packed RBCs.[4] Consequently, a patient with an acute 2-liter blood loss would likely need 6 liters of crystalloid solution to restore the PV and IFS deficits.

The crystalloid solution used for resuscitation should be a balanced electrolyte solution with the appropriate addition of sodium bicarbonate or lactate according to the concomitant acid-base status. This balanced electrolyte solution should not contain glucose, since the shock-induced release of glucagon and somatotropin augments the hyperglycemic response typically seen with the release of catecholamines.[20] When endogenous hyperglycemia from hemorrhagic shock is augmented by exogenous glucose in the crystalloid solution, the hyperglycemic response may exceed 1,000 mg/dl, which leads to inappropriate osmotic diuresis when optimal homeostasis calls for fluid conservation.[5,6]

The volume of crystalloid infusion is best guided by the response of the blood

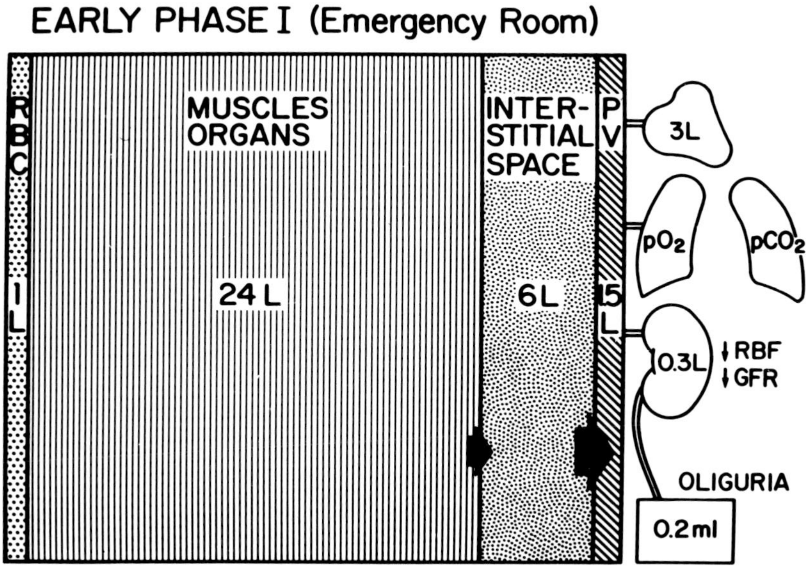

Figure 20.2. When a patient presents with severe or grade IV hemorrhagic shock, vasoconstriction and IFS matrix contraction lead to large salt and water deficits. Such deficits can be restored by infusing 3 liters of crystalloid solution for each 1 liter of estimated blood loss. Note the low renal perfusion (RBF) and filtration (GFR) with oliguria. (Reprinted from: Resuscitation Through the Three Phases of Hemorrhagic Shock After Trauma, with permission of the Canadian Medical Association, *CJS*, 33(6), 1990.)

pressure, pulse pressure, and urine output, whereas the volume of red cell replacement is best determined by the hemoglobin and hematocrit. With adequate crystalloid resuscitation, restoration and maintenance of the hematocrit at 30% should provide an adequate reserve against acute anemia from ongoing or recurrent bleeding, as well as adequate red cells for tissue perfusion and oxygen delivery. Maintaining the hematocrit at a preshock normal level of 45% may be counterproductive in this setting, where the slightly lower than normal hematocrit is associated with enhanced tissue perfusion and oxygen delivery because of a reduction in blood viscosity.[4,5]

Achievement of large-volume resuscitation in these acutely ill patients requires the establishment of at least two large-bore intravenous lines, one of which has the potential for measuring central venous pressure. Secure lines may be achieved by peripheral angiocatheters, by basilic or cephalic venous cutdown, or by percutaneous central vein cannulation of either the subclavian or internal jugular vein.[6,38] Each technique has specific advantages and disadvantages, so the decision must be based on the individual preference of the treating team. The authors prefer the rapid percutaneous subclavian vein approach, which is a quick and effective means of providing large-volume replacement and simultaneous measurement of central venous pressure. One disadvantage of this technique is the small incidence of pneumothorax or effusion, which requires thoracentesis and tube thoracostomy. Along with the volume expansion provided by crystalloid, rapid utilization of type-specific and then cross-matched blood is necessary to achieve appropriate blood replacement.

PHASE II—THERAPEUTIC CHALLENGES

After the bleeding has been controlled, the patient likely will enter into an obligatory extravascular fluid sequestration phase.[6,20] This fluid sequestration occurs in both the ICF and the IFS spaces (Figure 20.3). The ICF expansion is associated with changes in cell membrane potential due to decreased efflux of sodium and water from the cell; possibly this is due to a deficiency of adenosine triphosphate (ATP), which fuels the sodium-potassium ATPase pump.[15] The IFS expansion appears to be caused by the unraveling of the interstitial space matrix, which exposes the proteoglycans to albumin and other proteins.[39]

It was formerly believed that ICF and IFS expansion during phase II was due to increased capillary permeability. This implies an increase in the size of the small pores or in the number of large pores. The basis for this conclusion is the low serum proteins that were thought to result from leakage of these proteins into the IFS. This theory, however, discounts normal albumin and protein kinetics. Contrary to prior opinion, only 45% of the ECF albumin is in the PV; the remaining 55% is in the IFS in a dynamic equilibrium between the matrix proteoglycans and the sol portion of the IFS.[6,40] Furthermore, 7% of the 45% in the PV exits from the PV hourly, as an equal amount exits the IFS through the lymphatics to reenter the PV at a remote site. Thus, the PV and IFS are in a constant equilibrium with fluid and protein fluxes.

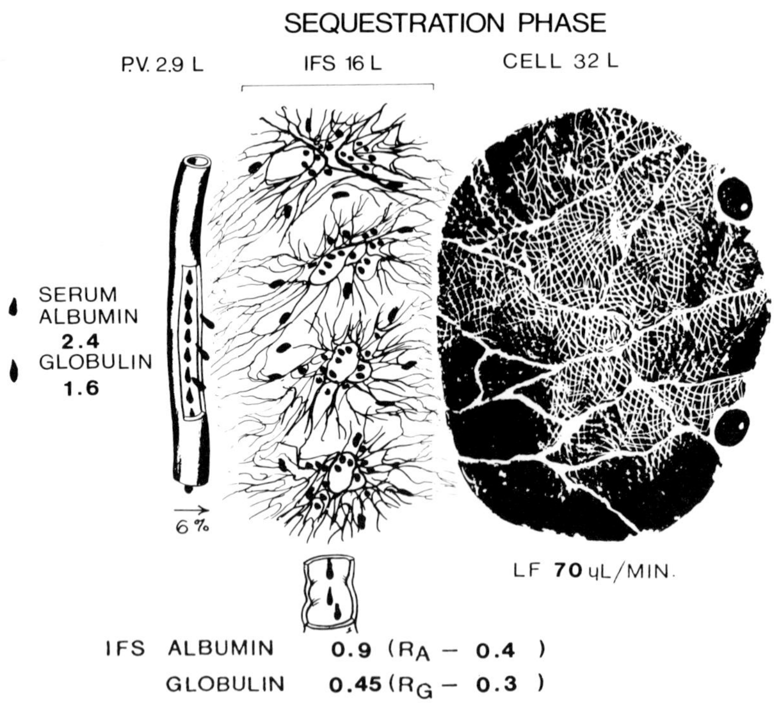

Figure 20.3. The cell and IFS expansion during phase II leads to extravascular protein relocation from the plasma, which has low albumin and globulin levels. Altered capillary permeability is *not* responsible for these changes. (Reprinted from: Resuscitation Through the Three Phases of Hemorrhagic Shock After Trauma, with permission of the Canadian Medical Association, *CJS*, 33(6), 1990.)

In contrast to the conclusions based on the *colloid leak* theory, prior studies from our laboratory show that the hourly loss of albumin from the PV in phase II is decreased to 6%.[39] Since the PV and serum albumin concentrations are both quite low in phase II, this 6% escape rate represents a very small amount of albumin flux from the PV to the IFS. Thus, the mechanisms by which phase II serum albumin levels fall must be related to an even lower amount of albumin return from the IFS to the PV (Figure 20.3). This decrease in the amount of albumin reentry into the PV would by necessity reflect albumin entrapment within the IFS matrix.[40] The conceptual and therapeutic implications of this phenomenon are enormous. Fluid shifts and protein changes consequent to hemorrhagic shock result more from hemodilution, from IFS matrix dynamics, and from cell membrane responses than from leaky capillaries.

Thus, therapy in phase II should be directed toward restoration of RBCV and PV, as judged by vital signs and not by total body fluid uptake or by serial weight changes.[4,5] During phase II, the weight gain often exceeds 10 kg in patients who require more than 10–15 transfusions during a single 24-hour bleeding episode. Loop diuresis given to prevent or correct ECF expansion is counterproductive and may be injurious due to the potential for additive PV contraction in a patient who is already in a PV-depleted state.[41] Exogenous diuresis in this setting may lead to renal shutdown, which is almost always fatal after hemorrhagic shock despite renal support capabilities like peritoneal dialysis and hemodialysis. Renal function during phase II is best maintained by a continuous aggressive regimen of fluid replacement following the above guidelines.

During late phase II, central pressures may rise precipitously. Rather than assuming that an elevated pulmonary capillary wedge pressure reflects inotropic failure, one may give a fluid bolus of 500 ml balanced electrolyte solution over a 30-minute interval and monitor the left ventricular stroke work to pulmonary capillary wedge pressure ratio[42,43] (Figure 20.4). When the slope created by this bolus infusion is steep, the elevated central pressure or pulmonary capillary wedge pressure must be due to some form of pulmonary failure and not to heart failure[44] (Figure 20.4). Oliguria and hypotension in this setting are treated by further fluid replacement despite the elevated central pressure. In contrast, when a flat curve results form the bolus infusion of a balanced electrolyte solution, one is dealing with inotropic failure and the patient needs inotropic support.[38]

PHASE III—THERAPY

Once the IFS and ICF spaces reach the full expansion typical of a specific hemorrhagic shock insult, the patient will enter into a fluid mobilization and diuretic phase. During phase III, the cell membrane potential returns toward normal as the sodium-potassium ATPase pump restores normal ionic fluxes. Concomitantly, the IFS matrix contracts, thereby increasing protein flux through the lymphatics back to the PV. During phase III, the PV and serum albumin concentrations rise, although the resultant serum albumin level remains well below normal[39] (Figure 20.5). The amount of albumin flux through the capillaries into the IFS is also increased during phase III, probably in response to the increased capillary hydrostatic pressure seen with PV expansion. Since the PV albumin efflux into the IFS is increased during phase III when the PV albumin concentration is rising, one must conclude that the IFS matrix is contracting, forcing the albumin into the lymphatic system and thence to the PV; this process is called *increased albumin exclusion*.[40]

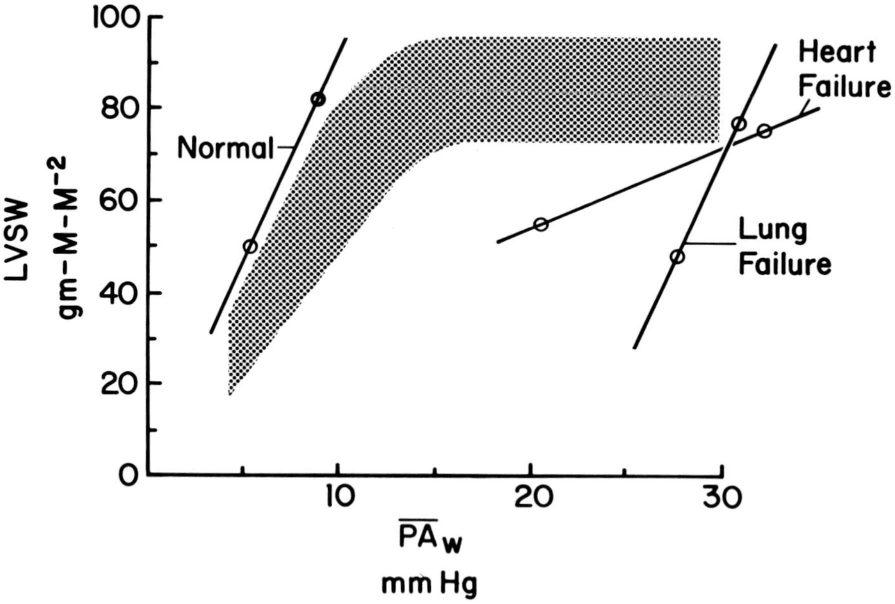

Figure 20.4. A high central pressure may result from shock-induced pulmonary failure. When a fluid bolus causes a steep rise in heart work (LVSW) with little change in central pressure (PAw), associated hypotension and oliguria are best treated by further volume expansion. (Reprinted from: Resuscitation Through the Three Phases of Hemorrhagic Shock After Trauma, with permission of the Canadian Medical Association, *CJS*, 33(6), 1990.)

Regardless of the physiological mechanisms, the hemodynamic responses during phase III necessitate an abrupt reduction in fluid infusion. The transition from phase II to phase III can be recognized by a gradual rise in blood pressure and pulse pressure, with cessation of the hypotensive episodes for which bolus infusions were previously needed to maintain adequate urine output.[4,5] When these subtle changes first appear, immediate restriction of fluid intake and cessation of any colloid therapy will reduce the likelihood of the development of postresuscitative hypertension.[4] The syndrome of postresuscitative hypertension is recognized by a sustained rise in systolic and diastolic blood pressures associated with an expansion of the PV and a significant expansion of the PV/IFS ratio. Therapy for this syndrome includes fluid restriction, avoidance of colloid, and loop diuresis using small doses (5–10 mg) of furosemide to decrease preload and prevent congestive heart failure.

Once the combination of decreased intravenous fluids, inotropic support, and pulmonary support (including ventilatory assistance as needed) facilitates homeostasis in the fluid mobilization phase, a full recovery can be expected; the diffuse, multiple organ insults will gradually disappear.

THE COLLOID CONTROVERSY

Starling in 1896 introduced the colloid controversy when he published the equation which now bears his name.[45] The Starling equation shows that the vascular efflux of water correlates directly with capillary conductivity (often inappropriately referred to as *permeability*) multiplied by the capillary surface area, with the magnitude of flow being

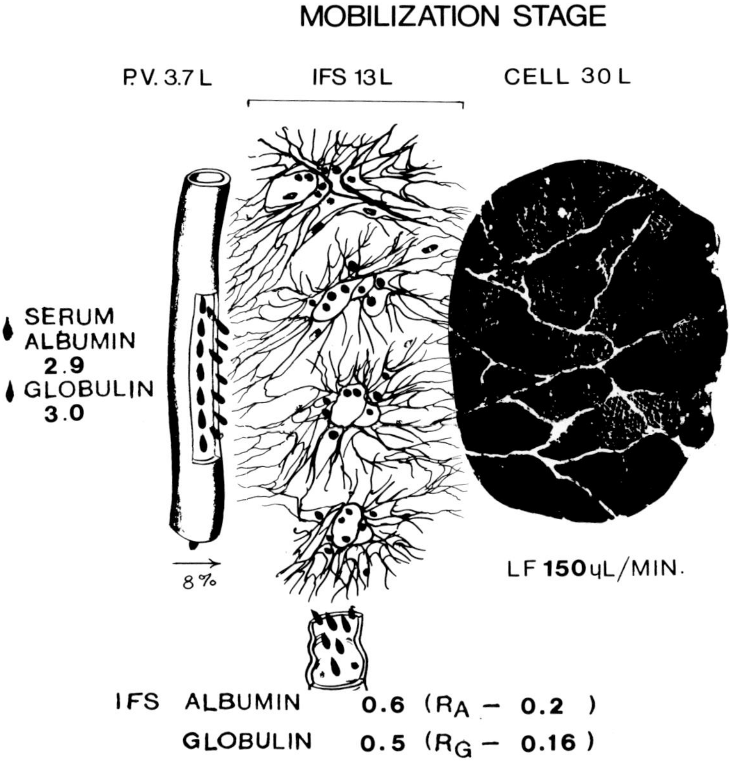

Figure 20.5. During phase III, cellular and IFS matrix contractions (increased albumin exclusion) restore plasma volume and increase plasma proteins. Concomitant diuresis circumvents acute heart and lung failure. (Reprinted from: Resuscitation Through the Three Phases of Hemorrhagic Shock After Trauma, with permission of the Canadian Medical Association, *CJS*, 33(6), 1990.)

influenced by the capillary hydrostatic pressure, the interstitial hydrostatic pressure, the capillary oncotic pressure, and the interstitial oncotic pressure. This equation shows that the flux of water from the PV is inversely related to capillary oncotic pressure if all other factors remain constant. Starling emphasized that this two-dimensional equation has limited application to mammals for three reasons: (1) mammals have a third fluid system, namely, the lymphatic system; (2) mammals have dynamic fluid fluxes between the IFS and the ICF; (3) changes in one component of the equation would lead to changes in the remaining components.[45] When prior retrospective nonrandomized studies from our laboratory suggested that supplemental albumin therapy increased pulmonary dysfunction, supplemental albumin therapy was stopped. When this decision brought about severe criticism, a prospective randomized analysis of the benefits of albumin supplementation was begun.

During a two-year interval, 94 injured patients with hemorrhagic shock were randomized to receive albumin or no albumin therapy. All patients had shock and received an average of 15 blood transfusions during phase I. The resuscitation regimens were similar, except that the 48 nonalbumin-treated patients received 20% more crystalloid. The amount of albumin supplementation was calculated to restore serum albumin levels and colloid oncotic pressure toward normal and was based upon multiple sequential measurements in similar patients.[46] The albumin-treated patients had an increase in the average capillary oncotic pressure (19.7 torr vs. 14.8 torr). The normal colloid oncotic pressure is 22–24 torr.

The albumin-treated patients had a higher serum albumin concentration, PV, and renal plasma flow (Figure 20.6). Despite the increase in renal perfusion, the albumin-treated patients had a lower filtration rate, sodium clearance, osmolar clearance, and urine output.[47,48] The fall in urine output was also seen by Carey and coworkers in injured Vietnam soldiers and by Siegel and coworkers in shocked baboons receiving albumin-supplemented resuscitation.[20,49] More recently, Ramsay and coworkers confirmed this oliguric effect of colloid supplementation in greyhound dogs subjected to a hemorrhage shock.[50]

The mechanism of decreased osmolar clearance and urine output following albumin supplementation probably involves an increase in both the oncotic and osmotic pressures within the glomerular tufts.[47] This encourages salt and water retention, thus explaining the fall in glomerular filtration. The plasma leaving the glomerular tuft via the efferent arterials remains hyperoncotic while perfusing the peritubular vessels within the inner medulla adjacent to the loops of Henle. The hyperoncotic plasma extracts fluid from the interstices of the inner medulla, thereby increasing the concentration gradient in the loops of Henle. This higher concentration gradient allows the permissive renal hormones, namely, ADH and aldosterone, to increase sodium and water reabsorption at the distal collecting tubules and in the collecting ducts (Figure 20.6). There is controversy regarding the mechanism by which albumin causes sodium retention, but our findings suggest

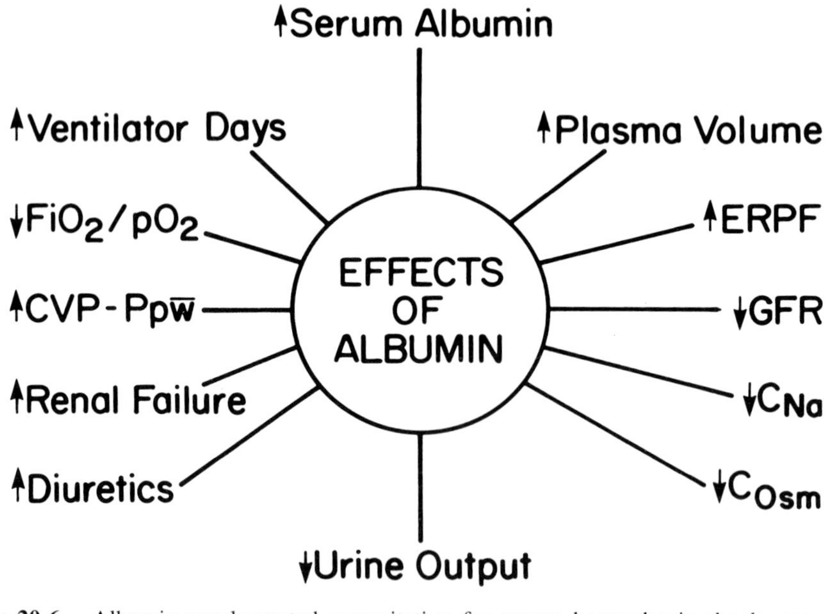

Figure 20.6. Albumin-supplemented resuscitation for severe hemorrhagic shock may increase plasma volume and renal flow (ERPF) but reduce filtration (GFR) and excretion of sodium (C_{Na}), osmoles (C_{osm}), and urine. The resultant weight gain increases central pressure (CVP-P_{pw}), impairs oxygenation (FiO_2/pO_2), and prolongs ventilatory needs. (Reprinted from: Resuscitation Through the Three Phases of Hemorrhagic Shock After Trauma, with permission of the Canadian Medical Association, *CJS*, 33(6), 1990.)

that the sodium retention after albumin supplementation is due to a sodium-potassium exchange at the distal nephron level.[48]

These renal effects of colloid supplementation disrupt the primary purpose of albumin or colloid infusion, namely, to exert an oncotic effect within the vascular system, thereby relocating IFS water to the PV for excretion by the kidneys. Unfortunately, the renal responses are counterproductive.[47] This leads to an increased need for diuretic therapy, a higher incidence of renal failure, and worse pulmonary function, as reflected by high central pressures, increased physiological shunting in the lungs, and a prolonged need for ventilatory support.[51] The mortality rate after colloid supplementation in injured patients with hemorrhagic shock also rises, as seen in this study and in the meta-analysis of all prospective randomized studies on the use of albumin supplementation for hemorrhagic shock.[51,52] There have been no prospective randomized studies on the use of colloid or albumin supplementation in the treatment of hemorrhagic shock in patients with gastrointestinal bleeding. Unpublished studies from our laboratory, however, suggest that the physiology of the hemorrhagic shock insult is comparable in patients with gastrointestinal bleeding.[53] We no longer use colloid supplementation in patients with severe, life-threatening gastrointestinal hemorrhage.

NONHEMODYNAMIC EFFECTS OF COLLOID THERAPY

Colloid-supplemented therapy for hemorrhagic shock may have nonhemodynamic disadvantages. Increased serum albumin causes a reciprocal fall in the non-albumin proteins including the immunoglobulins and coagulation proteins.[54] The fall in immunoglobulins may adversely affect the immune response, whereas the fall in coagulation proteins in man and in control animal models adversely affects coagulation and increases the need for blood replacement.[55-57] Successful resuscitation of hemorrhagic shock can be readily achieved without colloid supplementation. When a physician deems that colloid supplementation is necessary, the potential detrimental effects of each therapy should be anticipated and prevented.

REFERENCES

1. Clason AE, Macleod DAD, Elton RA: Clinical factors in the prediction of further hemorrhage or mortality in acute upper gastrointestinal hemorrhage. *Br J Surg* 73:985–987, 1986.
2. Katschinski BD, Logan RFA, Davies J, et al: Audit of mortality in upper gastrointestinal bleeding. *Post Med J* 65:913–917, 1989.
3. Sugawa C, Steffes CP, Ryuil N, et al: Upper GI bleeding in an urban hospital: Etiology, recurrence, and prognosis. *Ann Surg* 212:521–527, 1990.
4. Ledgerwood AM, Lucas CE: Postresuscitation hypertension: Etiology, morbidity, and treatment. *Arch Surg* 108:531–538, 1974.
5. Lucas CE: Resuscitation of the injured patient. The three phases of treatment. *Surg Clin North Am* 57:3–15, 1977.
6. Lucas CE, Ledgerwood AM: The fluid problem in the critically ill. *Surg Clin North Am* 63:439–454, 1983.

7. Lucas CE, Ledgerwood AM, Benishek DJ: Reduced oncotic pressure after shock. *Arch Surg* 117:675–679, 1982.
8. Mullins RJ, Bell DR: Permeability of rabbit skin and muscle microvasculature after saline expansion. *J Surg Res* 32:390–400, 1982.
9. Gann DS, Amarall JF: Pathophysiology of trauma and shock, in Zuidema GD, Rutherford RB, Ballinger WF (eds): The Management of Trauma, ed 4. Philadelphia, WB Saunders, 1985, pp 37–103.
10. Runciman WB, Skowronski GA: Pathophysiology of hemorrhagic shock. *Anaesth Intensive Care* 12:193–201, 1984.
11. Bond RF, Johnson GJ: Vascular adrenergic interactions during hemorrhagic shock. *Fed Proc* 44:281–289, 1985.
12. Byrnes GJ, Pirkle JC Jr, Gann DS: Cardiovascular stabilization after hemorrhage depends upon restitution of blood volume. *J Trauma* 18:623–627, 1978.
13. Dawson CW, Lucas CE, Ledgerwood AM: Altered interstitial fluid space dynamics and postresuscitation hypertension. *Arch Surg* 116:657–662, 1981.
14. Demling RH: Colloid or crystalloid resuscitation in sepsis, in Sibbald W, Sprung C (eds): *Perspectives on Sepsis and Septic Shock.* Los Angeles, Society of Critical Care Medicine, 1986, p 275.
15. Shires GT, Canizaro PC, Carrico CJ: Shock, in Schwartz SI, Shires GT, Spencer FC, et al (eds): *Principles of Surgery,* ed 4. New York, McGraw-Hill Book Co, 1984, p 116.
16. Wilson RF: The pathophysiology of shock. *Intensive Care Med* 6:89–100, 1980.
17. Green JF, Jackman AP: Mechanism of increased vascular capacity produced by mild perfusion hypothermia in the dog. *Circ Res* 44:411–419, 1979.
18. Pardy BJ, Dudley HAF: Sequential patterns of hemodynamic and metabolic changes in experimental hypovolemic shock: Responses to acute hemorrhage. *Br J Surg* 66:84–88, 1979.
19. Hechtman HB, Lonergan EA, Staunton PG, et al: Pulmonary entrapment of platelets during acute respiratory failure. *Surgery* 83:277–283, 1978.
20. Carey LD, Lowery BD, Cloutier CT: Hemorrhagic shock. *Curr Prob Surg* 8:1048–1058, 1971.
21. Hayes DF, Werner MH, Rosenberg IK, et al: Effects of traumatic hypovolemic shock on renal function. *J Surg Res* 16:490–497, 1974.
22. Lucas CE: Renal considerations in the injured patient. *Surg Clin North Am* 62:133, 1982.
23. Lowe RJ, Moss GS, Jilek J, et al: Crystalloid versus colloid in the etiology of pulmonary failure after trauma: A randomized trial in man. *Crit Care Med* 7:107–112, 1979.
24. Gann DS: Endocrine control of plasma protein and volume. *Surg Clin North Am* 56:1135–1145, 1976.
25. Pirkle JC Jr, Gann DS: Restitution of blood volume after hemorrhage: Mathematical description. *Am J Physiol* 228:821–827, 1975.
26. Lucas CE, Ledgerwood AM: Pulmonary response of massive steroids in seriously injured patients. *Ann Surg* 194:256–261, 1981.
27. Lucas CE, Sennish JC, Ledgerwood AM, et al: Parathyroid response to hypocalcemia after treatment of hemorrhagic shock. *Surgery* 96:711–716, 1984.
28. Gallick HL, Lucas CE, Ledgerwood AM, et al: Detrimental effect of recent thyroidectomy on hemorrhagic shock and resuscitation. *Circ Shock* 21:111–119, 1987.
29. McGonigal MD, Elliott L, Lucas CE, et al: Calcium homeostasis after parathyroidectomy in normal and shocked states. *Am Surg* 53:429–433, 1987.
30. Hekmatpanah J: The management of head trauma. *Surg Clin North Am* 53:47–57, 1973.
31. Lucas CE: Stress ulceration: The clinical problem. *World J Surg* 5:139–151, 1981.

32. Lucas CE, Sugawa C, Friend W, et al: Therapeutic implications of disturbed gastric physiology in patients with stress ulcerations. *Am J Surg* 123:25–34, 1972.
33. Ledgerwood AM, Lucas CE: Postoperative complications of abdominal trauma. *Surg Clin North Am* 70:715–731, 1990.
34. Ledgerwood AM: Hepatobiliary complications of sepsis. *Heart Lung* 5:621–623, 1976.
35. Champion HR, Jones RT, Trump BF, et al: Post-traumatic hepatic dysfunction as a major etiology in post-traumatic jaundice. *J Trauma* 16:650–657, 1976.
36. Dahn MS: Determinants of hepatic albumin production following injury and sepsis. PhD dissertation, Depts of Surgery and Biochemistry, Wayne State University, Detroit, Michigan, May, 1991.
37. Shires GT, Carrico CJ, Canizzaro PC: Response of the extracellular fluid, in Shires GT (ed): *Shock: Major Problems in Clinical Surgery,* Vol 13. Philadelphia, WB Saunders, 1973, p 15.
38. Lucas CE, Ledgerwood AM: Hemodynamic management of the injured, in Capan LM, Miller SM, Turndorf H (eds): *Trauma: Anesthesia and Intensive Care.* Philadelphia, JB Lippincott, 1991, pp 83–113.
39. Dawson CW, Lucas CE, Ledgerwood AM: Altered interstitial fluid space dynamics and postresuscitation hypertension. *Arch Surg* 116:657–662, 1981.
40. Lucas CE, Ledgerwood AM, Rachwal WJ, et al: Colloid oncotic pressure and body water dynamics in septic and injured patients. *J Trauma* 31:927–933, 1991.
41. Lucas CE, Zito JG, Carter KM, et al: Questionable value of furosemide in preventing renal failure. *Surgery* 82:314–320, 1977.
42. Johnston WE, Prough DS, Royster RL, et al: Pulmonary artery wedge pressure may fail to reflect left ventricular end-diastolic pressure in dogs with oleic acid-induced pulmonary edema. *Crit Care Med* 13:487–491, 1985.
43. Mammana RB, Hiro S, Levitsky S, et al: Inaccuracy of pulmonary capillary wedge pressure when compared to left atrial pressure in the early postsurgical period. *J Thorac Cardiovasc Surg* 84:420–425, 1982.
44. Alyono D, Ring WS, Chao RY, et al: Characteristics of ventricular function in severe hemorrhagic shock. *Surgery* 94:250–258, 1983.
45. Starling EH: On the absorption of fluids from the connective tissue spaces. *J Physiol (Lond)* 19:312–326, 1896.
46. Johnson SD, Lucas CE, Gerrick SJ, et al: Altered coagulation after albumin supplements for treatment of oligemic shock. *Arch Surg* 114:379–383, 1979.
47. Lucas CE, Ledgerwood AM, Higgins RF: Impaired salt and water excretion after albumin resuscitation for hypovolemic shock. *Surgery* 86:544–549, 1979.
48. Lucas CE, Ledgerwood AM, Higgins RF: Glomerulotubular sodium dynamics after supplemental albumin resuscitation. *Am Surg* 47:204–207, 1981.
49. Siegel DC, Cochin MS, Geocaris T, et al: Effects of saline and colloid resuscitation on renal function. *Ann Surg* 177:51–57, 1973.
50. Ramsay G, Ledingham M: Resuscitation in hemorrhagic shock—pulmonary and renal effects: An adverse effect of stabilized plasma protein solution on renal function. *Circ Shock* 22:261–268, 1987.
51. Lucas CE, Ledgerwood AM, Higgins RF, et al: Impaired pulmonary function after albumin resuscitation from shock. *J Trauma* 20:446–451, 1980.
52. Moss GS: Meta-analysis of albumin supplementation of resuscitation from hypovolemia. Personal Communication.
53. Lucas CE: Second Annual W.R. Ghent Lecture on Trauma: Abdominal organ injury: Diagnosis, treatment and education. *Can J Surg* 33:189–195, 1990.

54. Johnson SD, Lucas CE, Gerrick SJ, et al: Altered coagulation after albumin supplements for treatment of oligemic shock. *Arch Surg* 114:379–383, 1979.
55. Clift DR, Lucas CE, Ledgerwood AM, et al: The effect of albumin resuscitation for shock on the immune response to tetanus toxoid. *J Surg Res* 32:449–452, 1982.
56. Faillace DF, Ledgerwood AM, Lucas CE, et al: Immunoglobulin changes after varied resuscitation regimens. *J Trauma* 22:1–5, 1982.
57. Lucas CE, Ledgerwood AM, Mammen EF: Altered coagulation protein content after albumin resuscitation. *Ann Surg* 196:198–202, 1982.

V

TREATMENT OF NON-VARICEAL BLEEDING

21

MEDICAL TREATMENT FOR GASTROINTESTINAL BLEEDING

Jeffrey S. Wenger, M.D.
Jamie S. Barkin, M.D.

INTRODUCTION

Gastrointestinal (GI) blood loss continues to be one of the most challenging problems encountered by the physician. Over the past 40 years, progress has been made in the hemodynamic monitoring and interventional therapeutics used for control of GI hemorrhage. However, overall mortality rates from GI bleeding have not shown a significant improvement, probably because GI bleeding occurs more often now in an older population that has more associated systemic disease and thus may be more seriously ill. In addition, the use of nonsteroidal anti-inflammatory drugs (NSAIDs) is more frequent in this older group. Successful management of patients with upper GI bleeding requires a rapid yet accurate initial assessment of the severity and rapidity of blood loss, along with aggressive resuscitation and stabilization. This allows the physician time to utilize the advanced diagnostic and therapeutic modalities that will perhaps lead to decreased mortality. In this chapter we will review the medical management of patients with upper or lower GI bleeding prior to endoscopic, radiologic, or surgical intervention, emphasizing pharmacological therapy.

UPPER GASTROINTESTINAL BLEEDING

The common entities causing nonvariceal hemorrhage were delineated in a survey conducted by the American Society for Gastrointestinal Endoscopy (ASGE) of 2,225 patients with upper gastrointestinal (UGI) bleeding. This survey found that duodenal ulcers were the most common etiology of acute hemorrhage, occurring in 24.3% of patients, closely followed by gastric erosions (23.4%) and gastric ulcers (21.3%). Three relatively uncommon entities, Mallory-Weiss tear (7.2%), esophagitis (6.3%), and erosive duodenitis (5.8%), were next in order of frequency. Overall, these six conditions accounted for 88.3% of all cases of UGI bleeding.[1] The medical management of these clinically challenging disorders encompasses gastric lavage and pharmacological agents for gastric acid suppression and cytoprotection.

Gastric Lavage

Wangensteen and his colleagues in the late 1950s introduced the principle of gastric hypothermia for control of bleeding from the UGI tract. These authors proposed that a lower intragastric temperature would reduce gastric and hepatic blood flow, thereby promoting hemostasis.[2] Utilizing this principle, physicians have traditionally used iced solutions of saline or water for gastric lavage to slow bleeding. Ponsky et al. evaluated the effect of temperature on the hemostatic efficacy of saline irrigation and noted that solutions at room temperature produced the best results.[3] Bryant et al. compared the systemic effects of gastric lavage, using iced saline or water, and noted decreases in serum osmolality and potassium associated with the use of water solutions.[4] However, when this was combined with the administration of intravenous electrolyte solutions and careful monitoring of serum potassium, the authors concluded that the two solutions could be used interchangeably.[4] Therefore, since patients will be receiving intravenous electrolytes, and since the best temperature is room temperature, it is more efficient and cost effective to utilize tap water gastric lavage.

Regardless of the temperature or type of solution used, gastric lavage with a large-bore tube can reduce bleeding by several mechanisms. Aspiration reduces gastric distention, thereby reducing the diameter of exposed mucosal vessel lumens. Less distention also decreases gastrin release and the secretion of acid, a source of irritation at the bleeding site. Hemoglobin in the stomach will help buffer acid; however, the inherent fibrinolytic activity of retained blood outweighs this acid-neutralizing property. Merely removing retained blood from the stomach enhances clot formation at the bleeding site.[5] Thus, gastric decompression after initial irrigation with water serves to enhance hemostasis and should be utilized as part of the management of the bleeding patient.

Histamine 2 Receptor Antagonists

During gastric lavage, control of intragastric acidity appears beneficial. Several pharmacological agents have been developed to achieve this objective. The use of histamine 2 receptor antagonists (H_2RA) for the control and prevention of acute UGI bleeding caused by acid-peptic disorders (ranging from "itis" to ulcers) has been critically analyzed for two decades. H_2RA reduce gastric acid secretion by competitively inhibiting the binding of histamine to its receptor on the basolateral membrane of parietal cells. Consequently, intragastric pH is increased; when the pH rises above 3–4, pepsinogen secretion and the activity of pepsin are reduced.[6,7] Theoretically, this should lead to a reduction in the fibrinolytic action of pepsin and acid on the coagulum and, therefore, to an increase in platelet aggregation, with better control of bleeding and enhanced healing rates.

Active Bleeding and Rebleeding

In the actively bleeding patient with acid-peptic disease, extensive investigation has shown that, in fact, H_2RA do not lead to a cessation of hemorrhage or a reduction in bleeding rates. Zuckerman et al. found no significant difference between intravenous H_2RA therapy (i.e., cimetidine) and placebo in stopping UGI bleeding or reducing the rate of rebleeding during the same hospitalization.[8] Carr-Locke et al. studied the effect of H_2RA cimetidine on transfusion requirements, rebleeding rates, and the number of operations performed in patients with UGI bleeding secondary to either gastric or duodenal ulcers. They found no difference in these parameters compared with placebo.[9] This finding is not unexpected, as initial bleeding and rebleeding seem to be related to the presence of a visible vessel, and it is doubtful that basal acid suppression would make a significant difference in whether bleeding stops or not. These studies used H_2RA bolus therapy; however, more effective acid suppression with intragastric pH values above 7 can be accomplished by continuous intravenous infusion. By obtaining this level of pH, platelet aggregation and the formation of blood clots that are diminished in the presence of even small amounts of acid would be enhanced. Only at pH values greater than 7 can inactivation of pepsin occur completely, allowing clots to remain clotted and platelets to remain aggregated.[7,10] Fiorucci et al. found that administration by continuous infusion of cimetidine or ranitidine allowed more consistent control of intragastric pH, maintaining values above 6.[7] Thus, if our goal in treating patients with acid-related mucosal injury and consequent bleeding is to obtain a near-neutral intragastric pH, continuous intravenous infusion of H_2RA is the method of choice.[7,11] However, although H_2RA has achieved intragastric neutrality, it has not been reported to reduce active bleeding.

Initial cessation of UGI bleeding from a wide variety of sources occurs spontaneously in approximately 80% of patients. Unfortunately, recurrent bleeding occurs in as many as 25%. It is unclear whether H_2RA administration decreases rebleeding. Zuckerman et al. found no reduction in the rate of rebleeding from duodenal ulcers during the same hospitalization in patients who received intravenous H_2RA therapy with cimetidine at doses of 300 mg every 6 hours, adjusted for renal insufficiency. On the other hand, in two reports, oral ranitidine given in doses of 150 mg nightly was superior to placebo in preventing rebleeding.[8,12] Although it is well established that the H_2RA aid in rapid healing of ulcers and decrease their recurrence, there is still a paucity of published data showing that these agents are effective in preventing acute rebleeding.[13] To summarize, H_2RA therapy is useful for ulcer healing but will not stop active bleeding and may not prevent rebleeding.

Stress-Related Mucosal Disease

Increasing gastric pH via H_2RA therapy for the prophylaxis of bleeding from stress ulcers of the UGI tract is beneficial. Acute mucosal injury occurs in 75–100% of patients following a major physiological stress, and up to 50% of these lesions show endoscopic signs of recent or active bleeding. Clinically significant bleeding occurs in 5–20% of cases, and when this happens, mortality rates approach 50%.[14,15] Acute mucosal lesions that develop during severe illness can be attributed to several factors, including coagulopathy, reduced mucosal blood flow, inhibition of prostaglandin synthesis, bile reflux, reduced secretion of mucus and bicarbonate and, possibly, increased gastric acidity.[13,15,16] H_2RA therapy may decrease the occurrence of stress-related lesions by increasing mucosal blood flow and decreasing acid secretion. Overall, H_2RA have been found to reduce the formation of stress ulcers and may prevent progression of early mucosal lesions to deeper lesions that bleed.[17]

LaCroix et al., in their meta-analysis of 15 studies examining prophylaxis against UGI bleeding from stress mucosal lesions in patients in intensive care units (ICUs), found that cimetidine was effective in preventing UGI hemorrhage.[18] Therefore, continuous administration of H_2RA should be used in the ICU setting for patients who are at risk for stress-induced gastric mucosal injury.

Possible alternatives to the use of H_2RA for the prevention of stress ulcers are antacids or sucralfate. LaCroix et al. compared antacids to cimetidine in a meta-analysis and found that the two modalities were equally effective in preventing UGI bleeding from stress ulcerations.[18] Shuman et al. analyzed 16 prospective trials that suggested that antacids prevent stress ulcer bleeding more effectively than cimetidine, and found that antacids and cimetidine were equally efficacious, with the prevalence of overt bleeding approximating 3% in both groups of patients.[15] Furthermore, H_2RA and antacids were effective agents for the prophylaxis of stress-realted mucosal injury without the necessity for gastric pH monitoring. Cimetidine has been evaluated in this setting, without pH titration; overall bleeding rates of less than 5% have been reported, compared to placebo studies that have bleeding rates of approximately 20%. Similar results have been found when low-dose antacids were administered without titration to a specific pH goal.[15]

Sucralfate has the ability to protect ulcerated mucosa from the actions of gastric acid and pepsin, thereby preventing lesions from increasing their depth and reducing the incidence of bleeding. Cannon et al. studied the incidence of UGI bleeding in 62 mechanically ventilated patients, and compared the efficacy of sucralfate with that of cimetidine and antacids. Patients randomized to the cimetidine group received an intravenous dose of 300 mg every six hours, with adjustments made for creatinine clearance. The sucralfate group received 1 g dissolved in tap water by nasogastric tube every six hours. Titration to a specific pH was not performed in either of these groups. Patients randomized to receive antacids were initially given 30 ml via a nasogastric tube, with subsequent dosing dependent on a gastric pH equal to or exceeding 4.0. Only five patients (8%) developed clinically significant bleeding: four from the antacid group and one from the cimetidine group. No patients receiving sucralfate developed acute UGI bleeding. Cannon et al. believed that sucralfate was superior to both in preventing bleeding, as well as being less expensive and easier to administer.[16] However, there is no significant difference between these modalities of therapy. Laggner et al. compared ranitidine with sucralfate and found macroscopically visible bleeding in 18.7% of patients receiving sucralfate, 1 g six times a day via nasogastric tube, and in 43.7% of patients receiving 50 to 100 mg intravenously of ranitidine six times a day.[19] However, neither study used continuous infusions of the H_2RA, and gastric pH was often below 5 in those who bled, indicative of a less than aggressive approach to acid neutralization.

In summary, the H_2RA, antacids, and sucralfate all appear to be better than placebo in preventing stress ulcer–related bleeding. The ultimate choice, therefore, depends on the individual circumstances of each case, taking into account such factors as nursing time, cost, and potential side effects to the patient. The advantage of H_2RA, when given continuously via an intravenous route, is the simplicity of administration and therefore the reduced personnel costs, including nursing and pharmacy costs, compared to antacids, which require hourly administration, and sucralfate, which require administration every 6 hours.

NSAID-Induced Gastrointestinal Bleeding

Close to 100 million prescriptions for NSAIDs are written each year, nearly 50% of which are for patients over the age of 60. Approximately 15–25% of patients who take NSAIDs on a long-term basis develop peptic ulcerations, a circumstance that carries a twofold relative risk of bleeding.[20,21] Two types of lesions occur in the stomach and duodenum of patients who use aspirin and other NSAIDs. Acute topical mucosal lesions include petechiae, erosions and acute ulcers, and chronic solitary ulcers. Acute lesions result from dissolution of drug in the acidic contents of the stomach, allowing for entry into gastric cells, thereby resulting in mucosal damage. Compared with aspirin, NSAIDs cause less acute injury, as most are insoluble in the acidic environment of the stomach and are unable to penetrate directly the gastric mucosal cells.[22,23] Chronic focal ulcerations are the second type of lesion that occur in patients who ingest NSAIDs. The incidence of these lesions does not seem to be effected by preventing direct exposure of the drug to the gastric mucosa utilizing enteric-coated preparations, thus supporting a systemic effect of the drug as the cause of ulcerogenesis.[22,23] Overall, lesions occur more frequently in the stomach than in the duodenum, but complications can occur in both.

Prevention and effective treatment of NSAID-induced mucosal damage are available. Recent investigations have shown that misoprostol, a synthetic prostaglandin with cytoprotective features, significantly reduced the frequency of gastric ulcerations defined as lesions greater than 4 mm when administered with NSAIDs.[23] H_2RA and sucralfate were much less successful in the prevention of gastric ulcers caused by these drugs. H_2RA therapy does appear to be effective in reducing the frequency of duodenal ulcers in long-term NSAID users, whereas misoprostol has not been shown to be of benefit in the prevention of duodenal lesions in this setting.

Most studies evaluating the treatment for existing ulcers during continued NSAID therapy have shown that full-dose H_2RA leads to healing of both gastric and duodenal ulcers, though healing may be delayed. Similar results have been obtained with the use of antacids. Sucralfate has been effective in healing duodenal ulcers but not gastric lesions. Omeprazole was also effective for both duodenal and gastric lesions, without any apparent delay. Finally, misoprostol has not been shown to heal ulcers during continued NSAID therapy despite having antisecretory properties, nor has effective prophylaxis been documented in patients with recurrent gastric ulcers.[22-26]

To summarize, prophylaxis should be utilized in patients who must continue to use NSAIDs for prolonged periods and who have other associated risk factors for the development of peptic ulcers such as smoking, alcohol use, a history of peptic ulceration, or symptoms compatible with peptic ulcer disease (PUD). In patients without a history of acid-peptic disorders, or in those with a history of gastric ulceration, misoprostol at a dosage of 100 μg four times a day, rather than 200 μg four times a day, should be the initial dosage, as this is equally efficacious and results in less diarrhea. When the patient has a history of duodenal ulceration or PUD of unknown location, full-dose H_2RA should be used. NSAID therapy may be continued during treatment of acid-peptic disease unless complications such as hemorrhage or perforation occur. In this setting, NSAID therapy should be discontinued until complete healing occurs[22,23] (Table 21.1).

Omeprazole

Complete inhibition of acid secretion can be induced with omeprazole. Whether complete acid secretory inhibition will improve the outcome in patients with UGI bleeding is undetermined. Theoretically, complete inhibition should be superior to the partial inhibition seen with H_2RA, since small amounts of gastric acid are associated with antithrombotic effects. Omeprazole irreversibly binds to the enzyme H/K ATPase, located along the secretory canaliculi of the gastric parietal cell, thereby inhibiting its

TABLE 21.1. NSAID-Associated Ulcer Therapy

	Gastric Ulcer	*Duodenal Ulcer*
Discontinue NSAID	H_2RA Sucralfate Antacid Omeprazole	H_2RA Sucralfate Antacids Omeprazole
Continue NSAID	H_2RA High-dose antacid Omeprazole	H_2RA High-dose antacid Omeprazole Sucralfate
Prophylaxis	Misoprostol Omeprazole	H_2RA Omeprazole

activity. This results in the inability of parietal cells to secrete hydrogen in exchange for potassium ions. Secretion of acid can resume only after new H/K ATPase is synthesized, which takes approximately 72 hours.[27] Omeprazole administration heals duodenal and gastric ulcers faster than standard doses of H_2RA and can heal those ulcers resistant to higher doses of H_2RA.[27,28] Whether this more rapid healing, and healing of resistant ulcers, will lead to a reduced rate of bleeding from these lesions is unknown. Brunner and Chang recently compared high-dose, continuous intravenous ranitidine, at doses of 400 mg/day after a 50-mg bolus, to intravenous omeprazole, at doses of 40 mg every 12 hours after an initial bolus of 80 mg, in patients with UGI bleeding.[10] They found that 13 of 17 patients who continued to bleed with high-dose ranitidine therapy stopped bleeding when given omeprazole. Whether the difference in efficacy represents the effect of time or of the drug is unclear. After initial therapy with omeprazole, the bleeding stopped in 84% of the patients studied, whereas with initial administration of ranitidine, hemorrhage was controlled in only 15%.[10] While more effective reduction of gastric acidity by omeprazole holds promise for the patient bleeding from peptic ulcerations, reduction in bleeding complications and a decreased need for invasive endoscopic and surgical therapy are still unfulfilled hopes.

Daneshmond et al. compared omeprazole and placebo for the prevention of aspirin-associated gastric mucosal injury in 16 patients, and found a marked reduction in aspirin-induced mucosal damage, as measured by the quantity of mucosal bleeding in patients administered omeprazole.[29] Interestingly, the observed reduction in mucosal bleeding was closely related to the degree of anacidity created by omeprazole.[29] In addition, omeprazole has been shown to heal NSAID-induced gastric and duodenal ulcers more rapidly than H_2RA.[23,29] Therefore, use of medications such as proton pump inhibitors or high-dose H_2RA to markedly reduce acid secretion, as prophylaxis with aspirin and other NSAIDs, may be the most effective deterrent against mucosal damage and consequent bleeding due to these agents (Table 21.1). Further investigation is needed to evaluate this prevalent problem.

Antacids

Antacids are used extensively in a wide variety of acute states, including UGI bleeding, to prevent both recurrent ulcers and stress-induced mucosal injury. Tere et al.

assessed the hemostatic efficacy of antacids alone, or of antacids combined with cimetidine, in the prevention of further bleeding from acute mucosal lesions, gastric erosions, and gastric ulcerations.[30] They concluded that intravenous cimetidine combined with antacids was no more effective in stopping bleeding than were antacids alone. However, when given orally to patients who had already stopped bleeding, cimetidine along with antacids was more effective in the prevention of further bleeding than were antacids given as the sole treatment.[30] Antacids have been shown to be effective in preventing bleeding from stress-induced mucosal injury. However, compared with the H_2RA, these agents do not offer significantly better bleeding prophylaxis.[15,18]

To sum up, H_2RA, proton pump inhibitors, and antacids are effective, to varying degrees, in raising intragastric pH, preventing stress-induced bleeding, and promoting healing. Despite their frequent use, however, no agent has been shown to reduce active hemorrhage significantly. Consequently, the value of medications that raise intragastric pH in patients with active UGI bleeding rests not in their ability to cease bleeding, but rather to prevent recurrence of bleeding.

Sucralfate

The pathogenesis of UGI tract mucosal injury and subsequent bleeding involves disruption of the balance between aggressive and defensive mucosal factors and prostaglandin synthesis. Sucralfate, a sucrose sulfate-aluminum complex, is often used to treat and prevent UGI tract mucosal injury. Although its mechanism of action is not completely understood, sucralfate's effectiveness has been attributed to its ability to bind albumin and other surface proteins at the base of ulcerations or erosions, thereby exerting a cytoprotective effect against acid and pepsin.[16,31] Sucralfate also increases the production of prostaglandins, specifically PGE2, which may result in enhanced cytoprotective effects.[32-34] Furthermore, sucralfate binds bile acids and absorbs pepsin, thereby reducing two factors known to contribute to mucosal injury.[16,31] Goldfarb and Czaja compared sucralfate to cimetidine for terminating or preventing further bleeding from gastric or duodenal ulcers and found that both agents had equal benefit in 80% of patients.[34] This result was much better than that seen in historical controls.[34] Laggner et al. compared ranitidine to sucralfate for prevention of UGI bleeding in patients who required long-term mechanical ventilation and found sucralfate to be more effective in preventing minor bleeding.[19] However, caution should be used in interpreting these data, as all patients who bled required transfusions, regardless of the group to which they were "randomized."[19] To summarize, sucralfate is as effective as H_2RA and antacids in reducing bleeding from the UGI tract caused by stress-induced mucosal injury. Control of the acute bleeding episode with sucralfate, as with other agents, remains unproven.

Somatostatin (SST)

Despite numerous studies on its ability to stop UGI tract hemorrhage, SST use is infrequent and its role remains controversial. SST reduces splanchnic blood flow by constricting vascular smooth muscle, exerts a cytoprotective effect by promoting gastric mucus secretion, and inhibits both basal and stimulated acid secretion, as well as pepsin and gastric secretion. Its antisecretory effect may raise intragastric pH to as high as 7–7.5.[35-37] Corragio et al. found that both SST given by continuous infusion, 250 μg/

hour, and ranitidine given intravenously, 50 mg every 4 hours, were more effective than placebo for the control of UGI hemorrhage in actively bleeding patients.[35] Furthermore, all 25 patients receiving SST for moderately active bleeding stopped bleeding, whereas only 17 (65%) of 25 similar patients stopped bleeding with ranitidine. Of 27 patients with severe hemorrhage, 22 (81%) stopped bleeding with SST, compared to 13 of 26 patients (50%) who stopped bleeding with ranitidine during a 72-hour treatment period. Thus, SST in this small population was more effective than ranitidine or placebo in stopping active hemorrhage. Rebleeding rates and the necessity for surgery were also reduced.[35] Tulassay et al. noted improved control of hemorrhaging in patients with actively bleeding duodenal ulcers; 90% of bleeding ulcers stopped bleeding after 72 hours of SST therapy compared with 70% in the group given cimetidine.[37] Transfusion requirements were also less in the SST group; however, there was no significant difference in rates of rebleeding.[37] Obviously these are preliminary results. Further studies are required to learn what advantages SST therapy offers in a large patient population, particularly in regard to surgical intervention and, most important, mortality.

Another pharmacological agent utilized for the control of UGI bleeding is the antifibrinolytic agent tranxemic acid, which has been compared to cimetidine for treating patients with UGI bleeding. Decreased mortality was demonstrated in the small group of patients who received tranxemic acid, but there was no reduction in the frequency or severity of recurrent hemorrhage or in the need for surgery.[38] The explanation for this observed reduction in mortality rate was unclear.

PGE2 has been found to reduce bleeding from hemorrhagic gastritis and to prevent mucosal damage caused by aspirin.[39] Further investigation into prostaglandin cytoprotection should offer promising therapeutic possibilities.

The medical approach to UGI bleeding should be primarily concerned with the ulcer-healing process and the prevention of mucosal injury. Acid-peptic disease, NSAID damage, and stress-induced mucosal injury account for a large proportion of bleeding episodes, most of which, fortunately, with supportive management, will stop spontaneously. Because mortality has remained unchanged, physicians feel obligated to offer therapy despite the fact that none of these agents have been shown to terminate consistently the acute bleeding episode. On the other hand, prophylaxis against the development of various mucosal insults, and possibly the prevention of recurrent bleeding, can be effectively achieved. The agent used needs to be individualized to the patient because factors such as etiology, underlying medical illness, method of administration, side effects, and cost will influence management.

LOWER GASTROINTESTINAL BLEEDING

The medical management of lower gastrointestinal (LGI) bleeding presents a more challenging problem to the health care professional. Diverticular disease and angiodysplasia account for most cases of large-volume LGI hemorrhage in patients 60 years of age and older. Anorectal disorders are common causes for the passage of small amounts of blood. Meckel's diverticulum is the most common cause of lower intestinal bleeding in children, whereas inflammatory bowel disease is more prevalent in the adolescent group.[40] The initial management is similar to that for bleeding from an UGI source. Rapid, accurate assessment of the severity and rapidity of blood loss and resuscitative efforts to stabilize vital signs are followed by diagnostic and therapeutic intervention.

The initial diagnostic test for LGI bleeding is the nuclear bleeding scan, which can determine if the patient is actively bleeding and the intestinal site of bleeding. If the bleeding site is visualized by angiography, selective arterial infusion of vasopressin may have therapeutic application in the actively bleeding patient. This radiologically guided therapy may be considered a medical modality because a pharmacological agent is employed for local and systemic hemostatic effects. Browder et al. reported results of emergency angiography with selective arterial infusion of vasopressin for control of massive LGI bleeding.[41] Approximately 90% of patients in whom there was contrast extravasation from either angiodysplasia or diverticula stopped bleeding with vasopressin infusion. Control of bleeding by this angiographic technique allows patients who would have previously undergone emergency surgery to have an elective operation, thereby reducing mortality. Vasopressin infusion is generally continued for 24 hours; during this time, if the bleeding site in the colon has been identified, bowel preparation with oral lavage solution can be completed for colonoscopy. The success rate of the angiogram in determining the bleeding site depends upon its timing and the rate of bleeding. A delay of six hours or more between presentation and onset of angiography is the most important factor leading to failure to stop bleeding, probably due to reduced success in localizing the bleeding site.[41] Angiography with vasopressin infusion carries a risk of complications. Up to 7% of patients suffer major complications such as vascular thrombus, coronary ischemia, and lower extremity cyanosis, and 17% encounter minor problems such as catheter site hematomas.[42] Coronary ischemia can be reduced by simultaneous infusion of intravenous nitroglycerin, which has no effect on overall control of bleeding by vasopressin.

Estrogen

Pharmacological therapy directed at LGI hemorrhage is very limited and highly dependent on causal factors. Intestinal vascular lesions termed *angiodysplasia, vascular ectasia, arteriovenous malformation,* and *telangiectasia*[43] may be managed by heater probe or BICAP® ablation if the lesion is isolated. However, when many lesions are found or the source of bleeding is assumed to be from the small intestine, estrogen therapy may have a role in medical management.

Most of the clinical experience with estrogen therapy has focused on its efficacy in bleeding patients with vascular lesions associated with chronic renal failure and with Osler-Weber-Rendu syndrome or hereditary hemorrhagic telangiectasia. GI bleeding in patients with chronic renal failure is exacerbated by platelet dysfunction, prolongation of the bleeding time, and diminished von Willebrand factor. Furthermore, diffuse GI telangiectasias associated with chronic renal failure[44] in the setting of uremic coagulopathy pose an increased risk of bleeding. Cryoprecipitate and desmopressin, a synthetic analog of antidiuretic hormone (ADH) that increases autologous von Willebrand factor release, have been shown to decrease the bleeding time in uremic patients.[45] Based on studies showing that increased levels of estrogen during pregnancy corrected the bleeding in patients with von Willebrand's disease, Livio et al. investigated the influence of estrogen on clotting mechanisms.[45] Intravenous estrogen given to uremic patients shortened the bleeding time within 6 hours of infusion, and the improvement lasted for 14–16 days. Interestingly, the estrogen had no effect on the level of von Willebrand factor, indicating that some other factor is involved in the procoagulant effects of estrogen.[45]

Bronner et al. indicated that estrogen-progesterone therapy was associated with cessation of bleeding in a small group of uremic patients with GI telangiectasia. They cited several mechanisms that may be involved, including stasis in the mesenteric microcirculation and improved integrity of the vascular endothelial lining.[44] Flessa et al. noted that estrogen therapy may restore the endothelial continuity of abnormal vessels.[46] Bronner et al. caution, however, that the cessation of bleeding from the telangiectasias may have been spontaneous and not the actual effect of treatment.[44] Recent data show that approximately 50% of patients with presumed vascular ectasias stop bleeding spontaneously without treatment despite the need for many blood transfusions.[47,48] Van Cutsem et al. performed a double-blind crossover study using either ethinylestradiol (0.05 mg) plus norethisterone or placebo once daily by mouth for six months, at which time the drugs were crossed over to the other arm and continued for an additional six months. There was no bleeding in five of six patients who received active drug during the first six months of the trial, whereas all patients receiving placebo required transfusions. After crossover, all five patients had recurrent bleeding during placebo treatment, whereas only one patient who was crossed over to the active drug required a transfusion.[49] Potential side effects include thromboembolic disease with resultant pulmonary embolus, stroke, or myocardial infarction. Nausea, loss of libido, gynecomastia, and weight gain are less dangerous effects that have been reported.[46,48] Estrogen therapy should be considered for patients who are deemed poor surgical candidates, either because of the diffuse nature of the vascular ectasias or the concomitant medical illness, and for patients who are deemed poor endoscopic candidates because of either too many lesions or lesions beyond the reach of endoscopic ablation with laser or cautery.

Other Sites of LGI Bleeding

Bleeding from polyps and cancerous lesions is common but is rarely acute and massive. Hemorrhoidal bleeding is probably the most common cause of intermittent, less severe LGI hemorrhage. Conservative medical management includes a high-fiber diet and bulk agents, avoidance of straining while defecating, sitz baths, lubricating suppositories, and stool softeners. However, if significant bleeding or severe pain persists, definitive therapy with elastic banding or surgery may be required. Bleeding from inflammatory bowel disease is usually controlled by 5-aminosalicylic acid preparations or corticosteroids. Rarely, massive bleeding may require surgical intervention.

SUMMARY

This chapter has reviewed the medical management of GI bleeding, with an emphasis on noninterventional pharmacological therapy. Causes of bleeding are numerous, and the approach to the patient is dependent on many factors, including the manner of presentation, etiology, concurrent underlying illnesses, and available diagnostic and interventional technology. Despite continued advances in all aspects of management, from hemodynamic monitoring to diagnostic imaging to therapeutic intervention, morbidity and mortality remain significant. Further clinical investigation and laboratory research are essential to conquer this challenging and all too common problem.

REFERENCES

1. Silverstein FE, Gilbert DA, Tedesco FJ, et al: The National ASGE survey on upper gastrointestinal bleeding. *Gastointest Endosc* 27:80–93, 1966.
2. Wangensteen OH, Root HD, Salmon PA, et al: Depressant action of local gastric hypothermia on gastric digestion. *JAMA* 169:1601–1604, 1959.
3. Ponsky JL, Hoffman M, Swayogim DS: Saline irrigation in gastric hemorrhage: The effect of temperature. *J Surg Res* 28:204–205, 1980.
4. Bryant LR, Mobin-Uddin K, Dillon ML, et al: Corporation of ice water with iced saline solution for gastric lavage in gastroduodenal hemorrhage. *Am J Surg* 124:570–572, 1972.
5. Miller TA: Emergencies in acid peptic disease. *Gastroenterol Clin North Am* 17:303–315, 1988.
6. Feldman M, Burton ME: Histamine^{-2}-receptor antagonist. Standard therapy for acid acid-peptic diseases. *N Engl J Med* 323:1672–1680, 1990.
7. Fiorucci S, Clausi GC, Farinelli M, et al: Intragastric pH monitoring during antisecretory therapy in patients with gastrointestinal bleeding. *Am J Gastroenterol* 84:1416–1420, 1989.
8. Zuckerman G, Welch R, Douglas A, et al: Controlled trial of medical therapy for active upper gastrointestinal bleeding and prevention of rebleeding. *Am J Med* 76:361–366, 1984.
9. Carr-Locke DL, Traverner D, Wicks ACB: Cimetidine therapy does not prevent rebleeding from peptic ulceration. *Postgrad Med J* 60:400–403, 1984.
10. Brunner G, Chang J: Intravenous therapy with high doses of ranitidine and omeprazole in critically ill patients with bleeding peptic ulcerations of the upper intestinal tract: An open randomized controlled trial. *Digestion* 45:217–225, 1990.
11. Ostoa MJ, Russell JA, Seldin SJ, et al: Control of gastric pH with cimetidine: Boluses versus primed infusions. *Gastroenterology* 89:532–537, 1985.
12. Jensen DM, You S, Jensen ME, et al: Randomized controlled study of ranitidine maintenance for patients with a recent severe duodenal ulcer hemorrhage. *Gastroenterology* 98(Suppl):A65, 1990.
13. Feldman M, Burton ME: Histamine^{-2}-receptor antagonists. Standard therapy for acid-peptic diseases (part II). *N Engl J Med* 323:1749–1755, 1990.
14. Robert A, Kauffman GL: Stress ulcers, erosions and gastric mucosal injury, in Sleisenger MH, Fordtran JS (eds.): *Gastrointestinal Disease,* ed 4. Philadelphia, WB Saunders, 1989, p 772.
15. Shuman RB, Schuster DP, Zuckerman GR: Prophylactic therapy for stress ulcer bleeding. A reappraisal. *Ann Intern Med* 106:562–567, 1987.
16. Cannon LA, Heiselman D, Gardner W, et al: Prophylaxis of upper gastrointestinal tract bleeding in mechanically ventilated patients. A randomized study comparing the efficacy of sucralfate, cimetidine and antacids. *Arch Intern Med* 147:2101–2106, 1987.
17. Puera DA, Johnson L: Cimetidine for prevention and treatment of gastroduodenal mucosal lesions in patients in an intensive care unit. *Ann Intern Med* 103:173–177, 1985.
18. Lacroix J, Infante-Rivard C, Jenicek M, et al: Prophylaxis of upper gastrointestinal bleeding in intensive care units. A metaanalysis. *Crit Care Med* 17:862–869, 1989.
19. Laggner AN, Lenz K, Base W, et al: Prevention of upper gastrointestinal bleeding in long-term ventilated patients. Sucralfate versus ranitidine. *Am J Med* 86:81–84, 1989.
20. Peterson W: Bleeding peptic ulcer. Epidemiology and nonsurgical management. *Gastroenterol Clin North Am* 19:155–170, 1990.
21. Edelson JT, Tosteson ANA, Sax P: Cost effectiveness of misoprostol for prophylaxis against nonsteroidal anti-inflammatory drug-induced gastrointestinal tract bleeding. *JAMA* 264:41–47, 1990.

22. Graham D: The relationship between nonsteroidal anti-inflammatory drug use and peptic ulcer disease. *Gastroenterol Clin North Am* 19:171–182, 1990.
23. ACG Post-graduate Course Booklet, Section on NSAIDs 1990.
24. Graham DY, Agrawal N, Roth SH: Prevention of NSAID-induced gastric ulcer with the synthetic prostaglandin, misoprostol—a multi-center double-blind placebo controlled trial. *Lancet* 2:1277–1280, 1988.
25. Caldwell JR, Roth SH, Wu WC, et al: Sucralfate treatment of nonsteroidal anti-inflammatory drug-induced gastrointestinal symptoms and mucosal damage. *Am J Med* 82 (Suppl 3B):74–82, 1987.
26. McCarthy DM: Nonsteroidal anti-inflammatory drug-induced ulcer: Management by traditional therapies. *Gastroenterology* 96 (Suppl):662–674, 1989.
27. Matan PN: Drug therapy. Omeprazole. *N Engl J Med* 324:965–975, 1991.
28. Brunner G, Creutzfeldt W, Harke V, et al: Treatment with omeprazole in patients with peptic ulcerations resistant to extended high-dose ranitidine treatment. *Digestion* 39:80–90, 1988.
29. Daneshmond TK, Stein AG, Bhaskar NK, et al: Abolition by omeprazole of aspirin-induced gastric mucosal injury in man. *Gut* 31:514–517, 1990.
30. Tere J, Bordes JIM, Rimola A, et al: Cimetidine in acute gastric mucosal bleeding. Results of a double-blind randomized trial. *Dig Dis Sci* 25:92–96, 1980.
31. Hollander D: Efficacy of sucralfate for duodenal ulcers. A multicenter double-blind trial. *J Clin Gastroenterol* 3(Suppl 2):153, 1981.
32. Borrero E, Bank S, Margolis I, et al: Comparison of antacid and sucralfate in the prevention of gastrointestinal bleeding in patients who are critically ill. *Am J Med* 79(Suppl 2c):62–64, 1985.
33. Ligumsky M, Karmeli F, Rachmilewitz D: Sucralfate stimulation of gastric PGE2 synthesis—possible mechanism to explain its effective cytoprotective properties. *Gastroenterology* 86: 1164–1166, 1984.
34. Goldfarb JP, Czaja MJ: A comparison of cimetidine and sucralfate in the treatment of bleeding peptic ulcers. *Am J Gastroenterol* 80:5–7, 1985.
35. Coraggio F, Bertini G, Catalano A, et al: Clinical, controlled trial of somatostatin with ranitidine and placebo in the control of peptic hemorrhage of the upper gastrointestinal tract. *Digestion* 43:190–195, 1989.
36. Torres AJ, Landa I, Hernandez F, et al: Somatostatin in the treatment of severe upper gastrointestinal bleeding: A multicenter controlled trial. *Br J Surg* 73:786–789, 1986.
37. Tulassay Z, Gupta R, Papp J, et al: Somatostatin versus cimetidine in the treatment of actively bleeding duodenal ulcer: A prospective, randomized, controlled trial. *Am J Gastroenterol* 84:6–9, 1989.
38. Barer D, Ogilvie A, Henry D, et al: Cimetidine and tranxemic acid in the treatment of acute upper-gastrointestinal tract bleeding. *N Engl J Med* 308:1571–1575, 1983.
39. Konturek SJ, Kwiecien N, Obtulowicz W, et al: Comparison of prostaglandin E2 and ranitidine in prevention of gastric bleeding by aspirin in man. *Gut* 24:89–93, 1983.
40. Krevsky B: Evaluation of hematochezia. *Hosp Pract* 25:35–42, 1990.
41. Browder W, Cerise EJ, Litwin MJ: Impact of emergency angiography in massive lower gastrointestinal bleeding. *Ann Surg* 204:530–536, 1986.
42. Eckstein MR, Kelemouridis V, Athanasoulis CA, et al: Gastric bleeding: Therapy with intraarterial vasopressin and transcatheter embolization. *Radiology* 152:643–646, 1984.
43. Duray PH, Marcal JM, Livolsi VA, et al: Small intestinal angiodysplasia in the elderly. *J Clin Gastroenterol* 6:311–319, 1984.

44. Bronner MH, Pate MB, Cunningham JT, et al: Estrogen-progesterone therapy for bleeding gastrointestinal telangiectasias in chronic renal failure. An uncontrolled trial. *Ann Intern Med* 105:371–374, 1986.

45. Livio M, Mannuccio PM, Vigano G, et al: Conjugated estrogens for the management of bleeding associated with renal failure. *N Engl J Med* 315:731–735, 1986.

46. Flessa HC, Glueck HI: Heriditary hemorrhagic telangiectasia (Osler-Weber-Rendu disease). Management of epistaxis in nine patients using systemic hormone therapy. *Otolaryngology* 103:148–151, 1977.

47. Lewis BS, Kornbluth A, et al: Hormonal therapy for bleeding from angiodysplasia: Chronic renal failure. *Am J Gastroenterol* 85:1649–1651, 1990.

48. Richter J, Christensen M, Colditz G, et al: Angiodysplasia: Natural history and efficacy of therapeutic interventions. *Dig Dis Sci* 34:1542–1546, 1989.

49. Van Cutsem E, Rutgeerts P, Vantrappen G: Treatment of bleeding gastrointestinal vascular malformations with oestrogen-progesterone. *Lancet* 335:953–955, 1990.

22

ENDOSCOPIC COAGULATION THERAPY PART A: HEATER PROBE

Dennis M. Jensen, M.D.

INTRODUCTION

Severe gastrointestinal (GI) bleeding is a common and often serious medical and surgical problem, particularly in the ill or elderly. With careful endoscopic examinations, many bleeding lesions can be identified which are amenable to endoscopic treatment with heater probe. For adults with severe upper gastrointestinal (UGI) bleeding, the most prevalent diagnoses are peptic ulcers, GI angiomas, and Mallory Weiss tears.[1,2] For severe colonic or small bowel bleeding, GI angioma is the most frequent diagnosis in our referral hospitals.[3,4] Endoscopic coagulation with concomitant medical treatment often provides definitive hemostasis for these subgroups of patients. Before the advent of endoscopic hemostasis for control of active bleeding and prevention of rebleeding, surgery was the most common treatment of patients who had a high risk of continued bleeding or early rebleeding from these GI lesions. With significantly better drugs to accelerate ulcer healing or prevent rebleeding from GI angiomas, and with endoscopic hemostasis for control of GI hemorrhage, the role of resective surgery for primary treatment of nonvariceal bleeding has substantially changed in the last decade.

This chapter presents technical, laboratory, clinical, and randomized data on the use of the heater probe for endoscopic hemostasis of nonvariceal UGI bleeding lesions. Results and complications of endoscopic treatment with heater probe will be summarized for bleeding peptic ulcers, Mallory-Weiss tears, UGI angiomas, and watermelon stom-

The CURE studies cited in this chapter were supported in part by NIH Grants AM 17328 and 33273 and Veterans Administration Research Funds. For the CURE Hemostasis randomized studies, the author acknowledges the support of his coinvestigators Drs. T.O.G. Kovacs, G.A. Machicado, G.M. Randall, M. Sue, M.E. Jensen, and Hemostasis Research Nurses S. You and E. Pelayo. The animal studies could not have been completed without the assistance of G.A. Machicado and K. Hirabayashi.

ach. The techniques for heater probe treatment of each lesion differ significantly and should be referred to prior to undertaking the treatment of these different types of lesions.

METHODS

Heater Probe Equipment

The heater probe is a computer-controlled thermal cautery apparatus which delivers a predetermined amount of heat as a pulse to the tip of an endoscopic catheter for hemostasis.[5,6] Plate 29 shows the heater probe power unit, foot pedal, and large-diameter (3.2-mm) endoscopic catheter. A silicon chip in the probe tip generates the heat and controls the temperature to 250°C. In the tip of the endoscopic catheter, the chip is surrounded by a low-heat-capacity metal envelope which heats up in less than one-fifth of a second once the coagulation pedal is depressed. The current commercially available heater probe (from the Olympus Corporation) tip is coated with Silverstone, a nonstick, durable compound. Small-diameter (2.4-mm) and large-diameter (3.2-mm) probes are available for different applications (see Plate 30). When the heater probe is "fired," heat is conducted from the end or side of the tip into the patient's tissue without the flow of electrical current into the tissue. When the heater probe is held in firm contact with tissue such as an ulcer base and fired, the probe cools off in less than one-half of a second.[5]

An analog computer in the power unit is linked to the heater probe catheter to control the temperature and the total energy delivered to the tissue. This provides uniform coagulation of tissue. It is important that the temperature inside the tip does not increase above 250°C so that severe tissue damage or vaporization does not occur.[5] The temperature at the probe surface–tissue interface does not exceed 100°C, the boiling point of water.[5] Heat transfer to the tissue continues as long as pulses of heat are delivered.

Prior to endoscopic use, the heater probe power unit is programmed to deliver the desired amount of energy for effective coagulation of the particular endoscopic lesion, such as a peptic ulcer or angioma (Table 22A.1). From 5 to 30 joules (J) can be selected from the front of the power unit by pressing a corresponding number. The time for actual delivery of the heat to the tissue will vary with the joule setting, probe contact, and heat conductivity of the tissue or the medium surrounding the probe tip.[5,7] For example, a single 30-J pulse takes five to eight seconds to be delivered to the base of an ulcer when firm tamponade is applied.[7,8] In contrast, a 10-J pulse is delivered to an angioma in two to three seconds.

In the laboratory, 1-mm-diameter gut arteries required three or four pulses of 30 J each (a total of 90–120 J) to achieve coaptive coagulation.[7,8] Firm tamponade on the artery and application of the pulses in succession to the same site before moving the probe tip (i.e., tamponade station) were necessary to coagulate the arteries, which were 1–2.5 mm in diameter.[7-9] Two-millimeter arteries required five or six pulses (a total of 150–180 J) per tamponade station for coaptive coagulation. Large-diameter (3.2-mm) probes were more effective than small-diameter (2.4-mm) probes for coagulation of large arteries (Plate 30).

For washing during endoscopy, the heater probes have three water jets spaced distally around the periphery of the probe tip (Plate 31). These ports are recessed from the end of the probe so that washing can be performed when the probe is pressed (tamponaded) against the bleeding site. Irrigation while tamponading an active bleeder

TABLE 22A.1. CURE Hemostasis Research Group Techniques for Heater Probe Hemostasis

Lesion	*Tamponade Pressure*	*Setting (Joules)*	*Pulses/ Tamponade Station*	*Site of Hemostasis*
Chronic peptic ulcer*	Very firm	30	4	Only on visible vessel
Acute ulcer or Dieulafoy's disease†	Firm	25	3	Only on bleeding point
Mallory-Weiss tear†	Moderate	20	2–3	Only on bleeding point
GI angiomas‡	Gentle	10	1–2	Entire angioma

*Treatment of visible vessel (either actively bleeding or nonbleeding) only is recommended.
†Treatment of actively bleeding lesions only.
‡For treatment of all angiomas in the bowel segment causing GI bleeding.

will verify good probe placement, tamponade efficacy, and coaptation of the artery before initiating endoscopic coagulation.

PRINCIPLES OF ULCER HEMOSTASIS WITH HEATER PROBE

From studies of resection specimens, the histopathology of bleeding gastric ulcers has been well described.[10,11] The location, size, and histopathology of the arteries which bled were defined by gross examination, injection of barium into the feeding arteries, and careful histopathological examination of resected gastric ulcers removed at the time of urgent surgery for definitive hemostasis. The visible vessels seen at endoscopy correlated with an organizing clot in a side hole of the underlying artery or with a pseudoaneurysm of the penetrating artery. In the studies of Swain et al. of bleeding gastric ulcers,[10] the mean internal diameter of the artery which bled was only 0.7 mm (range, 0.3–1.8 mm). For the therapeutic endoscopist, an important finding was that the bleeding artery was closest to the surface of the ulcer crater at the point where the visible vessel was found. The penetrating artery had an unpredictable course below the visible vessel's location and often angulated steeply into the muscle layers or serosa. Most of the time, the artery was a secondary or tertiary branch rather than a main artery such as the left gastric artery.[10]

In more recent studies of patients with a fatal duodenal ulcer (DU) hemorrhage, Swain et al. reported similar anatomical and histopathological relationships.[12] However, about a third of the patients had arteries larger than 3 mm in diameter. Also, larger, deeper ulcers were evident for the fatal DU group than the previously studied group with gastric ulcers (GU)s which were resected at surgery.[10,12] Because DUs are not resected at the time of routine DU surgery (as for control of bleeding), there is little information on nonfatal DUs which bleed or on the size of their underlying arteries. Since endoscopic hemostasis with heater probe is successful for bleeding DUs most of the time, we assume that the arteries underlying nonfatal DUs which bleed are less than 2 mm in diameter.

Otherwise, endoscopic hemostasis would not be effective, at least with our current thermal or injection devices.[5,7]

Based on our current knowledge about the histopathology of bleeding ulcers and those with a nonbleeding, visible vessel, the goal of endoscopic hemostasis is to coagulate the underlying artery effectively.[1,2,7-9] On the basis of carefully controlled studies and treatments of ulcer patients with different stigmata of recent hemorrhage, endoscopic treatment should be considered for patients with major stigmata of recent hemorrhage (active arterial bleeding and a nonvisible bleeding vessel). However, patients with minor stigmata (adherent clots, flat spots) or no stigmata (clean ulcer base) are unlikely to benefit from this treatment because their rebleeding rates with medical management are very low.[2,13,14]

The general principles of arterial coagulation of ulcers are to apply firm tamponade with the heater probe via endoscopy directly upon the bleeding point or nonbleeding visible vessel in an attempt to interrupt blood flow in the underlying artery and then to apply enough heat to weld the walls of the artery together.[2,7-9] Very firm tamponade is possible en face and tangentially with the large heater probe because it is stiffer than most other probes, such as the currently available BICAP probe.[7] Intrinsic arterial hemostasis via the coagulation cascade will then occur in patients with normal platelet function. In CURE laboratory studies, this method enables the investigator to consistently weld together gut arteries as large as 2.5 mm in diameter.[7-9] Arterial hemostasis with the heater probe and other contact thermal devices will depend on tissue heating and coagulation, tissue edema, and arterial compression and coaptation.[1,7-9]

TECHNIQUES OF ULCER HEMOSTASIS WITH HEATER PROBE

Based upon CURE laboratory studies and extensive clinical experience,[5,7,9] we recommend firm tamponade of the actively bleeding site or visible vessel in a large or chronic-appearing ulcer base and coagulation with four 30-J pulses per tamponade station (total, 120 J) before repositioning the probe (Table 22A.1). Very firm tamponade and coagulation are feasible with either the tip (en face) or the side (tangential) of the heater probe catheter. If the bleeding ulcer can be identified at endoscopy even in a very tangential position, tamponade and coagulation with the heater probe will be possible because of its stiffness and its ability to coagulate with the side of the probe.

Bleeding small, shallow, or acute peptic ulcers (or Dieulafoy's anomaly) do not have a fibrotic base, and our treatment techniques with the heater probe differ from those of chronic ulcers. The CURE Hemostasis Research Group's techniques for heater probe treatment of small ulcers with active bleeding or nonbleeding visible vessels and actively bleeding Dieulafoy's anomaly are firm tamponade on the bleeding point, using 25-J pulses, and three pulses per tamponade station (total, 75 J) before moving the probe. Use of the large heater probe via a therapeutic endoscope is recommended for these lesions (Table 22A.1).

Good reproducible results will depend on the endoscopist's ability to find the bleeding point, access it with the heater probe, and use the stiffness of the heater probe to tamponade the bleeding site. This represents a major advance over the laser hemostatic devices or injection, which may be impossible to deliver to the underlying artery in tangential positions. Because of its superior coagulation and tamponade qualities in ulcer hemostasis, the large-diameter (3.2-mm) heater probe (Figure 22A.2) is recommended. For the diagnosis and treatment of patients with severe UGI hemorrhage and active ulcer bleeding, a two-channel therapeutic endoscope will facilitate endoscopy and will be necessary for simultaneous suctioning and coagulation[7,8] (Plate 32). This therapeutic endoscope also has the advantage of having two channels on opposite sides, so that the probe placement on bleeding lesions in different quadrants of the visualized field is much easier than with a single-channel instrument. Suctioning pooled blood from the treatment area will be necessary for adequate visualization during endoscopic treatment and for successful hemostasis.

Visualization of the bleeding site is facilitated by suctioning excess blood and fluid from the target area, positioning patients so that the blood flows away from the ulcer base (Plate 33), and performing target irrigation. At times, tamponade of the bleeding point while washing and suctioning will be necessary to localize a spurting or actively bleeding artery. Blind treatment around an ulcer base that has a bleeding point is usually not effective for coagulation of the bleeding point or the underlying artery. Plates 33 to 35 illustrate the treatment of an actively bleeding marginal ulcer with heater probe.

When clots obscure the active bleeding point, irrigation of the clots off the area may be possible with a high-volume wash setting. However, this is not recommended unless the patient has given informed consent for endoscopic hemostasis, the endoscopist is trained in the use of the heater probe (or other techniques), and the resuscitation is continuing in an intensive care unit (ICU) setting. Clots may be moved from the base of an ulcer by changing the position of the patient, by pushing the clot aside with the probe, or, on some occasions, by pulling small clots off the ulcer base with a polyp grasper. Since nonbleeding clots adherent to ulcers are a minor stigma of ulcer hemorrhage and are associated with a low frequency of early rebleeding in most studies, we do not recommend removing them forcibly unless the patient has previously bled from the same ulcer or is part of a randomized controlled study of nonbleeding clots.

RESULTS OF ULCER HEMOSTASIS WITH HEATER PROBE

Randomized Controlled Trials (RCTs)

Four RCTs of the heater probe from different countries have been reported.[15-18] Three reported significant benefits of the heater probe[16-18] compared to medical treatment, and one did not.[15] Table 22A.2 shows the results for the patients with major stigmata of ulcer hemorrhage (active bleeding or nonbleeding visible vessel).

Matthewson et al. reported an RCT of the heater probe versus the YAG laser versus standard medical-surgical management of patients with severe ulcer bleeding[15] (Table 22A.3). A total of 143 consecutive patients with stigmata of recent hemorrhage accessible to endoscopic diagnosis and treatment were randomized. At the time of initial endoscopy, patients were stratified for active bleeding, nonbleeding visible vessel, overlying clot, and flat red or black spots and were randomized to YAG laser treatment (44 patients), heater probe coagulation (57 patients), and control–no endoscopic treatment (42 patients). In their initial report, the authors analyzed all patients, together with major and minor stigmata, by different treatments.[15] For all the treatments of minor and major stigmata, they reported that the YAG laser was associated with a significantly lower

TABLE 22A.2. Randomized Controlled Trials of Ulcer Hemostasis with Heater Probe

Reference	*No. of Major Stigmata Patients*	*Rebleed Rate*		*Significant Benefit?*	*Other Significant Differences?*	*Compli-cations?*
		Med	*HP*			
Matthewson et al.[15]	105	42%	28%	No	No	Yes†
Lin et al.[16]	137	48%	18%*	Yes	Yes	No
Jensen et al.[17]	125	66%	25%*	Yes	Yes	No
Fullarton et al.[18]	43	22%	0%*	Yes	Yes	Yes†

Abbreviations: Med = medical treatment; HP = heater probe coagulation.
*$p < 0.05$ vs. medical group.
†One perforation was reported after heater probe treatment.

frequency of rebleeding than control treatment (20% vs. 42%), whereas the heater probe was not (28% heater probe vs. 42% control).

For the subgroups of patients with major or minor stigmata, there were no significant differences in outcome with the different treatments. The rebleeding rate for the 31 YAG patients with major stigmata was 26%, compared to 33% for the 42 heater probe patients and 47% for the 32 control patients.[15] Also, there were no significant differences for the 38 patients with minor stigmata of recent hemorrhage in terms of rebleeding rate: heater probe, 13%; YAG laser, 8%; and control, 30%.

There was one ulcer perforation among the heater probe–treated patients. With the YAG laser, bleeding was precipitated during treatment in about 20% of the patients with nonbleeding stigmata such as non-bleeding visible vessels or flat spots. In every case,

TABLE 22A.3. Randomized Studies of Heater Probe versus Other Treatments for Ulcer Hemostasis

Reference	*Patients with Major Stigmata*	*Rebleed Rates—Major Stigmata*					*Severe Compli-cations*
		HP	*Bipolar*	*YAG*	*Inject*	*Med*	
Matthewson et al.[15]	105	33%		26%‡		47%	Yes*
Lin et al.[16]	137	18%‡			33%	48%	No
Jensen et al.[17]	125	25%‡	39%			66%	No
Lin et al.[19]	128	12%			22%		No
Chung et al.[20]	(132) +	20%			21%		Yes†
Hui et al.[21]	(91) +	19%	10%		10%		No
	Ranges:	12–33%	10–39%	26%	10–33%	47–66%	

Abbreviations: HP = heater probe; YAG = Nd:YAG laser; Inject = injection therapy; Med = medical treatment without endoscopic treatment.

( )+ the Chung and Hui studies had a higher prevalence of oozing bleeding (69% and 89%, respectively) and a lower prevalence of severe active bleeding (31% and 11%, respectively).

*One perforation occurred after HP treatment. YAG precipitated bleeding in about 20% of patients with nonbleeding stigmata, which was controlled with further treatment.

†Two perforations were diagnosed after two treatments with heater probe in two ulcer patients.

‡$p < 0.05$ vs. medical.

Matthewson et al. were able to control the active bleeding by further YAG laser treatment.[15] They reported no perforations with the YAG laser.

In another RCT from Scotland, the heater probe significantly lowered the rebleeding rate in a study of 43 patients with either active ulcer bleeding or nonbleeding visible vessels.[18] Twenty patients were treated with the heater probe and 23 with medical therapy. Among the 18 patients with active ulcer bleeding in the heater probe group, 78% had initial hemostasis compared with none (0 of 21) in the medical group. The heater probe group had a significantly lower rebleeding rate (0%) than the medically managed group (22%). One perforation occurred three hours after heater probe treatment of an actively bleeding anterior wall duodenal ulcer. No deaths were reported in either treatment group.

In a large CURE RCT in Los Angeles, patients with active spurting bleeding (47) or nonbleeding visible vessels (73) were randomized to either heater probe, bipolar electrocoagulation (BICAP), or medical-surgical therapy.[17] Initial hemostasis rates with the heater probe and BICAP for spurting bleeding were 93% and 95% compared to 14% for the medical group. Yet, only the heater probe group benefited with significant reductions in postrandomization bleeding, units of red blood cells (RBCs) transfused, mean ICU days, and emergency surgery rates compared to medical patients.[17] For the group with nonbleeding visible vessels, heater probe treatment significantly decreased postrandomization rates of rebleeding, RBC transfusion, and emergency surgery. No major complications of the heater probe or BICAP occurred. CURE investigators observed that both the heater probe and BICAP were significant advances over lasers for emergency hemostasis in terms of portability, tamponade capability, ability to coagulate tangentially, washing capacity, efficacy, and expense.

Lin and his co-workers reported a fourth randomized controlled trial from Taiwan.[16] A total of 137 patients with clinically severe UGI hemorrhage and active bleeding (spurters and oozers, each about 26% and 32% of the total number randomized) or a nonbleeding visible vessel in an ulcer (30% and 40% of each treatment group) at initial endoscopy were randomized to medical-surgical treatment, heater probe coagulation, or injection with ethanol. After randomization, heater probe–treated patients had a significantly higher rate of permanent hemostasis than the medical group and lower rates of emergency surgery and mortality (Table 22A.4). The heater probe group also had fewer mean hospital days. The mean number of units of RBCs transfused was similar for all three treatment groups. Also, the injection group had significantly lower rates of emergency surgery and mortality than the medical group. No major complications of endoscopic hemostasis were described for patients treated once or twice (for severe rebleeding) with either alcohol injection or heater probe.

Lin et al. also stratified outcomes according to initial endoscopic stigmata: nonbleeding visible vessel, oozing, and spurting.[16] The permanent hemostasis rates are shown in Table 22A.5. The medical (control) group is important as a frame of reference of the severity of ulcer hemorrhage. For the spurting subgroup, heater probe treatment resulted in a significantly higher permanent hemostasis rate than injection with alcohol or medical treatment. Based primarily upon this difference, the authors concluded that the heater probe was superior to alcohol injection and should be the treatment of choice for ''massive'' ulcer hemorrhage.[16] The differences for the oozing subgroup were not as dramatic as those for the spurting subgroup, but the heater probe results were significantly different from the medical results.

Standardization of endoscopic treatment parameters such as probe size, tamponade

TABLE 22A.4. RCT of Patients with Major Stigmata of Ulcer Hemorrhage by Lin et al.

	Heater Probe	*Injection*	*Medical*
Total patients	45	46	46
More bleeding	18%*	33%	48%
Permanent hemostasis	91%*	67%	52%
Mean hospital days	6.2*	9.0	13.8
Emergency ulcer surgery	7%	4%	26%†
Mortality rate	2%	0%	15%†

Note: This was an RCT of 137 patients in Taiwan with severe ulcer hemorrhage and active bleeding (oozing or spurting) or nonbleeding visible vessels who received emergency endoscopy. Patients were randomized to heater probe coagulation, injection with ethanol, or medical-surgical management. Major outcomes are shown.

*$p < 0.05$ for heater probe vs. medical.

†$p < 0.05$ for medical vs. heater probe or injection.

Source: Reference 16.

pressure, site of application of treatment, and total energy applied may have influenced the results of these heater probe studies as much as inclusion of high-risk patients, experience and skill of the endoscopists, and size of the study.[8] For example, Matthewson et al. coagulated around the bleeding site or stigmata first, with firm pressure, whereas CURE investigators treated the visible vessel or active bleeding site directly after very firm tamponade. The small probe was used in 26% of Matthewson et al.'s cases but in less than 5% of CURE patients. The joules per tamponade station varied from 60–90 (London) to 120–150 (Los Angeles). These technical differences may account for some of the treatment results, especially with contact probes such as the heater probe or BICAP.[1-5,7-9]

Table 22A.2 summarizes the results of the four RCTs for patients with clinically severe ulcer bleeding and major stigmata of hemorrhage. These are relatively easy to put into perspective, because three out of four of them showed significant differences in rates of severe rebleeding and/or other outcomes compared to medically treated patients. Rarely, perforations were reported after heater probe treatment. Most experienced hemostasis investigators and the NIH Consensus Conference[13,14] concluded that patients with severe UGI hemorrhage and major stigmata of ulcer hemorrhage will benefit from heater probe hemostasis. However, technical skill and a standardized approach are required.[8]

TABLE 22A.5. RCT Hemostasis Results by Initial Bleeding Rate by Lin et al.

Stigmata	*Heater Probe*		*Injection*		*Medical*	
Nonbleeding visible vessel	88%	(16)	83%	(18)	68%	(22)
Oozing	100%*	(14)	80%	(15)	50%	(12)
Spurting	87%*	(15)	31%	(13)	25%	(12)
Totals	91%*	(45)	67%	(46)	52%	(46)

Note: See Table 22A.4 for details. The efficacy of permanent hemostasis was stratified by initial bleeding rates for endoscopic treatments (heater probe or alcohol injection once or twice) or medically treated patients. Shown are the percentage of hemostasis (and the number of patients treated).

*$p < 0.05$ for heater probe vs. medical group.

Source: Reference 16.

Other Prospective Comparative Studies of Endoscopic Treatments for Ulcer Hemostasis

Table 22A.3 summarizes the six comparative RCTs of heater probe and other techniques for ulcer hemostasis. The studies of Matthewson,[15] Lin,[16] and Jensen[17] and their colleagues included a control or medical treatment group. These were RCTs and were discussed in the previous section. Three other prospective studies did not include a control group[19-21] but are additional comparative studies of the heater probe and other endoscopic modalities.

Chung et al. randomized 132 patients with either oozing or spurting arterial bleeding from ulcers in a prospective comparative study of heater probe and injection sclerotherapy.[20] A total of 68 patients were treated with epinephrine injection and 64 with heater probe hemostasis. Twenty-four hours after randomization, all patients were reendoscoped, and those with any bleeding on endoscopy were empirically retreated with the same technique used initially. The majority of patients had duodenal ulcers (64% of the heater probe group and 74% of the injection group) and oozing-type bleeding (69% of both treatment groups). The minority of patients (31%) had spurting arterial bleeding. As an important point of reference, Chung et al. previously reported in an RCT that the definitive hemostasis rate (i.e., no severe rebleeding) for ulcer oozing on medical therapy was 71% and that for spurting ulcer bleeding was 30%.[22] The rebleeding rate for oozing ulcer places this stigma in the minor stigmata category, well below the nonbleeding visible vessel subgroup in rebleeding rate (about 50% on medical management).

When all the patients (oozers and spurters) were analyzed by treatment, the initial hemostasis rate was significantly higher for the injection group (96%) than for the heater probe group (83%). None of the other differences for injection vs. heater probe were significant, including the definitive hemostasis rate of 78% vs. 81%, the transfusion requirement of 4.5 units vs. 3.8 units, the emergency surgery rate of 20% vs. 22%, the median hospital stay of eight days vs. seven days, or the mortality of two vs. four. Table 22A.6 presents the results for oozing vs. spurting. Interestingly, injection appeared to be superior with oozing bleeders (definitive hemostasis rates of 87% vs. 80% for the heater probe–treated group). However, for the spurting group, the definitive hemostasis rate with the heater probe was better than the injection technique of epinephrine (75% vs. 62%). Chung et al. had difficulty accessing the oozing or spurting ulcers more frequently with the heater probe than with the injection technique.[20] Most other hemostasis investigators report the opposite results for chronic ulcers (more difficulty accessing with injection) because of the tamponade and tangential treatment capability of the heater probe compared to injection.

No major complications occurred in the injection patients. However, two perforations occurred in the heater probe group. Both of these patients had been empirically retreated at 24-hour endoscopy for endoscopically detected bleeding. The authors concluded that heater probe and epinephrine injection were equally effective for the control of active ulcer hemorrhage, but that injection was easier and may be safer if early retreatment is used.[20]

Lin et al. also reported a prospective randomized study of 78 patients with severe ulcer bleeding and major stigmata of recent hemorrhage who were randomized to endoscopic hemostasis with alcohol injection or heater probe.[19] All patients received similar medical management and were similar in background variables. The results are presented in Table 22A.7. In contrast to Chung et al.,[20] Lin and his co-workers had significantly

TABLE 22A.6. RCT Study of Active Ulcer Bleeding by Chung et al.

	Oozing		*Spurting*	
	Heater Probe	*Injection*	*Heater Probe*	*Injection*
Number of patients	44	47	20	21
Initial hemostasis	86%	100%	75%	86%
Difficult access	18%	4%	25%	14%
Retreatment	13%	9%	0%	0%
Definitive hemostasis	80%	87%	75%	62%
Emergency surgery	20%	13%	25%	38%
Mean RBC units transfused	4.0	4.0	3.4	5.7
Median hospital days	6	6	6	5
Mortality	5%	2%	10%	5%

Note: In this study from Hong Kong, 132 patients with severe ulcer hemorrhage and active bleeding (oozing and spurting) were randomized to injection with epinephrine or hemostasis with heater probe. Postrandomization results stratified by initial bleeding rate are shown. None of the differences are significant for these subgroups.
Source: Reference 20.

higher initial (100% vs. 81%) and permanent (95% vs. 71%) hemostasis rates with the heater probe patients than with the injection group.[19] The ease of tangential access with the heater probe facilitated ulcer hemostasis in some locations compared to the difficulty of injecting in tangential positions. Lin et al. reported that ulcers in the superior aspect of the duodenal bulb or on the lesser curvature of the stomach were easier to treat with the heater probe than injection. The resultant hemostasis rates in patients with ulcers in these locations were higher with the heater probe (100%, or 15 of 15 patients) than with injection (45%, or 5 of 11 patients). There were no complications with either treatment.

Hui et al. randomized 91 patients with clinically severe ulcer bleeding and oozing (89% of all patients) or spurting bleeding (11% of the patients) on initial endoscopy.[21] Similar numbers of patients were randomized to endoscopic treatment with the heater probe, BICAP, and the YAG laser. There were no significant differences in major outcomes. No major complications occurred with any treatment (Table 22A.3). However, the equipment cost per YAG laser–treated patient was significantly higher than that of either of the other two treatments. Perhaps because this particular trial included a large number of oozers and very few spurters, access and angulation were not factors determin-

TABLE 22A.7. Comparative Study for Patients with Major Stigmata by Lin et al.

	Heater Probe	*Injection*
Total patients	42	36
Initial hemostasis	100%*	81%
Rebleeding	12%	22%
Successful retreatment	75%	40%
Permanent hemostasis	95%*	71%

Note: All patients had active bleeding from an ulcer or a nonbleeding visible vessel.
*$p < 0.05$.
Source: Reference 19.

ing the outcomes. The authors concluded that all three endoscopic hemostasis methods were effective and safe for ''active ulcer bleeding.'' However, because BICAP and the heater probe were cheaper, these treatments were recommended for use.[21]

PRINCIPLES AND TECHNIQUES OF MALLORY-WEISS TEAR HEMOSTASIS WITH THE HEATER PROBE

Most patients with Mallory-Weiss syndrome stop bleeding spontaneously. From 37%[23] to 69%[24,25] of patients required no blood transfusions during their hospital course. The transfusion requirements for such patients averaged about 3.5 units.[23,26] In some of these patients, bleeding may not stop spontaneously. The reported frequency of continued bleeding varies from 21% (23) to 43%.[27] The natural history of the untreated, actively bleeding Mallory-Weiss tear is difficult to ascertain because very few RCTs have been reported. Laine's RCT of multipolar coagulation vs. sham therapy for active UGI tract hemorrhage included 17 patients with Mallory-Weiss tears.[28] Of the eight patients randomized to sham treatment, bleeding stopped in only one patient, transfusion requirements averaged 4.8 units, and urgent surgery was necessary in four patients.[28] Previously, active bleeding at endoscopy had been used as a guide for surgical intervention, but this was based on only a few cases and endoscopic therapies had not been previously used. In the CURE studies, continued bleeding occurred during the index hospitalization in 27% of patients with Mallory-Weiss tears without underlying portal hypertension compared to 88% of patients with Mallory-Weiss tears and portal hypertension.[29] All patients with continued bleeding required therapeutic endoscopy or surgery for hemostasis.

We modified our usual ulcer endoscopic coagulation techniques and guidelines[1,7] for patients with Mallory-Weiss tears by decreasing the tamponade pressure and reducing the power settings. This was done because the arteries under Mallory-Weiss tears are smaller than those usually seen under gastric or duodenal ulcers[10,12] and because the esophageal wall is thinner than the gastric or duodenal wall, especially after an acute tear. In comparative studies with BICAP or Gold probes (results discussed below), our technique included moderate tamponade directly on the actively bleeding Mallory-Weiss tear with the large (3.2-mm) probe, suctioning of excess blood and fluid, and coagulation with two to three 1-second pulses per tamponade station with a power setting of 3 to 4 on a 50-watt generator.[5,7] With the heater probe, we used moderate tamponade pressure directly on the bleeding site and coagulation with two to three 20-J pulses per tamponade station to control hemorrhage.

RESULTS OF MALLORY-WEISS TEAR HEMOSTASIS WITH THE HEATER PROBE

There are no RCTs of the heater probe for hemostasis of actively bleeding Mallory-Weiss tears. Laine reported one of the few RCTs of bleeding Mallory-Weiss tears, and described significant reductions in continued bleeding and urgent surgery for BICAP-treated patients.[28] Although stigmata of recent hemorrhage have been described for these tears, the rebleeding rates are extremely low for patients without active bleeding and without portal hypertension.[7,15] Therefore, except for actively bleeding Mallory-Weiss tears, endoscopic treatment is not routinely recommended unless rebleeding has occurred and a visible vessel is found.[30]

In CURE prospective RCT comparing multipolar electrocoagulation (BICAP or Gold probe) and the heater probe for the treatment of Mallory-Weiss tear hemorrhage in patients without underlying portal hypertension, we have shown similar efficacy and safety profiles.[29,30] In one study, BICAP was as effective as the heater probe in achieving hemostasis or preventing rebleeding in 12 patients with actively bleeding Mallory-Weiss tears or tears with visible vessels.[29] In another trial, the Gold probe and the heater probe had equal efficacy in six patients with actively bleeding Mallory-Weiss tears.[30] Active bleeding was controlled in every patient, and there were no rebleeding episodes.[29,30] No complications occurred during the trials with the power settings previously established.[29,30] There was no short-term recurrence.

PRINCIPLES AND TECHNIQUES OF ANGIOMA HEMOSTASIS WITH THE HEATER PROBE

The relative wall thickness of normal canine bowel, in decreasing order, is stomach > esophagus > duodenum > right colon > cecum.[7] These approximate the normal human bowel relationship. However, age, atrophy, or acute ulceration may decrease bowel wall thickness. Chronic inflammation, tumor, or edema may increase bowel wall thickness. Distention of the stomach during endoscopic coagulation, as well as distention of any hollow viscus, thins out the bowel wall and significantly increases the incidence of transmural thermal injury.[7] Not only is the relative thickness of the organ being treated important, but also the location of the angiomas and whether a perforation in the area could lead to a posterior penetration or a free perforation. In addition, the patient's age, overall medical condition, and operative risk need to be considered. A careful choice of endoscopic coagulation method and avoidance of distention are recommended.

Several important lessons about coagulation of the bowel wall have been learned from reported animal studies.[7] Histological studies in dogs have revealed that the relative depth of coagulation and the resultant histological damage of endoscopically treated gastric ulcers, in increasing order, is argon laser < biopolar coagulation < heater probe < YAG laser < monopolar coagulation. In CURE comparative studies, we found similar relative damage for treatment of normal mucosa (stimulating mucosal lesions such as angioma) for the canine stomach, duodenum, esophagus, right colon, and cecum.

The heater probe is commercially available (Olympus Corp) with small-diameter (2.4-mm) and large-diameter (3.2-mm) probes (Figures 22A.1 and 22A.2). For coagulation of GI angiomas (including watermelon stomach, Osler-Weber-Rendu syndrome, and UGI angiomas), we use 10 J per pulse. As with all other modalities, we test the probe on normal mucosa via endoscopy to adjust our settings prior to actual treatment of the angioma (Table 22A.1).

For elective coagulation, endoscopy with a large-channel (3.7-mm) or standard-channel (2.8-mm) instrument can be performed. When large lesions are suspected, large-channel instruments and large probes are preferred. Large probes coagulate better, cover more surface area, wash better, and often induce less bleeding because fewer pulses are required than in treatments with small probes.[7] Also, the heat per unit area of coagulation is less with the larger contact probes, thus reducing the risks of transmural injury or perforation in elderly patients with thin gut walls.[7] Occasionally, sticking and coagulum buildup on the probe occur. The probe should then be removed and mechanically cleaned with a wet gauze sponge. Further coagulation can then be done.

RESULTS OF PROSPECTIVE STUDIES FOR HEATER PROBE HEMOSTASIS OF UGI ANGIOMAS

There are no reported RCTs of heater probe endoscopic hemostasis for bleeding UGI angiomas or telangiectasias of Osler-Weber-Rendu syndrome. However, several prospective studies have been reported.[3,31] The CURE Hemostasis Group reported the largest prospective study of endoscopic treatment for bleeding UGI angiomas—104 patients.[3,31] Both UGI angiomas and Osler-Weber-Rendu telangiectasias were included. Criteria for a definitive diagnosis of angioma as the bleeding site were endoscopic active bleeding or stigmata of recent UGI bleeding on the angioma (clot, erosion, or spot) or hematemesis with clean angioma on endoscopy and no other UGI bleeding source.[3] "Incidental" angioma characterized the subgroup of patients with chronic GI bleeding and angioma on panendoscopy when the criteria for angioma as the definite bleeding source were not met. Treatment was given with the argon laser (22 patients), BICAP (50 patients), or the heater probe (37 patients). Patient outcomes were compared for a mean of 2.5 years before (on medical management) vs. after (on endoscopic treatment) coagulation. There were no major complications. Patients with documented UGI bleeding from Osler-Weber-Rendu telangiectasia or UGI angioma had good palliation with endoscopic hemostasis. There were significant increases in hematocrit, whereas transfusion requirements and hospitalizations for bleeding decreased significantly. Treatment of incidental angioma did not reduce GI bleeding or benefit those patients. Endoscopic treatment with heater probe or BICAP was technically easier than argon laser treatment, but all three methods were safe and equally effective. The CURE group also reported that the estimated cost of hospitalization and blood transfusions was reduced at least twofold by endoscopic hemostasis compared to medical management.[31]

ANTRAL VASCULAR ECTASIA

Antral vascular ectasias (watermelon stomach) have been recognized as gastric lesions which may be responsible for significant bleeding. Previous treatments for watermelon stomach have been blood transfusions, iron therapy, and surgical hemigastrectomy. However, endoscopic coagulation appears to be effective and safe in controlling hemorrhage from this lesion in patients without extensive gastric involvement.

Twelve patients who had watermelon stomach and GI bleeding were treated with heater probe by Petrini and Johnston.[32] These patients received a mean of four treatments and were followed for a mean period of 20 months. No further bleeding was evident in any of these patients during this period of follow-up. There were no complications.

Our CURE group had used bipolar coagulation (Gold probe or BICAP) or heater probe to treat six patients with watermelon stomach and severe anemia. The same settings were used as for heater probe treatment of angiomas (Table 22A.1). Bleeding was controlled in all patients, and hematocrits increased over a mean follow-up period of 12 months. There were no complications of treatment.

CONCLUSIONS

Over the last decade, the endoscopic treatment of nonvariceal bleeding has progressed significantly. The question "Which patients will benefit from endoscopic therapy?" has been addressed in several RCTs. For ulcers, the answer is: patients with clinically severe ulcer bleeding and major stigmata of recent hemorrhage (active bleeding or nonbleeding visible vessels). These are the patients who are at high risk for continued bleeding or rebleeding and who, in the past, had high rates of emergency surgery for hemostasis. Patients with actively bleeding Mallory-Weiss tears might also be considered as members of this group. Patients who are unlikely to benefit from endoscopic hemostasis are ulcer patients with either no stigmata or minor stigmata of recent hemorrhage (nonbleeding flat spots, clots, or slough). However, they are at significantly increased risk of an unnecessary therapeutic procedure (because of their low risk of rebleeding) and, as a result of the therapeutic procedure, are likely to have larger medical bills. Patients with documented GI bleeding from UGI angiomas or watermelon stomach will have good palliation of their chronic, recurrent bleeding from endoscopic hemostasis, and should be considered for endoscopic hemostasis and long-term follow-up.

In the hands of individual experts or experienced groups of investigators who have standardized endoscopic treatment and who have performed RCTs in high-risk patients with ulcer or Mallory-Weiss hemorrhage, heater probe coagulation via endoscopy has been shown to be effective and safe in three RCTs and three other prospective comparative studies. Significant reductions in rebleeding rates, transfusion requirements, need for emergency surgery, and/or direct costs have been reported. Heater probe hemostasis for bleeding UGI angiomas, Osler-Weber-Rendu telangiectasia, and watermelon stomach is safe. Control of active bleeding and recurrent bleeding is feasible when these lesions are the documented source of GI bleeding. Complication rates for heater probe coagulation are extremely low, but standardized techniques such as those of the CURE Hemostasis Research Group are recommended (Table 22A.1).

The newer endoscopic hemostasis devices (such as the heater probe) appear to have several major advantages over older devices (such as the argon or YAG laser, monopolar electrocoagulation) for emergency hemostasis of nonvariceal UGI lesions. These include tamponade and coaptation capabilities, the ability to coagulate tangentially as well as en face, portability, relative low cost, and absence of an erosive effect on tissue or arteries. Standardization and teaching of these techniques to trained endoscopists are essential. Injection sclerotherapy and bipolar electrocoagulation share many of these advantages over lasers or monopolar electrocoagulation.

Whether these technical advances, standardization of treatments, and/or endoscopic teaching will ultimately translate into better care for the nonvariceal bleeder is unknown. One could predict that a significant reduction in mortality from nonvariceal hemorrhage will depend upon more widespread training and application of standardized endoscopic techniques (such as heater probe treatment) to more patients at high risk for continued bleeding or rebleeding.

REFERENCES

1. Kovacs TOG, Jensen DM: Endoscopic control of gastroduodenal hemorrhage. *Ann Rev Med* 38:267–277, 1987.

2. Jensen DM: Recent developments in the diagnosis and treatment of severe upper gastrointestinal bleeding, in Tytgat GNJ, Van Blankenstein M (eds): *Gastrointestinal Emergencies.* In *Current Topics in Gastroenterology and Hepatology.* Stuttgart, Georg Thieme Verlag, 1990, pp 4–22.
3. Jensen DM, Machicado GA: Upper gastrointestinal angiomata: Diagnosis and endoscopic treatment, in Jensen DM, Brunetaud JM (eds): *Medical Laser Endoscopy.* Dordrecht, the Netherlands, Kluwer Academic Publishers, 1990, pp 71–91.
4. Jensen DM, Machicado GA: Techniques of hemostasis for lower GI bleeding. In Jensen DM, Brunetaud JM (eds): *Medical Laser Endoscopy.* Dordrecht, the Netherlands, Kluwer Academic Publishers, 1990, pp 99–107.
5. Jensen DM: Endoscopic control of non-variceal upper gastrointestinal hemorrhage, in Yamada T, Alpers D, Owyang C, et al (eds): *Textbook of Gastroenterology.* Philadelphia, JB Lippincott, 1991, pp 2618–2634.
6. Protell RL, Rubin CE, Auth DC, et al: The heater probe: A new endoscopic method for stopping massive gastrointestinal bleeding. *Gastroenterology* 74:257–262, 1978.
7. Jensen DM: GI endoscopic hemostasis and tumor treatment—experimental results and techniques, in Jensen DM, Brunetaud JM (eds): *Medical Laser Endoscopy.* Dordrecht, the Netherlands, Kluwer Academic Publishers, 1990, pp 45–70.
8. Jensen DM: Heat probe for hemostasis of bleeding peptic ulcers: Techniques and results of randomized controlled trials. *Gastrointest Endosc* 36 (Suppl):S42–S49, 1990.
9. Johnston JH, Jensen DM, Auth D: Experimental comparison of endoscopic yttrium-aluminum-garnet laser, electrosurgery, and heater probe for canine gut arterial coagulation: Importance of compression and avoidance of erosion. *Gastroenterology* 92:1101–1108, 1987.
10. Swain CP, Storey DW, Bown SG, et al: Nature of bleeding vessel in recurrently bleeding gastric ulcers. *Gastroenterology* 90:595–608, 1986.
11. Johnston JH: The sentinel clot and invisible vessel: Pathologic anatomy of bleeding peptic ulcer. *Gastrointest Endosc* 30:313–315, 1984.
12. Swain CP, Kalabakas A, Grandison A, et al: Size and pathology of vessel and ulcer in patients with fatal bleeding from duodenal ulcer. *Gastroenterology* 98:A133, 1990.
13. NIH Consensus Development Conference: Therapeutic endoscopy and bleeding peptic ulcers. *JAMA* 262:1369–1372, 1989.
14. Proceedings of the Consensus Conference on Therapeutic Endoscopy in Bleeding Ulcers. *Gastrointest Endosc* 36(Supp):S1–S65, 1990.
15. Matthewson D, Swain CP, Bland M, et al: Randomized comparison of Nd YAG laser, heater probe, and no endoscopic therapy for bleeding peptic ulcers. *Gastroenterology* 98:1239–1244, 1990.
16. Lin HJ, Lee FY, Kang WM, et al: Heater probe thermocoagulation and pure alcohol injection in massive peptic ulcer hemorrhage: A prospective randomized controlled trial. *Gut* 31:753–757, 1990.
17. Jensen DM, Machicado GA, Kovacs TOG, et al: Controlled randomized study of heater probe and BICAP for hemostasis of severe ulcer bleeding. *Gastroenterology* 94:A208, 1988.
18. Fullarton GM, Birnie GG, Macdonald A, et al: Controlled trial of heater probe treatment in bleeding peptic ulcers. *Br J Surg* 76:541–544, 1989.
19. Lin HJ, Tsai VT, Lee DS, et al: A prospective randomized trial of heater probe thermocoagulation versus pure alcohol injection in non-variceal peptic ulcer hemorrhage. *Am J Gastroenterol* 83:283–286, 1988.
20. Chung SCS, Leung JWC, Sung JY, et al: Injection or heat probe for bleeding ulcers. *Gastroenterology* 100:33–37, 1991.
21. Hui WM, Ng MMT, Lok ASF, et al: A randomized prospective study of the efficacy of laser,

heater probe, and bipolar electrocoagulation (BICAP) in active bleeding ulcers. *Gastroenterology* 96:A222, 1989.

22. Chung SCS, Leung JWC, Steele RJC, et al: Endoscopic injection of adrenaline for actively bleeding ulcers: A randomized trial. *Br Med J* 296:1631–1633, 1988.
23. Graham DY, Schwartz JT: The spectrum of the Mallory-Weiss tear. *Medicine* 57:307–313, 1977.
24. Pyper PC, Collins JSA, Beverland DE, et al: The Mallory-Weiss syndrome: A clinical review and follow-up. *J R Col Surg Edinburgh* 30:177, 1985.
25. Sugawa C, Benishek D, Walt AJ: Mallory-Weiss syndrome: A study of 224 patients. *Am J Surg* 145:30–33, 1983.
26. Knauer CM: Mallory-Weiss syndrome: Characterization of 75 Mallory-Weiss lacerations in 528 patients with upper gastrointestinal hemorrhage. *Gastroenterology* 71:5–8, 1976.
27. Papp JP: Electrocoagulation of actively bleeding Mallory-Weiss tears. *Gastrointest Endosc* 26:128–130, 1980.
28. Laine L: Multipolar electrocoagulation in the treatment of active upper gastrointestinal hemorrhage. *N Engl J Med* 316:1613–1617, 1987.
29. Jensen DM, Tung LA, You S, et al: Etiology and management of Mallory-Weiss bleeding in patients with or without portal hypertension. *Gastrointest Endosc* 34:A204, 1988.
30. Jensen DM, Kovacs TOG, Freeman M, et al: A multicenter randomized prospective study of gold probe versus heater probe for hemostasis of very severe ulcer or Mallory-Weiss bleeding. *Gastroenterology* 100:A92, 1991.
31. Jensen DM: Gastrointestinal angiomata, in *Gastrointestinal Endoscopy. Diagnostic and Therapeutic Procedures. An Information Resource Manual.* Manchester, Mass, American Society for Gastrointestinal Endoscopy, 1987, pp 11–15.
32. Petrini JL Jr, Johnston JH: Heat probe treatment of antral vascular ectasia. *Gastrointest Endosc* 35:324–328, 1989.

22

PART B: BIPOLAR/ MULTIPOLAR ELECTROCOAGULATION

Loren A. Laine, M.D.

In the last decade, a variety of endoscopic modalities for the treatment of gastrointestinal bleeding have been evaluated in clinical trials. These include both thermal methods and injection therapy. Thermal methods may be divided into contact methods (monopolar electrocoagulation, bipolar/multipolar electrocoagulation, and heater probe) and noncontact methods (YAG and argon lasers). The recent NIH Consensus Conference on therapeutic endoscopy and bleeding ulcers concluded that the two "most promising techniques" of endoscopic hemostasis, based on clinical efficacy and safety, were bipolar/ multipolar electrocoagulation and heater probe.[1] This review will provide a summary of the experimental background, equipment, technique, clinical trials, and complications of bipolar/multipolar electrocoagulation.

EXPERIMENTAL BACKGROUND

Bipolar electrocoagulation works by completion of an electrical circuit between two electrodes on the tip of a probe (in contrast to monopolar electrocoagulation, in which the circuit is completed between an electrode on the probe tip and a patient, or ground, electrode). The maximum temperature which can be achieved with bipolar electrocoagulation is 100°C. As the temperature rises toward 100°C, tissue water evaporates. Once the tissue is dry, the electrical flow is dramatically reduced because of high tissue resistance.[2] Unlike the monopolar generator, the bipolar generator output is too low to drive electrons across the region of desiccated tissue, effectively shutting off the bipolar probe at 100°C. Thus, the biophysics of bipolar electrocoagulation provides a safety feature to prevent severe tissue injury.

Bipolar electrocoagulation is effective in coagulating virtually 100% of arteries up to 2 mm in diameter in a canine model.[2] This size is important because Swain et al.[3] have shown that arteries in gastric ulcers with visible vessels that rebleed average 0.7

mm, with a range of 0.1 to 1.8 mm. The ability to compress a bleeding vessel with the bipolar probe before heat delivery (coaptive coagulation) appears to be the reason for its superior hemostatic efficacy—especially in arteries larger than 0.5 mm in diameter.[2] Hemostatic bond strengths as high as 2000 mm Hg have been reported with bipolar/multipolar electrocoagulation.[4]

EQUIPMENT

In the past, the BICAP (Circon-ACMI) was the sole form of bipolar/multipolar electrocoagulation commercially available, and all of the published clinical trials of bipolar/multipolar electrocoagulation employed it. Newer forms of bipolar probes have recently been introduced: the Gold probe (Microvasive) and the BiCOAG probe (Everest Medical) (Plate 36). Clinical experience with these probes is much more limited than that with the BICAP probe.

The BICAP probe is a multipolar probe; it has three pairs of electrodes on its side and tip. Electrocoagulation can be performed (the electrical circuit will be completed) as long as any pair of electrodes is in contact with the tissue. This allows for tangential application of the BICAP probe. The newer bipolar probes (Gold probe, BiCOAG probe) have the bipolar electrodes in a parallel spiral pattern along the length of the active portion of the probe. This also allows for tangential application.

A recent comparison of the BICAP and gold probes in an experimental setting[5] revealed that the only significant difference between them was that the Gold probe was stiffer. Since force of application is a factor in determining depth of coagulation (see below), the greater stiffness of the Gold probe may allow better coagulation, especially when the tip of the endoscope cannot be placed near the bleeding lesion (i.e., when a greater length of the probe must be extended outside of the endoscope) or when the probe is applied tangentially. However, the BICAP probe has just been stiffened, and the newly released probes allow a force of application similar to that of the Gold probe.

TECHNIQUE

Although bipolar electrocoagulation has been in clinical use for approximately 10 years, careful evaluation regarding optimal technique has only recently been undertaken. Important variables in the use of bipolar electrocoagulation include (1) appositional pressure applied to the bleeding lesion, (2) watt setting (1 to 10 or 5 to 50 watts on the BICAP generator), (3) duration of electrocoagulation, and (4) size of the probe (2.3 vs. 3.2 mm). Several investigators have evaluated the effects of these parameters in bipolar/multipolar electrocoagulation.

Johnston et al.[2] found that 10 or fewer two-second pulses at 25 watts (equivalent to a setting of 5 on the 50-watt BICAP generator) successfully coagulated all canine mesenteric arteries 0.25 to 1.5 mm in diameter as long as sufficient force was used to occlude the exposed arteries; if lighter application was used, treatment was not successful. Swain et al.[6] found that a strong force of application produced a greater surface area of coagulation than a weak force.

Jensen et al.,[7] assessing BICAP watt settings of 1 to 9 in a beef liver model, reported that a midrange setting of 5 produced the greatest depth of coagulation; in a follow-up abstract,[8] these authors indicated that the greatest coagulation depths for both BICAP and Gold probes occurred at watt settings of 3 and 5. In both reports, "firm tamponade" was used, but this parameter was not evaluated or quantified further.

Harrison and Morris[4] reported that a 20-second pulse duration with the BICAP produced a significantly greater hemostatic bond strength than a 2-second treatment, but they used 500 g in applying the probe tip—markedly higher than is achieved in clinical practice. Morris et al.[9] also have reported that the large (3.2-mm) BICAP probe is more effective in coagulating canine arterial hemorrhage than is the small (2.3-mm) probe. This difference was seen primarily in the larger arteries, those 1.5 mm or more in diameter.

Laine[5] recently evaluated the parameters of application force, watt setting, and treatment duration together in an encapsulated beef liver model in an attempt to determine which combination of parameters is most effective. The first question to address is, how much force can be applied with the bipolar probe placed through the biopsy channel of the endoscope? The maximal appositional force is just over 100 g,[5,10] and this number decreases significantly as the tip of the endoscope is moved farther from the bleeding lesion or the probe is applied tangentially. The maximal force of application for the bipolar probe is achieved when the tip of the endoscope is en face and as close as possible to the bleeding lesion.

Increasing the force of application (from 0 g to 50 g to 100 g) significantly increased the depth of coagulation; an increasing duration of coagulation (up to 10 or 14 seconds) was also associated with a greater depth of coagulation.[5] Interestingly, lower watt settings of 3 (15 watts) produced the greatest depths of coagulation—when combined with forceful application (100 g) and prolonged coagulation (14 seconds or seven consecutive 2-second pulses). Presumably, higher watt settings approach 100°C more quickly than low watt settings, leading to more rapid tissue desiccation and an earlier shutdown of thermal energy production.

In summary, the optimal technique for bipolar electrocoagulation should include (1) use of the large 3.2-mm probe, (2) positioning of the tip of the endoscope en face as close as possible to the bleeding lesion, (3) lower watt settings of 3 to 5 (15 to 25 watts), and (4) prolonged periods of coagulation (Plates 37 and 38). Multiple two-second pulses given in rapid succession appear to be as effective as a single long pulse of identical duration.[5]

CLINICAL TRIALS

Evaluation of clinical trials of endoscopic hemostasis requires assessment of the clinical and endoscopic criteria used by the investigators, as well as of the hemostatic technique employed. Clinical characteristics such as hemodynamic instability, bright red blood per os and per rectum, and significant transfusion requirements all indicate a large, acute bleed and are associated with an increased morbidity and mortality. Although increasing age and presence of concurrent illness are not clearly predictive of further bleeding, they are associated with an increased mortality.[1]

The appearance of an ulcer crater at endoscopy provides perhaps the best prognostic information available. Patients with active bleeding or a nonbleeding visible vessel have the worst prognosis: In our experience at the University of Southern California Medical Center (University of Southern California-U.S.C.), emergency surgery is required in almost two-thirds of patients with actively bleeding ulcers and one-third of those with ulcers containing nonbleeding visible vessels.[11,12] On the other hand, patients with a clean-based ulcer almost never rebleed or require emergency surgery, and those with stigmata of recent hemorrhage such as flat, pigmented spots or adherent clots also have a relatively low rate of rebleeding and emergency surgery.

Clinical trials of endoscopic hemostasis should include patients with clinical and endoscopic findings indicating a significant risk of persistent or recurrent bleeding. These patients are the ones most likely to benefit from intervention. Low-risk patients should not be included because hemostatic therapy is unlikely to improve the outcome in a group that rarely rebleeds or requires intervention. Significant differences therefore will be unlikely in trials which include a number of low-risk patients. It should be noted that the NIH Consensus Conference Panel also agreed that endoscopic therapy should be used only in patients at high risk for persistent or recurrent bleeding and death—those with clinical evidence of a large initial blood loss and with endoscopic evidence of active bleeding or a nonbleeding visible vessel (pigmented protuberance) in an ulcer crater.[1]

Two prospective, controlled trials from our institution have shown multipolar electrocoagulation (BICAP) to be effective.[11,12] Only patients with major upper gastrointestinal tract hemorrhage were eligible (bloody nasogastric aspirate, melena, or hematochezia; unstable vital signs, transfusion requirements of 2 or more units of blood in 12 hours, or a drop in hematocrit of at least 6% in 12 hours). The first study examined only patients with active bleeding at endoscopy (defined as persistent bleeding for at least five minutes of observation).[11] A total of 45 patients were included, and the results are shown in Table 22B.1. The second study included 75 patients with ulcers containing nonbleeding visible vessels[12] (Table 22B.2). Overall, these two studies show a significant benefit for multipolar electrocoagulation in all parameters except mortality. Electrocoagulation treatment not only decreased morbidity, it also led to a significant decrease in hospital charges.

Four controlled trials of multipolar electrocoagulation from the United Kingdom have been less positive.[13-16] The largest of the four trials did show a decrease in further bleeding and a trend toward lower transfusion requirements in the patients treated with multipolar electrocoagulation,[13] but the other three trials showed no benefit for this method.

Analysis of the clinical and endoscopic entry criteria for these trials and the hemostatic technique may provide an explanation for the differences in results between the

TABLE 22B.1. Multipolar Electrocoagulation for Active Upper Gastrointestinal Hemorrhage

	Sham Therapy (N = *23*)	*Electrocoagulation* (N = *21*)
Blood transfusions (units)	5.4 ± 0.9*	2.4 ± 0.9
Emergency surgery	57%*	14%
Hospital days	7.2 ± 1.1*	4.4 ± 0.8
Hospital charges ($)	7550 ± 1480*	3420 ± 750
Mortality	13%	0

*$p < 0.05$ for sham therapy vs. multipolar electrocoagulation (Wilcoxon rank sum and Fischer exact tests).
Source: Reference 11.

TABLE 22B.2. Multipolar Electrocoagulation for Ulcers with Nonbleeding Visible Vessels

	Sham Therapy (N = *37*)	*Electrocoagulation* (N = *38*)
Rebleeding	41%*	18%
Blood transfusions (units)	3.0 ± 0.6	1.6 ± 0.3
Emergency surgery	30%*	8%
Hospital days	6.2 ± 0.7*	4.3 ± 0.4
Hospital charges ($)	5730 ± 650*	3790 ± 410
Mortality	0	3%

*$p < 0.05$ for sham therapy vs. multipolar electrocoagulation (Wilcoxon rank sum and Fischer exact tests).
Source: Reference 11.

U.S.C. and British studies. Stringent clinical criteria were not used in the studies from the United Kingdom; rather, any patient with upper gastrointestinal hemorrhage or symptoms suggestive of it was eligible. In addition, three of the four studies included many patients with minor stigmata of recent hemorrhage,[13-15] while in the fourth trial, about 90% of the patients had nonbleeding visible vessels and the remainder had lesser stigmata.[16] Thus, these studies were not limited to patients with a high risk of further bleeding. Inclusion of low-risk patients decreases the chance that a significant benefit will be seen with hemostatic therapy, since the outcome in this group of patients is already relatively good without intervention.

Disparate techniques also may help explain at least some of the variability between the U.S.C. and U.K. studies. Laine, using a "scorched earth" technique,[11,12] applied the large (3.2-mm) BICAP probe with the maximal force possible to the vessel and the immediately surrounding area and treated for prolonged periods (mean, more than 40 seconds). In contrast, the investigators with less successful results applied coagulation for mean durations of less than 20 seconds[14-16] and did not report how forcefully they applied the probes to the bleeding sites. In addition, three of the four British studies used the small (2.3-mm) probes.

Preliminary results from a U.S. trial[17] that included only patients with active bleeding and nonbleeding visible vessels showed significantly better hemostasis with multipolar electrocoagulation than with no endoscopic treatment, but no significant improvement in other parameters (including further bleeding). However, these investigators have recently changed their technique (from 1- to 2-second pulses at a setting of 8 to 10- to 14-second pulses at a setting of 5), and their results have markedly improved.[18]

COMPARISON OF BIPOLAR/MULTIPOLAR ELECTROCOAGULATION WITH OTHER FORMS OF ENDOSCOPIC HEMOSTATIC THERAPY

Comparisons in the Experimental Setting

Bipolar/multipolar electrocoagulation and the heater probe are reported to be equally safe and effective in coagulating canine mesenteric arteries[2] and canine gastric ulcers.[19]

In addition, Johnston et al.[2] found that bipolar electrocoagulation and the heater probe were significantly more effective than the YAG laser in coagulation of canine arteries 0.5 mm in diameter or greater.

Swain et al.[6] compared four thermal probes (dry and liquid monopolar, multipolar, and heater probe) in experimental canine gastric ulcers and found that the multipolar and heater probes were safest based on the incidence of full-thickness damage. The multipolar and heater probes were comparable in all categories, except that multipolar electrocoagulation required 10.3 ± 7.6 pulses to achieve hemostasis versus 5.3 ± 2.3 pulses for the heater probe ($p < 0.02$). The authors therefore concluded that the heater probe was more effective than bipolar/multipolar electrocoagulation.

Although a number of differences exist between bipolar/multipolar electrocoagulation and the heater probe, the possibility of a difference in the hemostatic bond strength generated by the two methods may be the most important to consider. An abstract from 1985[20] states that the heater probe produces bond strengths significantly greater than those produced by multipolar electrocoagulation in 1-mm canine mesenteric arteries (~1400 vs. ~800 mm Hg). In contrast, Michaletz and Judge[10] reported mean coaptive bond strengths of 1154 mm Hg for multipolar electrocoagulation and 863 mm Hg for the heater probe (difference not statistically significant). Harrison and Morris[4] have recently shown that multipolar electrocoagulation produces a median bond strength of 1160 mm Hg (range, 500 to 2000 mm Hg) with a single prolonged application of 20 seconds. No studies have evaluated the maximal force of application which can be applied with the heater probe, but differences in the appositional force could explain variable results with these devices. Even if differences in hemostatic bond strength do exist between bipolar/multipolar electrocoagulation and the heater probe, we must question whether they are of clinical significance, since all the values reported are well above arterial pressure.

Rutgeerts et al.[21] recently compared multipolar electrocoagulation with injection therapy in the dog model. Thermal treatment successfully achieved hemostasis in all cases of bleeding ulcers and of spurting submucosal arteries, while injection therapy rarely stopped bleeding.

Prospective, Randomized Clinical Comparisons

Multipolar electrocoagulation has been compared to the YAG laser in three trials,[22-24] although all patients received injection therapy with epinephrine before thermal treatment in one of the trials.[22] No significant differences were seen in any parameter between the groups treated with multipolar electrocoagulation and YAG laser in any of the three studies (Table 22B.3).

Two prospective trials provide a comparison of multipolar electrocoagulation and the heater probe. Hui et al.,[24] studying only patients with actively bleeding ulcers, reported rebleeding in 7% of patients treated with multipolar electrocoagulation and in 19% of those treated with the heater probe; surgery was required for 7% of the electrocoagulation group and 15% of the heater probe group (differences not statistically significant) (Table 22B.3). In contrast, a preliminary report from Jensen et al.[17] comparing multipolar electrocoagulation, the heater probe, and no endoscopic treatment showed the heater probe to be significantly better than no treatment in terms of hemostasis, further bleeding, and rate of surgery, while electrocoagulation was significantly better than no endoscopic treatment only in terms of hemostasis (Table 22B.4). As mentioned earlier, since chang-

TABLE 22B.3. Comparison of Multipolar Electrocoagulation, YAG Laser, and Heater Probe for Actively Bleeding Ulcers

	Electrocoagulation (N = *27*)	*YAG Laser* (N = *18*)	*Heater Probe* (N = 27)
Primary hemostasis	89%	94%	96%
Rebleeding	7%	6%	19%
Blood transfusions (units)	2.3	1.5	1.9
Surgery for bleeding	7%	6%	15%
Hospital days	4.8	5.5	5.2
Mortality	7%	0	0

Source: Reference 24.

ing their technique, these investigators have had greatly improved results with multipolar electrocoagulation.

Two recent studies comparing multipolar electrocoagulation and injection therapy with absolute ethanol are available. In the first study,[25] all patients had clinical evidence of major upper gastrointestinal hemorrhage and endoscopic findings of an ulcer with active bleeding or a nonbleeding visible vessel. Results with both forms of treatment were excellent, and no significant differences were seen (Table 22B.5). Less than 10% of the patients in each group required urgent surgery for bleeding. Waring et al.[26] also found no significant differences between multipolar electrocoagulation and injection therapy: 20% of injected patients and 25% of patients given electrocoagulation rebled; surgery was performed in 6% of patients treated with injection versus 20% of those treated with multipolar electrocoagulation.

COMPLICATIONS OF BIPOLAR/ MULTIPOLAR ELECTROCOAGULATION

Although the relatively limited tissue injury caused by bipolar/multipolar electrocoagulation makes this device among the safest hemostatic methods, injury to at least the

TABLE 22B.4. Comparison of Multipolar Electrocoagulation, Heater Probe, and No Endoscopic Treatment for Ulcers with Active Bleeding or Nonbleeding Visible Vessels

	Control (N = *32*)	*Electrocoagulation* (N = *30*)	*Heater Probe* (N = *32*)
Hemostasis (active)	20%	90%*	93%*
Further bleeding	72%	44%	22%*
Surgery for bleeding	41%	33%	3%*
Blood transfusions (units)	3.5	3.7	1.3
Mortality	9%	3%	3%

*$p < 0.05$ vs. control (Wilcoxon rank sum and Fischer exact tests).
Source: Reference 17.

TABLE 22B.5. Comparison of Multipolar Electrocoagulation and Injection of Absolute Ethanol for Ulcers with Active Bleeding or Nonbleeding Visible Vessels

	Electrocoagulation (N = *31*)	*Injection* (N = *29*)
Further bleeding	6%	10%
Blood transfusions (units)	1.8 ± 0.6	1.3 ± 0.4
Surgery for bleeding	6%*	7%
Hospital days	5.8 ± 0.9	7.2 ± 2.5
Hospital charges ($)	7160 ± 1630	8520 ± 2960
Deaths	3%	3%

*One additional patient had emergency surgery for a perforated duodenal ulcer nine days after treatment.
Source: Reference 25.

mucosa and submucosa has been documented in man.[27] Thus, ulcers may be increased in size with endoscopic bipolar/multipolar electrocoagulation treatment, as well as with other hemostatic methods.

Induction of bleeding and perforation are the two major complications to evaluate in endoscopic hemostatic therapy. Bleeding may be induced by multipolar electrocoagulation in up to 35% of patients with nonbleeding visible vessels,[12,25] but it almost always can be controlled at the same endoscopy with continued electrocoagulation treatment.[12,25] Perforation has been reported immediately after multipolar electrocoagulation for upper gastrointestinal hemorrhage in only one patient (an 81-year-old female was treated conservatively without surgery and had an uncomplicated recovery).[16] Two cases of delayed perforation (4 days[22] and 9 days[25] after multipolar electrocoagulation for bleeding ulcers) also have been reported.

SUMMARY

Experimental data show that bipolar/multipolar electrocoagulation is effective in achieving hemostasis in vessels of the size encountered in bleeding peptic ulcers in man. Data from clinical trials indicate that bipolar/multipolar electrocoagulation is effective in improving the outcome in patients at high risk for persistent or recurrent bleeding—those with clinical evidence of major hemorrhage and endoscopic evidence of active bleeding or a nonbleeding visible vessel in an ulcer. Bipolar/multipolar electrocoagulation should be considered roughly comparable in efficacy to the heater probe and injection therapy. When using bipolar/multipolar electrocoagulation in the upper gastrointestinal tract to treat bleeding ulcers or Mallory-Weiss tears, the tip of the probe should be placed en face as close as possible to the bleeding lesion, the probe should be applied as forcefully as possible, a low watt setting should be used (3–5, 15 to 25 watts), and coagulation should be applied for prolonged periods.

REFERENCES

1. NIH Consensus Development Conference: Therapeutic endoscopy and bleeding ulcers. *JAMA* 262:1369–1372, 1989.

2. Johnston JH, Jensen DM, Auth D: Experimental comparison of endoscopic yttrium-aluminum-garnet laser, electrosurgery, and heater probe for canine gut arterial coagulation: Importance of compression and avoidance of erosion. *Gastroenterology* 92:1101–1108, 1987.
3. Swain CP, Storey DW, Bown SG, et al: Nature of the bleeding vessel in recurrently bleeding gastric ulcers. *Gastroenterology* 90:595–608, 1986.
4. Harrison JD, Morris DL: Does bipolar electrocoagulation time affect vessel weld strength? (abstract). *Gastroenterology* 96:A199, 1989.
5. Laine L: Determination of the optimal technique for bipolar electrocoagulation treatment: An experimental evaluation of the BICAP and Gold probes. *Gastroenterology* 100:107–112, 1991.
6. Swain CP, Mills TN, Shemesh E, et al: Which electrode? A comparison of four endoscopic methods of electrocoagulation in experimental bleeding ulcers. *Gut* 25:1424–1431, 1984.
7. Jensen D, Kirabayashi K, CURE Hemostasis Research Group: A study of coagulation depths with BICAP and heater probe to improve endoscopic hemostasis of bleeding peptic ulcers (abstract). *Gastrointest Endosc* 35:181, 1989.
8. Jensen DM, Kirabayashi K: A comparative study of coagulation depths and efficacy of arterial coagulation for Gold probe (abstract). *Am J Gastroenterol* 84:1161, 1989.
9. Morris DL, Brearley S, Thompson H, et al: A comparison of the efficacy and depth of gastric wall injury with 3.2- and 2.3-mm bipolar probes in canine arterial hemorrhage. *Gastrointest Endosc* 31:361–363, 1985.
10. Michaletz PA, Judge D: Microwave energy compared with heater probe and BICAP in canine models of peptic ulcer hemorrhage. *Gastroenterology* 97:676–684, 1989.
11. Laine L: Multipolar electrocoagulation in the treatment of active upper gastrointestinal hemorrhage: A prospective controlled trial. *N Engl J Med* 316:1613–1617, 1987.
12. Laine L: Multipolar electrocoagulation in the treatment of peptic ulcers with nonbleeding visible vessels: A prospective, controlled trial. *Ann Intern Med* 110:510–514, 1989.
13. O'Brien JD, Day SJ, Burnham WR: Controlled trial of small bipolar probe in bleeding peptic ulcers. *Lancet* 1:464–467, 1986.
14. Kernohan RM, Anderson JR, McKelvey ST, et al: A controlled trial of bipolar electrocoagulation in patients with upper gastrointestinal bleeding. *Br J Surg* 71:889–891, 1984.
15. Goudie BM, Mitchell KG, Birnie GG, et al: Controlled trial of endoscopic bipolar electrocoagulation in the treatment of bleeding peptic ulcers (abstract). *Gut* 25:A1185, 1984.
16. Brearley S, Hawker PC, Dykes PW, et al: Per-endoscopic bipolar diathermy coagulation of visible vessels using a 3.2 mm probe—a randomized clinical trial. *Endoscopy* 19:160–163, 1987.
17. Jensen DM, Machicado GA, Kovacs TOG, et al: Controlled randomized study of heater probe and BICAP for hemostasis of severe ulcer bleeding (abstract). *Gastroenterology* 94:A208, 1988.
18. Jensen D, Kirabayashi K, CURE Hemostasis Research Group: A study of coagulation depths with BICAP and heater probe to improve endoscopic hemostasis of bleeding peptic ulcers (abstract). *Gastrointest Endosc* 35:181, 1989.
19. Jensen DM, Tapia JI, Machicado GA, et al: Endoscopic heater and multipolar probes for treatment of bleeding canine gastric ulcers (abstract). *Gastrointest Endosc* 28:151, 1982.
20. Johnston J, Rawson S, Namihira Y: Experimental comparison of heater probe and BICAP for endoscopic treatment of gastrointestinal bleeding (abstract). *Gastrointest Endosc* 31:155–156, 1985.
21. Rutgeerts P, Geboes K, Vantrappen G: Experimental studies of injection therapy for severe nonvariceal bleeding in dogs. *Gastroenterology* 97:610–621, 1989.
22. Rutgeerts P, Vantrappen G, Van Hootegem P, et al: Neodymium-YAG laser photocoagulation

versus multipolar electrocoagulation for the treatment of severely bleeding ulcers: A randomized comparison. *Gastrointest Endosc* 33:199–202, 1987.

23. Goff JS: Bipolar electrocoagulation versus Nd-YAG laser photocoagulation for upper gastrointestinal bleeding lesions. *Dig Dis Sci* 31:906–910, 1986.
24. Hui WM, Ng MMT, Lok ASF, et al: A randomized prospective study of the efficacy of laser, heater probe (HP) and bipolar electrocoagulation (BICAP) in active bleeding ulcers (abstract). *Gastroenterology* 96:A222, 1989.
25. Laine L: Multipolar electrocoagulation versus injection therapy in the treatment of bleeding peptic ulcers: A prospective, randomized trial. *Gastroenterology* 99:1303–1306, 1990.
26. Waring JP, Sanowski RA, Woods CA, et al: Bicap versus injection sclerotherapy for bleeding ulcers: A randomized, controlled study (abstract). *Am J Gastroenterol* 84:1172, 1989.
27. Laine L, Weinstein WM: Multipolar electrocoagulation (MPEC)-induced gastric injury in man: A prospective study. *Gastrointest Endosc* 34:178–179, 1988.

22

PART C: LASER THERAPY

Pradeep K. Gupta, M.D.
David E. Fleischer, M.D.

Although lasers are now used in literally every medical subspecialty, as well as for the treatment of a wide variety of gastrointestinal (GI) diseases, their first GI application was for the management of bleeding. Although other nonlaser endoscopic therapies, which are less expensive and more portable, are more commonly used for acute GI bleeding, laser therapy in this area is important for several reasons. It was the first endoscopic therapy for hemostasis submitted to a large number of controlled clinical studies. In fact, the largest database from such studies is with lasers. Additionally, endoscopic laser therapy (ELT) has some unique features. It is the only modality using a nontouch technique (although it can be used by direct contact). Currently, most laser systems for bleeding utilize its thermal component, but because laser light is of one wavelength, its unique ability to be selectively absorbed may be critical in its application for future developments. This may involve laser light alone or a combination with tissue concentrated substances (e.g., photodynamic therapy).

HISTORICAL BACKGROUND

Maiman,[1] in 1960, first utilized the ruby laser and thus put to use the laser technology conceptualized by Einstein in 1917. In 1970, Goodale et al.[2] attempted to transfer the photocoagulative application used in ophthalmology to the digestive tract; utilizing a carbon dioxide laser, they reported obtaining control of bleeding gastric erosions. Three years later, Nath and coworkers,[3] working with the Kiefhaber group, first described transmission of a laser beam through a flexible fiber. In the mid 1970s, Dwyer et al.[4] in the United States and Kiefhaber[5] and Fruhmorgen and colleagues[6] in Germany successfully used endoscopic laser therapy to produce hemostasis in patients with upper GI bleeding.

PHYSICAL PRINCIPLES OF LASER THERAPY

The word *laser* is an acronym for ''light amplification by stimulated emission of radiation.'' This phenomenon occurs when an atom is excited to a higher energy state and stimulated to emit light as it returns to a lower energy state. When this occurs between two mirrors, the process is amplified. The beam can escape from the mirrored chamber if one of the mirrors is 100% reflective and the other is only partially reflective. The resulting laser light has several attributes: it is intense, monochromatic, and easily focused, hence its ease of use for endoscopic therapy.

The laser medium is the critical component of the laser system. It is a material which is capable of stimulating emission, that is, it is used to generate the beam. The wavelength produced is determined by the specific medium which imparts to the laser its specific properties. An electrical discharge can excite a gaseous medium (e.g., argon); a solid medium (e.g., neodymium:yttrium aluminum garnet [Nd:YAG]) requires an intense lamp light usually generated by an electrical supply; a liquid medium may be employed, as with a tuneable dye laser. The most commonly used lasers in medicine are the argon, carbon dioxide, Nd:YAG, and tuneable dye lasers. Laser light is differentiated from ordinary light by certain unique characteristics. Photons emitted are all of the same wavelength, that is, the beam is monochromatic. The beam is also temporally coherent, meaning that the photons are in phase. Finally, all the photons travel in the same direction; thus, there will be low divergence. It is the wavelength which determines whether the beam is visible or not, as well as the depth of penetration (Table 22C.1).

LASER–TISSUE INTERACTION

Laser–tissue interactions primarily consist of absorption and scattering.[7] Biological tissues have different laser–tissue interactions secondary to their proportionate volumes of water and hemoglobin. Light at short wavelengths is highly absorbed by hemoglobin, but within and beyond the red wavelength absorption by the hemoglobin molecule is low. Conversely, absorption by water is high with long wavelengths but low in the visible range. Thus, each type of laser has varying effects based on energy absorption according to wavelength. The energy produced by the argon laser (up to 10 watts, 514 nM), therefore, is highly absorbed by hemoglobin but the energy absorption is low for water. Both hemoglobin and water absorb to some extent the energy produced at the wavelength of the Nd:YAG laser (up to 100 watts at 1,064 nM and up to 30 watts at 1,318 nM).

Scattering is the second important factor.[8] As laser energy strikes a tissue surface, not all photons are absorbed. Some energy is dispersed at the point of contact; further dispersal occurs upon tissue penetration. This distribution of energy (scattering) occurs in many directions, resulting in either absorption or rescattering. Thus, laser–tissue interaction denotes more than straight-line penetration of the beam. Penetration of the

Table 22C.1. Characteristics of Medical Lasers Currently in Use

Type	*Wavelength (mm)*	*Penetration Depth*	*Visible*	*Adaptable to Flexible Endoscope*
Nd:YAG	1.06	Least superficial	No	Yes
Argon	0.05	Intermediate	Yes	Yes
Carbon dioxide	10.6	Superficial	No	No
Tuneable dye	0.5–0.75	Superficial	Yes	Yes

laser refers to the depth at which the energy level is only 10% of the initial energy level (Plate 39). The Nd:YAG laser has a penetration of approximately 4 mm, which means that at a tissue depth of 4 mm, the amount of energy remaining is 10% of the incident energy. Penetration of the argon laser is about 1 mm, and that of the carbon dioxide laser is about 0.1 mm.

The pattern of light intensities within the tissue is determined by the interdependent variables of absorption and scattering. The intensity with which incident light energy affects tissue is a function of wavelength, tissue constituents, and therapeutic spot size. The area of the tissue surface struck by the beam is the spot size. Spot size is proportional to the distance between the fiber and tissue for a given diameter with a fixed angle of beam divergence. Two other factors affecting tissue are the power output at which the machine is set and the pulse duration, which is the length of time the beam is applied to the tissue. Critical temperatures for endothelial damage, protein denaturation and coagulation, blood vessel constriction, and tissue vaporization are attained as heat is applied to tissue. These changes have associated endoscopic manifestations (Table 22C.2).

Clinically, the cellular effects of laser energy can be classified into two categories: coagulation and vaporization. The coagulative effect is that property which enables the endoscopist to achieve hemostasis in acute GI bleeding. It is the vaporizing effect by which tissue is ablated most rapidly. Tissue destruction occurs more slowly with coagulative necrosis. Both of these applications are dependent on the physical characteristics of the tissue and on the intensity and geometric configuration of the light beam. With the onset of laser therapy, thermal denaturation of tissue is initiated. The molecular structure of tissue is, to a great extent, determined by proteins. The configuration of the protein molecule is greatly affected by alterations in ambient temperature. By increasing the temperature to about 50°–60°C, the protein molecule undergoes a transition to a denatured state in which protein coagulates. Thus, a laser can achieve coagulation without surgical cutting and ablation. There is variability among the types of laser beams with respect to coagulative properties. The CO_2 laser is capable of sealing small vessels of capillary size or larger, since the distribution of thermal heat is narrow. Vessels of 0.25 mm can be sealed with the argon laser, whereas the Nd:YAG laser can seal vessels approaching 1 mm in diameter.[9] However, the Nd:YAG laser frequently will not stop bleeding in vessels

Table 22C.2. Relationship Between Temperatures and Tissue Events

Critical Temp (°C)	*Histologic Events*	*Endoscopic Manifestation*
45	Cell death, edema, endothelial damage, vasodilation	Erythema, edema cuff
60	Protein coagulates	Tissue turns gray-brown, blood turns black
80	Denatured collagen contracts, blood vessels constrict	Tissue ''puckers''
100	Tissue water boils	Vaporization causes divot
210+	Dehydrated tissue burns	Blackened tissue disappears, with or without glowing embers

larger than 1.0 mm in diameter due to rapid blood flow in larger vessels draining heat away.

HUMAN STUDIES—UPPER GI TRACT

Peptic Ulcer Disease

Dwyer,[4] Nath,[3] and Fruhmorgen[6] and their colleagues were the first to utilize the endoscopic laser for hemostasis in man. Although these were uncontrolled series, they are noteworthy. An initial report of the worldwide experience, summarized by Kiefhaber[10] in 1979, indicated that control of bleeding was achieved in 84% of 196 patients treated with argon lasers in seven centers. Of 1,533 patients treated in 31 centers, initial hemostasis was achieved in 90% utilizing the Nd:YAG laser. Since that time, the argon laser has fallen out of favor in most laser centers. The optical and physical properties of the Nd:YAG laser make it more versatile and, consequently, more suited for the treatment of active GI bleeding. Recently, Kiefhaber[11] summarized his 12-year experience with the Nd:YAG laser from 1975 to 1986. He reported an overall success rate of 94% in 1,144 patients with GI bleeding. Bleeding lesions included esophageal and gastric varices, Mallory-Weiss tears, ulcers, angiodysplasias, and tumors. Kiefhaber reported a reduction in mortality compared to surgical results.

Swain and associates[12] performed a controlled trial of YAG laser photocoagulation on 138 patients (70 in the treatment group and 68 in the control group) with ulcers and stigmata of recent hemorrhage (SRH). Patients were stratified into three groups: those with a visible vessel, those with other SRH, and those with clot that could not be washed off before therapy. They found that 7/70 laser-treated ulcers and 27/68 control ulcers rebled in the group as a whole. In the visible vessel group, rebleeding occurred from 6/39 treated and 23/43 control ulcers. Of those patients with other SRH, 0/17 treated and 1/13 controls rebled. Rebleeding occurred in 1/13 treated and 2/11 control ulcers with overlying clot. Only 10% of the treated population but 35% of the control population required emergency surgery. One treated patient and eight control patients died after an episode of rebleeding. The results of this study suggested that the use of the YAG laser significantly reduced the rebleeding rate, the need for emergency surgery, and mortality.

Rutgeerts et al.[13] divided 152 patients with hemorrhage in the upper GI tract into three groups: 23 patients with acute, spurting arterial bleeding were in group I; 86 patients with active bleeding but not spurting hemorrhage constituted group II; and 43 patients with recent bleeding made up group III. The finding related to group III was based on the presence of SRH but no active bleeding. A control group corresponding to group I was not included because the authors believed that this would be unethical. Initial hemostasis was achieved in 20/23 patients in group I, with 9/20 having permanent hemostatic control. There was recurrence of bleeding in 11 patients. Of the 23 patients in group I, 14 (62%) had to undergo surgery. The overall mortality rate for this group was 30%, with three of seven deaths (two postoperatively) being due to hemorrhage or shock. Forty-six patients in group II were treated by laser, and 40 were assigned to a control group. Of the laser-treated patients, 100% stopped bleeding compared to 77% of the control population. Bleeding recurred in 3/46 (7%) of the laser patients compared with 6/31 (20%) of the controls. One laser patient required surgery (2%) compared with five control patients (13%). The overall mortality, however, was similar in both groups, with six laser-treated patient deaths (13%) and six control patient deaths (15%). The incidence of recurrent bleeding and the need for surgery were reduced in group III, although not to a significant level, and overall mortality was insignificantly lower in the laser-treated group.

MacLeod et al.[14] conducted a single-blind controlled study on the use of the Nd:YAG laser for photocoagulation of single-vessel bleeding from peptic ulcers. Using endoscopy, 184 patients were determined to be bleeding from a single-vessel source in a peptic ulcer over a 20-month period. Patients were entered into the study if during the previous 24 hours they had had GI bleeding and had active arterial bleeding visualized at endoscopy or at least one of the following criteria: (1) shock as a result of blood loss on or after admission; (2) an initial or subsequent hemoglobin level of less than 10 g/dl; or (3) the need for a blood transfusion in the preceding 24 hours. Endoscopic criteria, in addition to the above entry criteria, also had to be fulfilled: (1) the presence of a gastric or duodenal ulcer with either an artery or a red, blue, or black spot in the ulcer base, thought to be the source of bleeding, or (2) the presence of a bleeding or nonbleeding solitary vessel, thought to be the source of blood loss. Of the original 184 patients, 130 failed to meet the study entry criteria. A total of 45 patients were entered into the study; of these, 25 were bleeding from ulcers with spots. Regardless of the treatment modality, all of these patients stopped bleeding. Twenty patients had arterial bleeding, with eight randomized to laser treatment and eight to the control group. Four others were allocated to laser treatment but did not receive it for various reasons. All eight patients in the control group required emergency surgery compared to only one of the eight laser-treated patients. The authors concluded that the incidence of continued bleeding and the need for emergency surgery are reduced with Nd:YAG laser coagulation therapy.

Ihre and coworkers[15] conducted a controlled randomized study on 135 patients with upper GI bleeding. All types of bleeding lesions, both active and inactive, were included. The laser group consisted of 66 patients, 23 of whom had acute bleeding. Of these, 15 were treated with the YAG laser and hemostasis was achieved in 14. However, seven of these patients rebled, with five ultimately requiring surgery. Of the 43 patients in the laser group without evidence of active bleeding, 9 rebled and 3 required surgery. The control group contained 69 patients; acute bleeding was evident at endoscopy in 19. Of those patients with acute bleeding sites, five required surgery. In the 50 nonbleeding patients, rebleeding occurred in 8. There was no statistical difference between the laser-treated patients and the control group with respect to continued or recurrent bleeding, the need for emergency surgery, and mortality.

Trudeau et al.[16] evaluated the Nd:YAG laser for patients with endoscopic SRH and visible vessels. Thirty-three patients were studied; 15 served as controls, with 18 receiving laser therapy. All of the patients (100%) in the laser-treated group stopped bleeding; 53% of the control group had initial control of bleeding. Mortality was 11% for the laser group and 33% for the control group. Only 5.5% of the laser group required surgery compared to nearly 27% of those in the control group. The authors concluded that YAG laser therapy reduces the need for urgent surgery and improves survival.

Krejs and associates[17] evaluated 174 patients with active bleeding or SRH due to peptic ulcer. They conducted a controlled randomized study, utilizing the YAG laser in 85 patients and randomizing 89 to the control group. The result was that 22% of the laser group and 20% of the controls had continued bleeding or rebleeding. Of those treated with the laser, 16% required urgent surgery compared to 17% of the controls.

There was no statistically significant difference in outcome between controls and actively bleeding patients. Among patients with visible vessels, 36% (5/14) of those undergoing laser therapy rebled, while 13% (2/15) of the control group rebled. The authors concluded that YAG laser photocoagulation was not beneficial in patients with acute upper GI bleeding from peptic ulcers.

An exceptional study by Swain et al.[18] evaluated 465 patients; the underlying cause of bleeding was peptic ulcers in 232. Of the 232, 147 had either active bleeding or SRH. Of the 147, 24 were excluded for defined criteria. Of the remaining 123 patients, 62 were treated with the YAG laser and 61 served as controls. Substratifications were made depending upon whether or not there was active bleeding, a nonbleeding visible vessel, an overlying clot, or other SRH. Overall, 5/62 laser-treated patients and 24/61 controls ($p < 0.02$) had continued bleeding. In those with active bleeding or visible vessels, the laser group fared better. Within the other substratifications, no significant differences in continued bleeding or recurrent bleeding existed. There was a reduction in mortality ($p < 0.02$) in the laser-treated group as well.

The results of three argon studies[19-21] were mixed. Vallon et al.[19] evaluated 136 patients with bleeding peptic ulcers. These patients were divided into three groups and randomized to laser therapy or control. Group I comprised 28 patients with actively bleeding ulcers; group II included 35 patients with nonbleeding visible vessels; and group III included 73 patients with nonbleeding ulcers without visible vessels but with a "central spot." Initial hemostasis was obtained in 10/15 laser-treated patients in group I; the remaining 5 required surgery. Of the controls in group I, 4/13 initially stopped bleeding. In groups II and III, consisting of patients with SRH but no active bleeding, argon laser therapy conferred no benefit with regard to prevention of recurrent bleeding or the need for surgery.

The study by Swain and coworkers[20] utilized the laser in 76 patients with actively bleeding peptic ulcers or SRH accessible to laser therapy. These patients were selected from a group of 330 patients presenting with acute upper GI hemorrhage. The 76 patients were divided into three groups. Group I consisted of those patients who, on endoscopy, had visible vessels; group II patients had other SRH; and group III patients had clots overlying the crater. Patients with active and inactive bleeding were included in all these groups. Hemostasis was better achieved in the laser-treated patients in group I; laser therapy also reduced the recurrence of bleeding and decreased mortality in this group. There were no differences between argon laser-treated and control patients in groups II and III.

Jensen et al.[21] conducted a small series on argon laser treatment. The overall outcomes in terms of transfusion requirements, need for emergency surgery, and mortality were lower in the argon laser-treated group.

To summarize, most of the controlled randomized studies support the beneficial effects of Nd:YAG laser use. This was best illustrated by Swain's[18] work. Four of the studies[13,15,22,23] concluded that there was no statistical difference between laser-treated and control groups with regard to continued bleeding, need for surgery, or mortality. Rhode et al.[23] included only active bleeders, with the authors concluding that laser therapy was not of benefit. Two of the studies[15,22] had design features which made it difficult to ascertain the benefits of laser therapy. The randomized controlled study by Krejs et al.[17] showed no advantage of laser photocoagulation. Critics of this and other studies point out that 221 patients were excluded from the study because they were deemed too medically unstable to be transported to the laser's location, and it may well have been these patients who would have gained the most benefit from the therapy. One can retort that the immobility of the laser is one of its drawbacks.

What can be gleaned from these data? Unfortunately, the amount of information from rigorously controlled scientific trials is scant. There is lack of uniformity regarding the lesions treated, as well as inclusionary/exclusionary criteria. This results in the dilemma of comparing apples to oranges. What is certain, however, is the safety of the Nd:YAG laser. No perforation was ever reported; thus, the safety afforded the patient and the operator is certain.

Other Arterial Sources

In addition to ulcer bleeding, there are other sources of arterial blood loss. The Nd:YAG laser has been used to treat Dieulafoy's lesion[24] and Mallory-Weiss tears.[25] In both cases, the technical approach is identical to that used with an ulcer. There are no large series with any of the endoscopic therapies for these two abnormalities.

VASCULAR ABNORMALITIES

Several vascular abnormalities of the digestive tract have been lumped under the category of arteriovenous malformations. The pathology of Kaposi's sarcoma is, of course, different from that of cavernous hemangioma or angiodysplasia. Angiodysplasia (often called *angioma, vascular ectasia,* and *telangiectasia*) and vascular ectasia will be considered here. These lesions may be found in the upper or lower GI tract or in both simultaneously. They may be either isolated or multiple. They may be associated with no known cause, or they may occur as part of a hereditary syndrome (Osler-Weber-Rendu) or be due to a nonhereditary etiology (chronic renal failure). A solitary angiodysplastic lesion is seen in Plate 40.

Angiodysplasia

These lesions are difficult to treat because of their tendency to rebleed and because they may be multiple or even inaccessible. Until recently, surgery was the major therapeutic intervention. Rutgeerts et al.[26] studied the effects of Nd:YAG laser photocoagulation on vascular malformations. Fifty-nine patients with a total of 482 lesions were entered into the study. Twenty-five patients had lesions localized to the upper GI tract, whereas 31 patients had lesions in the lower tract alone; only 3 patients had lesions in both the upper and lower GI tracts. These investigations showed a statistically significant reduction in bleeding rate, as well as a diminution of the transfusion rate at 1, 6, 12, and 18 months. The only groups of patients not demonstrating similar benefits were those with Osler-Weber-Rendu syndrome (four patients) and those with angiomas associated with Von Willebrand's disease; they all rebled. The overall success rate for the treatment of angiodysplasia in 49 patients was 82%.

Gostout et al.[27] evaluated 93 patients with vascular malformations; 83 had angiodysplasia and 10 had Osler-Weber-Rendu syndrome. All of the vascular malformations which could be identified were obliterated with the Nd:YAG laser. Successful control of bleeding was attained in nine patients with Osler-Weber-Rendu syndrome and in 72 patients with angiodysplasias. Three perforations and five instances of delayed bleeding occurred after a total 243 laser treatments. The authors concluded that careful use of endoscopic laser therapy can diminish blood loss from most GI malformations. Plate 41 shows an angiodysplastic lesion of the small intestine demonstrated at laparotomy and treated with intraoperative endoscopic laser therapy.

These favorable results have been reproduced by other investigators.[26-30] Naveau et al.[28] agreed with Rutgeerts et al.'s[26] observation that the number of lesions is closely related to the outcome. They added that, in their study, the presence of coagulation disorders and age were positively correlated with the recurrence of bleeding.

Antral Ectasia

Rider et al.[31] were the first to describe antral ectasia. As in their original report, "the gastroscopic findings were spectacular," but this impressive endoscopic abnormality was infrequently found. Jabbari et al.[32] coined the term *watermelon stomach* to describe the linear, erythematous "watermelon stripes" localized to the gastric antrum radiating in a spoke-like pattern from the pylorus. The typical endoscopic appearance is seen in Plate 42. The pathogenesis of this disorder is unknown, and treatment has generally been unrewarding. Steroids have been reported to be of value,[33] as has the heater probe;[34] however, a significant number of patients undergo antrectomy. In the hope of arresting bleeding and avoiding surgery, the Nd:YAG has been employed, with good results.[35,36] The group at the Mayo Clinic[37] treated 13 patients with endoscopic evidence of watermelon stomach. Transfusion requirements were eliminated and no major complications were encountered. The treatment of antral ectasia with laser therapy is still in its infancy; critics may say that patients have not had long-term follow-up to fully determine the effects of photocoagulation, but preliminary reports indicate a reduction in transfusion requirements.[33-37] Clearly, the vast number of patients associated with laser treatment of peptic ulcer disease has not been approached with the photocoagulative therapy of angiodysplasia, but initial reports showing elimination of the need for transfusions and surgery are certainly encouraging.

OTHER BLEEDING LESIONS

Radiation Proctitis

With increasing use of radiation therapy for various tumors, particularly abdominopelvic neoplasia, there has been a concomitant rise in radiation-induced rectal bleeding. Bleeding usually arises from fragile mucosal vascular lesions (Plate 43). Traditional medical therapy has included steroid retention enemas, oral sulfasalazine, sitz baths, stool softeners, and antispasmodics, all of which have generally been unsatisfactory. Ahlquist et al.[38] treated four patients with chronic hematochezia and transfusion-dependent anemia secondary to radiation-induced mucosal changes with the Nd:YAG laser. All four patients had a favorable response to coagulation phototherapy, with symptomatic, hematological, and endoscopic improvement. Similarly, Alexander and Dwyer[39] treated eight patients with rectal bleeding induced by radiation therapy. After an average follow-up period of 21 months from the time of the first laser treatment, transfusion requirements markedly diminished, but three major complications (ileus) and one minor (pain) complication occurred. The authors concluded that radiation-induced bleeding of the lower GI tract can be treated safely and effectively with Nd:YAG laser photocoagulation.

In the authors' experience, about 50% of patients who undergo laser treatment benefit. Usually bleeding is not completely abated, but it is significantly reduced. If the patient does not improve with the first series of laser treatments (usually one or two sessions), further therapy is seldom helpful.

Bleeding Neoplasms

There is little published information about endoscopic laser therapy for bleeding tumors in the upper GI tract. In large series from Europe where laser treatment has been used for colon carcinoma, bleeding from the tumor was a frequent indication. Mathus-Vliegen and Tytgat reported benefit in 88% of 32 patients whose main complaint was blood loss.[40] In one series reported by Lambert and another by Brunetaud et al., similar results were achieved.[41,42] Plates 44 & 45 show a bleeding colon cancer before and after laser treatment.

In some patients with gastric cancer and in others with metastatic carcinoma to the stomach and duodenum, laser therapy has been used to reduce the transfusion requirement. Often metastatic lesions originate from the breast, the kidney, or a primary melanoma. In contrast to ulcer bleeding, it is laser therapy that is most effective. The ability to ''spray paint'' broader areas and the deeper penetration to seal feeding vessels give the laser the advantage. Laser therapy is most beneficial for lesions measuring 5 cm or less.

TECHNIQUE

Conventional laser therapy is a noncontact method; the laser waveguide does not come into contact with the tissue. This is advantageous in that it is much easier to aim a noncontact device.

Once the ulcer is located and an en face view is obtained, the laser fiber is extended just beyond the tip of the endoscope (Plate 46). To obtain the most effective coagulation, the tip should be 1–2 cm from the target, with short-duration (0.3–0.5 second) pulses of high power (70–90 watts). The beam is aimed circumferentially around a visible vessel. The endoscopist should wait until edema becomes visible. Then the vessel itself is treated. The approach to an actively bleeding lesion is similar. Since the Nd:YAG laser is not absorbed by hemoglobin, any clots overlying an ulcer need not be removed, since the laser will pass through them.

Tangential orientation of the laser beam is a less favorable position in treating bleeding lesions. There is variability in thermal effects with areas closest to the laser receiving large amounts of energy; erosive effects and induced bleeding may occur.

The treatment principles of vascular malformations are similar to those of ulcers. Treatment is easiest when the lesion is not actively bleeding. An en face view makes therapy technically easier. A distinction should be made between small (2 mm or less) and large lesions (greater than 4 mm). This differentiation is important because of the tendency for large lesions to have induced bleeding, thus making a mental image of the lesion prior to its treatment is of paramount importance. If bleeding is provoked with treatment, endoscopic therapy can be continued in the immediate postbleed period. Small vascular malformations can be treated directly, with the beam aimed at the entire lesion. With larger angiodysplasias, circumferential treatment of the lesion precedes advancement to the center. Powers of 50–90 watts are used with 0.3- to 0.5-second durations.

Special attention should be paid to the technical aspects of treating colonic vascular malformations. The colon, particularly the cecum and ascending colon, is the thinnest section of the GI tract. Thus, distention, which further thins the wall, should be minimized when insufflating air. If multiple lesions are evident, the process is simplified when smaller lesions are treated first, since the incidence of provoked bleeding is lessened. Treating distal lesions first has the added benefit of preserving the ability to coagulate proximal lesions, since blood flows distally. It has been suggested that standard endoscopic medications lower blood pressure sufficiently to reduce perfusion of the vascular malformation. When an expected malformation is not seen, some experienced endoscopists recommend reversing the hypotensive effect with a narcotic antagonist, allowing the malformation to be more apparent. The authors have not found this to be of value.

When treating neoplastic lesions, the goal is to treat as much of the surface as possible. These lesions tend to ooze from numerous dysplastic tumor vessels. If the divergent beam is farther from rather than closer to the tumor, the spot size will be larger and a larger area can be treated with each pulse. The power will need to be adjusted according to the distance, and settings may vary from 50 watts (if the fiber is close to the tumor) to 100 watts (if it is far away). Pulse durations as long as 10 seconds may be used.

Limitations

The major drawback to laser therapy for acute bleeding is the fact that the laser is not portable. Since a large percentage of patients with bleeding ulcers are treated in the intensive care unit (ICU), a device is not likely to be commonly employed if it cannot be easily transported to the ICU. However, a new design allows high power output from single phase electricity and a better cooling system so that portability is improved.[43]

Although comparative studies show equivalent efficacy and safety when the laser is compared to other thermal devices, some investigators believe that the noncontact aspect is a disadvantage. Those who favor the heater probe or multipolar coagulating probes believe it is advantageous to tamponade the lesion at the time of therapy. Additionally, they believe that it is easier to treat lesions tangentially with the contact devices, and that this offers an advantage for lesions located high in the stomach or in the duodenum which cannot always be viewed en face. Finally, some endoscopists feel that it is valuable to be able to wash the area being treated. This is not possible with standard laser fibers, but it is possible with the other two thermal modalities.

The high initial cost (>$100,000) is viewed as a deterrent to laser use. However, when we consider the versatility of the device, this is not an unreasonable outlay for most medical centers.

THE FUTURE

Where will the laser fit in terms of future applications for GI bleeding? Unless the laser becomes a portable device, it offers little advantage over other devices for the treatment of ulcers. The laser is more advantageous for the treatment of some lesions—watermelon stomach, radiation proctitis, and some bleeding GI tumors; since such patients are usually treated electively, the laser will have a key role here.

The promise of laser therapy for the future lies in whether its unique advantages are harnessed. Today the laser is used as a thermal device. The potential to use laser energy in a nonthermal capacity has not been tapped. Because it is a monochromatic form of light, it can be selectively absorbed (Plate 47). With selective absorption, only a specific tissue will absorb the laser energy, and the effect on the tissue is not dependent on thermal injury. Therefore, the ability to target abnormal tissue (ulcer, cancer, etc.) exists. One may use the laser as a single modality or couple it with a substance that is concentrated in the pathological area (photodynamic therapy). The future of laser therapy for GI bleeding depends on whether or not this capacity to deliver energy selectively is developed. As just another thermal device, the expense and lack of portability are major drawbacks. The untapped potential of this treatment modality represents an exciting path to be traveled.

REFERENCES

1. Maiman TE: Stimulated optic radiation ruby. *Nature (Lond)* 187:493–494, 1960.
2. Goodale RL, Okada A, Gonzales R, et al: Rapid endoscopic control of bleeding gastric erosions by laser radiation. *Arch Surg* 101:211–214, 1970.
3. Nath G, Gorisch W, Kiefhaber P: First laser endoscopy via a fiberoptic transmission system. *Endoscopy* 5:208, 1973.
4. Dwyer RM, Yellin AE, Craig J, et al: Gastric hemostasis by laser phototherapy in man. A preliminary report. *JAMA* 236:1383–1384, 1976.
5. Nath G, Gorisch W, Kreitmair A, et al: Transmission of a powerful argon laser beam through a fiberoptic flexible gastroscope for operative gastroscopy. *Endoscopy* 5:213, 1973.
6. Fruhmorgen P, Reidenbach J, Bodem R, et al: Experimental examinations on laser endoscopy. *Endoscopy* 6:116, 1974.
7. Cummins L: Laser tissue interaction, in Fleischer D, Jensen D, Bright-Asare P (eds): *Therapeutic Laser Endoscopy in Gastrointestinal Disease*. Boston, Martinus Nijhoff, 1983, pp 9–38.
8. Enderby CE: Medical laser fundamentals, in Fleischer D, Jensen D, Bright-Asare P (eds): *Therapeutic Laser Endoscopy in Gastrointestinal Disease*. Boston, Martinus Nijhoff, 1983, pp 1–8.
9. Auth D: Fundamentals of laser for endoscopy and laser tissue interactions, in Jensen DM, Brunetano JM (eds): *Medical Laser Endoscopy*. Dordrecht, the Netherlands, Kluwer Academic Publishers, 1990, pp 1–15.
10. Kiefhaber P: International experience with lasers for gastrointestinal bleeding. Proceedings III International Laser Congress, Detroit, 1979.
11. Kiefhaber P: Indications for endoscopic neodymium-YAG laser treatment in the gastrointestinal tract. Twelve years experience. *Scand J Gastroenterol* 22(Suppl 139):53–63, 1987.

12. Swain CP, Kirkham JS, Salmon P, et al: Controlled trial of Nd-YAG laser photocoagulation in bleeding peptic ulcers. *Lancet* 1:1113–1117, 1986.
13. Rutgeerts P, Van Trappen G, Broeckaert L, et al: Controlled trial of YAG laser treatment of upper digestive hemorrhage. *Gastroenterology* 83:410–416, 1982.
14. MacLeod IA, Mills PR, Mac Denzie JF, et al: Neodymium yttrium aluminium garnet laser photocoagulation for major haemorrhage from peptic ulcers and single vessel: A single blind controlled study. *Br Med J* 286:345–348, 1983.
15. Ihre T, Johansson C, Seligsson U, et al: Endoscopic YAG-laser treatment in massive upper gastrointestinal bleeding. Report of a controlled randomized study. *Scand J Gastroenterol* 16:633–640, 1981.
16. Trudeau W, Siepler JK, Ross K, et al: Endoscopic neodymium:YAG laser photocoagulation of bleeding ulcers with visible vessels (abstract). *Gastrointest Endosc* 31:138, 1985.
17. Krejs GJ, Little KH, Westergaard H, et al: Laser photocoagulation for the treatment of acute peptic ulcer bleeding: A randomized controlled clinical trial. *N Engl J Med* 316:1618–1621, 1987.
18. Swain CP, Bown SG, Salmon P, et al: Controlled trial of Nd:YAG laser photocoagulation in bleeding peptic ulcers. *Lasers Surg Med* 3:111, 1983.
19. Vallon AG, Cotton PB, Laurence BH, et al: Randomized trial of argon laser photocoagulation in bleeding peptic ulcers. *Gut* 22:228–233, 1981.
20. Swain CP, Storey DW, Northfield TC, et al: Controlled trial of argon laser photocoagulation in bleeding peptic ulcers. *Lancet* 2:1313–1316, 1981.
21. Jensen DM, Machicado GA, Tapia JI, et al: Endoscopic argon laser photocoagulation of patients with severe upper gastrointestinal bleeding (abstract). *Gastrointest Endosc* 28:151, 1982.
22. Escourrou J: Nd:YAG laser therapy for acute gastrointestinal hemorrhage, in Atsumi, Nimsakul (eds): *Laser Tokyo 1981*. Tokyo, Intergroup Corp, 1981.
23. Rhode H, Thon K, Fischer M, et al: Results of a defined therapeutic concept of endoscopic neodymium-YAG-laser therapy in patients with upper gastrointestinal bleeding (abstract). *Br J Surg* 67:360, 1980.
24. Al-Kawas FH, O'Keefe JO: Nd:YAG laser treatment of a bleeding Dieulafoy's lesion. *Gastrointest Endosc* 33:38–39, 1987.
25. Kiefhaber P, Kiefhaber K, Huber F, et al: Usefulness of Nd:YAG laser applications in acute gastrointestinal hemorrhage. *Lasers Surg Med* 3:111, 1983.
26. Rutgeerts P, Van Gompel F, Geboes K, et al: Long term results of treatment of vascular malformations of the gastrointestinal tract by neodymium Yag laser photocoagulation. *Gut* 26:586–593, 1985.
27. Gostout CJ, Bowyer BA, Ahlquist DA, et al: Mucosal vascular malformations of the gastrointestinal tract; clinical observations and results of endoscopic neodymium. Yttrium-aluminum-garnet laser therapy. *Mayo Clin Proc* 63:993–1003, 1988.
28. Naveau S, Aubert A, Poynard T, et al: Long term results of treatment of vascular malformations of the gastrointestinal tract by neodymium YAG laser photocoagulation. *Dig Dis Sci* 35:821–826, 1990.
29. Bown SG, Swain CP, Storey DW, et al: Endoscopic laser treatment of vascular anomalies of the upper gastrointestinal tract. *Gut* 26:1338–1348, 1985.
30. Cello JP, Grendell JH: Endoscopic laser treatment for gastrointestinal vascular ectasias. *Ann Intern Med* 104:352–354, 1986.
31. Rider JA, Klotz AP, Kirsner JB: Gastritis with venocapillary ectasia as a source of massive gastric hemorrhage. *Gastroenterology* 24:118–123, 1953.

32. Jabbari M, Cherry R, Lough JO, et al: Gastric antral vascular ectasia: The watermelon stomach. *Gastroenterology* 87:1165–1170, 1984.
33. Calam J, Walker RJ: Antral vascular lesion, achlorhydria, and chronic gastrointestinal blood loss: Response to steroids. *Dig Dis Sci* 25:236–239, 1980.
34. Petrini JL, Johnston JH: Heater probe therapy for vascular ectasia of the antrum (abstract). *Gastrointest Endosc* 32:174–175, 1986.
35. Frager JD, Brandt LJ, Frank MS, et al: Treatment of a patient with watermelon stomach using transendoscopic laser photocoagulation. *Gastrointest Endosc* 34:134–137, 1988.
36. Tsai HH, Smith J, Danesh BJ: Successful control of bleeding from gastric antral vascular ectasia (watermelon stomach) by laser photocoagulation. *Gut* 32:93–94, 1991.
37. Gostout CJ, Ahlquist DA, Radford CM, et al: Endoscopic laser therapy for watermelon stomach. *Gastroenterology* 96:1462–1465, 1989.
38. Ahlquist DA, Gostout CJ, Viggiano TR, et al: Laser therapy for severe radiation-induced rectal bleeding. *Mayo Clin Proc* 61:927–931, 1986.
39. Alexander TJ, Dwyer RM: Endoscopic Nd:YAG laser treatment of severe radiation injury of the lower gastrointestinal tract: Long-term follow-up. *Gastrointest Endosc* 34:407–411, 1988.
40. Mathus-Vliegen E, Tytgat GNJ: Laser photocoagulation in the palliation of colorectal malignancies. *Cancer* 57:2212–2216, 1986.
41. Lambert R: Photodestruction par laser des tumeurs colorectales. *Gastroenterol Clin Biol* 7:59A, 1983.
42. Brunetaud JM, Maunoury V, Ducrotte P, et al: Palliative treatment of rectosigmoid carcinoma by laser endoscopic photo ablation. *Gastroenterology* 92:663–668, 1987.
43. Swain CP: Nd:Yag laser: The pro approach. *Gastrointest Endosc* 36:S30–S31, 1990.

Editor's Note: Additional confirmation of Swain's results can be found in two more recent references:

Matthewson K, Swain CP, Bland M, et al: Randomized comparison of Nd-YAG laser, heater probe (HP) and no endoscopic therapy for bleeding peptic ulcer. *Gastroenterology* 92:1522, 1987.

Matthewson K, Swain CP, Bland M, et al: Randomized comparison of Nd:YAG laser, heater probe, and no endoscopic therapy for bleeding peptic ulcers. *Gastroenterology* 98:1239–1244, 1990.

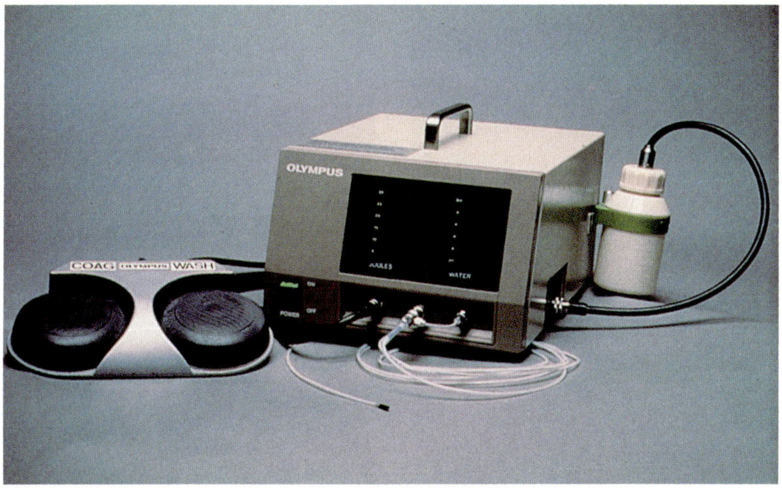

Plate 29. Heater probe power unit with foot pedal and large probe (Olympus Corp.).

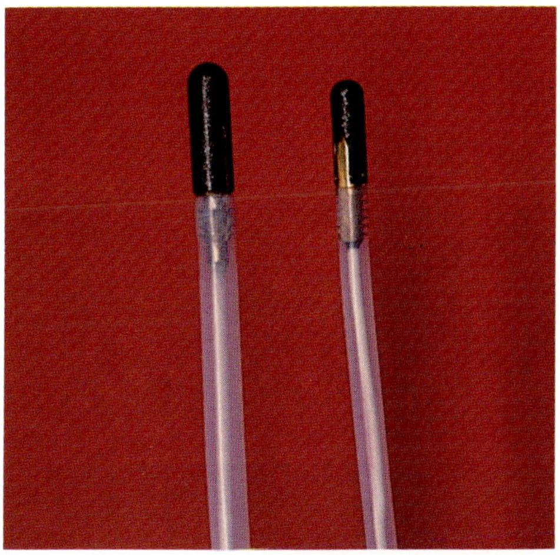

Plate 30. Large (3.2 mm—left) and small (2.4 mm—right) diameter endoscopic heater probes.

Plate 31. Irrigation from the tip of a heater probe with a curtain of water. Simultaneous tamponade and washing of a bleeding arterial lesion are feasible with the heater probe.

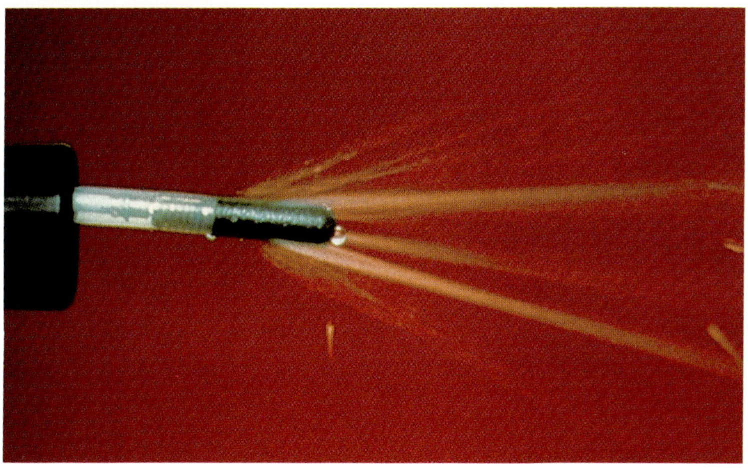

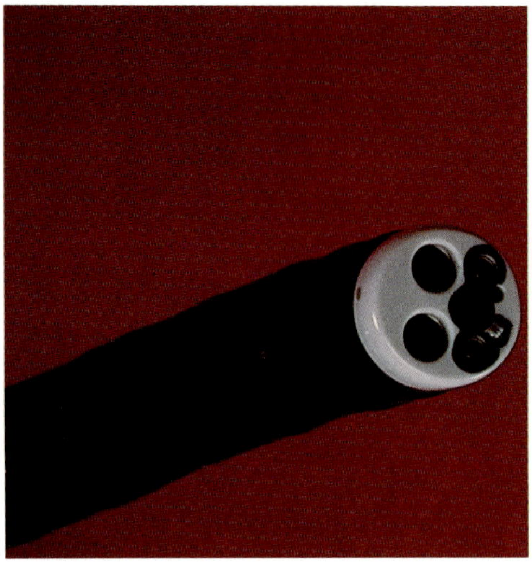

Plate 32. A dual-channel therapeutic endoscope with two 3.7-mm-diameter suction channels (Olympus Corp.) facilitates simultaneous suctioning and hemostasis of actively bleeding ulcers, Mallory-Weiss tears, and esophageal varices.

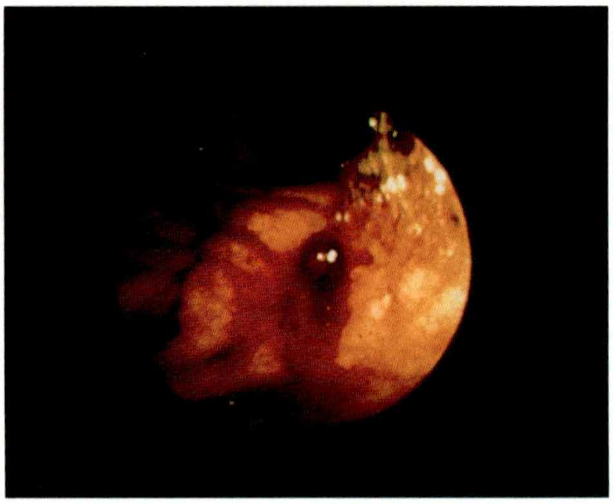

Plate 33. A marginal ulcer with an actively bleeding visible vessel was identified in a patient with severe UGI hemorrhage. The patient is positioned so that blood flows away from the ulcer. (Picture courtesy of G. Machicado, M.D.)

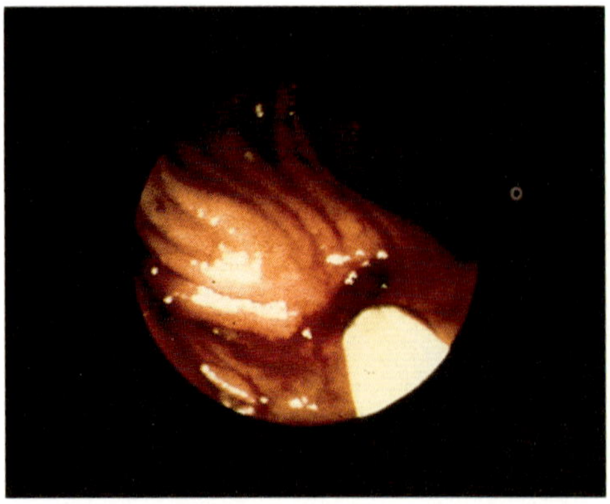

Plate 34. Firm tamponade is applied directly upon the bleeding visible vessel to control active bleeding with a large heater probe. Excess blood is suctioned and four 30-J pulses are delivered without moving the probe tip. (Picture courtesy of G. Machicado, M.D.)

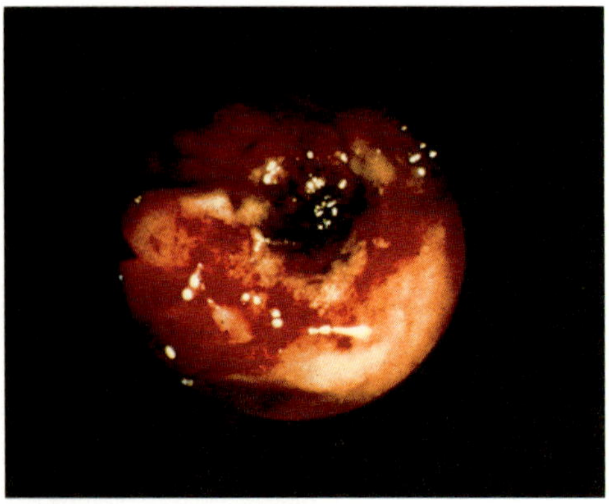

Plate 35. Ulcer appearance immediately after coagulation and hemostasis. Such ulcers heal readily with H2 receptor antagonists and supportive care. (Picture courtesy of G. Machicado, M.D.)

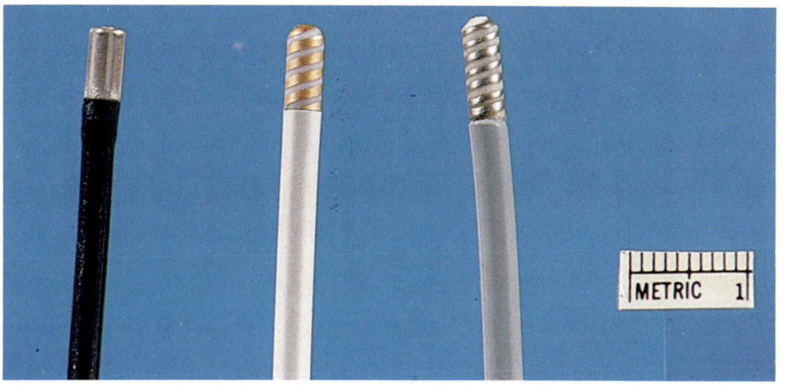

Plate 36. The three bipolar probes: BICAP, Gold, and BiCOAG.

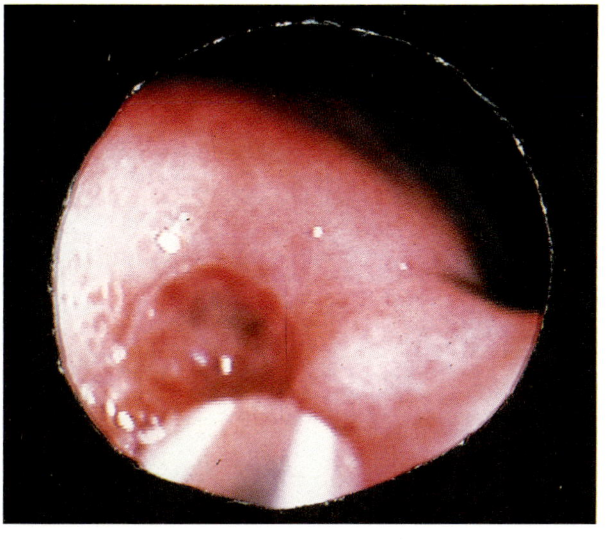

Plate 37. The BICAP probe is seen approaching a nonbleeding visible vessel in an ulcer for application of electrocoagulation.

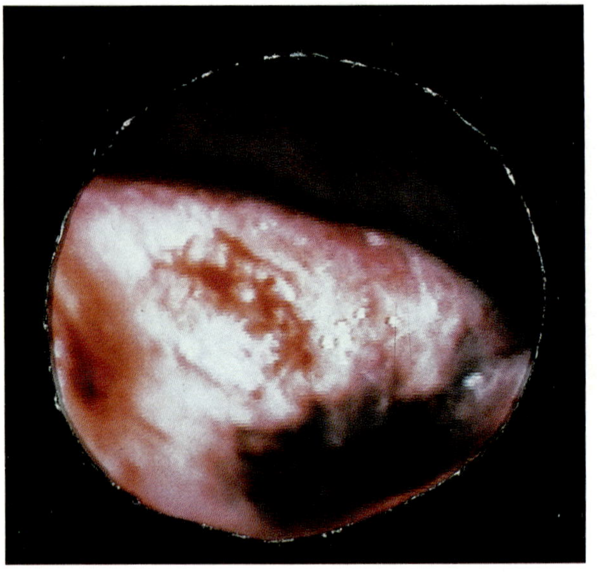

Plate 38. Appearance of the ulcer base after endoscopic treatment with the BICAP probe.

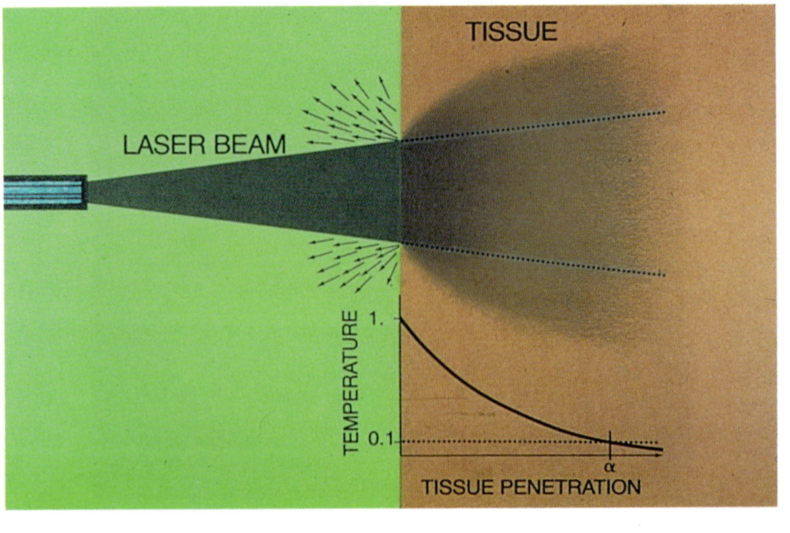

Plate 39. Schematic showing a divergent laser beam. Penetration with the Nd:YAG laser is greatest at the surface.

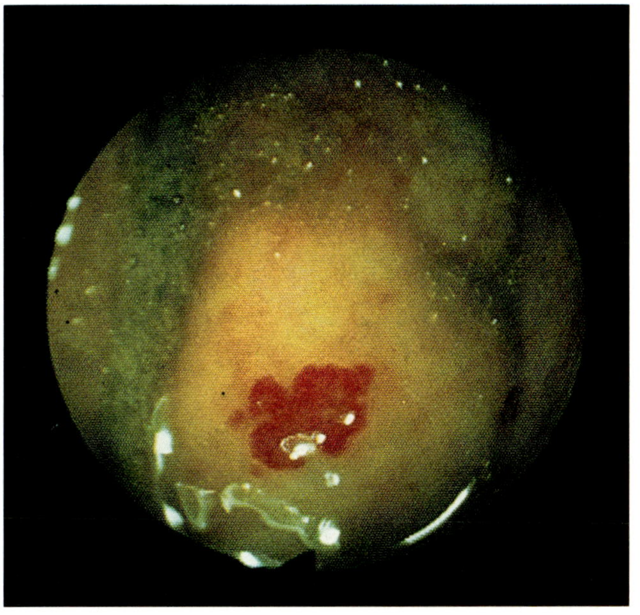

Plate 40. Cecal angiodysplasia.

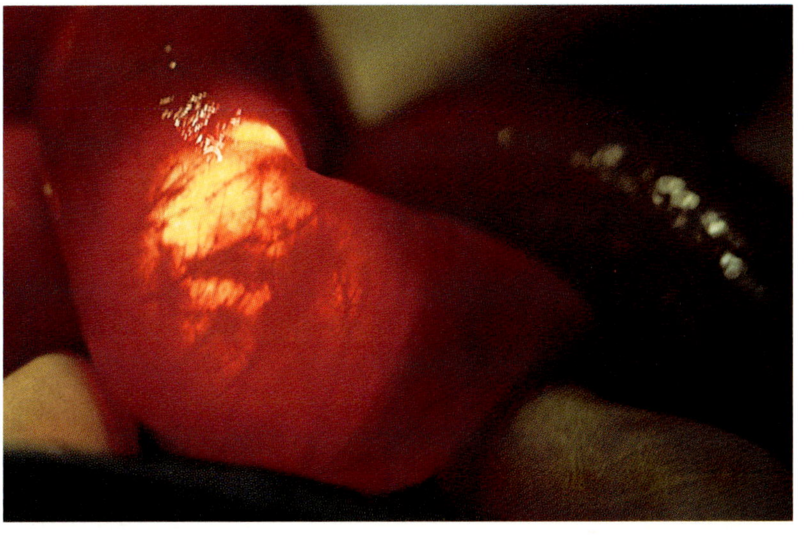

Plate 41. Jejunal angiodysplasia. Small bowel lesion identified at the time of laparotomy. The endoscopic light shines through from within the lumen of the bowel to highlight the lesion. Later, endoscopic laser therapy was utilized to coagulate the lesion.

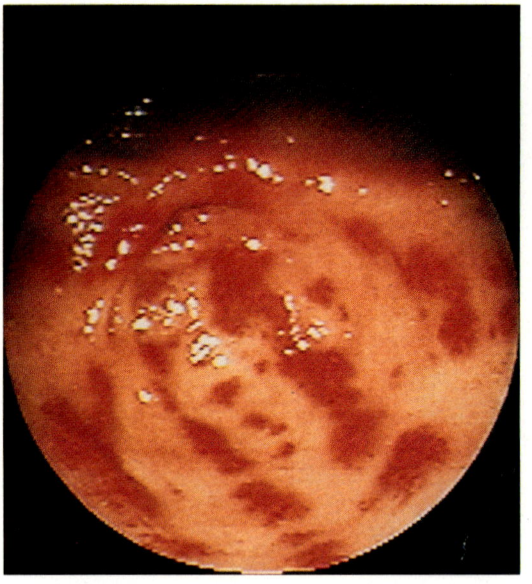

Plate 42. Typical endoscopic appearance of antral ectasia (watermelon stomach). Ectatic lesions form stripes.

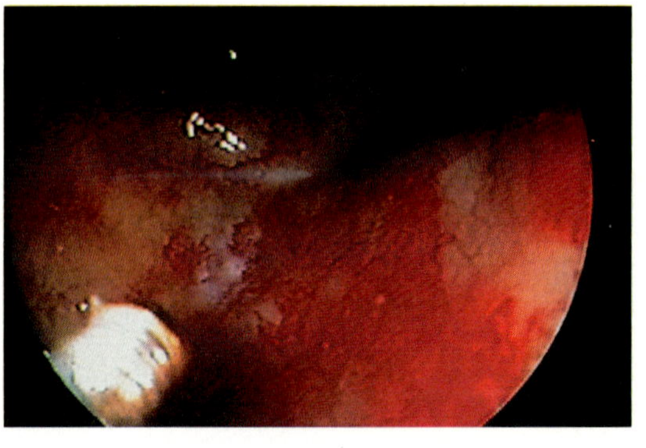

Plate 43. Confluent area of abnormal vessels in the rectum induced by radiation injury. The laser fiber is in place for treatment.

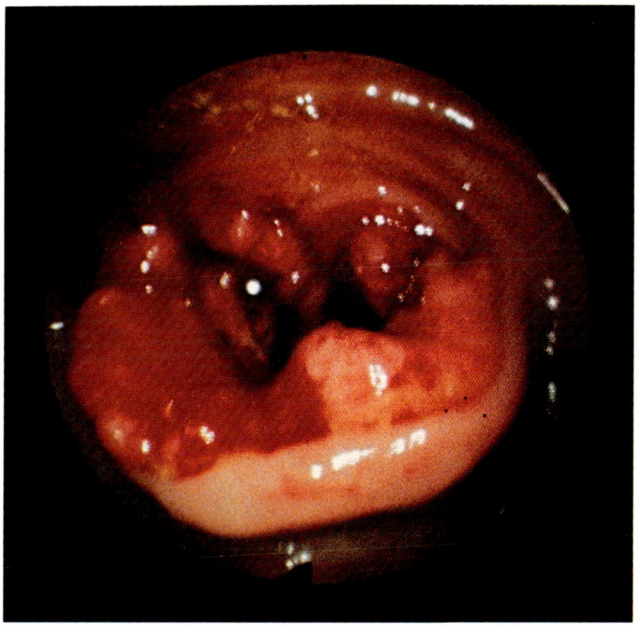

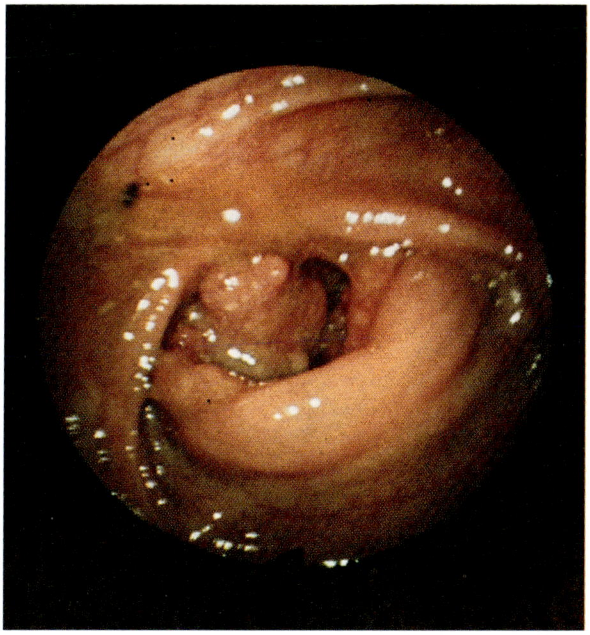

Plate 44 & 45. Carcinoma of the descending colon which caused slowly progressive blood loss. Before laser; after therapy.

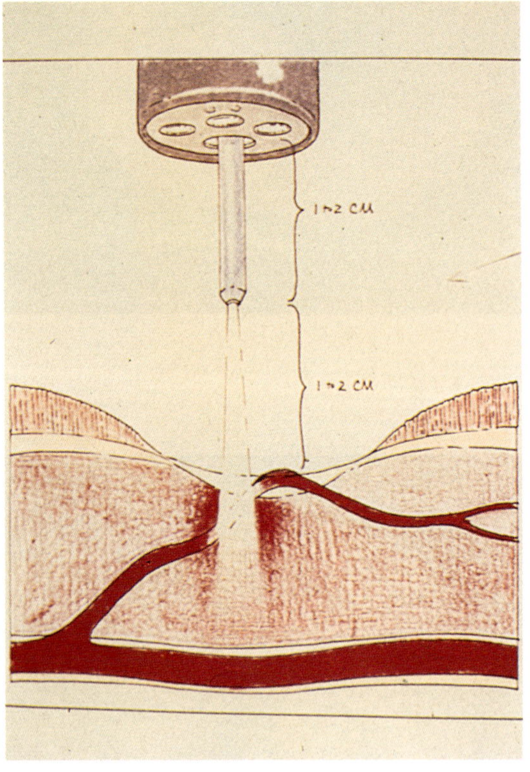

Plate 46. Schematic of a laser fiber extending from the tip of the endoscope 1 cm above the surface aimed to treat a vessel in an ulcer bed. (From Fleischer D: Endoscopic therapy of GI neoplasms, in Waye J, Geenan J, Fleischer D (eds): *Techniques in Therapeutic Endoscopy*. Philadelphia and New York, Sanders/Gower Publishing Co, 1987. Used with permission.)

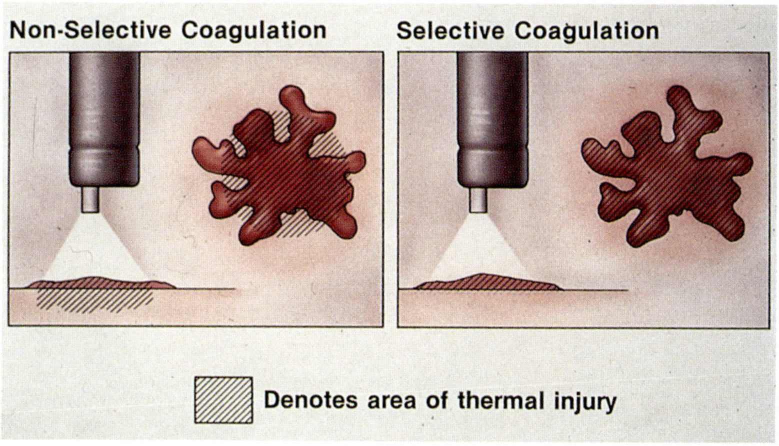

Plate 47. Nonselective absorption injures the vessel due to thermal energy and may cause injury to adjacent tissue. With selective absorption, the vessel is coagulated without injury to surrounding tissue.

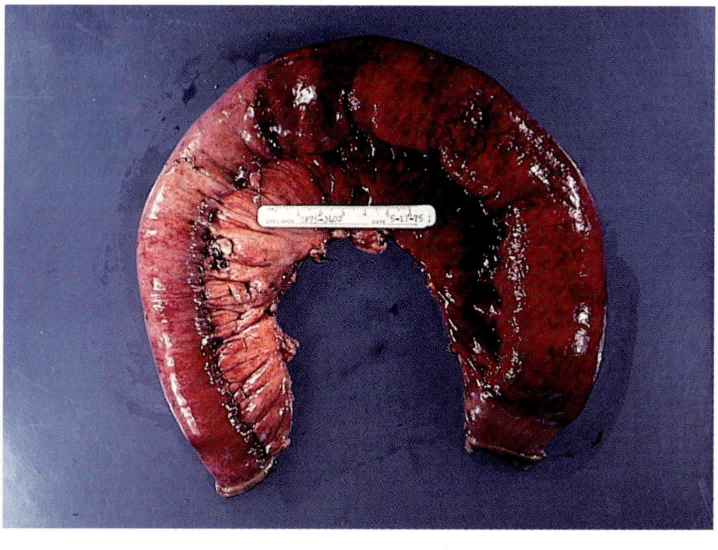

Plate 48. Intramural hematoma of the jejunum causing gastrointestinal bleeding in a patient who was taking anticoagulants.

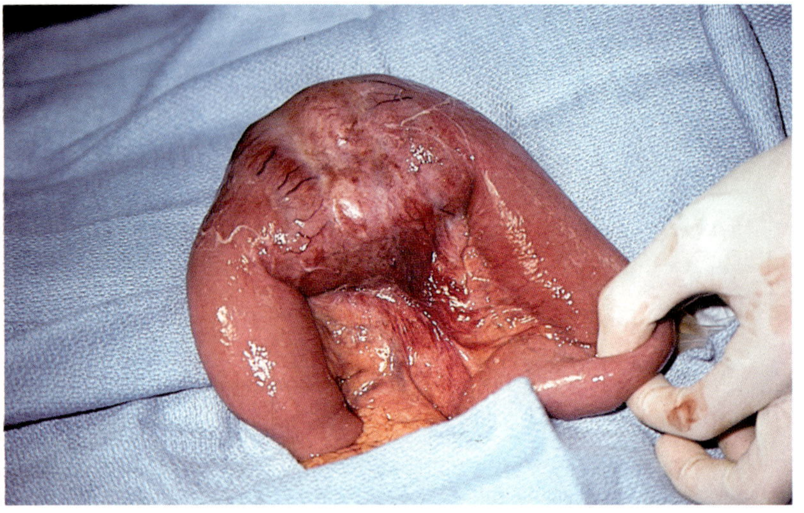

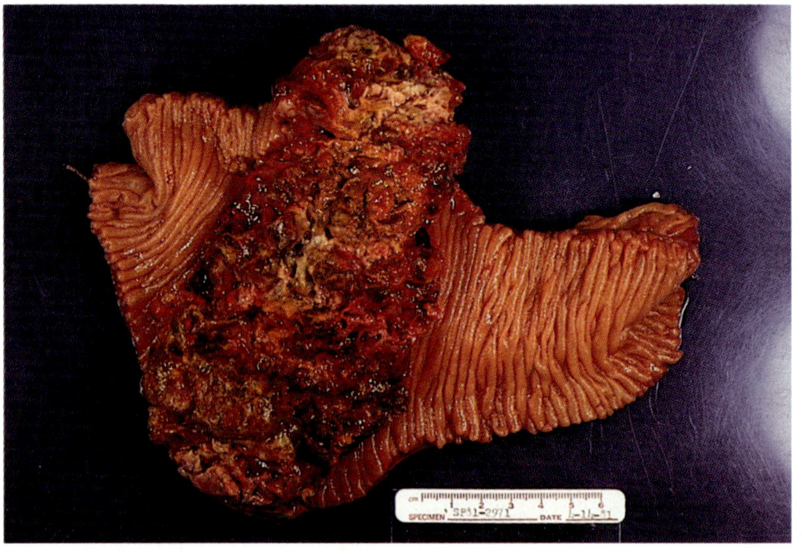

Plates 49 & 50. Adenocarcinoma of the lung metastatic to the ileum caused chronic gastrointestinal bleeding. Appearance at operation. Opened specimen.

23

ENDOSCOPIC INJECTION THERAPY

Choichi Sugawa, M.D.
Bernard M. Schuman, M.D.

INTRODUCTION

Several endoscopic techniques have been developed to control active upper gastrointestinal tract bleeding.[1-4] Injection sclerotherapy has been shown to be relatively safe and effective in the control of esophageal varices.[4] For nonvariceal bleeding lesions, thermal devices such as heater probes,[5] bipolar circumactive probes (BICAP),[6] and lasers[7] have been used. Recently, injection therapy has been expanded to treat nonvariceal gastrointestinal hemorrhage.[8,9] Injection therapy is a simple, inexpensive, and readily available means of treating active bleeding from the gastrointestinal tract. This method has been applied in Japan and Europe and is rapidly gaining popularity in the United States.[10-12] Sclerosants or vasoconstrictors have been used, alone or in combination. Effective initial hemostasis has been achieved in about 90% of patients in over 800 cases reported in the literature. No deaths from the procedure have been reported. In this chapter, we review the indications, techniques, various sclerosing agents, results, and complications of injection therapy.

INDICATIONS

The indication for endoscopic injection hemostasis is active bleeding from accessible lesions, including peptic ulcers, acute gastric mucosal lesions, esophagitis, Mallory-Weiss tears, and arteriovenous malformations (AVMs).[4,9,10] Nonbleeding, so-called visible vessels also warrant injection hemostasis. Prophylactic therapy of AVMs is also indicated in patients with multiple lesions.

TECHNIQUE

Endoscopic hemostasis should be attempted only when the precise bleeding site is visible, when hemostatic devices can be placed accurately at the bleeding area, and when hemorrhage is not torrential.[4] The technique and volume of injection therapy for bleeding lesions varies, depending on the type of sclerosing agent. A plastic sclerotherapy catheter, or a metal injector with a retractable 3-, 4-, or 5-mm 23- to 25-gauge needle, is used. Sclerosant is injected at three or four sites around an exposed bleeding vessel about 1 to 3 mm from the vessel. The volume of sclerosant should be minimized in order to avoid extending tissue damage, and differs with the type of sclerosing agent.

Most bleeding from peptic ulcers occurs from a single artery just below the ulcer base.[13,14] The visible vessel seen endoscopically on the ulcer base is actually a sentinel clot from a side hole in the underlying artery.[15,16] It is important to understand the pathological anatomy of a sentinel clot. Endoscopic hemostasis should aim at the underlying artery and not the overlying sentinel clot.[17] Acute gastric mucosal lesions, esophagitis, and Mallory-Weiss tears rarely bleed persistently, but when massive bleeding occurs, it is usually related to arterial bleeding or a sentinel clot. AVMs are located in the mucosa and submucosa; endoscopic injection should be aimed at the submucosal level at the same time, avoiding full-thickness injury.

SCLEROSING AGENTS AND MECHANISM OF ACTION

Hypertonic Saline-Epinephrine Solution

Saline (3.6%, 3 ml) and epinephrine (1:20,000) solution is injected in three or four sites at the base of a bleeding vessel,[18] with a total dose of 9 to 12 ml. For bleeding lesions with extensive fibrosis, 1 ml of saline (7.2%) and epinephrine solution is similarly injected, with a total dose of 3 to 4 ml. Repeat prophylactic injections are made at the site of any visible vessel 24 to 48 hours after initial hemostasis.[18] The mechanism of hemostasis with hypertonic saline and epinephrine solution is ascribed primarily to the vasoconstrictive action of epinephrine and secondarily to the physicochemical properties of the hypertonic sodium chloride solution.[18,19] In addition to allowing prolonged action of epinephrine, a hypertonic sodium chloride solution has been shown to cause such alterations as tissue swelling, fibrinoid degeneration of the vascular wall, and consequent thrombosis in the vascular lumen.

Epinephrine Alone (1:10,000) or Diluted (1:10,000) with Normal Saline

This solution is made by mixing epinephrine (1:1,000, 1 ml) with normal saline (0.9%, 9 ml). Between 1 and 3 ml of epinephrine (1:10,000) is injected into multiple sites around the bleeding vessel, as well as into the bleeding point itself. The total volume ranges from 6 to 12 ml, with the larger volume used to stop spurting vessels. Repeat prophylactic injections are also made at any visible vessel 24 or 48 hours after initial hemostasis. The hemostatic mechanism for epinephrine (1:10,000) consists of vasoconstriction of the submucosal arterioles of the stomach and creates a local tamponade effect on the bleeding vessel.[19] Epinephrine also causes platelet aggregation and may promote thrombus formation within the bleeding vessel. All of these factors are likely to contribute to definitive hemostasis.

Absolute Ethanol

Dehydrated ethanol (98%, Abbott Laboratories) is injected, using a 1-ml disposable plastic tuberculin syringe, with a total dose of 0.6 to 1.0 ml.[11,20] The ethanol is injected slowly, in amounts of 0.1 to 0.2 ml per injection, at three or four sites surrounding the bleeding vessel and 1 or 2 mm from the vessel. Because of its stiff shaft, the Olympus injector NM1-K is best suited for ethanol injection therapy.

The mechanism of hemostasis obtained by absolute ethanol injection is dehydration and fixation of the exposed blood vessel wall, as well as the surrounding tissue.[21] The resulting local vasoconstriction, vascular wall degeneration, and endothelial cell destruction lead to local thrombosis.

Epinephrine Followed by BICAP, Neodynium: Yttrium Argon Garnet (Nd:YAG) Laser, Monopolar Electrocoagulation, or Polidocanol

Epinephrine (1:10,000, 5 to 12 ml) is injected submucosally around the blood vessel to obtain initial hemostasis or to decelerate bleeding by volume compression and vasoconstriction. To achieve definitive hemostasis by obliterating the vessel, BICAP, Nd:YAG laser,[22] monopolar electrocoagulation,[23] or polidocanol[24] (1%, 5 ml) is applied into the same area.

Thrombin in Normal Saline

Thrombin (100 IU) in normal saline (0.9%, 3 cc) is injected into and around the bleeding vessel until bleeding stops.[25] This usually requires 10 to 15 ml of the solution. Initial hemostasis is accomplished by volume compression. Additionally, thrombin injection enhances solid fibrin network formation due to the accelerated conversion of fibrinogen to fibrin.

Other Sclerosing Agents

Sodium morrhuate (5%) is used mainly for the treatment of esophageal varices. Adams[26] used a mixture of sodium morrhuate (5%, 3 ml), thrombin (2 ml) and dextrose (50%) to sclerose and thrombose the bleeding vessel. For sclerotherapy of esophageal varices, one of us (C.S.) has been using a thrombosclerosant mixture (a total of 18 ml) consisting of sodium tetradecyl sulfate (1%, 12 ml), thrombin (1,000 units/ml 3 ml) and cephazolin (1 g in 3 ml). Two milliliters of this cocktail, using canine gastric serosal blood vessel models, has been found effective.[19] However, long term historical effects of this cocktail have not been studied.

RESULTS

Hypertonic Saline-Epinephrine Solution

In 1985, Hirao et al.[18] of Japan published results of hypertonic saline and epinephrine injection. They treated 158 patients (72% had gastric ulcers and 9.5% had duodenal ulcers), achieving permanent hemostasis in 93%. Only 1 out of 128 patients who received prophylactic repeat injections required emergency surgery. No complications were reported.

Epinephrine Alone (1 : 10,000) or Diluted (1 : 10,000) with Normal Saline

In 1987 Leung and Chung,[27] from Hong Kong, treated 37 patients with actively bleeding ulcers (27 duodenal and 10 gastric) by injecting 0.5 ml of 1 : 10,000 epinephrine alone into multiple sites around the bleeding vessels and into the bleeding point itself. The total volume used ranged from 1.5 to 10 ml (mean, 4.1 ml), with the larger volume required to stop spurting vessels. All patients had initial hemostasis, but five patients rebled four hours to four days later; one patient stopped bleeding spontaneously; one patient's bleeding was controlled by repeat epinephrine injection; and three patients underwent emergency surgery. There was no morbidity or mortality due to the local or systemic effects of epinephrine.

Chung et al.[28,29] also reported their results of a randomized controlled study of epinephrine injection for actively bleeding ulcers. Sixty-eight patients with active bleeding (spurting or oozing) from ulcers were divided into two groups. The *injection group* consisted of 34 patients, of whom 9 were bleeding from a spurter. In the *control group* of 34 patients, 10 were bleeding from a spurter. Endoscopy was performed 24 hours later, and repeat injection was carried out for patients in the *injection group* if active bleeding was again seen. All patients receiving injection therapy had initial hemostasis. The mean amount of blood transfusions was 3.8 units in the *injection group* and 5.9 units in the *control group* ($p < 0.05$). Emergency surgery was necessary in 5 patients (15%) in the *injection group* and in 14 patients in the *control group* ($p < 0.02$). The authors concluded that endoscopic epinephrine injection was effective in stopping bleeding and decreased the transfusion requirement, as well as the need for emergency surgery.

Steele et al.,[30] from England, reported that endoscopic injections of 1 : 10,000 epinephrine alone controlled initial arterial bleeding from ulcers in 15 patients; rebleeding in 3 patients was also controlled by repeat elective injection 24 hours later.

Absolute Ethanol

Asaki and coworkers, in Japan, have the largest reported clinical experience. In a multicenter study[31] they treated 332 patients, of whom 90% had peptic ulcers and 52% had exposed blood vessels. Initial hemostasis was obtained in 330 patients (99%), rebleeding occurred in 20 (6%), and 3 patients developed perforation, which was not considered to be due directly to ethanol injection.

At Wayne State University, we treated 75 patients with upper gastrointestinal bleeding, including 53 patients with peptic ulcer. Ethanol injection was successful in 73 patients. Of 56 lesions actively bleeding at the time of endoscopic treatment, 52 were initially controlled. Rebleeding occurred in three of these patients. Final hemostasis was obtained in 50 of 56 actively bleeding lesions (89%).

Pascu and coworkers,[32] from Romania, in a randomized prospective study, treated 145 patients who had nonvariceal upper gastrointestinal hemorrhage with either active bleeding (Forrest I) or stigmata of recent hemorrhage (Forrest II). These patients were divided into two comparable groups according to the day of the week on which emergency endoscopy was performed: Group A (78 patients), in which conventional treatment was applied; and Group B, in which endoscopic hemostasis with absolute alcohol was performed. Absolute alcohol injection achieved hemostasis in all the cases of active hemorrhage and prevented recurrence in 24 out of 25 cases with a clot or visible vessels. Emergency surgery was not necessary in any of the patients in Group B. The mortality rate was significantly lower in Group B than in Group A (10 deaths in Group A, 2 in Group B; $p < 0.05$).

Permanent hemostasis with the use of absolute ethanol injection reportedly has a success rate of about 90%.[31,33,34]

Epinephrine followed by BICAP, Nd:YAG Laser, Electrohydrocoagulation, or Polidocanol

Rutgeerts et al.,[22] from Belgium, carried out a randomized trial, comparing the efficacy of BICAP and YAG laser in the treatment of bleeding peptic ulcers. All 50 bleeding lesions in each group were injected with 4 to 8 ml of epinephrine (1:10,000) before BICAP or laser application. Definitive hemostasis occurred in 72% after one treatment in both the BICAP and laser groups. After two sessions, the cumulative success rate was 86% in the BICAP group and 88% in the laser group. One perforation occurred in each treatment (2%). The authors concluded that both treatments are highly and equally effective in the treatment of severe bleeding from peptic ulcers.

Boix et al.,[23] from Spain, combined injection of epinephrine with electrohydrocoagulation (simultaneous distilled water irrigation and monopolar coagulation), followed by injection of polidocanol (1%). They controlled 26 of 28 (92.8%) actively bleeding ulcers initially, and 23 of 28 (82.1%) permanently in an uncontrolled study. No complications were reported.

There are many reports from Europe on injection therapy, using epinephrine (1:10,000) followed by polidocanol (1%). Soehendra and colleagues[24] treated 114 bleeding lesions, including 60 peptic ulcers, 50 described as pulsating and 64 as oozing, with good results. They achieved permanent hemostasis in 42 (84%) of the pulsating lesions and in 59 (92%) of the oozing lesions without complications. Panes et al.,[35] from Spain, reported the results of a controlled trial of 113 patients. Fifty-five patients with actively bleeding peptic ulcers were treated with injection of epinephrine, polidocanol, and an H_2 blocker. Fifty-eight patients were treated with only an H_2 blocker as a control. There were no complications. Major recurrent hemorrhage during the hospital stay occurred in three injected patients (5.5%) and 25 control patients (43.1%) ($p < 0.001$). Requirements of emergency surgery (5% in the treated group, 34% in the control group), transfusion requirements, and the length of the hospital stay were significantly reduced in the injection group. However, mortality was not significantly reduced. Another controlled study by Balanzo et al.,[36] from Spain, showed a reduction in the rebleeding rate and in transfusion requirements in 36 patients with bleeding ulcers who were treated with local injection of epinephrine-polidocanol, compared with 36 patients without injection therapy. Kortan et al.,[37] in Canada, using the same combination, treated 56 massively bleeding lesions. They obtained hemostasis in 90% of the pulsating lesions and in 100% of the oozing lesions, with no major morbidity.

Thrombin in Normal Saline

Fuchs and colleagues,[25] from Germany, switched from polidocanol to thrombin because polidocanol caused injection-related ulcers in 8%, and partial necrosis of the gastric wall in 1% of 200 patients treated with polidocanol. They treated another group of 47 patients who had upper gastrointestinal bleeding with thrombin in normal saline. Thirty-one of 47 lesions (66%) were ulcers of the stomach, and 17 (14%) were duodenal ulcers. Spurting bleeders were successfully treated in 7 out of 10 cases (70%). Ten of 13 oozing lesions (85%) were permanently controlled. The rate of initial hemostasis in the overall group of acute hemorrhage was 96%. The injection method proved ultimately successful in 75% of the cases. No complications were observed.

Other Sclerosing Agents

Adams,[26] from the United States, reported successful hemostasis of bleeding peptic ulcers in eight patients following endoscopic injection of a mixture of sodium morrhuate (5%, 3 ml), thrombin (2 ml), and 50% dextrose (50%, 5 ml). There were no complications.

Comparison of Different Methods

Chen and associates,[38] from Taiwan, compared the hemostatic effects of hypertonic saline-epinephrine (HS-E) solution and pure ethanol (PE) in 67 patients with nonvariceal gastrointestinal bleeding. Thirty-three patients had HS-E and 34 patients had PE injection. The hemostatic effect was permanent in 29 cases (88%) but failed in 4 cases (12.1%). The hemostatic effect of PE was permanent in 31 cases (91%), temporary in 1 case (3%), and failed in 2 cases (5.9%). There were no complications. This study suggested that the hemostatic effect was more effective by PE injection in the group of patients with stigmata of recent hemorrhage, while HS-E injection showed better results in patients with active bleeding.

Lin et al.,[39] also from Taiwan, in a prospectively randomized trial, compared injection of ethanol to heater probe in 78 patients with peptic ulcer hemorrhage. The initial and ultimate success rates of the heater probe group were better than those of the ethanol group. The rebleeding rates for the heater probe and ethanol groups were similar. The heater probe controlled spurting bleeding in all 15 patients treated, whereas injection controlled only 5 of 12 patients. The authors concluded that the heater probe is the treatment of choice if the bleeding is a spurter or is located over the lesser curvature of the stomach or the superior wall of the duodenal bulb, since the lesions are easily accessible to the heater probe.

Chung et al.,[40] from Hong Kong, randomized 122 patients with actively bleeding ulcers to heater probe or epinephrine (1 : 10,000 up to 10 ml) injection therapy had found no difference in the number of emergency operations, the transfusion requirements, mortality, or median hospital days. They concluded that heater probe and epinephrine injection are equally efficacious in controlling ulcer bleeding but that epinephrine injection may be technically easier to perform.

Woods et al.,[41] from the United States, prospectively compared BICAP and ethanol injection in 21 male patients. They concluded that both types of therapy are equivalent endoscopic hemostatic modalities, and both are less successful in patients with large ulcers (>20 mm) or with significant orthostatic hypotension on admission.

Laine[42] randomized patients with severe ulcer bleeding into two groups: those with ethanol injection and those with BICAP therapy. Ethanol injection and BICAP therapy appeared equally effective and safe in 60 randomized patients who had ulcers with active bleeding ($N = 26$) or nonbleeding visible vessels ($N = 34$).

Experimental Studies

Using a canine gastric and colonic blood vessel model, the Detroit group[43] found that (1) ethanol injection had no effect on bleeding from larger gastric vessels unless the injection was made 24 hours and 48 hours prior to vessel transection; (2) ethanol injection was effective in hemostasis immediately after injection of the small vessels (colonic group), and 24 hours and 48 hours after injection of the large vessels (gastric group); (3) gastric submucosal injection led to ulcers which extended into the muscle layer at one week and were completely healed by three weeks, with no perforation or bleeding. These data support the potential efficacy of therapeutic ethanol injection for the control of small-vessel bleeding, as well as the potential prophylactic value against rebleeding from larger vessels. Our recent experimental study[19] showed that injection of hypertonic saline-epinephrine or epinephrine alone is more effective than injection of absolute ethanol in achieving hemostasis of active bleeding from canine gastric serosal vessels. This is probably due to the more significant local tamponade effect on the bleeding vessel by the injection of hypertonic saline-epinephrine or epinephrine alone. It was also found that injection therapy in general is not as effective as the thermal method in controlling active severe bleeding from canine gastric serosal vessels.[44]

Randall et al.,[45] from the United States, using canine gut arteries, predicted that absolute ethanol and TES (a mixture with a final concentration of 1% tetradecyl sulfate, 32% ethanol, and 0.3% normal saline) are more effective in arterial coagulation but cause more severe tissue injury than epinephrine (1:10,000) or saline (7.6% 3.6%, and normal). Rutgeerts et al.,[46] using the Protell ulcer maker in dogs, concluded that the acute hemostasis effect of injection therapy depends largely on the injected volume. Thrombosis of vessels after alcohol or ethoxysclerol injection may contribute to long-term hemostasis. They also concluded that injection therapy, using epinephrine, is not as effective as the thermal method to control spurting bleeding.

COMPLICATIONS

Asaki et al.[20] originally reported perforations with ethanol injection in 1 of 84 patients. In a multicenter study using ethanol, they reported three perforations out of 332 patients. Fuchs and associates[25] reported two perforations (1%) with polidocanol (1%) injection. DiFelice[47] reported that 1 out of 40 patients had surgery 24 hours after injection of epinephrine-polidocanol for a large acute gastric ulcer in the process of perforation and died of pulmonary embolism four days later. Rutgeerts et al.[22] treated 100 patients with bleeding ulcers by epinephrine injection, followed by either BICAP or Nd:YAG laser. One perforation occurred in each treatment group of 50 patients (2%).

Treatment-induced bleeding has been reported to be a major problem with laser therapy.[48] Reactivation of bleeding can also occur by heater probe[17] or BICAP. Reactivation of bleeding is very rare in injection therapy. One case of treatment-induced bleeding has been reported so far. Panes et al.[35] reported that 1 out of 18 patients with nonbleeding visible vessels had uncontrolled hemorrhage following injection with epinephrine and polidocanol.

SUMMARY

Injection therapy for the control of nonvariceal gastroduodenal bleeding is effective in stopping active bleeding. Endoscopists in the United States find injection therapy appealing because needles and medications are inexpensive, are readily available, and can be brought to the bedside easily. This therapy can be done at the time of diagnostic endoscopy and can be repeated if bleeding recurs. Injection therapy is relatively easy to perform, and reported complications are few. Endoscopic injection therapy can be invaluable as definitive therapy for patients unable to tolerate an operative procedure or as a temporizing measure to control active bleeding, so that a definitive operative procedure may be performed electively with less morbidity and mortality.[49,50] Several controlled studies showed that injection therapy led to fewer transfusions, less need for surgery, a shorter hospital stay, and less cost. Nishioka and Richter[51] reported that significant savings (up to $2,500 per patient) could be achieved by laser hemostasis of peptic ulcers with visible vessels. Injection therapy is the most cost-effective hemostatic modality, compared with Nd:YAG laser, heater probe, and BICAP. However, peptic ulcer disease is usually recurrent, and the cost analysis for the treatment of this disease cannot be measured by one single admission.

Hemostatic effects appear to be better with hypertonic saline-epinephrine or epinephrine alone in patients who are actively bleeding.[19,38] Absolute ethanol is more effective in patients with stigmata of recent hemorrhage[38,43] (including nonbleeding visible vessels or slow hemorrhage). Tissue damage is significant with absolute ethanol[43] and 1% polidocanol.[25] Precise injection of a small amount of ethanol around the exposed blood vessel is sometimes technically difficult. Twelve milliliters of epinephrine (1 : 10,000) does not seem to cause tissue damage. In cases of active bleeding, we are currently using epinephrine, followed by heater probe or BICAP. Prophylactic injection, after initial hemostasis or repeat treatment for rebleeding, is effective and improves the ultimate results of endoscopic therapy.[18,52] Additional randomized clinical trials of injection therapy, heater probe, and BICAP with controls are needed to assess the true effectiveness and safety of these modalities.

REFERENCES

1. Castell DO, Blankenbaker RG, Bozymski EM, et al: Consensus statement on therapeutic endoscopy and bleeding ulcers. *Gastrointest Endosc* 36:S62–S65, 1990.

2. Pitcher JL: Therapeutic endoscopy and bleeding ulcers: Historical overview. *Gastrointest Endosc* 36:S2–S7, 1990.
3. Sugawa C, Lucas C: Endoscopic control of upper gastrointestinal tract bleeding, in Dent TL (ed): *Surgical Endoscopy*. Chicago, Year Book Medical Publishers, 1985, p. 23.
4. Sugawa C: Endoscopic diagnosis and treatment of upper gastrointestinal bleeding. *Surg Clin North Am* 69:1167–1183, 1989.
5. Jensen DM: Heat probe for hemostasis of bleeding peptic ulcers: Techniques and results of randomized controlled trials. *Gastrointest Endosc* 36:S42–S49, 1990.
6. Laine L: Bipolar/multipolar electrocoagulation. *Gastrointest Endosc* 36:S38–S41, 1990.
7. Swain CP: Nd:YAG laser: The pro approach. *Gastrointest Endosc* 36:S30–S31, 1990.
8. Schuman BM: Endoscopic injection therapy for nonvariceal upper gastrointestinal hemorrhage: Is it too good to be true? *Gastrointest Endosc* 33:121–122, 1987.
9. Sugawa C: Injection therapy for the control of bleeding. *Gastrointest Endosc* 36:S50–S52, 1990.
10. Sanowski RA, Waring JP: Editorial: Endoscopic injection therapy for nonvariceal bleeding lesions of the upper gastrointestinal tract. *J Clin Gastroenterol* 11:247–252, 1989.
11. Sugawa C, Fujita Y, Ikeda T, et al: Endoscopic hemostasis of bleeding of the upper gastrointestinal tract by local injection of ninety-eight per cent dehydrated ethanol. *Surg Gynecol Obstet* 162:159–163, 1986.
12. Sugawa C, Bradley SJ: Endoscopic sclerosis of nonvariceal gastroduodenal hemorrhage. *Probl Gen Surg* 7:43–48, 1990.
13. Swain CP, Storey DW, Brown SG, et al: Nature of the bleeding vessel in recurrently bleeding gastric ulcers. *Gastroenterology* 90:595–608, 1986.
14. Swain CP: Pathophysiology of bleeding lesions. *Gastrointest Endosc* 36:S21–S22, 1990.
15. Johnston JH: The sentinel clot/visible vessel revisited. *Gastrointest Endosc* 32:238–239, 1986.
16. Johnston JH: Endoscopic hemostasis for bleeding peptic ulcers. *Gastrointest Endosc* 33:260–261, 1987.
17. Johnston JH: Endoscopic thermal treatment of upper gastrointestinal bleeding. Overview and guidelines. *Endosc Rev* 2:2–20, 1985.
18. Hirao M, Kobayashi T, Masuda K, et al: Endoscopic local injection of hypertonic saline-epinephrine solution to arrest hemorrhage from the upper gastrointestinal tract. *Gastrointest Endosc* 31:313–317, 1985.
19. Whittle T, Sugawa C, Lucas C, et al: Effect of hemostatic agents in canine gastric serosal blood vessels. *Gastrointest Endosc* 37:305–309, 1991.
20. Asaki S, Nishimura T, Satoh A, et al: Endoscopic hemostasis of gastrointestinal hemorrhage by local application of absolute ethanol: A clinical study. *Tohoku J Exp Med* 141:373–383, 1983.
21. Asaki S, Nishimura T, Satoh A, et al: Endoscopic control of gastrointestinal hemorrhage by local injection of absolute control: A basic assessment of the procedure. *Tohoku J Exp Med* 140:339–352, 1983.
22. Rutgeerts P, Vantrappen G, Van Hootegem PV, et al: Neodynium-YAG laser photocoagulation versus multipolar electrocoagulation for the treatment of severely bleeding ulcers: A randomized comparison. *Gastrointest Endosc* 33:199–202, 1987.
23. Boix J, Planas R, Humbert P, et al: Endoscopic hemostasis by injection therapy and electrohydrocoagulation in high risk patients with active duodenal bleeding ulcer. *Endoscopy* 6:225–227, 1987.
24. Soehendra N, Grimm H, Kempeneers I: Sclerosing therapy in gastrointestinal hemorrhage. *Acta Endosc* 16:47–53, 1986.

25. Fuchs KH, Wintz HJ, Schaube H, et al: Initial experience with thrombin as injection agent for bleeding gastroduodenal lesions. *Endoscopy* 18:146–148, 1986.
26. Adams W: Endoscopic sclerosis of bleeding duodenal and antral ulcers. *Gastrointest Endosc* 30:A149, 1984.
27. Leung JW, Chung SC: Endoscopic injection of adrenalin in bleeding peptic ulcers. *Gastrointest Endosc* 33:73–75, 1987.
28. Chung SCS, Leung JWC, Steele RJC, et al: Epinephrine injection for actively bleeding ulcers: A randomized controlled study. *Gastrointest Endosc* 33:146, 1987.
29. Chung SCS, Leung JWC, Steele RJL, et al: Endoscopic injection of adrenaline for actively bleeding ulcers: A randomized controlled study. *Br Med J* 296:1631–1633, 1988.
30. Steele RJC, Logie JRC, Munro A, et al: Endoscopic haemostasis in non-variceal upper gastrointestinal haemorrhage using adrenaline injection. *J R Coll Surg Edinb* 34:133–135, 1989.
31. Asaki S: Endoscopic hemostasis by local absolute ethanol injection for upper gastrointestinal tract bleeding—a multicenter study, in Okabe H, Honda T, Ohshiba S (eds): *Endoscopic Surgery*. New York, Elsevier, 1984, p 105.
32. Pascu O, Draghici A, Acalovchi B: The effect of endoscopic hemostasis with alcohol on the mortality rate of nonvariceal upper gastrointestinal hemorrhage. A randomized prospective study. *Endoscopy* 21:53–55, 1989.
33. Hajiro K: Japanese experience with local injection and hemoclips. Symposium on endoscopy in upper GI bleeding. *The XIIth International Gastroenterology Congress—The Vth European Gastrointestinal Endoscopy Congress*. Lisbon, September 1984.
34. Miller FR, Stark B, Greenberg RE: Use of absolute alcohol injection for control of upper GI bleeding. *Gastrointest Endosc* 35:A155, 1989.
35. Panes J, Forne M, Marco C, et al: Controlled trial of endoscopic sclerosis in bleeding peptic ulcers. *Lancet* 2:1292–1294, 1987.
36. Balanzo J, Sainz S, Such JC, et al: Endoscopic hemostasis by local injection of epinephrine and polidocanol in bleeding ulcer. A prospective randomized trial. *Endoscopy* 20:289–291, 1988.
37. Kortan P, Haber G, Maron N: Endoscopic injection therapy for non-variceal bleeding lesions of the upper gastrointestinal tract. *Gastrointest Endosc* 32:A145, 1986.
38. Chen PC, Wu CS, Liaw YF: Hemostatic effect of endoscopic local infection with hypertonic saline-epinephrine solution and pure ethanol for digestive tract bleeding. *Gastrointest Endosc* 32:319–323, 1986.
39. Lin HJ, Tsai YT, Lee SD, et al: A prospective randomized trial of heat probe thermocoagulation versus pure alcohol injection in non-variceal peptic ulcer hemorrhage. *Am J Gastroenterol* 83:283–286, 1988.
40. Chung SCS, Leung JWC, Sung JY, et al: Heat probe or epinephrine injection for actively bleeding ulcers: A randomized comparison. *Gastrointest Endosc* 35:A152, 1989.
41. Woods A, Sanowski RA, Waring JP, et al: Endoscopic therapy for gastric and duodenal ulcer bleeding: A comparison of BICAP coagulation versus ethanol sclerotherapy. *Gastrointest Endosc* 34:A209, 1988.
42. Laine L: Multipolar electrocoagulation versus injection therapy in the treatment of bleeding peptic ulcers. A prospective, randomized trial. *Gastroenterology* 99:1303–1306, 1990.
43. Sugawa C, Fujita Y, Lucas C, et al: Hemostatic effect of local intramural injection of dehydrated ethanol in the canine gastrointestinal tract. *Gastrointest Endosc* 35:28–32, 1989.
44. Sugawa C, Hasuyama H: Comparison of endoscopic electro-surgical hemostasis in canine gastric serosal vessels. *Gastrointest Endosc* 31:A169, 1985.
45. Randall GM, Jensen DM, Hirabayashi K, et al: Controlled trial of sclerosing agents for hemostasis of canine gut arteries. *Gastroenterology* 96:1274–1281, 1989.

46. Rutgeerts P, Geboes K, Vantrappen G: Experimental studies of injection therapy for severe nonvariceal bleeding in dogs. *Gastroenterology* 97:610–621, 1989.
47. DiFelice G: Endoscopic injection treatment in patients with shock and gastrointestinal bleeding or stigmata of recent hemorrhage. *Endoscopy* 19:185–189, 1987.
48. Krejs GJ, Little KH, Westergaard H, et al: Laser photocoagulation for the treatment of acute peptic ulcer bleeding. *N Engl J Med* 316:1618–1621, 1987.
49. Pimpel W, Boeckl O, Heinerman M, et al: Emergency endoscopy: A basis for therapeutic decisions in the treatment of severe gastroduodenal bleeding. *World J Surg* 13:592–597, 1989.
50. Sugawa C, Steffes CP, Nakamura R, et al: Upper GI bleeding in an urban hospital. Etiology, recurrence, and prognosis. *Ann Surg* 212:521–527, 1990.
51. Nishioka NS, Richter JM: Endoscopic therapy of bleeding peptic ulcers: A cost-benefit analysis. *Gastrointest Endosc* 33:277–283, 1987.
52. Panes J, Viver J: Endoscopic sclerosis in bleeding ulcers. Can results be improved? *Endoscopy* 21:196, 1989.

24

TOPICAL THERAPY

Stephen E. Silvis, M.D.

PREFACE

There is no topical therapy for gastrointestinal bleeding which is in widespread use throughout the world. Only the therapy with fibrinolytic inhibitory agents is supported by positive controlled studies. This chapter will review the status of the topical therapies currently being evaluated.

INTRODUCTION

With modern fiberoptic endoscopy, excellent visualization of the entire gastrointestinal tract is available. The vast expanse of small intestinal mucosa remains difficult to examine. Fortunately, most gastrointestinal bleeding occurs above the ligament of Treitz or below the ileoceal valve; these areas can be readily examined in superb detail.

Endoscopic therapy for upper gastrointestinal bleeding discussed in other chapters has been shown to have a significantly positive effect when appropriate groups of patients are treated by heater probe, electrocoagulation, laser coagulation, or injection therapy. However, all of these methods fall significantly short of being an ideal endoscopic therapy for gastrointestinal bleeding. For example, none of these methods can be utilized for diffuse bleeding, and all of them produce additional tissue destruction.

Topical therapy has an unfulfilled promise of being a nearly ideal therapy. If proven effective, endoscopic administration of topical agents to control gastrointestinal bleeding has a number of advantages. These agents produce little or no tissue damage at the bleeding site. They can be applied to large areas of the gastrointestinal tract, thus being applicable for diffuse as well as focal lesions. Administration would not necessarily require precise visualization of the bleeding point or direct contact with that specific area. The topical materials are usually inexpensive, and the portable delivery systems can be used through standard endoscopic instruments. Human and animal data on evaluated topical therapy are limited, and few clinical control trials have been performed. Agents that have been studied include compounds which depress the fibrinolytic system, cyanoacrylate tissue glues, microcrystalline collagen hemostat (MCH, Avitene), and various clotting factors. Gastric cooling, gastric freezing, and topical application of vasoconstricting agents have been tried but were found ineffective. These modalities are no longer being studied, and they will not be reviewed in this chapter.

THE USE OF FIBRINOLYTIC INHIBITORY AGENTS

Controlled trials of tranexamic acid with either intravenous or oral therapy in acute upper gastrointestinal bleeding have been performed. Endoscopic application of these agents has not been made because the duration of action of the compound is so short, necessitating frequent endoscopic intubation. In addition, adequate therapeutic levels can be obtained by oral use of the agent. Henry and O'Connell[1] reviewed six double-blind controlled studies of upper gastrointestinal bleeding that included 1,286 patients.[2-7] The tranexamic acid treatment was associated with a 20–30% reduction in the rate of rebleeding, a 30–40% reduction in the need for surgery, and a 40% reduction in mortality. Although tranexamic acid generally has low toxicity, there were 11 thrombotic events in the treated group compared to 4 in the placebo group. These differences were not significant, but the trend is a cause for concern. The authors caution about drawing conclusions from these six studies because each of them had a somewhat different design. The problem of publication bias, that is, the preferential publication of positive studies, remains a threat to all meta-analysis. This review reinforces the need for a large, well-controlled study of fibrinolytic inhibitory agents in the treatment of upper gastrointestinal bleeding.

CYANOACRYLATE TISSUE ADHESIVE IN THE TREATMENT OF UPPER GASTROINTESTINAL BLEEDING

Cyanoacrylate tissue adhesives are attractive as topical agents because they polymerize rapidly and form a dense, durable film over the treated lesions. Trifluoroisopropyl cyanoacrylate (MBR 4197, Flucrylate) applied topically has been studied in two animal experimental ulcers. Martin and Silvis[8] and Silvis[9] showed decreased bleeding from chronic canine ulcers, while Protell et al.[10] did not demonstrate control of bleeding in an acute ulcer model. In an open study, Martin et al.[11] and Silvis[9] treated 18 patients with topical MBR 4197. Of the 18, 4 were technical failures; however, treatment was effective in 12 of 14 patients in whom it was satisfactorily administered. This study prompted a control trial, reported by Peura et al.,[12] in which 52 patients (24 given MBR 4197 and 28 controls) were evaluated. Six of the 24 treated patients had continued bleeding or rebled and required surgery. Four of the 28 control patients continued bleeding, and 3 required surgery. Technical problems with the delivery system and premature polymerization caused failure of delivery in many instances. The currently available tissue glues for topical administration are certainly safe but are not being studied at present in the United States. Investigation of topically applied tissue adhesives has continued in China[13] with a compound that was identified as α-cyanoacrylate (V-1 Gel). The Chinese investigators are apparently using a propylene cyanoacrylate and are adding a stabilizing gel which controls the rate of polymerization. Preliminary studies in both dogs and patients reveal positive results, with no evidence of tissue damage. Control studies have not been performed.

Butyl cyanoacrylate (Histoacryl)[14-19] has been used in Europe to inject esophageal varices. It is generally mixed with Lipiodal in varying proportions to delay the rate of polymerization and to make the injection opaque. No controlled studies have been done. However, it appears to be useful in the obturation of very large varices, particularly bleeding gastric varices. The Lipiodal makes the injected polymer radiopaque, allowing it to be followed radiographically. In some patients the polymer has produced necrosis of the vein and the overlying mucosa. The polymer casts erode into the gastrointestinal tract, but they have not produced obstruction or bleeding when passed through the intestinal tract. There has been one reported case[20] of necrosis of the duodenum following injection of Histacryl into a bleeding duodenal ulcer. In that case, the patient also had an injection of polidocanol at the same time, so it is difficult to determine what produced the necrosis. Histacryl is not available for clinical use in the United States.

MICROCRYSTALLINE COLLAGEN HEMOSTAT (MCH, AVITENE)

MCH is a virtually nontoxic salt of bovine collagen. MCH activates the intrinsic clotting system, attracts platelets, and swells on contact with blood to form a patch which seals blood vessels. Abbott and Austin[21] demonstrated that MCH stopped experimentally induced carotid artery bleeding in normal, heparinized, and thrombocytopenic dogs. Wilkinson et al.[22] demonstrated a decrease in capillary bleeding from skin graft donor sites in humans. Klein et al.[23] observed a marked decrease in bleeding from standard ulcers in a canine model when either MCH powder or slurry was applied. Complete cessation of bleeding occurred in none of 14 controls in 13 of 28 treated patients. In 23 of the 28 patients, bleeding was decreased by more than 75%. Feld et al.[24] did not confirm these results in similar canine experiments. Klein et al.[23] treated nine patients who had bled for more than 72 hours and had required transfusions. Eight of these patients stopped bleeding after endoscopic administration of MCH slurry, but there is no mention of rebleeding in the report. MCH is practical to administer and is associated with no adverse effects. A prospective controlled clinical study using MCH slurry was discontinued because of lack of clinical resources.[25] MCH might be useful in treating diffuse bleeding lesions of the upper gastrointestinal tract, but studies confirming this have not yet been performed. To my knowledge, no controlled studies for the treatment of gastrointestinal bleeding with MCH are being performed at the present time.

CLOTTING FACTORS

Smith et al.[26] developed a unique technique to hold a thrombin-containing material against a bleeding lesion by mixing it into a ferromagnetic slurry. The material was then forced into the ulcer with a powerful electromagnet. The investigators were able to stop "severe bleeding" from experimentally produced gastric ulcers and from arteries opened in the mesentery or omentum. In addition, they stopped active clinical bleeding in two duodenal ulcers, a gastric ulcer, and two Mallory-Weiss tears. Carlson et al.[27] and Jensen et al.[28] found that ferromagnetic tamponade did not control bleeding from experimental ulcers or esophageal varices produced in the canine model. Peura[29] evaluated five patients using this technique. The trial was terminated due to technical problems, primarily because of the difficulty in applying the thick ferromagnetic mixture to the ulcer base. In addition, holding the mixture in the ulcer base with the magnet was a problem due to patient movement. Peura did not believe that the magnetic technique holds much promise because cumbersome, large, expensive electromagnets are required and the patient must be totally immobilized for successful therapy.

Linscheer and Fazio[30,31] developed a system to deliver cryoprecipitate thrombin spray via a four-lumen catheter. The four channels delivered (1) saline to wash the lesion, (2) CO_2 to dry the lesion, (3) a syringe with 10 ml of cryoprecipitate, and (4) a syringe with 5 ml of thrombin. Bleeding patients with an average need for 12 units of blood were treated endoscopically with this system, which produced immediate cessation of bleeding. There was no evidence of rebleeding in the one week follow-up period. There is one report of massive bleeding from a Crohn's disease–related fistula in the duodenum successfully treated with a fibrin glue.[32] Nakajima and Himeno[33] reported on the use of liquid thrombin, W14859, compared to topical thrombin in the treatment of 29 patients with upper gastrointestinal bleeding. One patient received oral thrombin after direct application of thrombin. Another eight received either a direct application or oral administration. Treatment was effective in 86% of the patients who had not received blood transfusions and in 80% of those who had been transfused. The data given are not adequate to allow evaluation of the severity of the bleeding. Multiple etiologies for the bleeding were present and there was no control group in these studies. These factors make it very difficult to evaluate the study.

Groitl and Scheele[34] reported on 16 patients who were treated with a fibrin tissue adhesive made by combining fibrinogen, thrombin, factor XIII, calcium iodide, and aprotine. Four of the patients were treated for anastomotic leaks, and six patients were treated for gastrointestinal bleeding. The bleeding in all patients was controlled by the treatment. Follow-up endoscopy showed firm, clean granulation tissue in the ulcer bases. The authors believed that the main advantages of this treatment were the absence of any additional damage and the induction of fibroblasts and granulation tissue. The treatment was useful in chronic bleeding lesions in very elderly patients with high surgical risks.

Barker and Leicester[35] devised a unique therapy for a patient with severe hemorrhagic esophagitis. They wrapped a 10 × 12-cm sheet of collagen hemostat around the esophageal balloon of a Sengstaken-Blakemore tube and tied it in place with catgut sutures. After 72 hours the sutures had dissolved and the balloon was removed. The bleeding stopped and did not recur. Although severe bleeding from diffuse esophagitis is rare, the available treatments are very unsatisfactory. This therapy of tamponading collagen directly on oozing esophagitis seems rational and, indeed, in the reported patient was apparently effective. Further utilization in other patients with severe hemorrhagic esophagitis seems warranted.

Ederle et al.[36] treated 16 bleeding patients with human fibrin sealant (Tissucol). The bleeding lesions were five duodenal ulcers, four gastric ulcers, one anastomotic ulcer, one ulcerating cancer, two Mallory-Weiss tears, and one erosive gastritis. All of the lesions were controlled, and only one patient rebled.

Valenzuela et al.[37] reported on nine patients treated with either fibrin glue or sham treatment. One of the six treated patients rebled compared to two of the three sham-treated patients. The authors found this "treatment of potentially bleeding ulcers a cumbersome procedure" and are not continuing the study.

Because clotting factors carry the risk of transmitting infection, they are of questionable utility at present in view of the acquired immune deficiency syndrome (AIDS) epidemic. In addition, other methods of treatment are available to treat focal lesions. It would seem that if clotting factors are to be evaluated further, this should be done in patients with diffuse bleeding where other methods of therapy are not available. However, these bleeding problems will be very difficult to study because severe bleeding from diffuse lesions tends to be unpredictable and because sizable numbers of patients will be required to show a treatment effect.

A major disadvantage of topical therapies has been the delivery system. For these agents to work well, excess fluid, mucus, and bloody debris must be removed. In addition, gentle pressure on the application site would probably improve effectiveness, but no means for doing this has been devised. Topical therapies show promise of providing a simple, inexpensive approach to the treatment of diffuse bleeding areas, as well as supplemental treatment to current techniques to prevent rebleeding. Evaluation of topical therapy modalities will require very large multicenter studies, which are not underway at the present time, so that answers will not be forthcoming in the near future.

REFERENCES

1. Henry DA, O'Connell DL: Effects of fibrinolytic inhibitors on mortality from upper gastrointestinal haemorrhage. *Br Med J* 298:1142–1146, 1989.
2. Cormack F, Chakrabarti RR, Jouhar AJ, et al: Tranexamic acid in upper gastrointestinal haemorrhage. *Lancet* 1:1207–1208, 1973.
3. Biggs JC, Hugh TB, Dodds AJ: Tranexamic acid and upper gastrointestinal haemorrhage—A double blind trial. *Gut* 17:729–734, 1976.
4. Engqvist A, Brostrom O, Feilitzen F, et al: Tranexamic acid in massive haemorrhage from the upper gastrointestinal tract: A double blind study. *Scand J Gastroenterol* 14:173–178, 1979.
5. Bergqvist D, Dahlgren S, Hessman Y: Local inhibition of the fibrinolytic system in patients with massive upper gastrointestinal haemorrhage. *Ups J Med Sci* 85:173–178, 1980.
6. Barer D, Ogilvie A, Henry D, et al: Cimetidine and tranexamic acid in the treatment of acute upper gastrointestinal tract bleeding. *N Engl J Med* 308:151–155, 1983.
7. Stael von Holstein C, Eriksson SB, Kallen R: Tranexamic acid as an aid to reducing blood transfusion requirements in gastric and duodenal bleeding. *Br Med J* 294:7–10, 1987.
8. Martin TR, Silvis SE: The endoscopic control of GI blood loss with a tissue adhesive (MBR 4197). *Gastroenterology* 72:A1098, 1977.
9. Silvis SE: Topical therapy: Cyanoacrylate and other modalities, in Papp J (ed): *Endoscopic Control of Gastrointestinal Hemorrhage*. Boca Raton, Fla, CRC Press, 1981, pp 111–127.
10. Protell RL, Silverstein FE, Gulacsik C, et al: Failure of cyanoacrylate tissue glue (flucrylate, MBR 4197) to stop bleeding from experimental canine gastric ulcers. *Dig Dis* 23:903–908, 1978.
11. Martin TR, Onstad GR, Silvis SE: Endoscopic control of massive upper gastrointestinal bleeding with a tissue adhesive (MBR 4197). *Gastrointest Endosc* 24:74–76, 1977.

12. Peura DA, Johnson LF, Burkhalter EL, et al: Use of trifluoroisopropyl cyanoacrylate polymer (MBR 4197) in patients with bleeding peptic ulcers of the stomach and duodenum: A randomized controlled study. *J Clin Gastroenterol* 4:325–328, 1982.
13. Zeng-lie L, Hui-chuan Y, Xi-ping B, et al: Endoscopic hemostasis in upper GI hemorrhage with tissue adhesion. *Chin Med J* 101:823–827, 1988.
14. Soehendra N, Nam V Ch, Grimm H, et al: Endoscopic obliteration of large esophagogastric varices with bucrylate. *Endoscopy* 18:25–26, 1986.
15. Loperfido S: Endoscopic treatment of bleeding gastric varices with bucrylate. *Endoscopy* 19:87, 1987.
16. Feretis C, Tabakopoulos P, Benakis P, et al: Endoscopic hemostasis of esophageal and gastric variceal bleeding with histoacryl. *Endoscopy* 22:282–284, 1990.
17. Rauws EAJ, Jansen PLM, Tytgat GNJ: Endoscopic sclerotherapy of gastric varices with bucrylate. Treatment of acute bleeding and long term follow-up. *Gastrointest Endosc* 37:242, 1991.
18. Grimm H, MayDeo A, Noar M: Bleeding esophago-gastric varice: Is endoscopic treatment with cyanoacrylate the final answer? *Gastrointest Endosc* 37:275, 1991.
19. Loperfido S: Endoscopic hemostasis of gastric bleeding from Dieulofoy's ulcer with histoacryl. *Endoscopy* 21:199–200, 1989.
20. Vallieres E, Jamieson C, Haber GB, et al: Pancreatoduodenal necrosis after endoscopic injection of cyanoacrylate to treat a bleeding duodenal ulcer: A case report. *Surgery* 106:901–903, 1989.
21. Abbott WM, Austin W: The effectiveness and mechanism of collagen-induced topical hemostasis. *Surgery* 78:723–729, 1975.
22. Wilkinson TS, Tenery JH, Zufi D: The skin graft donor site as a model for evaluation of hemostatic agents. *Plast Reconstr Surg* 51:541–544, 1973.
23. Klein FA, Drucek C, Breuer RI, et al: Control of upper gastrointestinal bleeding with a microcrystalline collagen hemostat. *Dig Dis Sci* 27:981–985, 1982.
24. Feld AD, Silverstein FE, Keegan MD: Failure of microfibrillar collagen hemostat (MCH, Avitene^{R}) to stop bleeding from experimental canine ulcers. *Gastrointest Endosc* 27:132, 1981.
25. Breuer RI, Craig RM: Topical agents in the management of gastrointestinal bleeding, in Silvis SE (ed): *Therapeutic Gastrointestinal Endoscopy*. New York, Igaku-Shoin, 1990, pp 212–224.
26. Smith FW, Heinonen LA, Peterson EC, et al: The use of a strong magnetic field in the control of gastrointestinal bleeding. *Gastroenterology* 78:1264, 1980.
27. Carlson D, Jensen DM, Machicado G, et al: Treatment of experimental bleeding gastric ulcers and erosions with ferromagnetic tamponade. *Gastroenterology* 78:1147, 1980.
28. Jensen DM, Silpa ML, Tapipa JI, et al: Comparison of different methods for endoscopic hemostasis of bleeding canine esophageal varices. *Gastroenterology* 84:1455–1461, 1983.
29. Peura DA: Topical therapy for the control of gastrointestinal bleeding. *Gastrointest Endosc* 36:S53–S55, 1990.
30. Linscheer WG, Fazio TL: Control of upper gastrointestinal hemorrhage by endoscopic spraying of clotting factors. *Gastroenterology* 77:642–646, 1979.
31. Linscheer WG, Fazio TL: Endoscopic control of upper gastrointestinal bleeding: Alternate spraying of thrombin and fibrinogen. *Gastrointest Endosc* 23:233–234, 1977.
32. McCarthy PM, Frazee RC, Hughes RW, et al: Barium-impregnated fibrin glue: Application to a bleeding duodenal sinus. *Mayo Clin Proc* 62:317–319, 1987.
33. Nakajima T, Himeno S: Clinical evaluation of W14859 (liquid thrombin) on upper gastro-

intestinal haemorrhage: Comparative study of W14859 versus topical thrombin. *J Int Med Res* 17:479–485, 1989.

34. Groitl H, Scheele J: Initial experience with the endoscopic application of fibrin tissue adhesive in the upper gastrointestinal tract. *Surg Endosc* 1:93–97, 1987.
35. Barker P, Leicester RJ: Collagen overcoat: An approach to haemorrhagic oesophagitis. *Br J Surg* 75:1111, 1988.
36. Ederle A, Scattolini C, Vantgini I, et al: Human fibrin sealant in upper GI tract bleeding (letter). *Endoscopy* 21:112, 1989.
37. Valenzuela GA, Lind CD, Pambianco DJ, et al: Fibrin glue: Is it practical in the treatment of acute upper gastrointestinal bleed? *Gastrointest Endosc* 36:77–78, 1990.

25

ANGIOGRAPHIC MANAGEMENT

Ernest J. Ring, M.D.

In 1963, Nusbaum and Baum recognized that, regardless of etiology or location, bleeding follows a disruption in the wall of a blood vessel and, therefore, like other types of vascular pathology, can be demonstrated angiographically.[1] Experimentally, they found that blood loss at rates as low as 0.5 cc/min is readily visualized at angiography because the radiopaque contrast medium extravasates from the bleeding site along with the blood.[2,3] They then accumulated extensive clinical evidence which documented the value of selective arteriography in localizing bleeding throughout the gastrointestinal tract.

Nusbaum and Baum subsequently began to use the angiographic catheter to treat bleeding by introducing agents that selectively reduced or stopped flow in the bleeding vessel.[4] Over the past 25 years these methods have been refined, and the role of transcatheter therapy for bleeding at specific sites has been thoroughly investigated.[5-14] This chapter reviews the current status of these transcatheter therapies and their role in the management of patients with gastrointestinal hemorrhage.

ANGIOGRAPHIC LOCALIZATION OF A BLEEDING SITE

Although selective angiography is only one of several methods of locating a source of gastrointestinal blood loss and has several limitations, this modality continues to play an important diagnostic role in complex cases. The procedure may be performed on severely ill patients and requires little patient cooperation. No special preparation is necessary, and an accurate diagnosis can be made despite the presence of a large amount of blood in the gastrointestinal tract. The radiographic diagnostic criteria are straightforward, and the localization is readily established with minimal interobserver variation.

Radiographic Appearance of Bleeding

Typically, bleeding is first detected during the arterial phase of selective arteriography when a localized collection of contrast material begins to appear. As filming continues, the extravasation becomes increasingly apparent and is especially obvious at the end of the angiographic series, when all of the intravascular contrast has washed out. The radiographic appearance of extravasated contrast material varies with the rate of bleeding and the nature of the space in which the blood is collecting. Very brisk, continuous bleeding produces the largest, most easily seen collections and may even provide excellent opacification of the mucosa of the gastrointestinal tract (Figure 25.1). Small amounts of extravasation appear as localized collections; usually the collections are amorphous, but occasionally they outline an ulcer crater or a colonic diverticulum (Figure 25.2). Within a few minutes, most of the contrast material which has extravasated into the gastrointestinal tract is diluted and carried distally by peristalsis, so that it does not persist between sequential injections.

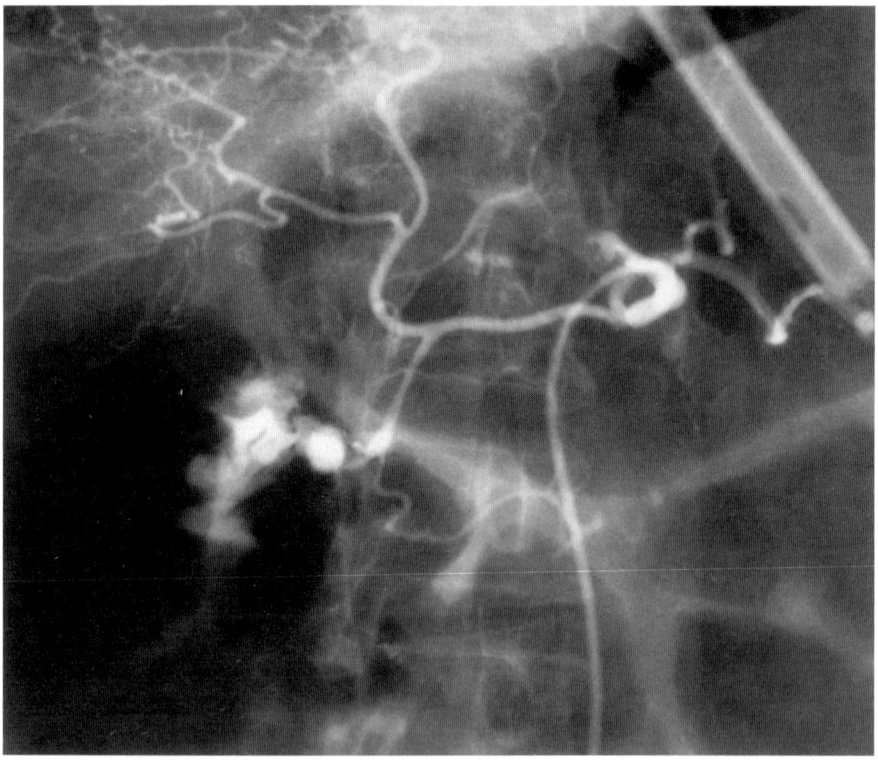

A

Figure 25.1. Massive bleeding from a duodenal ulcer. (*A*) Early film from a hepatic arteriogram shows extravasation from the gastroduodenal artery. (*B*) Later in the angiographic series, the extravasation outlines the duodenal mucosa. (*C*) After all of the intravascular contrast medium has washed out, the entire descending duodenum is opacified by extravasated contrast medium.

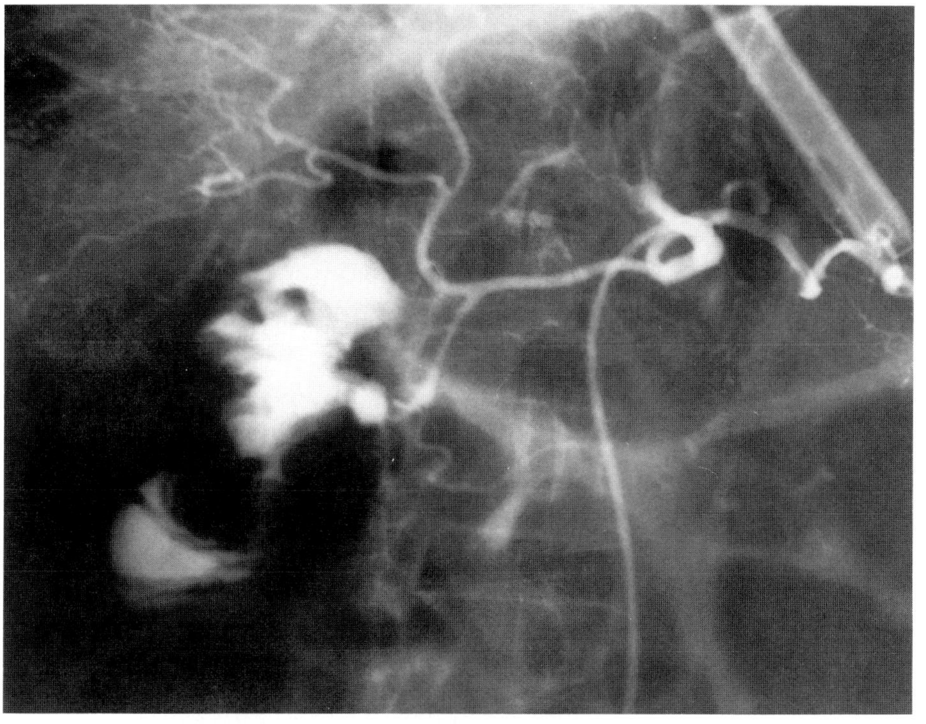

B

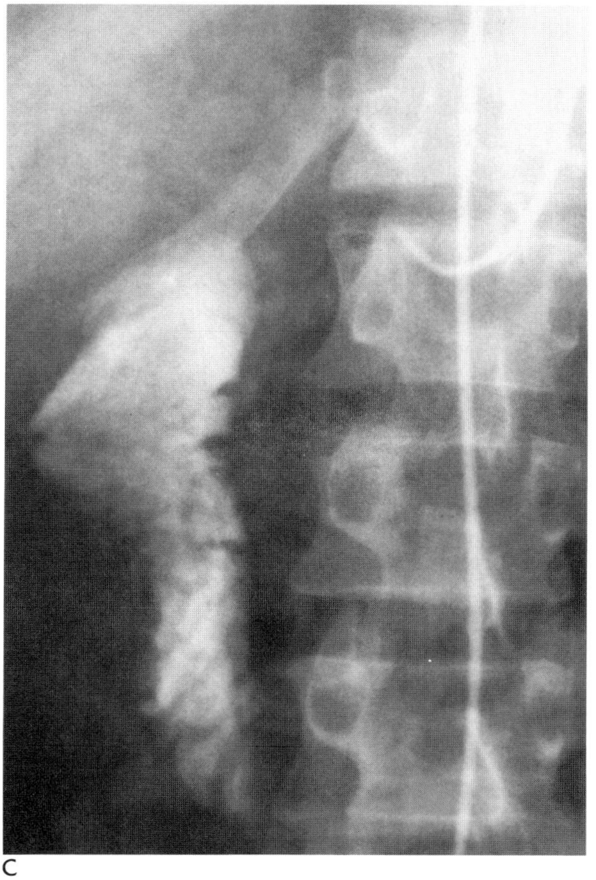

C

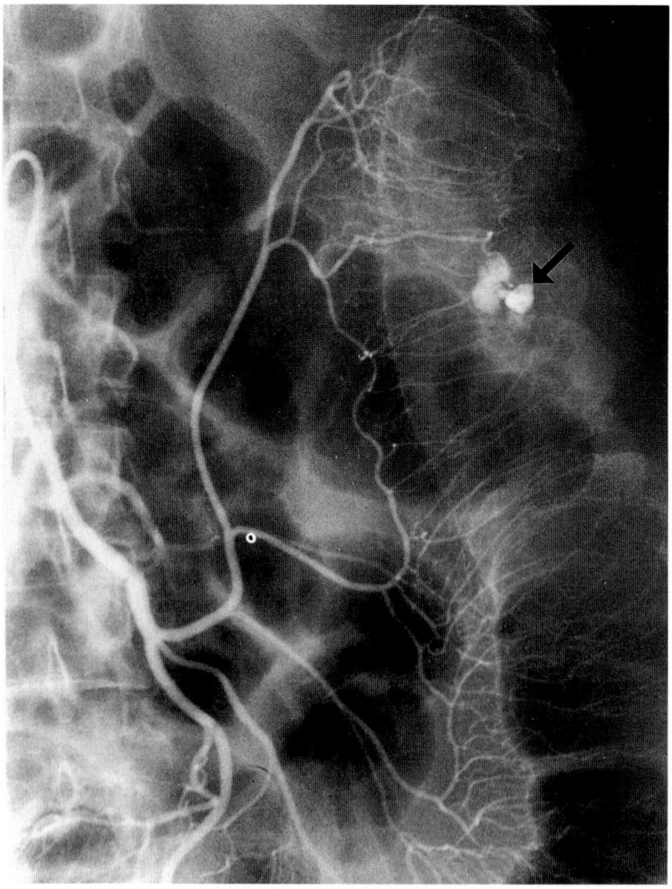

Figure 25.2. Bleeding from a colonic diverticulum. A radiograph obtained during an inferior mesenteric arteriogram shows extravasated contrast medium filling a colonic diverticulum (*arrow*).

Rate of Detectable Bleeding

In their early experimental studies, Baum and Nusbaum showed that selective arteriography could demonstrate arteriocapillary bleeding at rates greater than or equal to 0.5 ml/min.[1-3] Interestingly, this rate, which has been so widely quoted in the literature as the lower limit of angiographically detectable bleeding, actually reflected a limitation of Baum and Nusbaum's laboratory method. Since their experimental model was incapable of consistently maintaining blood loss at less than 0.5 ml/min, and since they were able to identify extravasation at this rate, it is likely that even lower rates of blood loss might actually be detectable.

False-Negative Examinations

Considering the known sensitivity of angiography in localizing bleeding, it is disappointing that clinical experience with this method has not been more consistently successful and that false-negative examinations are common. However, in order to localize hemorrhage, the angiographic injection must coincide with an episode of active blood loss. In many patients, hemorrhage is intermittent and, if the arteriogram is performed between spurts of blood loss, there are no positive findings.

Unnecessary false-negative examinations for upper gastrointestinal tract bleeding can usually be avoided, since the presence of active blood loss can generally be determined by observing the nasogastric aspirate. Thorough irrigation of the stomach should be performed immediately before arteriography is begun, and the examination should be withheld unless there is evidence of continued blood staining of the irrigant. Intermittent gastric aspiration should also be performed during the course of arteriography. Occasionally, after bleeding has stopped, old clots in the stomach may continue to color the nasogastric aspirate, thus mimicking active hemorrhage. Any uncertainty can usually be resolved by placing a large-bore tube in the stomach to evacuate all remaining clots.

Determining when angiography is appropriate for patients with lower gastrointestinal tract bleeding is a much more complicated clinical problem. The extent and severity of colonic hemorrhage are frequently difficult to evaluate using clinical criteria alone, since blood often continues to pass through the rectum for several hours after bleeding has actually ceased. In addition, lower gastrointestinal tract bleeding commonly affects patients who are elderly and difficult to stabilize, so that ongoing vital signs may overestimate the degree of active blood loss. Radioisotopic examinations can demonstrate active hemorrhage and are useful in selecting those patients with lower gastrointestinal tract bleeding who are most likely to benefit from angiography.[15,16] The technique is simple and noninvasive, and is capable of demonstrating venous bleeding at rates as low as 0.1 ml/min.

ANATOMICAL LOCALIZATION OF BLEEDING

Since the angiographic demonstration of bleeding is specific to the vessel injected, precise localization is possible only if the vessel supplies one anatomical area. Bleeding that originates from the gastroepiploic artery, for example, is easily localized to the greater curvature of the stomach. On the other hand, anatomical localization is less specific when the extravasation comes from a branch of the gastroduodenal artery which provides blood flow to both the gastric antrum and the proximal duodenum.

Because of the overlapping of small bowel loops and mesenteric arterial branches, it is usually difficult to transpose the findings of superior mesenteric arteriography to the surgical field. If subselective catheterization of the bleeding branch is performed prior to surgery, the catheter can be left in place to facilitate intraoperative localization of the bleeding site. After the small bowel has been surgically exposed, a blue dye is injected through the catheter to visibly stain the area of bowel to be removed.

ANGIOGRAPHIC TECHNIQUES OF CONTROLLING BLEEDING

Vasopressin Infusion

Angiographic control of bleeding is achieved by selectively introducing agents through a catheter that locally reduce the blood flow to the bleeding site. Originally, pharmacological methods were used for this purpose. Vasopressin has had the widest clinical acceptance as a relatively safe, reliable intra-arterial vasoconstrictor. Selective infusion of vasopressin into a visceral artery causes constriction of small, peripheral branches at low dosages and progressively affects larger, more proximal vessels at increasingly higher dosages. The effect of vasopressin is neither antagonized by adrenergic blocking agents nor prevented by vascular denervation, but it may be reversed with nitroglycerin. Vasopressin's action is direct and immediate, and a repeat arteriogram performed 15 to 20 minutes after the beginning of an infusion will accurately determine the effectiveness of therapy. The principal advantage of vasopressin therapy is that the dosage can be modified to produce varying degrees of vasoconstriction and, consequently, a more controlled and reversible ischemic effect than that of embolic therapy.

Catheter Position for Vasopressin Therapy

Generally, the more selectively the catheter tip can be placed, the better the chance of controlling bleeding. However, subselective infusions into branches of the mesenteric artery are not considered necessary to control bleeding from the bowel, since main mesenteric artery infusions have been shown to be safe and highly effective and are not technically difficult to perform. Subselective catheterization of the gastroduodenal artery is not usually necessary for the treatment of bleeding duodenal ulcers. Direct infusion of vasopressin into the common hepatic artery is considered safe because, experimentally, flow in the hepatic artery is not reduced[17] and, clinically, considerable experience has shown that damage to the liver does not occur.[18] When bleeding occurs in the distribution of the left gastric artery, direct infusion of vasopressin into that vessel is much more likely to control hemorrhage than is celiac axis infusion. Because of the proximal origin of the left gastric artery, it is usually impossible to anchor an infusion catheter securely in the celiac axis without having its tip extend beyond the left gastric artery's origin. Therefore, most celiac axis infusions deliver the vasoconstrictor only to the splenic and hepatic branches, and are ineffective for gastric fundal bleeding.

Method and Rate of Vasopressin Infusion

Although other schemes have been devised, Baum's original protocol for infusing vasopressin has persisted both in the literature and in clinical practice.[4] Once the bleeding site has been demonstrated and the catheter appropriately positioned, the infusion is started at a rate of 0.2 unit/min. The drug is diluted with either saline or dextrose solution and is delivered continuously by an infusion pump at a rate of at least 0.5 ml/min. After the infusion is begun, the patient is observed closely for signs of any systemic reactions. A post-therapy angiogram is obtained 15 to 20 minutes after the vasopressin infusion is begun by injecting contrast material at the same rate and in the same volume used in the original arteriogram (Figure 25.3). Immediately before the post-therapy arteriogram, the

Figure 25.3. Bleeding hepatic flexure diverticulum treated with infusion of vasopressin into the superior mesenteric artery. (*A*) A superior mesenteric arteriogram shows extravasation from a branch of the right colic artery (*arrow*). (*B*) Twenty minutes after an infusion of vasopressin through the catheter was begun, a repeat superior mesenteric arteriogram was performed. This shows moderate constriction of the mesenteric artery branches and no further extravasation.

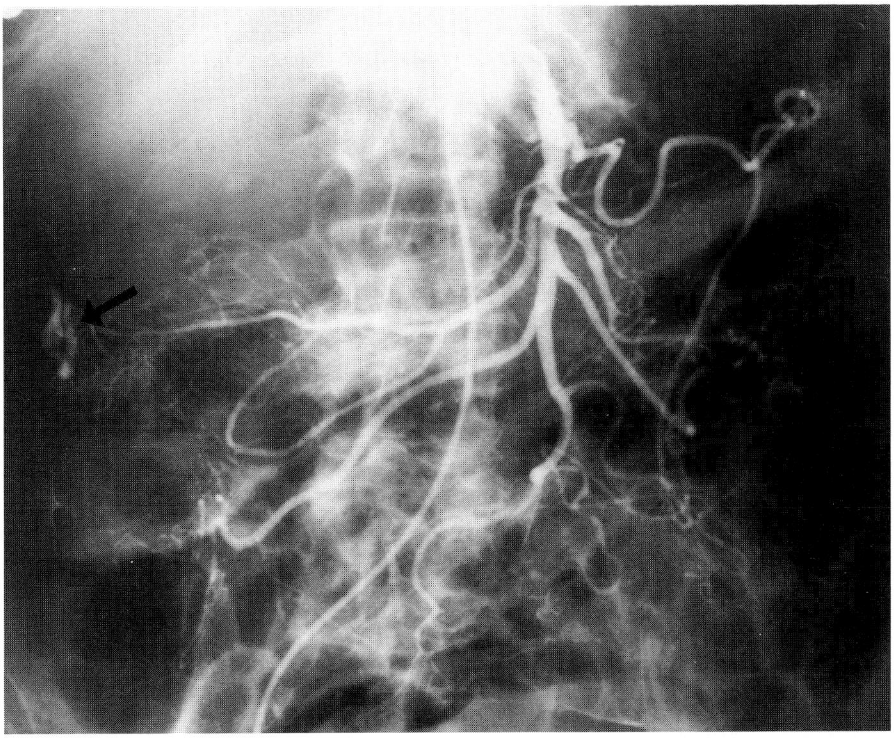

A

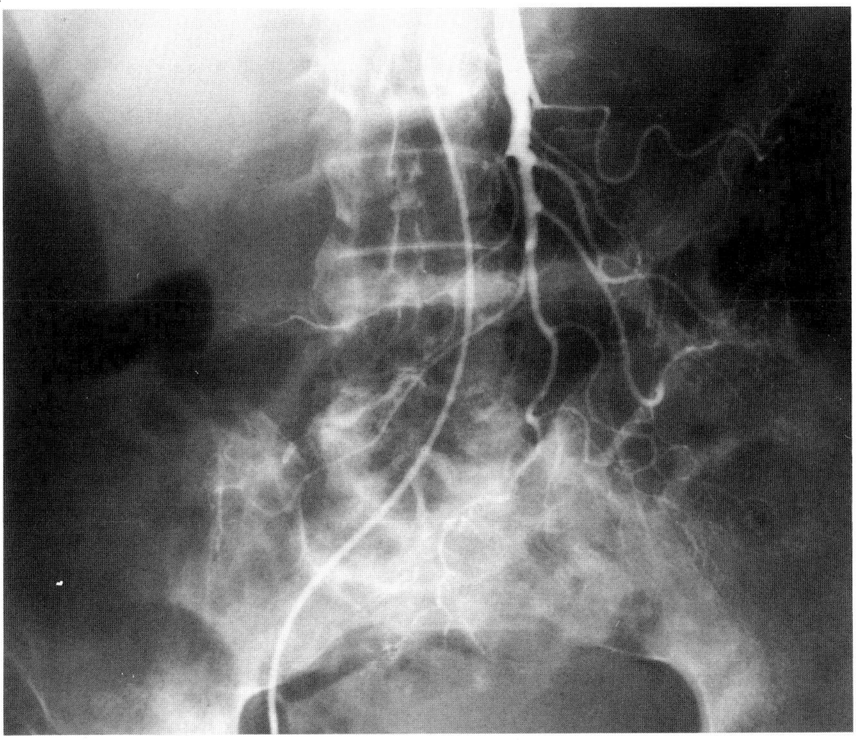

B

vasopressin in the catheter is removed so that a bolus of vasoconstrictor is not administered along with the contrast medium. The post-therapy angiogram is analyzed to ensure that

1. There is a moderate reduction in the caliber of the infused vessels, with preservation of good forward flow into the capillary and venous phases.
2. There is still filling of branches in the vicinity of the bleeding point.
3. There is no further extravasation.

If all these criteria have been met, a pressure dressing is applied around the catheter entry site and the patient is transferred to an intensive care unit. If there is no clinical evidence of recurrent bleeding, the initial infusion rate is continued for 24 to 36 hours and then reduced by 50% for an additional 24 hours. The vasopressin infusion is then stopped, but the catheter is kept in place and patency is maintained by infusing plain saline or dextrose solution for 8 to 12 hours more. If the patient remains clinically stable during that time, the catheter is removed.

Systemic Reactions to Vasopressin

Minor abdominal cramping and diarrhea are common and insignificant sequelae of vasopressin therapy. Abdominal pain which persists for more than 20 or 30 minutes suggests the possibility of bowel ischemia, and the catheter's position should be checked. Almost all patients develop a systemic antidiuretic hormone (ADH) effect for a variable period; water retention and electrolyte imbalance are managed with diuretics and electrolyte replacement. In a small number of patients, non-dosage-dependent cardiotoxic effects may occur; hypertension, bradycardia, and arrhythmias are the ones most commonly seen.

If a vasopressin infusion initially controls bleeding, the effect should continue as long as the same dosage rate is maintained. Unlike other vasoconstrictors, vasopressin is not associated with an escape phenomenon or tachyphylaxis. Whenever renewed bleeding occurs during the course of an infusion, some change in the vasopressin delivery system should be suspected. Most commonly, bleeding recurs because the angiographic catheter has become dislodged from the bleeding vessel. The catheter's position can be readily checked by obtaining a portable abdominal radiograph while simultaneously hand-injecting contrast through the catheter. The infusion should also be checked; the infusate may have been prepared at the wrong concentration or even with the wrong agent. Rebleeding can also result from mechanical malfunctions of the catheter and the infusion pump system.

If recurrent bleeding develops while the dosage of vasopressin is being tapered, hemostasis can be achieved by reverting to the original dosage rate and maintaining that rate for another 24 to 36 hours before again attempting to taper. If the patient cannot be weaned from vasopressin and has renewed bleeding after a second attempt at dosage reduction, some other form of therapy should be attempted.

SELECTIVE OCCLUSION TECHNIQUES FOR CONTROL OF BLEEDING

Selective embolization and other mechanical occlusive techniques have become increasingly popular methods of treating acute hemorrhage. Embolic therapy can be accomplished rapidly. This avoids the possible systemic effects of vasopressin and the need for long-term catheterization of the femoral artery. However, the flow reduction produced by embolic particles is less controllable than that of vasoconstrictive therapy, and, once injected, emboli are irretrievable and their effects irreversible. To minimize the risk of tissue ischemia, a great deal of technical expertise is required to deliver the emboli to a specific bleeding branch. Most authors consider embolic therapy the angiographic treatment of choice for bleeding duodenal ulcers; many also believe it to be the best angiographic way to treat bleeding from branches of the left gastric artery. Despite some recent controversy, embolization for mesenteric arterial bleeding is not usually recommended, except for patients who are not surgical candidates and who fail to respond to vasoconstrictors. Hemorrhage from organs with vascular beds not responsive to vasoconstrictors (e.g., liver and pancreas) is always managed angiographically by mechanical occlusion of the bleeding branches.

Methods of Transcatheter Embolization

Gelfoam, a slowly absorbed gelatin sponge, is probably the most widely used embolic agent. Individual emboli are cut or torn from sterile 3 × 5-cm pads of surgical Gelfoam. If very small fragments are used initially, occlusions will occur in small end arteries, decreasing the potential for collateral reconstitution. To perform the embolization, several small pieces of Gelfoam are placed in a contrast-filled syringe and slowly injected. Since the Gelfoam floats in the contrast material, the syringe is inverted during the injection. As the occlusion progresses more proximally, increasingly larger emboli are used. Large emboli are injected individually by rolling the moistened Gelfoam into a cigar-shaped plug and placing it directly into the hub of the stopcock or catheter. Gelfoam's extreme compressibility allows relatively large embolic plugs to be delivered through small catheters. If the Gelfoam will not pass through the catheter, a guidewire is used to push and fragment the material until it can be injected easily.

As long as there is good forward flow in the catheterized vessel, emboli will be carried antegrade but, as occlusion is approached, the flow pattern of injected emboli becomes unpredictable. Gelfoam delivered after this point may remain in an unstable position in the proximal portion of the vessel or may reflux into the aorta. Embolic reflux can be prevented by injection through a balloon occlusion catheter. The progress of the occlusion should be closely followed fluoroscopically by injecting contrast material after each embolization. If small emboli are used initially, occlusions will be evidenced by slowing of forward flow. If progressively larger emboli are injected, abrupt cutoff of the arterial branches will be seen. The occlusion produced by Gelfoam is not permanent; most vessels recanalize in periods ranging from 10 days to several weeks. Following Gelfoam embolization, patients commonly develop a fever of up to 38°C, which may persist for as long as 24 to 36 hours and then subside spontaneously.

Coiled pieces of guidewire with attached thrombogenic fibers can be passed through an angiographic catheter to occlude an arterial lumen permanently. Unlike other embolic materials, the coils are radiopaque, permitting a more controlled embolization. The coils can be obtained in several diameters for use in different vessels. Very small coils that can pass through coaxial catheters are now available for occlusion of peripheral branch vessels. Detachable balloon catheters are also used to create permanent local occlusions, but they are expensive and somewhat cumbersome, so their use has been limited to specific problems such as intra-arterial aneurysms.

Ivalon, a polyvinyl alcohol foam, is also a permanent occluding agent. The material is stored in formalin and must be thoroughly washed with saline solution before being cut into small pieces for embolization. Ivalon can be difficult to inject through polyethylene catheters because of its high coefficient of friction. The material is physiologically inert and, once lodged in the vessel, becomes incorporated into dense fibrous tissue without inducing inflammatory changes in the vessel itself.

The rich arterial collateral blood supply to most regions considered for embolization usually provides sufficient blood flow to prevent ischemic infarction after transcatheter occlusion therapy. This is especially true in the pelvis, duodenum, and stomach, all of which can be embolized safely under most circumstances. The mesenteric arterial anatomy offers less opportunity for collateral blood supply, and iatrogenic bowel infarction after mesenteric embolization may sometimes occur. The spleen and kidney have very poor intrinsic collateral arterial anastomoses and, in these organs, tissue loss invariably follows successful occlusion therapy. To some extent, the efficacy of transcatheter occlusion therapy in controlling bleeding is inversely related to its safety. The same collaterals which prevent ischemic injury can reconstitute flow to a bleeding vessel and permit continued blood loss. After a vessel has been occluded in an area rich with potential collaterals, it is important to demonstrate the alternative blood supplies to ensure that hemostasis has actually been achieved. If repeat angiography shows continued extravasation through a collateral branch, further therapy is warranted.

THE ROLE OF ANGIOGRAPHIC THERAPY FOR BLEEDING FROM SPECIFIC SITES

Esophageal Arterial Bleeding

Proximal esophageal bleeding is rarely demonstrated angiographically because the upper two-thirds of the esophagus derives its blood supply from small branches of the thoracic aorta. The distal esophagus, however, receives arterial flow from left gastric artery branches, so that bleeding from lesions such as esophagitis and Mallory-Weiss tears can be demonstrated by left gastric arteriography and successfully treated with either selective vasopressin infusions or embolic therapy (Figure 25.4).

Gastric Mucosal Bleeding

Massive bleeding from the gastric mucosa seldom presents as an isolated problem but usually occurs in patients debilitated by a variety of underlying conditions, such as (1) prolonged stress (often following surgery or major trauma), (2) drug or alcohol ingestion, (3) severe burns (Curling's ulcers), or (4) uremia. Clinically, the bleeding is massive and often not responsive to conservative measures. Successful surgical management usually requires extensive gastric resection, and the operative mortality is high.

Figure 25.4. Arterial bleeding from the distal esophagus. (*A*) A left gastric arteriogram shows extravasation from branches in the distal esophagus (*arrows*). (*B*) Twenty minutes after beginning an infusion of vasopressin, the arteriogram was repeated. The gastric and distal esophageal branches are constricted, and there is no longer any extravasation.

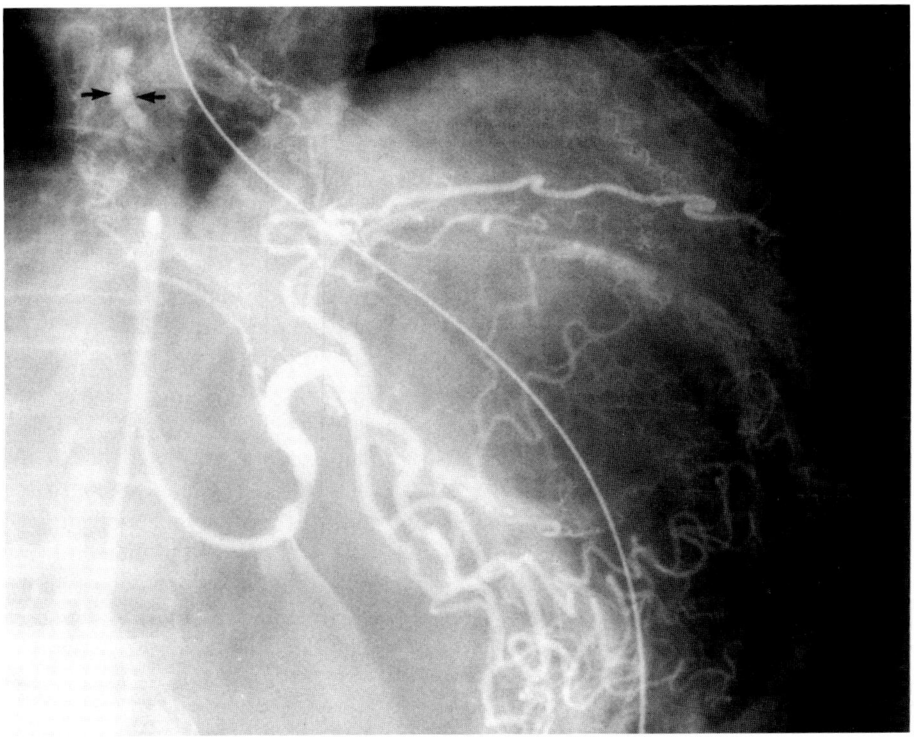

A

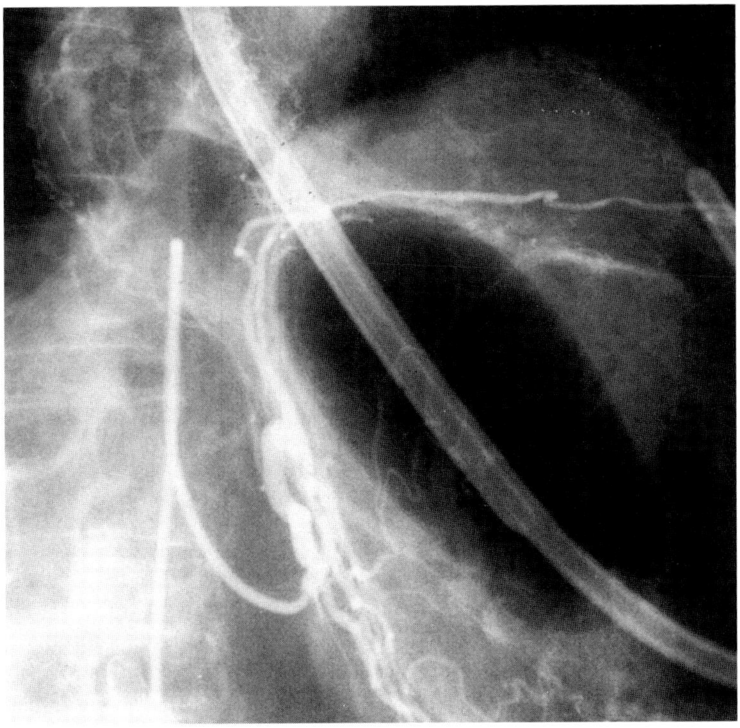

B

Fortunately, this type of bleeding occurs much less often than it did a few years ago. Advances in prophylaxis with antacids and histamine^{-2} blockers have sharply reduced the incidence of stress-induced gastric bleeding following major surgery or trauma.

The low morbidity and high success rate of angiographic therapy have made it a primary form of treatment of patients with any type of gastric bleeding[9,19] (Figure 25.5). Gastric hemorrhage may originate from a single ulceration or from diffuse oozing at numerous sites. Bleeding from stress gastritis is usually very responsive to selective infusions of vasopressin into the left gastric artery and, after initial hemostasis is achieved, surgery can be avoided in over 80% of patients. Recurrent bleeding develops in only about 15% of these patients.[19] In isolated instances, bleeding originates from a vessel other than the left gastric or gastroepiploic artery. Infusing vasopressin into the appropriate vessel supplying one of these branches will control bleeding in most cases.

Embolization of bleeding gastric vessels is now being used with increasing frequency as an alternative form of transcatheter therapy. Rapid control of bleeding can be achieved in most patients, and complications from gastric embolizations are infrequent. This approach avoids the problems of long-term arterial catheterization and vasopressin side effects. Several reports have shown that embolization of the left gastric artery is as effective as selective vasopressin infusion in controlling most types of bleeding (Figure 25.6). Excessive embolization has reportedly caused gastric infarction in patients with previous partial gastrectomy.[20] The choice of transcatheter therapy must be made on an individual basis; it depends on variations in vascular anatomy that may make embolization impractical and on associated diseases that may be contraindications to vasopressin infusion.

Duodenal Ulcer Bleeding

Unlike patients with gastric mucosal bleeding, those with duodenal ulcer disease are usually in good general health. Duodenal bleeding is also more likely to be self-limited but, when it proves refractory to medical therapy, angiography has been used to locate and control the bleeding. In most patients, bleeding duodenal ulcers are easily demonstrated by celiac or hepatic arteriography. Occasionally, the bleeding originates from a branch of the inferior pancreaticoduodenal artery and is shown only by superior mesenteric arterial injections. Transcatheter therapy of bleeding duodenal ulcers has been disappointing. Vasopressin infusions successfully control duodenal hemorrhage in less than 50% of cases.[13] This poor result is partly related to the fact that blood vessels are less responsive to the effects of vasoconstrictors in areas of chronic ulceration. More importantly the multiplicity of blood supply to the duodenum creates complex hemodynamics and allows the flow to be redirected to the bleeding site from an alternative source during the vasopressin infusion.

Embolization of the bleeding duodenal branch artery will often stop blood loss when vasoconstrictors are ineffective. However, emboli must be carefully placed to prevent rebleeding from collateral vessels. The dual blood supply to the duodenum through the pancreaticoduodenal arcades from both the celiac and superior mesenteric arteries provides extensive collateral pathways which can continue to bring blood to the bleeding branch. For embolic therapy to be effective, the actual peripheral bleeding branch usually must be superselectively occluded (Figure 25.7) or the supplying arcade "double-

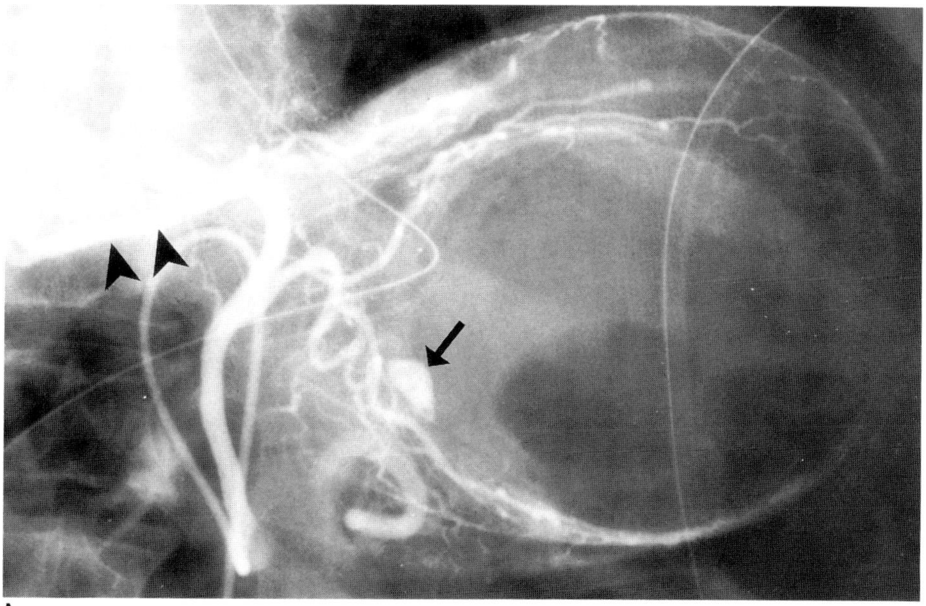

A

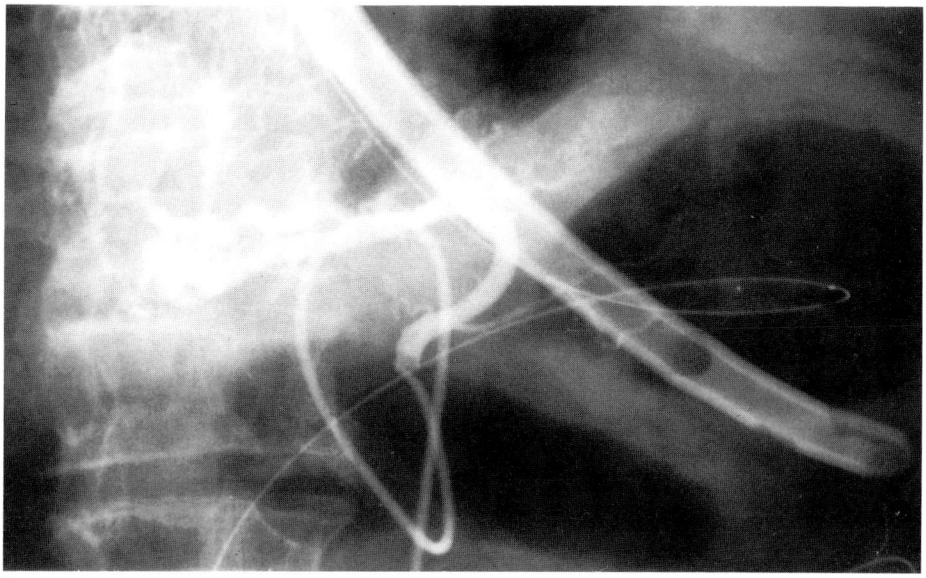

B

Figure 25.5. Bleeding stress ulcer treated with vasopressin infusion into a combined left gastric/left hepatic trunk. (*A*) A selective left gastric arteriogram shows a localized collection of contrast (*arrow*). The left hepatic artery is a branch of the left gastric artery (*arrowheads*). (*B*) After vasopressin infusion, the gastric branches are intensely constricted. There is no change in the size of the left hepatic artery branch.

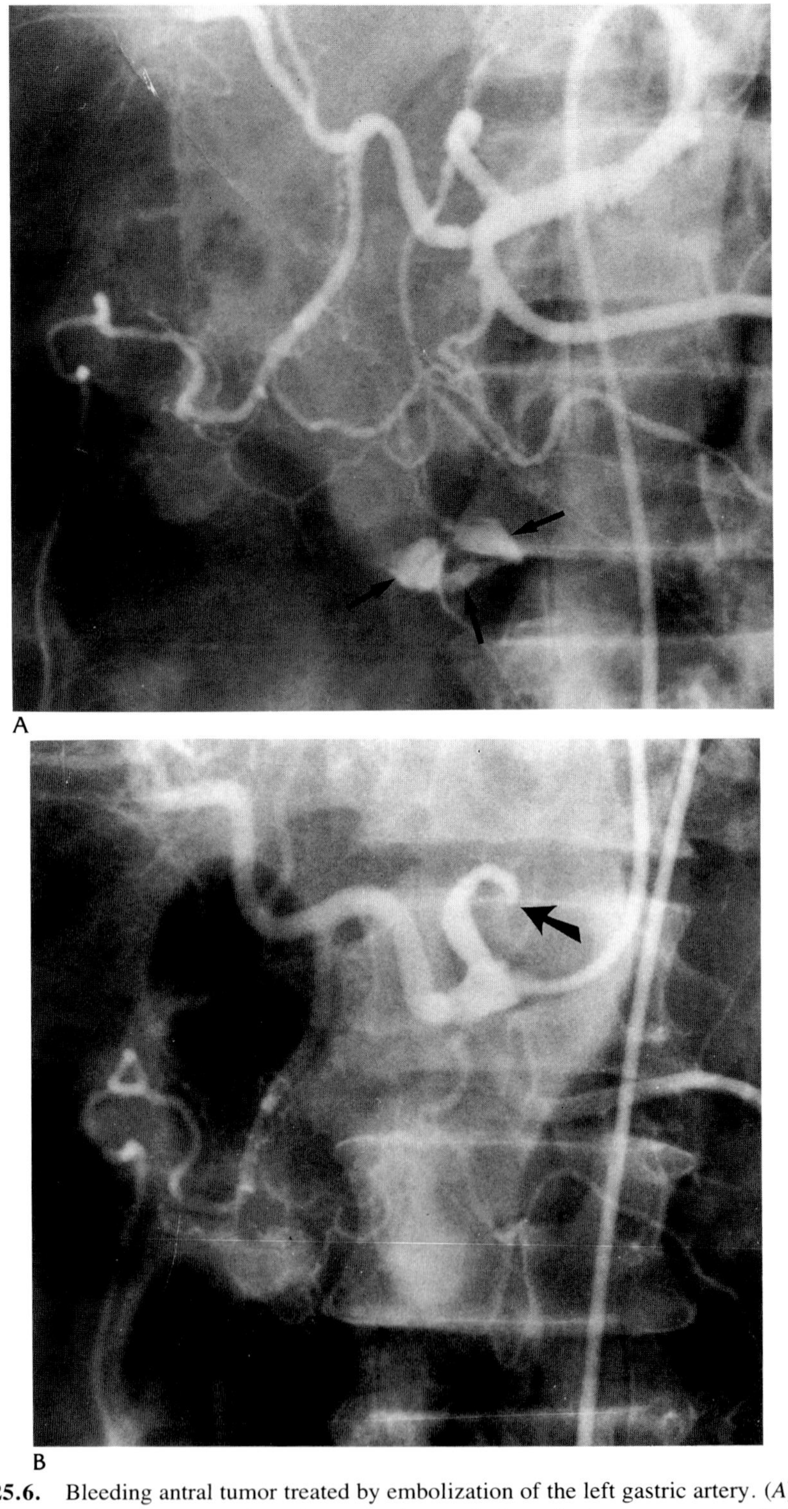

Figure 25.6. Bleeding antral tumor treated by embolization of the left gastric artery. (*A*) A celiac axis arteriogram shows extravasation of contrast (*arrows*) along the lesser curvature. (*B*) A repeat celiac axis arteriogram after embolization of the left gastric artery shows it to be occluded (*arrow*). There is no further extravasation.

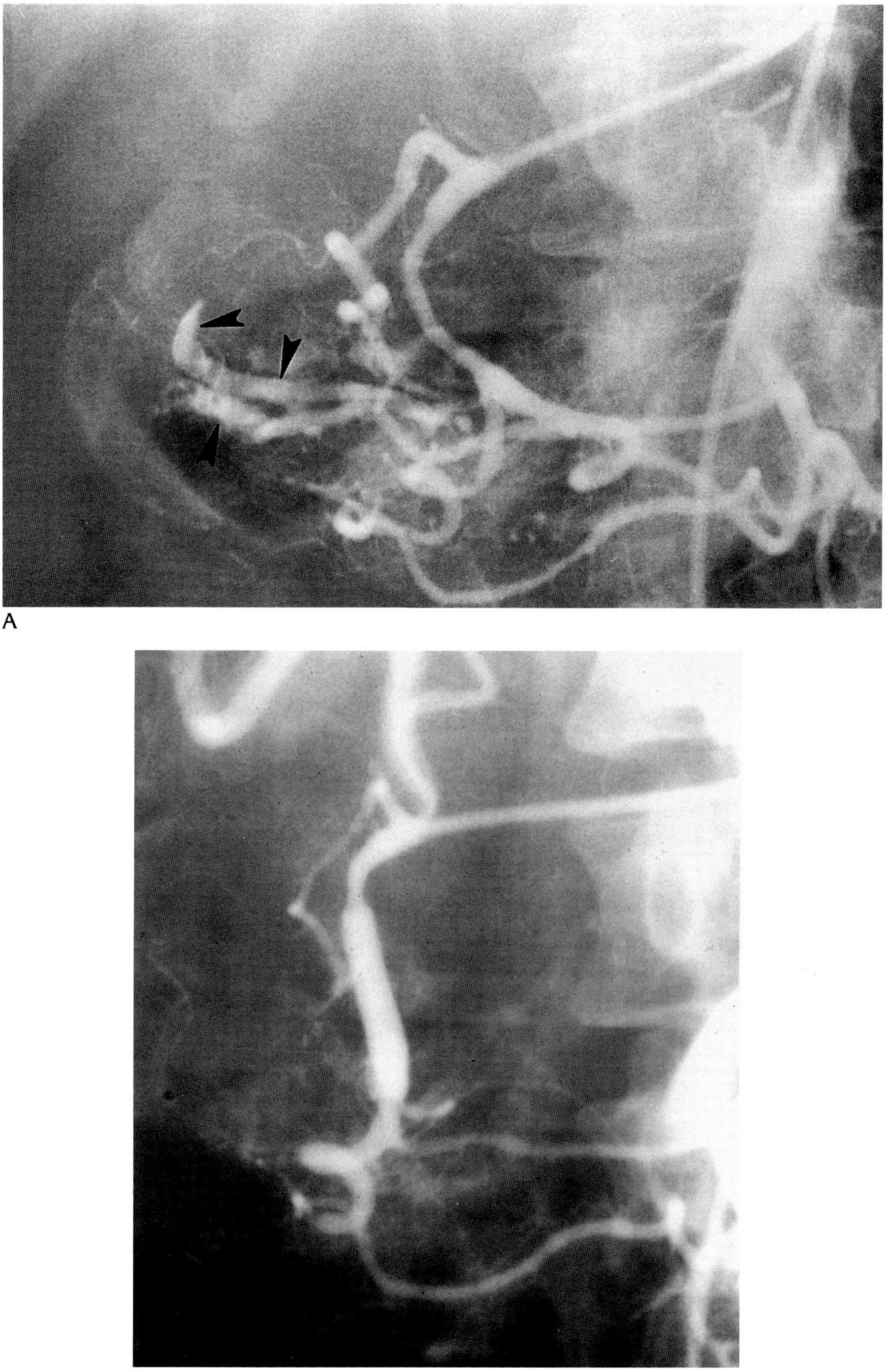

A

B

Figure 25.7. Superselective embolization of bleeding branches of the gastroduodenal artery in a patient bleeding from a duodenal ulcer. (*A*) A gastroduodenal arteriogram shows bleeding from a branch of the superior pancreaticoduodenal artery (arrows). (*B*) The specific bleeding branch was catheterized and occluded with a plug of Gelfoam. A repeat gastroduodenal arteriogram shows that the vessel has been occluded, and there are no collaterals resupplying the bleeding branch.

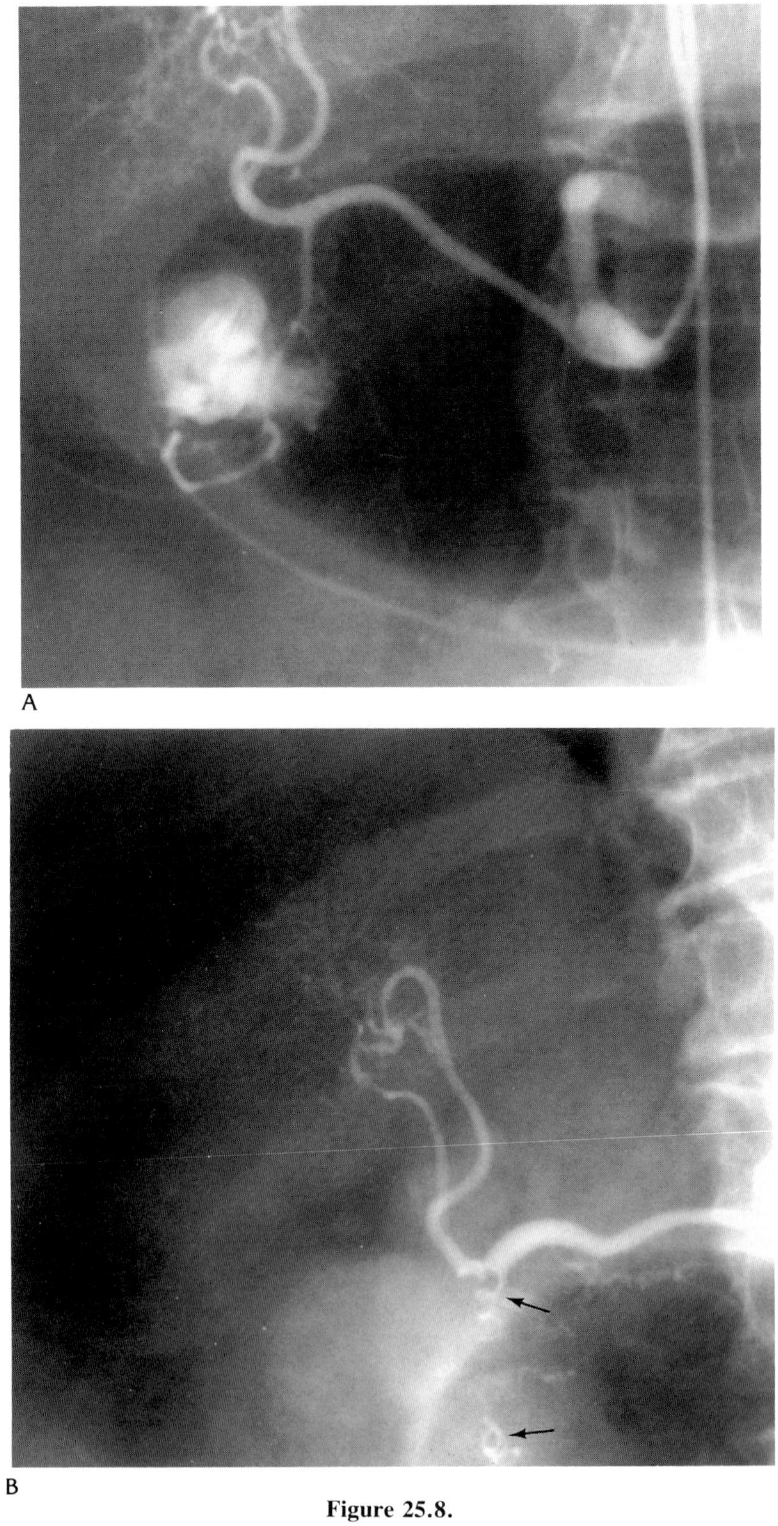

Figure 25.8.

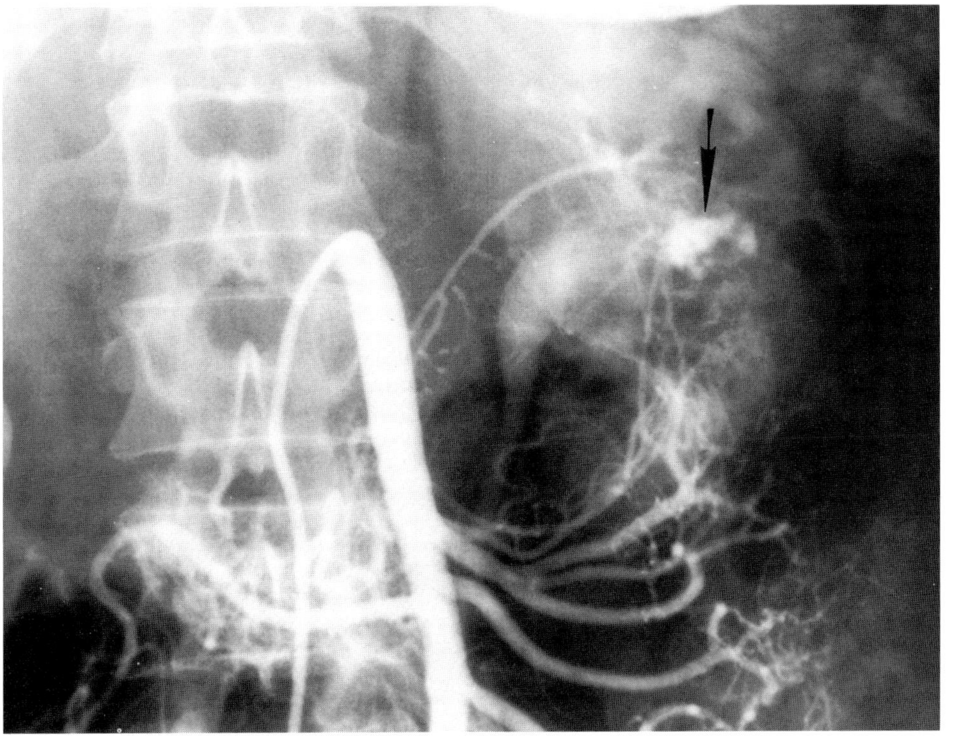

Figure 25.9. Bleeding from an anastomotic ulcer following partial gastrectomy and Billroth II anastomosis. After a left gastric arteriogram failed to demonstrate a bleeding site, the superior mesenteric artery was catheterized and an arteriogram was performed. This showed a bleeding site (*arrow*) from a proximal jejunal branch connected with the anastomotic loop.

ligated,'' with the embolic occlusion placed both proximal and distal to the site of extravasation (Figure 25.8).

If the embolic therapy proves ineffective and surgery is required, prolonged delays in the angiography suite can considerably worsen the prognosis. Furthermore, even when it successfully stops the bleeding, angiographic therapy is only a temporary measure. In most cases, an operation is still required to deal with the underlying problem. Because of the chronicity of the underlying disease process and the difficulty of controlling bleeding with transcatheter techniques, angiographic therapy is generally considered inappropriate for bleeding duodenal ulcers except when the patient has other problems that are considered contraindications to surgery.

Figure 25.8. ''Double ligation'' for bleeding originating directly from the gastroduodenal artery. (*A*) A hepatic arteriogram shows extravasation originating directly from the gastroduodenal artery. (The hepatic branches show changes of advanced liver cirrhosis.) (*B*) A coaxial catheter was advanced down the gastroduodenal artery beyond the point of extravasation, and a stainless steel coil was deployed. The catheter was then withdrawn proximal to the extravasation, and a second coil was placed (*arrows*). (Without the distal coil, it is likely that the bleeding would have recurred through collateral vessels.)

Anastomotic Ulcer Bleeding

Bleeding from recurrent ulceration after gastroenterostomy usually originates from jejunal branches of the superior mesenteric artery and can often be controlled by direct infusions of vasopressin into the superior mesenteric artery (Figure 25.9). If the bleeding originates from the gastric remnant, angiographic therapy may be more hazardous, since many of the potential collateral vessels have been ligated during a prior operation.

Small Bowel Bleeding

Gastrointestinal bleeding only occasionally originates in the ileum or jejunum. Small bowel bleeding is usually secondary to infection, tumor, arteriovenous malformation, or inflammatory bowel disease. Because many of these lesions are associated with abnormal

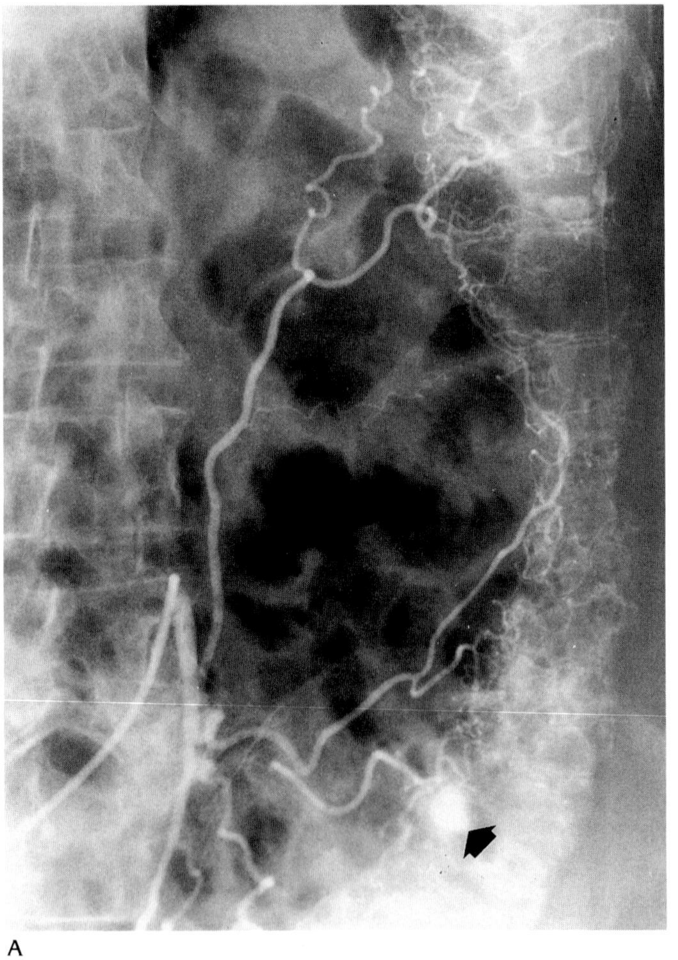

A

Figure 25.10. Bleeding sigmoid diverticulum. (*A*) An inferior mesenteric arteriogram demonstrates extravasation (*arrow*) into a diverticulum in the sigmoid colon. (*B*) After a vasopressin infusion, the bleeding was controlled.

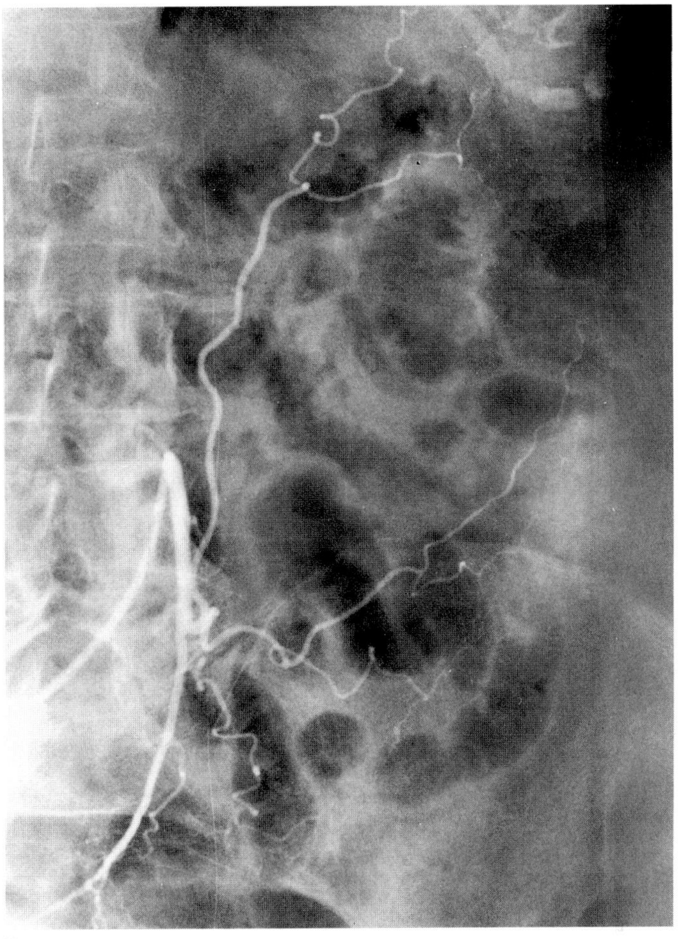

B

vessels, vasopressin therapy is frequently ineffective. Superselective embolic therapy has occasionally been used for patients who are not candidates for surgery, but only when there is life-threatening hemorrhage that does not respond to vasopressin.

Colonic Bleeding

Massive bleeding from the colon is usually secondary to diverticular disease or angiodysplasia and resolves with conservative measures in 90% of patients.[21] Patients bleeding from diverticular disease are usually elderly and have other associated diseases, so that the mortality for those requiring an operation to control bleeding may be as high as 30 to 50%.[21] Mesenteric arteriography can localize the site of bleeding to the right or left colon. Angiographically demonstrated bleeding occurs to the right of the splenic flexure in roughly 65% of all patients studied.[22] Severe diverticular bleeding can be controlled with selective mesenteric arterial infusions of vasopressin in 80 to 90% of patients[23] (Figure 25.10). Rebleeding after successful therapy is uncommon, and the prognosis for patients whose bleeding can be controlled angiographically is similar to that for patients whose bleeding stops spontaneously.

Pancreatic Bleeding

Massive bleeding from the pancreas occurs as a complication of pancreatitis, pseudocyst, abscess, or surgery. Selective embolization of the responsible pancreatic branch can usually stop the hemorrhage acutely, but because of the nature of these lesions and the arterial anatomy of the pancreas, rebleeding from collateral vessels or from another site is common (Figure 25.11).

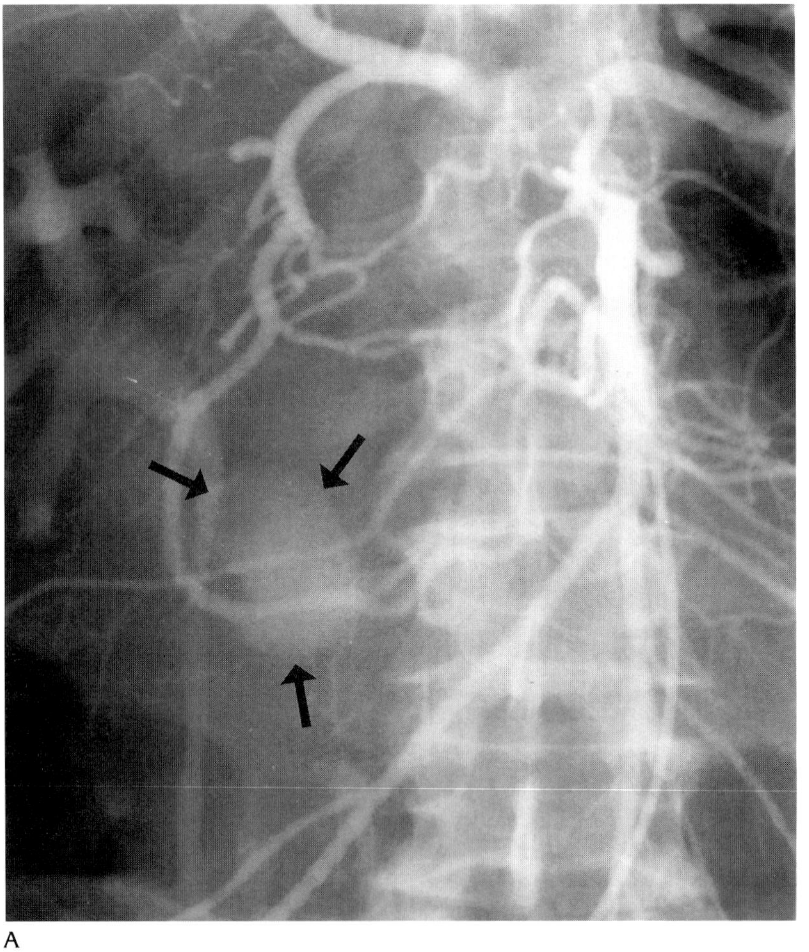

A

Figure 25.11. Bleeding from a false aneurysm secondary to pancreatitis and pseudocyst. (*A*) A superior mesenteric arteriogram shows stretching of the pancreatic head branches around a large false aneurysm (arrows). (*B*) The inferior pancreaticoduodenal artery was selectively catheterized and injected to show the site of the false aneurysm (*arrow*). (*C*) The vessel associated with the false aneurysm was subselectively catheterized, and coils were placed to occlude the artery on either side of the aneurysm.

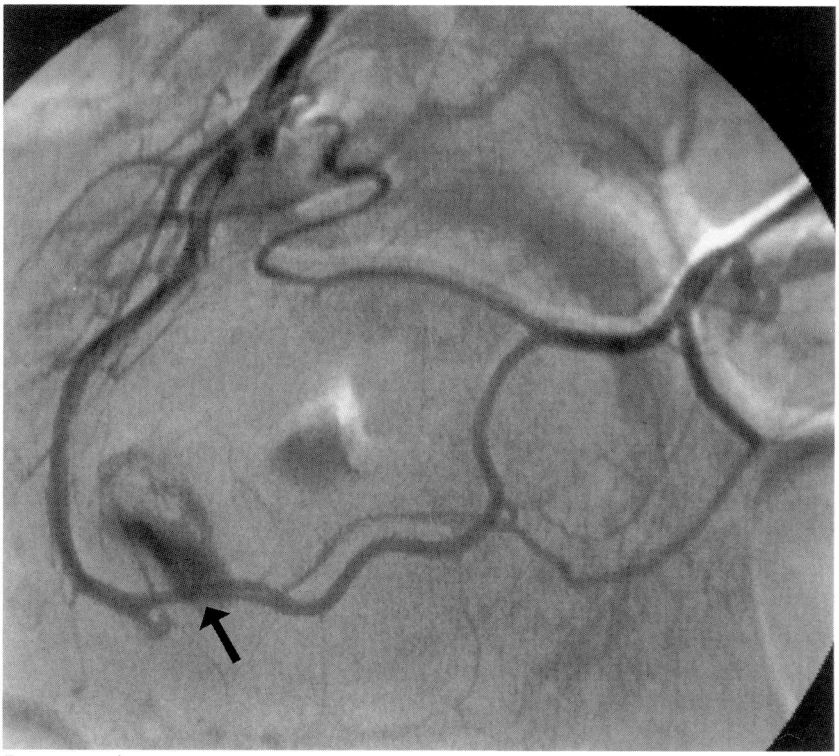

B

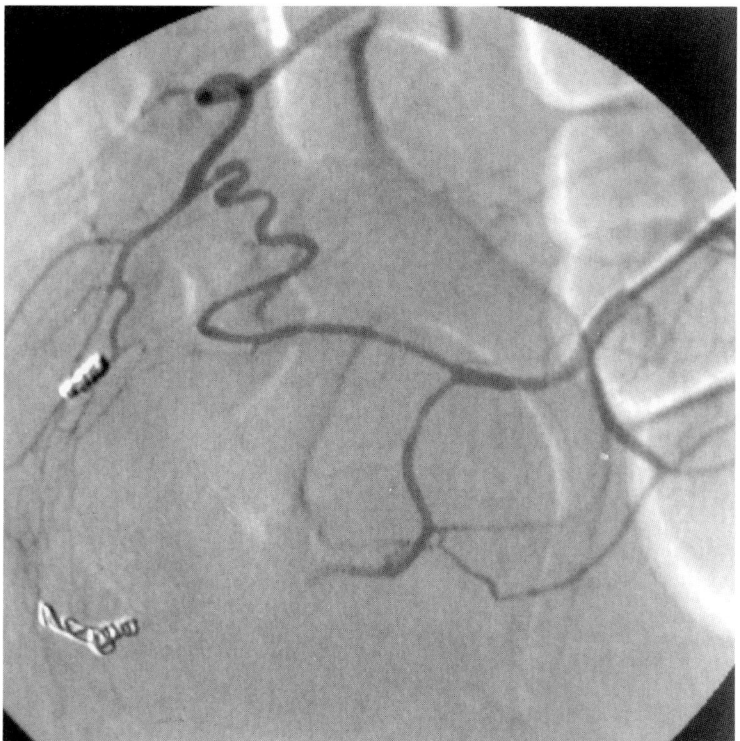

C

Hemobilia

Hemobilia after trauma or percutaneous intervention is especially well suited for transcatheter embolization therapy (Figures 25.12, 25.13). Modern superselective catheterization techniques using small coaxial catheters generally limit the extent of the occlusion to the single involved bleeding branch. However, major hepatic artery branches can

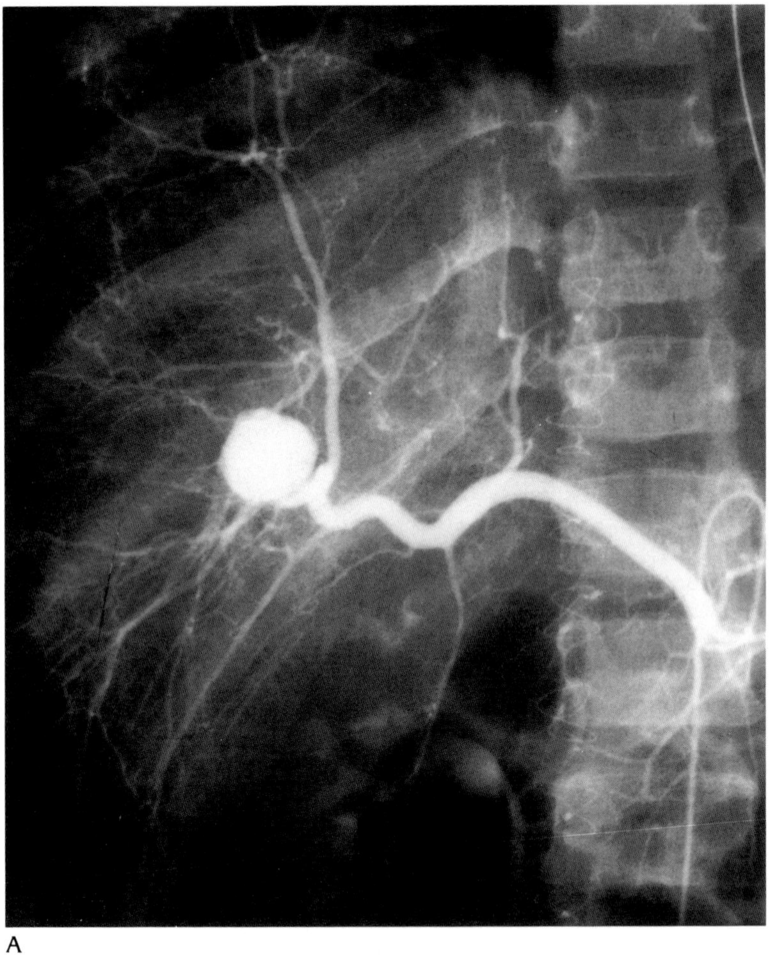

A

Figure 25.12. Embolization of the hepatic artery for traumatic hemobilia. (*A*) A hepatic arteriogram shows a false aneurysm of a branch of the right hepatic artery. (*B*) The hepatic artery was embolized with pieces of Gelfoam, and the false aneurysm was occluded.

Figure 25.13. Hemobilia after percutaneous liver biopsy. (*A*) A hepatic arteriogram shows a fistula between a hepatic artery branch and a peripheral biliary radical (*arrows*). (*B*) A late film from the arteriogram shows opacification of the duct, which is distended by clot (*arrows*). (*C*) The specific bleeding branch was catheterized and occluded with a stainless steel coil (*arrow*).

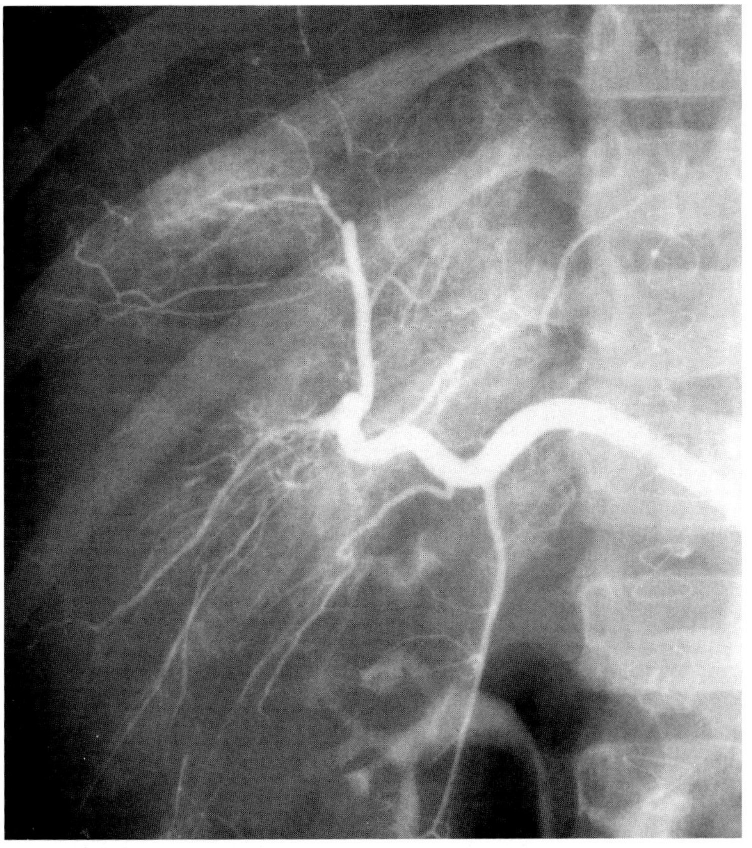

B

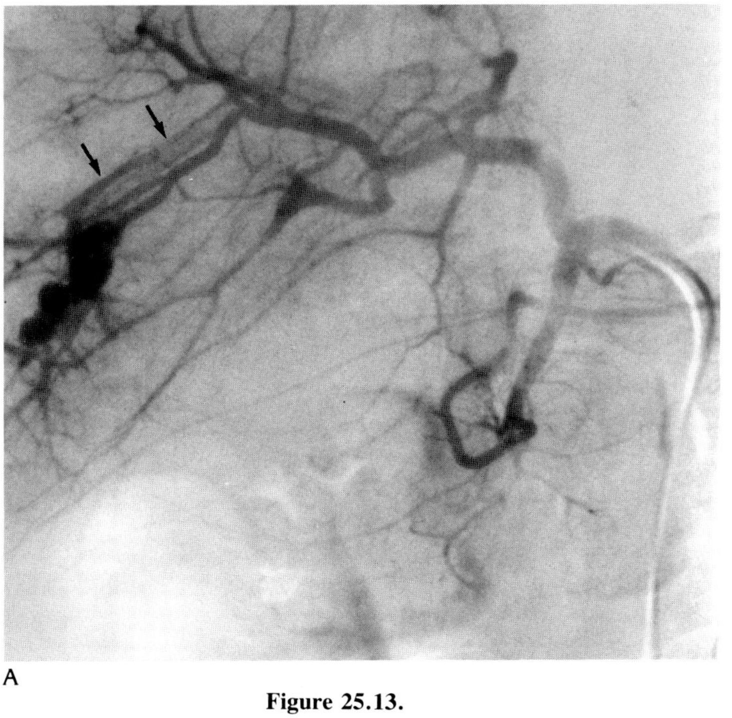

A

Figure 25.13.

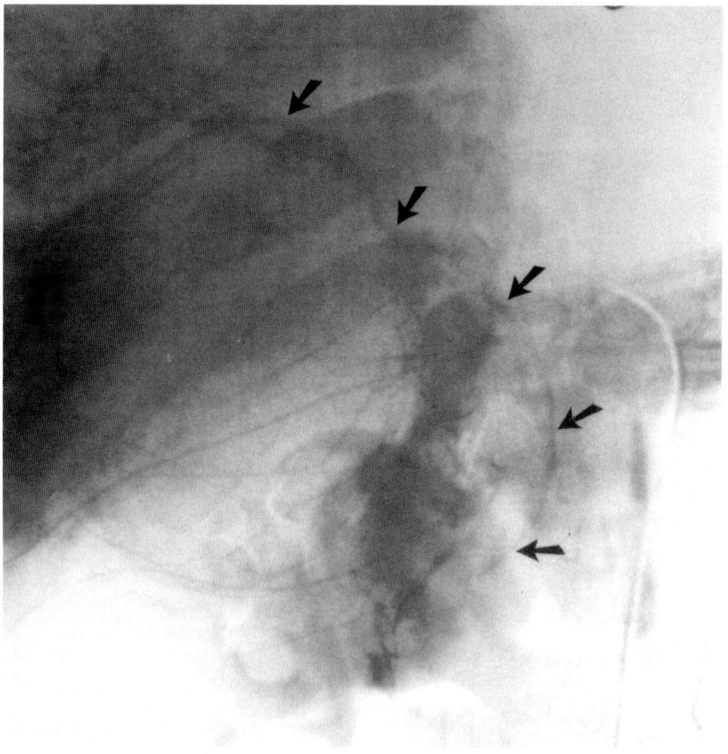

B

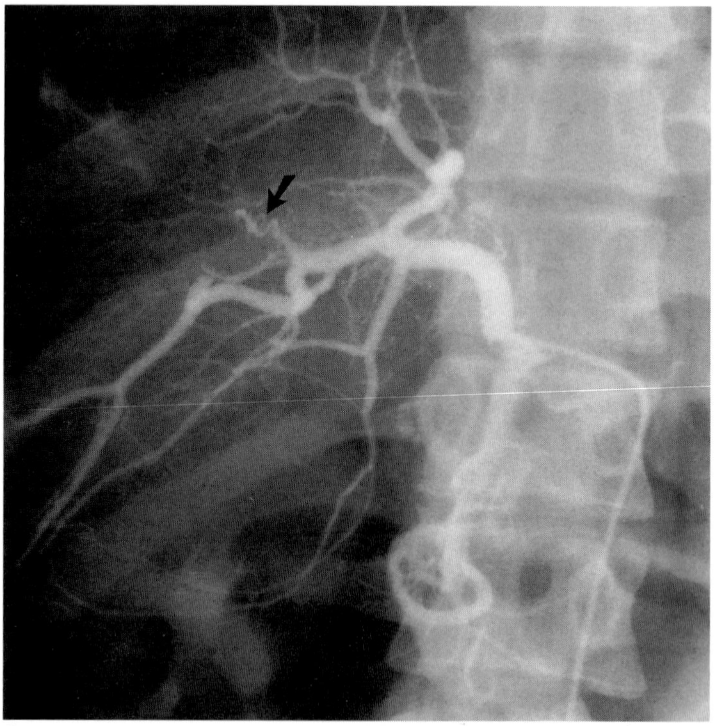

C

Figure 25.13. (Continued)

be safely embolized as long as portal vein flow is normal.[24] Dearterialization of the liver is remarkably safe because the portal venous flow provides adequate nutrients.

REFERENCES

1. Nusbaum M, Baum S: Radiographic demonstration of unknown sites of GI bleeding. *Surg Forum* 14:374, 1963.
2. Baum S, Nusbaum M, Blakemore WS, et al: The pre-operative radiographic demonstration of intra-abdominal bleeding from undetermined sites by percutaneous selective celiac and superior mesenteric arteriography. *Surgery* 58:797, 1965.
3. Nusbaum M, Baum S, Blakemore WS, et al: Demonstration of intra-abdominal bleeding by selective arteriography: Visualization of celiac and superior mesenteric arteries. *JAMA* 191:389–390, 1965.
4. Nusbaum M, Baum S: The control of gastrointestinal hemorrhage by selective mesenteric arterial infusion of vasopressin. *Radiology* 98:497–505, 1971.
5. Nusbaum M, Baum S, Blakemore WS, et al: Clinical experience with selective intra-arterial infusion of vasopressin in the control of gastrointestinal bleeding from arterial sources. *Am J Surg* 123:165–172, 1972.
6. Baum S, Athanasoulis CA, Waltman AC, et al: Angiographic diagnosis and control. *Adv Surg* 7:49, 1973.
7. Carsen GM, Casarella WJ, Spiegel RM: Transcatheter embolization for treatment of Mallory-Weiss tears of the esophagogastric junction. *Radiology* 128(2):309–313, 1978.
8. Waltman AC, Greenfield AJ, Novelline RA, et al: Pyloroduodenal bleeding and intra-arterial vasopressin: Clinical results. *AJR* 133:643, 1979.
9. Athanasoulis CA: Therapeutic applications of angiography. *N Engl J Med* 302(20):1117–1125, 1980.
10. Rosch J, Dotter CT, Antonovic R: Selective vasoconstrictor infusion in the management of arterio-capillary gastrointestinal hemorrhage. *AJR* 116:279, 1972.
11. Chuang VP, Reuter ST: Selective arterial embolization for control of traumatic splenic bleeding. *Invest Radiol* 10(1):18–24, 1975.
12. Waltman AC, Greenfield AJ, Novelline RA, et al: Pyloroduodenal bleeding and intra-arterial vasopressin: Clinical results. *AJR* 133:643, 1979.
13. White RI, Harrington DP, Novak G, et al: Pharmacologic control of hemorrhagic gastritis: Clinical and experimental results. *Radiology* 111:549–557, 1974.
14. Gold RE, Grace M: Gelfoam embolization of the left gastric artery for bleeding ulcer. *Radiology* 116:575–580, 1975.
15. Alavi A: Radionuclide localization of gastrointestinal hemorrhage [Letter]. *Radiology* 142:801–803, 1982.
16. Miskowiak J, Nielsen SL, Munck O: Scintigraphic diagnosis of gastrointestinal bleeding with 99m-Tc-labeled blood-pool agents. *Radiology* 141:499, 1981.
17. Simmons JT, Baum S, Sheehan BA, et al: The effect of vasopressin on hepatic arterial blood flow. *Radiology* 124:637–640, 1977.
18. Conn HO, Ramsby GR, Sterer EH: Hepatic arterial escape from vasopressin induced vasoconstriction: An angiographic investigation. *AJR* 24:399, 1973.
19. Athanasoulis CA, Baum S, Waltman AC, et al: Control of acute gastric mucosal hemorrhage; intra-arterial infusion of posterior pituitary extract. *N Engl J Med* 290:597–603, 1974.

20. Bradley EL 3d, Goldman ML: Gastric infarction after therapeutic embolization. *Surgery* 79:421–424, 1976.
21. Behringer GF, Albright NL: Diverticular disease of the colon: A frequent cause of rectal bleeding. *Am J Surg* 125:419–423, 1973.
22. Cassarella WJ, Kanter TE, Seaman WB: Right-sided colonic diverticula as a cause of acute rectal hemorrhage. *N Engl J Med* 286:450, 1972.
23. Baum S, Rosch J, Dotter CT, et al: Selective mesenteric arterial infusions in the management of massive diverticular hemorrhage. *N Engl J Med* 288:1269–1272, 1973.
24. Tegtmeyer CJ, Besidjian DR, Gerguson WW: Transcatheter control of iatrogenic hemobilia. *Cardiovasc Intervent Radiol* 4:88, 1981.

26

SURGICAL TREATMENT FOR MASSIVE NON-VARICEAL UPPER GASTROINTESTINAL HEMORRHAGE

Christopher Steffes, M.D.
David Fromm, M.D.

DEFINITION OF MASSIVE HEMORRHAGE

There is no uniform definition of massive hemorrhage. This is largely related to the difficulty of accurate assessment of the magnitude of bleeding when the patient is first seen, as opposed to retrospective criteria (e.g., 40% loss of blood volume, hemoglobin below 8 g/dl). The problem is compounded by the fact that the bleeding may occur over several days before meeting given criteria of massive bleeding. However, most clinicians would agree that major blood loss has occurred when vital (including postural) signs are unstable.

LESIONS

Peptic ulcer disease is the most common cause of significant upper gastrointestinal hemorrhage. Esophageal varices, the second most frequent cause, is considered in detail in Part VI. Peptic ulcer (27–47%), acute gastric mucosal lesions (23–33%) Mallory-Weiss syndrome (2–11%), and esophagitis (3–13%) constitute the majority of causes in large series.[1-4] The variability reflects differences in community and urban hospital populations. However, bleeding peptic ulcers are the most frequent lesions requiring surgery.[1]

INDICATIONS AND TIMING FOR SURGERY

The indications for and optimum timing of surgery remain controversial. Most of the information comes from patients with bleeding peptic ulcers. Thus, a certain degree of extrapolation to other lesions is presently unavoidable. Several reports suggest that an aggressive policy of early operation leads to a decrease in mortality, particularly in patients older than 60 years.[5-8] For example, a threefold decrease in mortality (from 12 to 3.9%) has been reported with the use of an aggressive but selective policy of management.[9] However, this has not been a uniform observation.[10,11] The problem is that there are reports of increased, decreased, or unchanged mortality associated with surgery.[10] The confounding variables in these reports include differences in the threshold for emergency surgery and in the study populations, as well as patient exclusion criteria and the fact that most bleeding stops spontaneously. An aggressive policy increases operative rates,[5,12] and in one sense some patients will undergo an unnecessary operation (at least at that particular time), since they might have stopped bleeding spontaneously.[5,13] However, minimizing both the short- and long-term risks of transfusion should not be underestimated.

An important factor relating to the timing of an operation is the general agreement that an elective operation for bleeding is associated with a lower postoperative mortality. However, blind subscription to this tenet in an attempt to stabilize the patient by giving an excessive number of transfusions leads to unnecessary exclusion of an emergent operation. For example, a high-risk patient can become an even worse risk if allowed to undergo additional periods of hemodynamic instability and/or given an excessive number of transfusions. Recommendations for the timing of surgery are further complicated by difficulties in meaningful comparisons of published mortality data for peptic ulcer because of variable patient selection in retrospective studies.[14]

The necessity for emergent operation is obvious in the presence of uncontrolled bleeding, but the key in proceeding with surgery for other patients lies in the identification of those who are at high risk for continuing bleeding or rebleeding. Delaying an operation until a second bleed occurs may increase the mortality.[8] The principal factors predicting the risk of continued or recurrent bleeding are age, magnitude of blood loss (including shock), and endoscopic appearance of the ulcer.[15,16]

There is considerable disagreement about basing the decision to operate on the magnitude of the bleed or the occurrence of rebleeding.[6,7,13,17,18] Traditional criteria include a transfusion requirement of more than 5 units,[9] or more than 1 unit every eight hours, or the presence of shock. Selection for surgery is a problem in some cases when successful resuscitation is followed by stability, which is generally indicative of (at least temporarily) cessation or diminution of bleeding. However, the presence of shock on admission has been found to carry a 70% risk of rebleeding. Thus, many surgeons consider shock as an indication for operation[16] even though hemodynamic stability has been achieved. A prospective study (without the aid of endoscopic diagnosis) found that immediate operation for patients presenting in shock reduced the overall mortality from 23% to zero.[8]

Some advocate operation for the first episode of in-hospital rebleeding,[9] but others wait until after the second episode of rebleeding in a patient under 50 years of age.[19] A repeat admission for hemorrhage is considered an indication for surgery, as is a history of repeated small bleeds.[20] A prohibitive operative risk would deter one from operating but this should be a truly inordinate risk, since many series indicate that elderly patients benefit from early surgery.[7]

Certainly, an immediate operation is required in the presence of refractory shock, where the blood pressure does not respond to fluid and blood administration. Bleeding of such magnitude is due to erosion of the ulcer into a major artery. If a spurting vessel is seen and is not controlled by available endoscopic means, emergent surgery is necessary. If the bleeding is controlled by endoscopic means, it has been recommended that surgery should be performed within 24 hours, as soon as the patient is stabilized.[20] Our results suggest that an early aggressive operative approach after attempted or temporizing endoscopic control is associated with a favorable outcome.[1]

The presence of stigmata of recent hemorrhage associated with rebleeding, such as a visible vessel/sentinel clot, an oozing ulcer base, or a black spot or fresh clot, is a strong consideration for surgery.[6,7] Absence of such stigmata is reassuring.[16] The location of the ulcer is another consideration.[21] Prepyloric ulcers, in contrast to typical more proximal (type I) gastric ulcers, rarely bleed.[16] The incidence of rebleeding is also reported to be significantly greater when the ulcer is located high along the lesser curve of the stomach in the vicinity of the left gastric artery or in the duodenum in the vicinity of the gastroduodenal artery.[21] The majority of patients with combined ulcers have an element of pyloric stenosis and the gastric ulcers tend to be large and deep, making them prone to hemorrhage.

Certain clinical variables are believed to influence the outcome and should be considered in the decision to operate. Rebleeding is significantly associated with age greater than 60 years, admission hemoglobin less than 8.0 g/dl, and hematemesis on admission, along with endoscopic stigmata of recent hemorrhage.[22,23] The presence of melena on admission may represent an increased risk. Shock combined with endoscopic findings of a visible vessel or clot predicted rebleeding in several studies.[22,24] However, others find that endoscopically observed stigmata add little value to shock in predicting rebleeding.[16,25] Still others report that age greater than 60 years, admission hemoglobin less than 10 g/dl, shock, previous ulcer surgery, a history of medication use, the presence of a gastric ulcer, and endoscopic stigmata of recent hemorrhage are all associated with an increased risk of rebleeding.[15]

Several of the indications for operation for bleeding ulcer are listed in Table 26.1. A protocol that we have found useful calls for *emergent* operation if 3 units of blood initially given do not restore hemodynamic stability or if 3 units achieved hemodynamic stability but maintenance of the latter requires more than one transfusion in any subsequent eight-hour period. This approach has been shown to be associated with the same mortality as that for patients operated on immediately after resuscitation and thus avoids, to some degree, unnecessary emergent operation.[26]

OTHER FACTORS INFLUENCING SURGICAL MANAGEMENT

Coagulation abnormalities should be corrected before a decision to operate is made. Platelet function abnormalities, manifested by a prolonged bleeding time, can occur with the use of aspirin or nonsteroidal anti-inflammatory drugs. Bleeding from drug-induced erosions or associated ulcers may stop precipitously after platelet transfusion if the bleeding time is prolonged. A history of anticoagulant use or underlying hematological disease is sometimes overlooked initially. Thrombocytopenia is more frequent with the increasing use of chemotherapy. Deficiencies in vitamin K–dependent clotting factors and clinically significant thrombocytopenia can occur in the presence of liver disease. Cryoprecipitate or 1-deamino-8-D-arginine vasopressin (especially in uremic gastritis[27]) are useful in specific clotting factor deficiencies.

TABLE 26.1. Various Reported Indications for Operation for Bleeding Peptic Ulcer

- Uncontrolled bleeding
- First episode of rebleeding (age >60 years)
- In-hospital rebleeding
- Second episode of in-hospital rebleeding (age <60 years)
- Previous admission for bleeding
- Repeated small bleeds
- Bleeding while receiving optimal nonoperative treatment
- Refractory shock
- Shock on arrival (age >60 years)
- Endoscopic appearance
  - Spurting artery
  - Oozing base
  - Visible vessel
  - Sentinel clot
  - Fresh clot
- Location near gastroduodenal or left gastric artery
- Previously documented ulcer
- Two-year history of dyspepsia
- Age >60
- Therapy
  - >3 units initial blood replacement
  - 3 units initial blood replacement restoring hemodynamic stability, but then requires >1 unit in any 8-hour period
  - >5 units of blood transfusion and/or 1 unit blood every 6 hours
  - 8 units of blood or colloid replacement in 48 hours (age >60 years)
  - 8 units of blood or colloid for initial replacement or 12 units in 48 hours (age <60 years)

Source: Reference 14.

Significant underlying medical illness is often used as a reason to avoid early operation. However, this argument should take into account the prognosis of the illness in question. The problem is that the patient with significant underlying illness is the one who can least tolerate the stress of bleeding, which may be greater than the stress of a carefully done operation.

Cirrhotic patients with bleeding unrelated to portal hypertension also present a problem. In these patients, mortality approaches that predicted by the Child's classification for portasystemic shunts.

The mortality due to bleeding from either a duodenal or gastric ulcer more than doubles after age 60. Some physicians continue to be less aggressive about advising early operation for bleeding duodenal ulcer as opposed to gastric ulcer. This is based on the erroneous belief that the mortality for bleeding gastric ulcer is twice that for bleeding duodenal ulcer. However, this does not appear to be the case when age and other factors are matched. An aggressive approach leading to operation in patients over age 60 is supported by a prospective study in which the criteria for early operation included 4 units of blood or plasma expander within 24 hours, or one rebleed, or endoscopic evidence of recent bleeding, or a previous episode of bleeding and a two-year history of dyspepsia.[6]

Using this scheme, the mortality was 2% compared to 13% with less stringent criteria. It is the elderly patient with significant other disease(s) who is least likely to withstand an episode of hypovolemic shock. While there is little doubt that younger patients tolerate hemodynamic instability better, one should not underestimate the morbidity of this event or the morbidity in such patients.

GASTRIN

The incidence of gastrinoma and antral G cell hyperfunction (or antral G cell hyperplasia) is rare relative to that of ordinary peptic ulcer disease. Yet, significant morbidity occurs as a result of incorrect treatment. Less than complete removal of the antral mucosa is insufficient for the treatment of antral G cell hyperfunction, and not knowing that the patient has a gastrinoma usually leads to inaccurate exploration and operation, even though the approach to such patients is controversial.

Serum gastrin measurements are frequently neglected in patients who present with an acute complication of peptic ulcer disease such as bleeding. Waiting for the result of this measurement will unnecessarily delay an urgent or emergent operation. However, full treatment with an H_2 receptor antagonist can be continued postoperatively until the gastrin value is known.

SPECIFIC SITUATIONS

Esophagitis

Esophagitis rarely is a source of massive bleeding requiring operative intervention. Nonoperative treatment is effective in the majority of cases. However, if an operation is required, a so-called valvuloplastic procedure (e.g., Nissen fundoplication) frequently is all that is necessary to control the diffuse oozing.[28]

Mallory-Weiss Syndrome

The Mallory-Weiss syndrome occurs in 8 to 15% of patients with acute upper gastrointestinal bleeding.[29,30] Up to 86% of patients have a history of antecedent vomiting, retching, coughing, or straining.[29,30] More than 80% of the mucosal tears are located on the lesser gastric curve at the esophagogastric junction and mostly involve the gastric mucosa, extending to the submucosa. The tears are multiple in 17% of patients. Other lesions frequently coexist with the Mallory-Weiss tear, especially gastric erosions[29,30] due to ingestion of aspirin, nonsteroidal anti-inflammatory agents, or alcohol.

More than 90% of tears stop bleeding spontaneously, and many can be controlled by endoscopic means. Surgery has been recommended after the transfusion of approximately 6 units of blood[29] in patients of acceptable risk, but the actual number of required transfusions before undertaking an operation is not established. An anterior gastrotomy with oversewing of the bleeding mucosa is sufficient for hemostasis. Mortality in Mallory-Weiss syndrome is reported to be 3 or 4%, but many of the deaths occur in cirrhotic patients.

Acute Gastric Mucosal Lesions

Stress ulcers are superficial and occur on a background of mucosal inflammation. Unlike peptic ulcer, stress ulcer is not a primary disease of the upper gastrointestinal tract but rather an indication of severe underlying illness. Sepsis, shock, trauma, and burns are predisposing conditions.

The major manifestation of stress gastritis and ulceration is hemorrhage. Uncontrolled bleeding from stress ulcer rarely occurs today, provided that there is rapid resuscitation and attention to metabolic care and prophylaxis. Upper gastrointestinal bleeding has been almost completely eliminated in burn patients receiving aggressive control of gastric luminal pH.[31] A number of nonoperative methods have been proposed to deal with uncontrollable bleeding from stress ulcers.

Surgical intervention is rarely necessary but is obviously indicated when nonoperative methods fail. The operation of choice is controversial because of high incidence of rebleeding. The operative mortality also is high, ranging from 17 to 34% in some series.[32] The procedures most frequently performed have been vagotomy with drainage, vagotomy with gastrectomy, and subtotal gastrectomy. There is a role for total gastrectomy, which probably is the procedure of choice if bleeding persists despite rigorous control of gastric pH. Alternatively, the stomach can be devascularized by ligating both gastroepiploic and both gastric arteries, leaving only the short gastric vessels intact.[33] In all operative procedures with the exception of total gastrectomy, the mucosal bleeding points may be suture-ligated. The operative management of bleeding stress ulcer must be accompanied by continued prophylaxis (if total gastrectomy was not done) and continued efforts to correct the underlying illness which led to the stress ulcers.

Bleeding as a result of alcohol- or drug- (aspirin and nonsteroidal anti-inflammatory drugs) associated gastritis rarely requires operation. Here too, the operative approach remains controversial, but the same principles applicable to stress gastritis generally apply.

While the gastric mucosal changes due to stress ulcer in the majority of instances are similar to those associated with intracranial disease or trauma, the latter (referred to as *Cushing's ulcers*) are associated with hypersecretion of acid,[34] which may be real or relative to that observed for stress ulcer. The classic Cushing's ulcer involves a greater area of mucosal erosion than a stress ulcer, but many patients with cerebral trauma also have hypotension due to other concomitant injuries. While there may be a crossover effect between stress and Cushing's ulcers in such patients, classic Cushing's ulcers are rarely seen today. Gross mucosal changes identical to stress ulcers occur in patients with severe trauma restricted to the brain and in the absence of corticosteroid treatment. Prophylactic treatment directed at the hypersecretion of acid is effective in preventing hemorrhage. In the rare event that operation for continuing hemorrhage is required, suture ligation of the bleeding points and vagotomy with drainage are effective, according to anecdotal reports.

Penetrating Duodenal Ulcer

Most cases of massive hemorrhage from a peptic duodenal ulcer involve penetration of the gastroduodenal arterial complex.[35] Three-point ligation that encompasses the gastroduodenal artery proximal and distal to the area of penetration, as well as the transverse pancreatic artery originating from the gastroduodenal arterial complex, is an important maneuver for preventing rebleeding in the immediate postoperative period. Use of a stout needle is required to pierce the scar tissue deep enough to secure the blood vessels. A definitive operation is also done to facilitate healing of the ulcer and prevent rebleeding.

The type of definitive operation (vagotomy with drainage, vagotomy with antrectomy, subtotal gastrectomy, or proximal gastric vagotomy) done for bleeding duodenal ulcer depends on the operative approach to the bleeding site, the anatomical circumstances, and the experience of the surgeon. No matter which operation is favored, it is not necessary to excise the ulcer; to do so invites complications.

The majority of patients will stabilize once control of hemorrhage is obtained. The decision to do a definitive procedure in the relatively unstable patient must be weighed against the concept that this is precisely the patient who cannot tolerate a future hemorrhage. This is not always prevented by intensive treatment with medication(s), and the overall risk of rebleeding is substantial.

If proximal gastric vagotomy is favored, some thought must be given to this procedure before opening the duodenum. The general tendency is to make a longitudinal duodenotomy that cuts across the pylorus. While the latter can be repaired, this does not guarantee satisfactory pyloric function. Thus, a transverse duodenotomy is favored to gain access to the bleeding ulcer if proximal vagotomy is to be done. The duodenotomy can be closed in the same direction it was made without compromising the lumen.

If a longitudinal duodenotomy is performed and, in haste, it is made too long or there is significant scarring, there may be luminal compromise from a Heinecke-Mickulicz pyloroplasty. In this case, it is safer to close the duodenum securely, without regard to preservation of the luminal diameter, and perform a gastrojejunostomy.

There are no substantive data indicating that one type of drainage procedure is better than another. Both the Finney and Jaboulay procedures are cumbersome (both are side-to-side gastroduodenostomies, but in Finney's operation the pylorus is transsected as well). Thus, most surgeons favor either the Heinecke-Mickulicz pyloroplasty or gastroenterostomy.

If gastrectomy is favored (either antrectomy with truncal vagotomy or subtotal gastrectomy), thought must be given to the quality of the duodenal stump for either closure or anastomosis to the residual stomach. There are no substantive data indicating that a gastrojejunal approach (Billroth II) is a better procedure for bleeding duodenal ulcer than a gastroduodenal reconstruction (Billroth I). One must determine if safe transection of the duodenum can be performed and if the circumstances are optimal for healing. Several situations pose problems in dealing with the proximal duodenum (Table 26.2). The long axis of the duodenum can be shortened by fibrosis, thus drawing the ampulla of Vater proximally close to the distal edge of the ulcer. A posterior ulcer may encompass the accessory pancreatic duct (Santorini) or cause considerable fibrotic reaction from burrowing into the pancreas. The fibrosis associated with a superiorly situated ulcer can draw the pylorus distally, placing it in even closer proximity to the common bile duct without apparent distortion of the pylorus; on rare occasions, the ulcer may appear to penetrate or actually penetrate the wall of the common bile duct. Periduodenal fibrosis may also distort the course of the common hepatic artery, making it vulnerable to injury during dissection. Fibrosis resulting from an inferiorly situated ulcer may encompass the transverse mesocolon, making the middle colic vessels susceptible to injury. Edema of

Table 26.2. Technical Hazards of Operating on the Difficult Duodenum

Shortening of the long axis, drawing the ampulla of Vater close to the ulcer
Ulcer encompassing the accessory pancreatic duct
Ulcer penetrating the pancreas
Fibrosis drawing the pylorus in proximity to the common bile duct
Ulcer penetrating the common bile duct
Distortion of the common hepatic artery
Fibrosis encompassing vessels of the transverse mesocolon
Scarred duodenum resulting in imperfect suture placement or healing

the duodenum and fibrosis in general are situations that can result in imperfect placement of sutures and/or healing. Thus, when problems with the duodenum can be anticipated, it is best to avoid transection of the duodenum and settle for a less adventurous operative procedure.

It is insufficient merely to transect the right and left vagal trunks during truncal vagotomy. The esophagus must also be circumferentially cleared of tissue immediately adjacent to its muscularis for a distance of 5 to 7 cm. This is necessary to ensure division of vagal branches that originate from the vagal trunks proximal to their sites of transection and innervate the proximal stomach. Such stripping of the esophagus also is an essential part of proximal gastric vagotomy.

In the presence of transmural esophagitis, the inflamed, softened esophageal wall can be easily perforated or torn. If the esophagus is perforated (as may occur during passage of a finger around the esophagus posteriorly), immediate repair is done. The injured esophagus should be sutured and the suture line may be protected (or reinforced) with a fundoplication.

The patient with portal hypertension presents two major problems. First, the bleeding ulcer may be missed because, in these patients, the ulcer is occasionally situated on the duodenal side of the pyloric ring. Second, varices in the vicinity of the esophagus may preclude safe vagotomy. Thus, preference is given to a subtotal gastrectomy if hemodynamic stability is achieved following control of the ulcer bleeding site.

Gastric Ulcer

Treatment of bleeding gastric ulcer is associated with different anatomical hazards and fewer options for definitive control of the disease than duodenal ulcer. After controlling the hemorrhage in an elderly, unstable patient, one must determine the merits of continuing the operative procedure by doing something definitive for the ulcer disease. In such patients, some surgeons prefer just to excise a bleeding gastric ulcer locally. If the ulcer lies on the lesser curve and is externally excised without regard for the nerves of Latarjet, the patient is at risk for functional gastric outlet obstruction as a result of antral denervation. Thus, it is safer to perform a gastrotomy, suture-ligate the bleeding site, and excise the ulcer from within the gastric lumen, leaving the submucosa or at least the serosa intact. The resulting defect is closed within the gastric lumen. If the ulcer is just excised, it is imperative to continue prophylactic treatment for the ulcer disease with medication. This has been anecdotally successful in short-term follow-up but there is question about long-term efficacy, especially in patients taking nonsteroidal anti-inflammatory agents.

The standard operative approach for a type I gastric ulcer is antrectomy without vagotomy. The effectiveness of removing all of the antrum lies in the fact that this procedure removes the transitional zone lying at the junction of parietal-cell-bearing and antral-cell-bearing mucosa or ulcer-bearing area,[36] while at the same time reducing acid secretion. In the case of combined (gastric and duodenal) ulcer disease (type II), antrectomy (for the gastric ulcer) with vagotomy (for the duodenal ulcer) is the procedure of choice. The same approach is used for prepyloric or pyloric ulcers (type III), which appear to respond better to antrectomy with vagotomy than to either procedure alone.[37]

Definitive surgery for gastric ulcer requires removal of all of the antral mucosa,[37] which is not necessarily accomplished by hemigastrectomy per se. The antral mucosa may extend to the area near the cardioesophageal junction along the lesser curve, giving preference to a Schoemaker resection, which involves resection of more of the lesser than the greater curve.[36] There has been some enthusiasm for a nonresective procedure, either truncal vagotomy with drainage or proximal gastric vagotomy. However, most reports indicate that these procedures are associated with higher rates of ulcer recurrence.[37]

Patients with a lesser curve ulcer near the esophagogastric junction (type IV) have extension of the antral mucosa to this level. Type IV ulcers comprise 4 to 5% of gastric ulcers and have a propensity to present with bleeding. The curious nature of ulcers in this location is that Kelling in 1918 and Madlener in 1923 both demonstrated that resection of as little as 5 cm of distal stomach results in prompt healing. Some report healing after vagotomy with drainage, while others find a 12% recurrence when gastrectomy is not done. A delay in gastric emptying of liquids has been observed in patients with type IV ulcers. This may account for the efficacy of destruction or excision of the pylorus while leaving the transitional zone intact.

The hazard of antrectomy for a high-lying lesser curve ulcer is that it may result in compromise of the cardioesophageal junction. This is easily avoided by doing antrectomy without clamps in a ''freehand'' fashion using an electrosurgical instrument. An esophageal bougie is placed per os into the stomach if there is concern about compromising the cardioesophageal junction during resection or closure of the proximal aspect of the gastric stump. If there is compromise of the cardioesophageal junction during excision of a proximal lesser curve ulcer, the situation is remedied by a Roux-en-Y jejunal reconstruction that includes the cardioesophageal junction in the suture line.

Patients should be advised postoperatively to avoid aspirin-containing compounds and nonsteroidal anti-inflammatory drugs. The latter are believed to be a major factor in 25% of patients with gastric ulcer, in 39% of patients with prepyloric ulcers, and in 20% of postoperative ulcer recurrences.[37]

Gastrinoma

If a patient is known to have a gastrinoma and suffers from a massively bleeding ulcer while receiving therapy for the Zollinger-Ellison syndrome, serious consideration must be given to a total gastrectomy.

POSTOPERATIVE COMPLICATIONS

Wound Infection

Due to unavoidable contamination of the operative field by blood emanating from the gastrointestinal lumen, some authors report a wound infection rate as high as 30%. This has prompted several surgeons to leave the skin and subcutaneous tissues open for at least the immediate postoperative period.

Aspiration Pneumonia

Many patients have experienced a greater than expected incidence of aspiration pneumonia diagnosed in the immediate postoperative period. This is most likely not a consequence of surgery per se, but rather is due to vomiting while an oro- or nasogastric tube is in place preoperatively and/or is a complication of endoscopy.

Hemorrhage

A few patients will have recurrent upper gastrointestinal bleeding postoperatively. If a nasogastric tube is used, a small amount of bleeding may be noted in the immediate postoperative period. This ceases spontaneously and essentially can be ignored. In contrast, some patients (1% or less) will have significant bleeding from the suture line in the face of normal coagulation parameters within 24 hours of the operation. Anastomotic bleeding rarely requires reoperation, since it almost always stops spontaneously, even though transfusion may be required. Bleeding may also be noted on about the seventh postoperative day. This rarely requires transfusion and probably is related to dissolution of the internal absorbable anastomotic sutures or, more likely, mucosal necrosis at the suture line. While these considerations generally apply, there is a danger in making an assumption about the cause of postoperative bleeding. Another lesion may have been overlooked or suture ligation of the original bleeding site may not be secure. Endoscopy is frequently helpful in resolving the dilemma.

Dysphagia

An occasional patient may complain of dysphagia, presumably related to edema or an intramural hematoma of the esophagus resulting from vagotomy. Dysphagia generally subsides spontaneously over a one- to two-month period. Troublesome dysphagia is easily treated by swallowing a mercury-weighted bougie (such as a Maloney dilator). More rarely, periesophageal fibrosis may occur and require operative treatment.[38]

Suture Line Disruption and Pancreatitis

Disruption of the duodenal stump suture line occurs more often than leaks from a gastrojejunal or gastroduodenal anastomosis, pyloroplasty, or gastrotomy. Leakage from the duodenal stump occurs in about 2 to 3% of Billroth II gastrectomies for duodenal ulcer and has been associated with a 40 to 80% mortality.[39] Most often, but not invariably, the disruption occurs after a difficult dissection involving the duodenum and thus implies difficulty in obtaining proper closure of the stump. About half of the leaks are clinically evident on the second through fourth days, and the remainder are recognized on the fifth through seventh postoperative days.[40] The time that this occurs during the first postoperative week does not appear to influence survival.[41]

The presentation of suture line disruption can be difficult to distinguish from acute pancreatitis. Pancreatitis occurring as a result of operative trauma usually is manifested within the first 24 hours (at least retrospectively) of operation, and thus a diagnosis of pancreatitis made later should be suspected.

Difficulty may occur in establishing an early diagnosis, as well as in distinguishing between leakage from a suture line and the onset of acute pancreatitis. Satisfactory radiographic demonstration of all suture lines using a water-soluble contrast medium helps to differentiate between a leak and pancreatitis. However, radiographs demonstrating intact suture lines can be misleading, because the leakage initially may be quite small and may subsequently progress. If contrast cannot be made to reflux into the afferent limb of a gastrojejunal anastomosis, it must be assumed that duodenal stump disruption occurred as a result of afferent limb obstruction.

Treatment of a free anastomotic leak involves those principles used in the treatment of an enteric fistula: control of the leak, control of the sepsis, and maintenance of nutrition. The patient is prepared for surgery (restitution of plasma volume, administration of antibiotic(s), etc.) as soon as the diagnosis of free leakage is established. The abdomen is reentered through the previous incision. It is essential that the anastomotic sites are gently manipulated, if at all, in order to avoid further injury. The temptation to merely place a few sutures at the site of disruption should be avoided, since these sutures generally are ineffective and may even enlarge the fistula as further breakdown occurs. Dismantling of a gastroduodenal or gastrojejunal anastomosis in the face of gross peritonitis also creates a problem, because one is dealing with abnormal tissue in a patient who generally is quite ill.

The primary purpose of surgery is to provide drainage (control of the leak and sepsis). It is unusual for the suture line breakdown to be large enough and the surrounding tissue reaction minimal enough to clearly see the site of disruption in order to insert a catheter into the lumen. The precise placement of drains is predicated upon the anatomical extent of the leak and the location of collection(s). Even with what appears to be good drainage, the patient remains at risk for subsequent development of intra-abdominal abscess.

A contained suture line disruption usually presents with persistent fever (often initially attributed to another cause, such as atelectasis) and delayed gastric emptying, the symptoms of which initially can be somewhat subtle (e.g., mild esophageal reflux). A leak which is contained need not be drained, provided that there is good communication with the lumen. Antibiotic treatment for this circumstance usually suffices. Nasogastric suction may be necessary because of attendant peristomal edema.

Gastric Outlet (Stomal) Obstruction

Stomal obstruction occurs in about 5% of patients and usually is not recognized until after the fifth postoperative day.[42] Well-recognized causes include anastomotic edema, stenosis, angulation, leak, adhesions, perianastomotic abscess, intramural hematoma, an improperly placed suture occluding the stoma, pancreatitis compressing the stomal region, compression of the jejunum by the transverse mesocolon in a retrocolic anastomosis, jejunogastric intussusception, and retroanastomotic hernia. However, the cause of obstruction does not appear to be clear in the majority of patients. Endoscopy may show edema of the gastric folds, leading toward an eccentric stoma. These folds, but not the distorted center of the stoma, are often seen in retrospect on upper gastrointestinal radiographs. Just beyond the enlarged mucosal folds the endoscope may pass more or less readily through the anastomosis, yet barium fails to pass or passes very slowly through the stoma. In this case, passage is often dependent upon the position of the patient.

In the absence of a perianastomotic abscess, occluding suture, free anastomotic leak, hernia, or intussusception, the preferred initial approach is nonoperative treatment with nasogastric suction and maintenance of nutrition. This treatment and patience are generally effective. Opinions vary about the duration of nonoperative treatment before reoperation is undertaken when a specific or clear cause of obstruction is not apparent. Our preference is to wait for four to six weeks, since the majority of problems due to edema or hematoma will subside by that time. If resolution has not occurred by then and no obvious external cause is evident, it is a frustrating experience at reoperation to find an anastomosis through which a finger can be easily passed, even though "functional" obstruction remains. The preferred treatment in this situation is to resect and redo the anastomosis or, in the case of a Billroth I anastomosis, pyloroplasty, or proximal gastric vagotomy, convert it to a gastrojejunostomy. A "plastic" procedure on the anastomosis generally is associated with a high incidence of failure.

Acute Afferent Loop Obstruction

One must avoid the trap of confusing the diagnosis of acute pancreatitis with acute afferent loop obstruction. Although patients with a Billroth II gastrectomy may have pancreatitis due to other causes, an increase in serum amylase is more likely due to afferent loop obstruction. The importance of this distinction is that closed afferent loop obstruction will progress to gangrene and peritonitis. While the finding of bile in the gastric aspirate tends to favor a diagnosis of pancreatitis due to another etiology, the obstruction may be high grade but incomplete. With appropriate positioning and sufficient contrast, the afferent loop will generally fill radiographically if it is normal.

The outcome of surgery for acute obstruction has been almost uniformly good, provided that there is no delay in treatment. If the diagnosis of acute obstruction remains in doubt, it is safest to do an exploratory laparotomy because of the high mortality associated with the obstruction. The procedure performed depends upon the operative findings.

Lesser Curve Necrosis

Necrosis of the lesser curve of the stomach is a unique and rare complication of proximal gastric vagotomy, occurring in 0.15% of patients.[43] Clinical manifestations of necrosis may not appear until the fourth or fifth postoperative day and include gastrointestinal hemorrhage, ileus, abdominal distention, shock, or wound infection due to a gastric fistula.[44] Some instances of necrosis are localized to a small (2- to 3-cm) area, whereas others are more extensive. The etiology of this situation is unclear, but proximal gastric vagotomy results in sacrifice of the right and left gastric arterial arcades, even though the short gastric arcade and both epiploic arcades remain intact. Early recognition of necrosis is facilitated by gastroscopy. Subtotal gastrectomy will most likely be necessary for survival.[45]

OUTCOME AND PROGNOSIS

In spite of advances in medical and surgical treatment, endoscopy, and critical care, several studies suggest that the overall mortality of upper gastrointestinal bleeding, is still about 10%.[46] The explanation appears to lie in the advancing age of the population,[46,47] but variations in mortality figures also appear as a consequence of the predominant disease of the particular patient population. While the mortality of variceal bleeding has changed little, survival rates have improved for other entities. An overall mortality of 8.9% for upper gastrointestinal bleeding was reported in 1970,[48] but this varied from 41% for varices to 5.5% for duodenal ulcer. The 1980 American Society for Gastrointestinal Endoscopy survey found the overall mortality to be 10.8%, but 8.7% for those less than 60 years of age and 13.4% for those more than 60 years of age.[49] Recent large series including a small number of patients with bleeding varices report overall mortality to range from 3 to 9%.[50,51] Others continue to report mortalities of up to 23%.[52] Actual exsanguination occurs in about 25 to 33% of deaths.[1,53]

Broad differences exist among patient groups and diagnoses. Meaningful comparisons of mortality should be based on the diagnosis,[54] discounting for a morbid clinical status where the deaths are unrelated to bleeding per se but are a manifestation of severe underlying disease.[51] Recent reports find a mortality of 1 to 4% for duodenal ulcer when limited to those not dying of another disease.[1,50,55] Gastric ulcer carries a slightly higher risk, from 1 to 9%, probably because the affected patients are older.[1,50,51] Mortality for Mallory-Weiss tears has been as high as 10%, but many of these patients have portal hypertension. The more typical figure is 2%.[51,55] Acute gastric mucosal lesions carry a 3 to 7% death rate, but almost all of these are confined to patients with significant underlying disease.[1,55]

Mortality increases four- to fivefold if hemorrhage occurs during hospitalization. The death rate has been reported to be 23 to 30%,[1,52] but as many as 64%[56] are due to underlying disease. Others report an even greater difference in mortality: 70% for massive bleeding during hospitalization compared to 22% for those admitted for upper gastrointestinal bleeding.[56]

Prognostic factors associated with morbidity include age,[57] cirrhosis, organ failure, bleeding site, and the magnitude of blood loss. Mortality increases from 8.5% to 30.7% with continued bleeding or rebleeding.[54] Shock on admission was associated with a 32% mortality in 1970[48] and continued with a 28% risk in 1990.[1] Low-risk variables, which can be gathered within the first hour of presentation, include age less than 75 years, no unstable comorbid illness, a normal prothrombin time, no ascites, systolic blood pressure greater than 100 mm Hg on admission, and a nasogastric aspirate free of fresh blood.[58]

Overall mortality following a surgical procedure also varies with the diagnosis and clinical status. Death rates as high as 45% are reported by some series involving mostly emergent operations,[57] but more typical figures range from 12 to 17%.[59] Several series report no major decrease in operative mortality over the last several decades, presumably due to the increasing age of patients.[47,59,60] However, a low mortality has been reported for some subgroups. Recent series indicate that the surgical mortality for ulcers is as low as 0 to 3.7%, and almost all deaths are limited to those who bleed while hospitalized.[1,25,61] Decreases in overall surgical mortality may be due to protocols involving early diagnosis and early aggressive intervention that require a greater intensity of overall care.[62] In a prospective trial of such management, which included defined indications for surgery, overall mortality for all upper gastrointestinal bleeding fell from 9% to 2.4%, and surgical mortality fell from 16–20% to 1.6%.[25] A broader application of such approaches may decrease the overall number of deaths from upper gastrointestinal bleeding.

Older reports emphasize a high incidence of recurrent bleeding within five years of definitive treatment for bleeding peptic ulcer disease.[36] These figures should be interpreted cautiously, since reports do not always distinguish among the causes. More recent accounts indicate that definitive treatment is indeed effective in preventing recurrent bleeding.

REFERENCES

1. Sugawa C, Steffes CP, Nakamura R, et al: Upper GI bleeding in an urban hospital. *Ann Surg* 212:521–527, 1990.
2. Silverstein FE, Gilbert DA, Tedesco FJ, et al: The national ASGE survey on upper gastrointestinal bleeding. I. Study design and baseline data. *Gastrointest Endosc* 27:73–79, 1982.
3. Sugawa C: Endoscopic diagnosis and treatment of upper gastrointestinal bleeding. *Surg Clin North Am* 69:1167–1183, 1989.
4. de Dombal FY, Clarke JR, Clamp SE, et al: Prognostic factors in upper G.I. bleeding. *Endoscopy* 18(Suppl 2):6–10, 1986.
5. Hellers G, Ihre T: Impact of change on early diagnosis and surgery in major upper gastrointestinal bleeding. *Lancet* 2:1250–1251, 1975.
6. Morris DL, Hawker PC, Brearley S: Optimal timing of operation for bleeding peptic ulcer: Prospective randomized trial. *Br Med J* 288:1277–1280, 1984.
7. Wheatley KE, Snyman JH, Brearley S: Mortality in patients with bleeding peptic ulcer when those age 60 or over are operated on early. *Br Med J* 301:272, 1990.
8. Read RC, Huebl HC, Thal AP: Randomized study of massive bleeding from peptic ulceration. *Ann Surg* 162:561–577, 1965.
9. Hunt PS, Korman MG, Hansky J: Bleeding duodenal ulcer: Reduction in mortality with a planned approach. *Br J Surg* 66:633–635, 1979.
10. Dronfield MW, Atkinson M, Langman MJS: Effect of different operation policies on mortality from bleeding peptic ulcer. *Lancet* 1:1126–1128, 1979.
11. Vellacott KD, Dronfield MW, Atkinson M, et al: Comparison of surgical and medical management of bleeding peptic ulcers. *Br Med J* 284:548–550, 1982.
12. Kim U, Rudick J, Aufses AH: Surgical management of acute upper gastrointestinal bleeding. *Arch Surg* 113:1444–1447, 1978.
13. Koff RS: Benefit of endoscopy in upper gastrointestinal bleeding in patients with liver disease. *Dig Dis Sci* 26(Suppl):12S–16S, 1981.
14. Steffes C, Fromm D: The current diagnosis and management of upper gastrointestinal bleeding, in Cameron JL (ed): *Advances in Surgery*, Vol 25. Mosby Year Book, Inc., St. Louis 25: 331–361.
15. Brearley S, Hawker PC, Morris DL, et al: Selection of patients for surgery following peptic ulcer hemorrhage. *Br J Surg* 74:893–896, 1987.

16. Hunt PS: Bleeding gastroduodenal ulcer: Selection of patients for surgery. *World J Surg* 11:289–294, 1987.
17. Yajko RD, Norton LW, Eiseman B: Current management of upper gastrointestinal bleeding. *Ann Surg* 181:474–480, 1975.
18. Murray WR: Surgical management of hemorrhage from peptic ulceration (editorial). *Br J Surg* 73:947–948, 1986.
19. Darle N: Operative treatment in massive peptic ulcer bleeding. *Scand J Gastroenterol* 29(Suppl 110):109–111, 1985.
20. Roher HD, Thon K: Impact of early operation on the mortality from bleeding peptic ulcer. *Dig Surg* 1:32–36, 1984.
21. Swain CP, Salmon PR, Northfield TC: Does ulcer position influence presentation or prognosis of acute gastrointestinal bleeding? (abstract). *Gut* 27:A632, 1986.
22. MacLeod IA, Mills PR: Factors identifying the probability of further hemorrhage after acute upper gastrointestinal hemorrhage. *Br J Surg* 69:256–258, 1982.
23. Clason AE, MacLeod DAD, Elton RA: Clinical factors in the prediction of further hemorrhage or mortality in acute upper gastrointestinal hemorrhage. *Br J Surg* 73:985–987, 1986.
24. Bornman PC, Theodorou NA, Shuttleworth RD, et al: Importance of hypovolemic shock and endoscopic signs in predicting recurrent hemorrhage from peptic ulceration: A prospective evaluation. *Br J Med* 291:247–249, 1985.
25. Hunt PS, Hansky J, Korman MG: Mortality in patients with hematemesis and melena: A prospective study. *Br Med J* 1:1238–1240, 1979.
26. Enquist IF, Karlson KE, Dennis C, et al: Statistically valid ten-year comparative evaluation of three methods of management of massive gastroduodenal hemorrhage. *Ann Surg* 162:550–571, 1965.
27. Juhl A, Jorgensen F: DDAVP and life-threatening diffuse gastric bleeding in uremia. *Acta Chir Scand* 153:75–77, 1987.
28. Safaie-Shirazi S, Hardy BM: Treatment of reflux esophagitis resulting in massive esophageal bleeding. *Arch Surg* 111:365–367, 1976.
29. Hastings PR, Peters KW, Cohn I: Mallory-Weiss syndrome: Review of 69 cases. *Am J Surg* 142:560–562, 1981.
30. Sugawa C, Benishek D, Walt AJ: Mallory-Weiss syndrome—a study of 224 patients. *Am J Surg* 145:30–33, 1983.
31. Counce JS, Cone JB, McAlister L, et al: Surgical complications of thermal injury. *Am J Surg* 156:556–557, 1988.
32. Wilson WS, Gadacz AT, Olcott C III: Superficial gastric erosions. *Am J Surg* 126:133–140, 1973.
33. Richardson JD, Aust JB: Gastric devascularization. *Ann Surg* 185:649–654, 1973.
34. Norton L, Greer J, Eiseman B: Gastric secretory response to head injury. *Arch Surg* 101:200–204, 1970.
35. Berne CJ, Rosoff L: Peptic ulcer perforation of the gastroduodenal artery complex. *Ann Surg* 169:141–144, 1969.
36. Fromm D: Ulceration of the stomach and duodenum, in Fromm D (ed): *Gastrointestinal Surgery*. New York, Churchill Livingstone, New York, 1985, chapter 9.
37. Dulchavsky S, Fromm D: The management of benign gastric ulcer, in Cameron JL (ed): *Current Surgical Therapy*, Vol 4. Philadelphia, BC Decker, in press.
38. Suleiman SI, Maglad SA, Hobsley M: Dysphagia following selective vagotomy. *Br J Surg* 66:607–608, 1979.
39. Weaver DW, Fromm D: Dudodenal stump problems, in Levine BA (ed): *Perspective in General Surgery*, Vol 1. St Louis, Quality Medical Publishing, 1990, pp 82–88.

40. Larsen BB, Foreman RC: Syndrome of the leaking duodenal stump. *Arch Surg* 63:480–485, 1951.
41. Pearson SC, MacKenzie RJ, Ross T: The use of catheter duodenostomy in gastric resection for duodenal ulcer. *Am J Surg* 106:194–205, 1963.
42. Fromm D, Resitarits D, Kozol R: An analysis of when patients eat after gastrojejunostomy. *Ann Surg* 207:14–20, 1988.
43. Johnston D: Operative mortality and postoperative morbidity of highly selective vagotomy. *Br Med J* 4:545–547, 1975.
44. Hoile RW, Turner JCD: Gastric fistula after proximal gastric vagotomy. *Br Med J* 3:282–283, 1975.
45. Moore FP, Wyllie JH: Ischaemic necrosis of lesser curve after proximal gastric vagotomy. *Br Med J* 4:328, 1975.
46. Allan R, Dykes P: A study of the factors influencing mortality rates from gastrointestinal hemorrhage. *Q J Med* 45:533–550, 1976.
47. Darle N, Haglund U, Larsson I, et al: Management of massive gastroduodenal hemorrhage. *Acta Chir Scand* 146:277–282, 1980.
48. Schiller KFR, Trvebve SC, Williams DG: Hematemesis and melena, with special reference to factors influencing the outcome. *Br Med J* 2:7–14, 1970.
49. Silverstein FE, Gilbert DA, Tedesco FJ, et al: The national ASGE survey on upper gastrointestinal bleeding. II. Clinical prognostic factors. *Gastrointest Endosc* 27:80–93, 1982.
50. Nikolopoulou P, Andrikopoulos P, Dougenis D: Emergency endoscopy in upper gastrointestinal hemorrhage: Evaluation of 885 patients. *J R Coll Surg Edinb* 33:121–123, 1988.
51. Katschinski BD, Logan RFA, Davies J, et al: Audit of mortality in upper gastrointestinal bleeding. *Postgrad Med J* 65:913–917, 1989.
52. Larson G, Schmidt T, Gott, J, et al: Upper gastrointestinal bleeding: Predictors of outcome. *Surgery* 100:765–772, 1986.
53. Dagradi AE, Ruiz RA, Weingarten ZG: Influence of emergency endoscopy in the management and outcome of patients with upper gastrointestinal hemorrhage—analysis of 500 cases. *Am J Gastroenterol* 72:403–415, 1979.
54. de Dombal FY, Clarke JR, Clamp SE, et al: Prognostic factors in upper G.I. bleeding. *Endoscopy* 18(Suppl 2):6–10, 1986.
55. Morgan AG, Clamp SE: OMGE international upper gastrointestinal bleeding survey, 1978–1986. *Scand J Gastroenterol* 23(Suppl 144):51–58, 1988.
56. Chojkier M, Laine L, Conn HO, et al: Predictors of outcome in massive upper gastrointestinal hemorrhage. *J Clin Gastroenterol* 8:16–22, 1986.
57. Nilsson F, Wahlberg J: Survival and emergency surgery on upper gastrointestinal bleeding. *Acta Chir Scand* 147:555–559, 1981.
58. Bordley DR, Mushlin AI, Dolan JG, et al: Early clinical signs identify low-risk patients with acute upper gastrointestinal hemorrhage. *JAMA* 253:3282–3285, 1985.
59. Kim B, Wright HK, Bordan D, et al: Risks of surgery for upper gastrointestinal hemorrhage 1972 versus 1982. *Am J Surg* 194:474–476, 1985.
60. Welch CE, Rodkey GV, Gryska PVR: A thousand operations for ulcer disease. *Ann Surg* 204:454–467, 1986.
61. Fullarton GM, Birnie GG, MacDonald A, et al: The effect of introducing endoscopic therapy on surgery and mortality rates for peptic ulcer hemorrhage—a single center analysis of 1125 cases. *Endoscopy* 22:110–113, 1990.
62. Gostout CJ: Acute gastrointestinal bleeding—a common problem revisited. *Mayo Clin Proc* 63:596–604, 1988.

27

SURGICAL MANAGEMENT OF INTESTINAL BLEEDING

Theodore R. Schrock, M.D.

Surgical management of intestinal bleeding properly encompasses all aspects of diagnosis and treatment, including endoscopic procedures. For the purposes of this chapter, however, surgical management is more narrowly defined as preparation for and conduct of an open abdominal operation. The discussion here is limited further to bleeding that is known or suspected to arise at sites distal to the ligament of Treitz.

INDICATIONS

The need for surgical intervention depends on the acuteness and rate of bleeding, the volume of blood lost, the nature and location of the bleeding lesion, availability and success of radiographic or endoscopic forms of treatment, and the presence of associated medical conditions. Any of these factors may so dominate the clinical picture that a decision for or against operation may be made on that basis alone. In most patients, all of these factors are integrated in the exercise of surgical judgment.

The acuteness of bleeding and the rate of bleeding are related but separable parameters. One may bleed acutely at a rapid rate (e.g., from diverticula) or a slow rate (e.g., from hemorrhoids), and one may bleed chronically (intermittently) at a rapid rate (e.g., from vascular ectasia) or a slow rate (e.g., from colonic cancer). An operation may be required in patients in any of these categories, but the timing of the procedures varies.

The volume of blood lost is an important factor. A patient who requires 3 or more units of blood to stabilize hemodynamic parameters initially is bleeding massively.[1,2] With this degree of hemorrhage, diagnostic evaluation to locate the bleeding site should be aggressive because it is likely that an operation will be necessary. Volume and rate determine the need for an operation in patients with persistent bleeding; if a unit of blood is transfused every eight hours to maintain stability, surgical intervention is obligatory in the majority of cases. The issue should be decided when 4 to 6 units of blood have been given or are anticipated to be given. The volume of blood loss becomes a concern in chronic persistent or intermittent bleeding. As transfusion requirements mount, the probability increases that surgery will be needed.

The nature and location of the bleeding lesion(s) are strong determinants of the need for an operation. Some lesions almost invariably are treated surgically (e.g., colonic cancer), others sometimes require operation (e.g., diverticular disease), and still others infrequently need laparotomy (e.g., acute infectious diseases). For obvious surgical lesions, it is preferable to operate electively after the bleeding has stopped, but emergency operation may be compelled by persistent bleeding. The location of the lesion in the small intestine, colon, or anorectum is important, and it is essential to determine if the process is discrete or diffuse. Inability to localize the bleeding site is a major concern. The formidable difficulties of operating under these circumstances are well known. If the patient's condition permits, it is prudent to invest sufficient time and effort in diagnostic evaluation to establish the area of bleeding rather than operating with inadequate information. These decisions can be very difficult and, in some individuals, it may be necessary to explore the abdomen for acute or chronic bleeding despite the lack of localizing data.

The availability and success of radiographic or endoscopic treatment have become increasingly important in determining which patients should undergo surgery. In some circumstances, endoscopic treatment makes operation for intestinal bleeding unnecessary.[3] In others, endoscopic or radiographic control is temporary and should be followed by definitive operation. Finally, some situations mandate surgery. Recurrence of bleeding after spontaneous or therapeutic hemostasis is an indication to intervene surgically, especially if the bleeding site is known.

The patient's general condition and the presence of associated medical conditions influence the decision to operate. If a patient is in good general condition, a necessary operation should be carried out promptly if other methods fail. A major medical problem such as disseminated cancer, acute myocardial ischemia, or a combination of less serious conditions denotes a substantial operative risk. Some of these patients should have surgery sooner rather than later because they are unable to tolerate persistent bleeding, but the tendency is to delay surgery in high-risk patients. When finally called upon, the surgeon must deal with the combined impact of the bleeding lesion, the associated medical conditions, and the consequences of large blood loss.

Statistics on the need for operation for intestinal bleeding vary according to the definitions used, the patient population, the aggressiveness of alternative types of intervention, and other factors. In one recent study, an operation was performed in only 7 of 107 (6.5%) patients who were admitted to a surgical unit with significant lower gastrointestinal bleeding requiring at least 2 units of blood transfusion.[2] Bleeding stopped spontaneously in 90% of these patients before transfusions exceeded 2 units, but if a patient required more than 4 units of blood in the first 24 hours, there was a 50% chance that surgery would be necessary. In an earlier report, emergency laparotomy and colon resection for acute colonic hemorrhage was performed in 9.6% of 292 patients admitted with bleeding.[1] In still another series, the average number of transfusions required for severe hematochezia ranged from 2.4 units in nonsurgical patients to 9.5 units in the surgical group.[4] Four or more units were given to 68% of patients who underwent an operation. Of interest, 58% of patients subjected to operation in this report had been hospitalized previously for bleeding.[4]

PREOPERATIVE MANAGEMENT

Finding the bleeding site is a decidedly important aspect of preoperative management. If the bleeding rate is slow, there should be ample time to obtain the necessary studies, prepare the patient, and perform a semielective or elective operation. With threatened exsanguination, localizing studies may be impossible. Many patients fall between these extremes; their operations are urgent, but there is time to do endoscopy or angiography or both.

Patients who undergo surgery for massive intestinal bleeding tend to be elderly, and they often have associated medical conditions that need to be identified and treated. In one series, the age range was 46 to 87 years.[4] Hypertension was present in 57% of these patients, heart disease in 40%, cerebrovascular disease in 17%, and diabetes mellitus in 17%. Intestinal bleeding may be associated with hemophilia, renal failure, immunosuppression from organ transplantation, cancer chemotherapy, and various other disorders.

Blood volume should be replenished preoperatively and during the operation. Transfusions of blood and blood products are given cautiously and only on demonstrated need in today's environment of anxiety about transmissible disease. When active bleeding occurs, concerns about these issues should not allow patients to remain hypotensive and underperfused. This misguided practice exacts a high price in terms of postoperative complications.

The bowel should be prepared if the operation is elective or semielective. Oral polyethylene glycol solutions act quickly and effectively. If the patient is bleeding actively, there may not be time to cleanse the colon. Fortunately, the blood acts as a cathartic and provides partial cleansing. Antibiotic administration orally and/or intravenously follows standard practice in elective cases. Emergency patients certainly should receive intravenous antibiotics.

Obtaining informed consent can present a problem if the location of the bleeding point is unknown. The patient should be counseled about the possibility of a stoma, although an ileostomy or colostomy is required in very few patients.

OPERATION

Position

If the bleeding site has been pinpointed unequivocally to the small intestine on preoperative studies, the supine position for laparotomy is acceptable. If there is any question about the bleeding site, however, as is the case for the majority of emergent patients, it is preferable to place the patient in the lithotomy position to gain access to the anus for intraoperative colonoscopy.

Incision

A vertical midline incision is optimal for patients with active intestinal bleeding. Precise localizing information may suggest that some other type of incision be used, but the midline approach is the most flexible.

Exploration

The abdomen is explored in the hope of finding the bleeding site. One should be wary of preoperative localizing information, because it may be incorrect or there may be multiple lesions.[5] Studies that suggest a lesion in the small intestine usually do not pinpoint the site precisely along the intestinal length. The endoscopist may be in error regarding the position of a colonic lesion; sometimes the actual site is quite different than was thought during endoscopy.

On occasion, one is fortunate and a bleeding lesion is obvious (Plate 48). More often, however, there is blood in part or all of the small intestine and colon, so that the source is not apparent. Bilious material can closely resemble blood when seen through the intact intestinal wall, and the inexperienced surgeon may be misled.

Intraoperative Localization

Methods of finding the bleeding site during operation are listed in Table 27.1.

Gross Inspection

The stomach and duodenum, small intestine, colon, and rectum should be inspected thoroughly. The retroperitoneal portions of the colon and both flexures must be mobilized if the bleeding site is not apparent. One should avoid trauma to the intestinal wall because ecchymoses and small hematomas can confuse the issue. In the past, surgeons routinely applied noncrushing clamps to isolate segments of the small bowel or colon in the hope that blood would fill one segment and thus reveal the site. This technique is unrewarding and traumatic.

Transillumination

The small intestine should be transilluminated to look for small vascular lesions. A strong, focused light is essential. One of the operating room lights, a headlight on an assistant, or a flexible fiberoptic light meets this need. Transillumination is facilitated by intraoperative endoscopy, as described elsewhere. As suspicious lesions are encountered, they are marked with sutures.[6]

Table 27.1. Methods of Intraoperative Localization of Intestinal Bleeding

Gross inspection
Transillumination
Compression
Enterotomy
Endoscopy
Angiography
Methylene blue
Scintigraphy
Doppler ultrasound
Venous oxygen

Compression

The small intestine can be compressed between two glass slides to better display vascular lesions and small tumors. This method is not used much today because intraoperative endoscopy is more effective.

Enterotomy

Gastrotomy or gastroduodenotomy is performed when there is evidence of bleeding from the stomach or duodenum. In patients who are believed to be bleeding from lesions distal to the ligament of Treitz, however, unguided enterotomies or colotomies usually do not help locate the bleeding area and they contaminate the operative field with bacteria. At one time, surgeons favored making a colotomy in the midtransverse colon to observe whether blood welled up from a proximal or distal site. This procedure is futile and has been abandoned.

Endoscopy

Intraoperative endoscopy is the procedure of choice if inspection and transillumination are inconclusive. Before flexible endoscopy became available, a rigid sigmoidoscope was inserted into the lumen through one or more enterotomies or colotomies in the hope of finding the bleeding points.[7] The short instrument, its rigidity, and the unsatisfactory optics were factors that limited the success of this procedure. Extensive peritoneal contamination was common and infections were frequent.

A flexible endoscope can be inserted into the lumen of the small intestine through an enterotomy. An exteriorized loop is covered with a sheet of plastic to exclude the nonsterile instrument from the surgical field. This type of intraoperative endoscopy is seldom required because the entire small bowel and colon can be inspected by instruments passed orally or per rectum in most patients.

It is preferable to do intraoperative colonoscopy first if the colon is suspect. Intraoperative colonic cleansing can be achieved by irrigation of saline through a Foley catheter inserted directly into the cecum[8] or through the appendix.[9] Three liters of solution usually is sufficient. Often the colon is clean enough without this step because of the cathartic action of blood.

The colonoscope is inserted per rectum and advanced quickly with the help of the surgeon; it should pass through the ileocecal valve into the distal ileum. As the colonoscope is moved farther into the ileum, the small bowel is examined serially in 10- to 15-cm segments.[10] It is important to inspect on insertion rather than on withdrawal because the inevitable trauma creates artifacts in the form of tears and hematomas. A suture is placed to mark the limit of the intraoperative endoscopy from below.

Peroral intraoperative enteroscopy is described elsewhere in this book (see Chapter 18). The method can be applied to patients with chronic or acute bleeding.[11-13] In a recent study of patients with chronic occult intestinal bleeding, intraoperative enteroscopy found specific mucosal abnormalities in 67% of patients, but only 49% of survivors after resection never rebled.[13]

Angiography

Intraoperative angiography is most useful in patients who have preoperative angiographic demonstration of a bleeding site in the small intestine. It can be difficult to identify the involved segment of bowel at operation if there is no gross lesion, and empiric resection of intestine should be avoided. With advance planning and with the patient in a suitably equipped operating room, intraoperative angiography can be very helpful.

Intraoperative angiography is performed most commonly through a percutaneous femoral arterial catheter that is inserted before operation and is left in place. Heparin flushes maintain patency.[14,15] The catheter is placed as selectively as possible into the vessel feeding the bleeding site. One technique requires that a very small catheter be passed through the outer catheter and advanced far distally to the point where the vessel pierces the bowel wall, if that is possible. With this extremely selective approach, magnification arteriography through the small inner catheter confirms the precise catheter position in relation to the small bowel lesion.[14] At this point, the patient is taken to the operating room, where 1 ml of methylene blue is injected through the small inner catheter, thus marking the segment for resection.[14]

An alternative technique is required if the preoperative angiogram is positive but a catheter cannot be placed as selectively as described above. At operation, the approximate position of the bleeding site is identified based on properative angiograms, and the intestinal mesenteric border is marked with radiopaque clips that serve as reference points.[15,16] Groups of clips are placed at intervals of 12 inches, and angiography of each segment is done. An active bleeding site is checked against the reference clips as a guide for resection.[15] If bleeding is not active, the vascular pattern of the preoperative angiogram is compared with the intraoperative films which have the metal clips as markers.[15] It may be possible to localize the lesion in this way.

Another method of intraoperative angiography avoids the morbidity of a transfemoral catheter and instead relies on direct injection of segmental arterial branches.[17] An x-ray cassette with a sterile cover is placed behind the segment of bowel in question. Metal clips are placed at the mesenteric border, and a segmental arterial branch feeding this section of intestine is isolated. A 21-gauge butterfly needle is directly into the artery, contrast (7–12 ml) is injected, and films are exposed. The procedure can be repeated at several sites until the bleeding lesion is identified. The potential for causing mesenteric hematomas is a disadvantage of this technique.

Methylene Blue

Intraoperative injection of methylene blue through an extremely selective angiographic catheter was described above.[14] An earlier method based on observation of the clearing time of the dye was thought to be a guide to the presence of an arteriovenous malformation, but it is not widely used.[18]

Scintigraphy

Preoperative demonstration of active intestinal bleeding may be followed by intraoperative scintigraphy to identify the bleeding point precisely.[19] If bleeding is documented on preoperative endoscopy or angiography, ^{99m}technetium-labeled erythrocytes are injected into the patient just before the operation is performed. If bleeding is seen on standard preoperative ^{99m}technetium-labeled erythrocyte scan, the patient may proceed directly to laparotomy.

Atraumatic clamps are placed every 30 cm on loops of the small intestine. Segments are imaged sequentially with a mobile gamma camera for a period of three minutes each, and the segments with the most intense tracer activity are then resected.[19]

Doppler Ultrasound

It has been reported that intraoperative Doppler ultrasound successfully detects arteriovenous malformations in the intestine.[20,21] Little data have appeared on this method since the initial reports.

Venous Oxygen

Selective measurement of mesenteric venous pressure and pO_2 may help identify an arteriovenous malformation, according to some reports.[21,22]

Preparation of the Specimen

If a resected specimen of intestine is simply handed to the pathologist for routine examination, small bleeding lesions are likely to be missed. As a minimum, the surgeon should open and wash the bowel in segments, using gentle compression to find areas where blood is expressed.[23] These areas are then marked with sutures to guide the pathologist.

Specimen angiography can be performed by injecting contrast into the feeding artery and taking a radiograph. A more elaborate technique of injection and clearing permits detection of tiny lesions by both angiography and pathologic examination.[14,24] After a specimen of small intestine is resected, the vessels are injected immediately with radiopaque silicon rubber, a radiograph of the injected specimen is obtained, and the presence of the lesion within the specimen is confirmed. The specimen is then immersed in increasing concentrations of alcohol and, finally, in absolute alcohol followed by a solution of methyl salicylate. Vessels in the cleared specimen can be examined and photographed under the dissecting microscope. The dehydration process is subsequently reversed, and a specimen is submitted for histological examination.

LESIONS OF THE SMALL INTESTINE

Causes of bleeding from the small intestine are described elsewhere in this book. All of these lesions are uncommon, and some are rare indeed. The main problem is locating the lesion. Once it is found, the surgical treatment consists of resection and primary anastomosis in nearly all patients. Decisions are not difficult in patients with focal disease—primary or metastatic tumors (see Plates 49 & 50), Meckel's diverticulum, jejunal diverticula, and duplication cysts.

Extensive Crohn's disease can present a dilemma in deciding how much to resect. Aortoenteric fistulas are challenging because the infected graft must be dealt with and the blood supply to the lower body preserved.[25] Various other situations are problematic because of the nature of the bleeding lesion and/or the patient's underlying condition.

LESIONS OF THE LARGE INTESTINE

Before modern diagnostic methods became available, surgeons were forced to operate for severe colonic bleeding in very unfavorable circumstances—in elderly patients; in the presence of exsanguinating hemorrhage; in a blood-filled, unprepared colon; and with no information about the source of bleeding. Intraoperative maneuvers included application of bowel clamps, colotomies, and intraoperative colonoscopy with a rigid sigmoidoscope. Empiric ("blind") segmental colectomy was performed in many patients. A left colectomy was done if the patient had diverticula, and a right colectomy was carried out if there was some reason to suspect bleeding on that side. Soon it was learned that colonic bleeding occurs about equally from the right and left colons.[7] Empiric segmental resection is associated with a high rebleeding rate (30–50%) and a prohibitively high operative mortality rate (30–40%).[1,26] Total abdominal colectomy (subtotal colectomy—resection of the completed colon but not the rectum) was found to have a lower mortality rate (11%), and the rebleeding rate was greatly reduced—to zero in one large series of patients.[26] With more experience, however, the errors associated with empiric total colectomy became apparent.[27] They include failure to consider the contribution of systemic diseases to bleeding and overlooking the presence of bleeding lesions in the upper tract, small bowel, or rectum.

Angiography and colonoscopy have greatly altered the surgical management of bleeding lesions of the intestine.[28-31] Knowledge of the bleeding site from preoperative studies spells the difference between empiric resection and directed resection, limited resection and extensive resection, less morbidity and more morbidity, and lower mortality and higher mortality.

The choice of operation for colorectal bleeding depends on the nature of the lesion, its location, acuteness of bleeding, severity of bleeding, the patient's age and general condition, and the presence of other intestinal abnormalities. Table 27.2 lists the most common types of operations that are performed for bleeding from the large intestine. The choice of operation in different reports reflects many variables. Total colectomy is still performed in about one-half of resected patients, but the trend is toward greater selectivity.[2,32,33] If the location of a colonic bleeding site is unknown and bleeding is not life-threatening, it may be wise to defer the operation until the source is identified rather than perform total colectomy. When it is necessary, total colectomy usually is completed with a primary ileoproctostomy.[34]

Vascular Ectasias

If the bleeding is known to be limited to the right colon based on angiography or colonoscopy, cannot be controlled by colonoscopic methods, and bleeding persists, an operation should be undertaken.[35] Debate continues as to whether patients who bleed

Table 27.2. Operations for Bleeding from the Large Intestine

Operation	*Patients Undergoing This Operation (%)**
Right hemicolectomy	11–89
Left hemicolectomy	11–33
Other segmental colectomy	0–17
Total colectomy	20–79

*References 2, 9, 28, 32, 33, and 35.

transiently from ectasias and then stop should undergo elective resection; the decision may hinge on the patient's general condition. Elective operation certainly should be performed in patients who bleed repeatedly.[36]

An extended right hemicolectomy is recommended for vascular ectasias.[36-38] The resection should include the entire right colon and the transverse colon to its midpoint. Resection of the ileum is not required. There has been controversy over the need for resection of the left colon in patients who apparently are bleeding from right-sided vascular ectasias but also have extensive diverticulosis of the left colon.[39] If the left colon is not resected, as many as 20% of patients rebleed, but the risk associated with recurrent bleeding may be lower than the morbidity and mortality of total colectomy.[35,36] As a rule, it is probably best to avoid resecting the left colon in these circumstances.

Although the preoperative diagnosis of bleeding colonic vascular ectasias may seem secure, one should look for a second source at operation. In one series of 40 patients who underwent operation for angiodysplasia, 9 patients (22.5%) were discovered to have additional lesions of the small bowel, either at the original laparotomy or subsequently when bleeding recurred.[5] A Meckel's diverticulum was discovered in four patients, carcinoid of the ileum in one, multiple jejunal arteriovenous malformations in one, and an ulcerated duodenal diverticulum in one.

Diverticular Disease

During the 1960s, colonic diverticula were believed to be responsible for most cases of severe lower gastrointestinal hemorrhage.[7] The description of vascular ectasias pushed diverticular disease into the background to some extent, and the importance of diverticula as sources of bleeding was questioned.[40] There is no doubt that colonic diverticula are capable of bleeding, but one should not attribute bleeding to diverticula without convincing evidence.[40] If the diagnosis is persuasive and the diverticula are confined to left colon, a left hemicolectomy is adequate surgical treatment. Resection should extend at least to the proximal descending colon. Primary anastomosis is performed if conditions permit.

Other Lesions

A large variety of lesions of the colon, rectum, or anus can be responsible for bleeding from the lower gastrointestinal tract. Arteriovenous malformations, telangiectasias, Dieulafoy's ulcer, cecal ulcer, and neoplasms can be resected. Cavernous hemangiomas of the rectum are managed by sphincter-preserving procedures.[41] Diffuse intestinal hemangiomatosis is very challenging; if endoscopic control is not possible, identifiable lesions should be excised at operation through enterotomies or by segmental resections.[36] Recurrent bleeding and repeated operations are the rule.

RESULTS

Farrands and Taylor reported that a policy of aggressive diagnostic evaluation, endoscopic therapy, and operation when needed have lowered the overall mortality rate to 2% among patients with acute lower gastrointestinal bleeding who required at least 2 units of transfused blood.[2] Eaton reported an overall mortality rate of 15% in patients who required more than 2 units.[1] Higher overall mortality rates are reported in patients with massive lower hemorrhage—reaching 21% in one series.[33]

Operative mortality rates depend on the patient mix, the acuteness and severity of bleeding, and the urgency of operation. At one extreme are patients with elective or semielective right colectomy for vascular ectasias; the operative mortality rate ranged from zero in one series[42] to 10% in another.[28] At the other extreme, the mortality rate for emergency operations for active bleeding still reaches 20%.[28,32]

The relationship of preoperative angiography to operative mortality rates is a subject of discussion. In one study, unsuccessful angiographically directed treatment delay operation and contribute to a mortality rate of 38%. In addition, angiographic treatment led directly to two fatal complications, one from cardiac arrest during the procedure and the second from intestinal infarction as a consequence of transcatheter embolization.[33] Other authors, however, point to the benefits of angiography. One group reported two postoperative deaths in 14 patients (14%) with positive arteriographic findings who underwent emergency operation compared to five deaths in 10 patients (50%) undergoing emergency operation without preoperative arteriography.[31] These patients likely were bleeding more massively and therefore were poorer risks than those who underwent successful arteriography. Seven patients with negative arteriography had emergency laparotomy, and there were no deaths in this group. The authors point out that the actual bleeding site was seen by extravasation in 50% of patients who underwent arteriography and this finding allowed the surgeon to perform segmental resection.[31] Clearly, angiography or any other diagnostic study in bleeding patients should be performed expeditiously to avoid undue delays that contribute to morbidity and mortality.

SUMMARY

Finding the bleeding site is the key to successful surgical management of intestinal bleeding. Operation is undertaken if endoscopic or angiographic management is unsuccessful or if the nature of the lesion demands that an operation be performed in any event. Careful evaluation and treatment of associated medical conditions, bowel preparation whenever possible, and intravenous antibiotics are important preoperative steps.

At operation the abdomen is explored systematically, and obvious bleeding lesions are treated. Useful intraoperative methods to localize bleeding include transillumination, endoscopy, angiography, and scintigraphy. Resected specimens should be prepared for the pathologist in a manner that is likely to increase the yield of diagnostic information.

Most lesions of either the small or the large intestine are not difficult to manage. Vascular ectasias of the colon require extended right hemicolectomy. If the bleeding site is found in the left colon, left colectomy is sufficient. Total abdominal colectomy is reserved for patients with bleeding that is limited to the colon but cannot be pinpointed further.

Results of surgery reflect a low mortality rate in favorable cases. Results in the high-risk cases remain unfavorable despite modern methods of evaluation and treatment. The patient population is the strongest determinant of the outcome.

REFERENCES

1. Eaton AC: Emergency surgery for acute colonic haemorrhage—a retrospective study. *Br J Surg* 68:109–112, 1981.
2. Farrands PA, Taylor I: Management of acute lower gastrointestinal haemorrhage in a surgical unit over a 4-year period. *J R Soc Med* 80:79–82, 1987.
3. Schrock TR: Does endoscopy affect the surgical approach to the patient with upper gastrointestinal bleeding? *Dig Dis Sci* 26:27S–30S, 1981.
4. Newhall SC, Lucas CE, Ledgerwood AM: Diagnostic and therapeutic approach to colonic bleeding. *Am Surgeon* 47:136–142, 1981.
5. Steger AC, Galland RB, Hemingway A, et al: Gastrointestinal haemorrhage from a second source in patients with colonic angiodysplasia. *Br J Surg* 74:726–727, 1987.
6. Richardson JD: Management of acute and chronic gastrointestinal bleeding distal to the ligament of Treitz. *Perspect Gen Surg* 1:3–24, 1990.
7. Klein RR, Gallagher DM: Massive colonic bleeding from diverticular disease. *Am J Surg* 118:553–557, 1969.
8. Batch AJG, Pickard RG, De Lacey G: Peroperative colonoscopy in massive rectal bleeding. *Br J Surg* 68:64–67, 1981.
9. Scott HJ, Lane IF, Glynn MJ, et al: Colonic haemorrhage: A technique for rapid intra-operative bowel preparation and colonoscopy. *Br J Surg* 73:390–391, 1986.
10. Flickinger EG, Stanforth AC, Sinar DR, et al: Intraoperative video panendoscopy for diagnosing sites of chronic intestinal bleeding. *Am J Surg* 157:137–144, 1989.
11. Apelgren KN, Vargish T, Al-Kawas F: Principles for use of intraoperative enteroscopy for hemorrhage from the small bowel. *Am Surgeon* 54:85–88, 1988.
12. Lau WY, Wong SY, Yuen WK, et al: Intraoperative enteroscopy for bleeding angiodysplasias of small intestine. *SGO* 168:341–344, 1989.
13. Ress A, Benacci J, Sarr MG: Intraoperative enteroscopy for chronic occult gastrointestinal bleeding of presumed small bowel origin: Is it worthwhile? Presented to the Society of Surgery of the Alimentary Tract, 1991. New Orleans, Digestive Disease Week.
14. Athanasoulis CA, Moncure AC, Greenfield AJ, et al: Intraoperative localization of small bowel bleeding sites with combined use of angiographic methods and methylene blue injection. *Surgery* 87:77–84, 1980.
15. Fazio VW, Zelas P, Weakley FL: Intraoperative angiography and the localization of bleeding from the small intestine. *SGO* 151:637–640, 1980.
16. Hines JR, Stryker SJ, Neiman HL, et al: Intraoperative angiography in intestinal angiodysplasia. *SGO* 152:453–460, 1981.
17. Robertson HD, Gathright JB Jr: The technique of intraoperative segmental artery arteriography to localize vascular ectasias. *Dis Colon Rectum* 28:274–276, 1985.
18. Fogler R, Golembe E: Methylene blue injection, an intraoperative guide in small bowel resection for arteriovenous malformation. *Arch Surg* 113:194–195, 1978.
19. Biener A, Palestro C, Lewis BS, et al: Intraoperative scintigraphy for active small intestinal bleeding. *SGO* 171:388–392, 1990.
20. Pinkerton JA Jr: Intraoperative Doppler localization of intestinal arteriovenous malformation. *Surgery* 85:472–474, 1979.
21. Cooperman M, Martin EW Jr, Evans WE, et al: Use of Doppler ultrasound in intraoperative localization of intestinal arteriovenous malformation. *Ann Surg* 190:24–26, 1979.
22. Evans WE, O'Dorsio TM, Molnar W, et al: Intraoperative localization of intestinal arteriovenous malformation. *Arch Surg* 113:410–412, 1978.

23. Hagihara PF, Chuang VP, Griffen WO: Arteriovenous malformations of the colon. *Am J Surg* 133:681–687, 1977.
24. Aldabagh SM, Trujillo YP, Taxy JB: Utility of specimen angiography in angiodysplasia of the colon. *Gastroenterology* 91:725–729, 1986.
25. Champion MC, Sullivan SN, Coles JC, et al: Aortoenteric fistula. Incidence, presentation recognition, and management. *Ann Surg* 195:314–317, 1982.
26. Drapanas T, Pennington DG, Kappelman M, et al: Emergency subtotal colectomy: Preferred approach to management of massively bleeding diverticular disease. *Ann Surg* 177:519–526, 1973.
27. Gianfrancisco JA, Abcarian H: Pitfalls in the treatment of massive lower gastrointestinal bleeding with "blind" subtotal colectomy. *Dis Colon Rectum* 25:441–445, 1982.
28. Colacchio TA, Forde KA, Patsos TJ, et al: Impact of modern diagnostic methods on the management of active rectal bleeding. Ten year experience. *Am J Surg* 143:607–610, 1982.
29. Schrock TR: Conceptual developments through colonoscopy. *Surg Endosc* 2:240–244, 1988.
30. Jensen DM, Machicado GA: Diagnosis and treatment of severe hematochezia. The role of urgent colonoscopy after purge. *Gastroenterology* 95:1569–1574, 1988.
31. Udén P, Jiborn H, Jonsson K: Influence of selective mesenteric arteriography on the outcome of emergency surgery for massive, lower gastrointestinal hemorrhage. A 15-year experience. *Dis Colon Rectum* 29:561–566, 1986.
32. Browder W, Cerise EJ, Litwin MS: Impact of emergency angiography in massive lower gastrointestinal bleeding. *Ann surg* 204:530–536, 1986.
33. Leitman IM, Paull DE, Shires GT III: Evaluation and management of massive lower gastrointestinal hemorrhage. *Ann Surg* 209:175–180, 1989.
34. Scott HW Jr, Weaver FA, Fletcher JR, et al: Is ileoproctostomy a reasonable procedure after total abdominal colectomy? *Ann Surg* 203:583–589, 1986.
35. Roberts PL, Schoetz DJ Jr, Coller JA: Vascular ectasia. Diagnosis and treatment by colonoscopy. *Am Surgeon* 54:56–59, 1988.
36. Dickstein G, Boley SJ: Vascular lesions of the colon, in Condon RE (ed): *Shackelford's Surgery of the Alimentary Tract,* ed 3. Philadelphia, WB Saunders, 1991, pp 70–83.
37. Boley SJ, Sammaratano R, Brandt LJ, et al: Vascular ectasias of the colon. *SGO* 149:353–359, 1979.
38. Farnell MB, Larson DE: The investigation and management of gastrointestinal bleeding, in Irving MH, Beart RW Jr (eds): *Gastroenterological Surgery,* ed 3. Boston, Butterworths, 1983, pp 118–157.
39. Welch CE, Athanasoulis CA, Galdabini JJ: Hemorrhage from the large bowel with special reference to angiodysplasia and diverticular disease. *World J Surg* 2:73–83, 1978.
40. Spencer J: Lower gastrointestinal bleeding. *Br J Surg* 76:3–4, 1989.
41. Aylward CA, Orangio GR, Lucas GW, et al: Diffuse cavernous hemangioma of the rectosigmoid—CT scan, a new diagnostic modality, and surgical management using sphincter-saving procedures. Report of three cases. *Dis Colon Rectum* 31:797–802, 1988.
42. Wright HK, Pelliccia O, Higgins EF jr, et al: Controlled, semielective, segmental resection for massive colonic hemorrhage. *Am J Surg* 139:535–538, 1980.

28

APPROACH TO POSTOPERATIVE BLEEDING (REBLEEDING) AFTER SURGERY FOR GASTROINTESTINAL BLEEDING OR GENERAL ABDOMINAL PROCEDURES

Philip E. Donahue, M.D.

INTRODUCTION

The prevention of gastrointestinal rebleeding postoperatively is a most important responsibility for all surgeons, especially for those who operate in and around the gastrointestinal tract. If bleeding becomes sustained, there are substantial risks to the patient, both immediately and postoperatively.[1]

Since the signs and symptoms of bleeding are often subtle, they are frequently confused with ordinary postoperative sequelae. The patient who has already undergone a major surgical trauma, whether as an elective event or as an urgent intervention, is not an ideal candidate for another operation. The second procedure is an urgent or emergent procedure, with morbidity risks which exceed those of an elective procedure by a factor of 10 or more. Even when an operation is not required, there is substantial potential morbidity associated with additional blood transfusions. The prevention and/or appropriate treatment of postoperative bleeding is an extremely relevant aspect of surgical practice.

Despite hopes to the contrary, an experienced surgeon will have to deal with postoperative bleeding. When the occasional rebleeding episode occurs, much to the distress of the patient, family, and caregivers, a realistic plan of action, based on facts and not on wishful thinking, will usually be successful. If the original surgical problem was gastrointestinal bleeding, management of postoperative bleeding is based upon the same principles which led to the first operation: namely, optimal resuscitation and attempts to localize the site of bleeding, keeping in mind the initial operation and treatment.

Occasionally, reoperation is necessary because of extraintestinal sites of bleeding unrelated to the primary operation. While the unligated vessel is universally feared as a cause of bleeding, reoperation may not reveal a discrete bleeding site. If an injured mesenteric vessel, splenic capsular tear, or other organ damage is found to be the cause of bleeding, only surgical treatment will be curative.

NONSPECIFIC SITE (REACTIVE) HEMORRHAGE

At times, reexploration for postoperative hemorrhage does *not* identify a specific bleeding site; the usual explanation given for this type of bleeding is "reactive" or secondary bleeding due to granulation tissue within or near the operative field. This type of bleeding is aggravated by coagulopathy, massive transfusion, or hypothermia. If reoperation is necessary and no specific bleeding site is identified, the unsatisfying diagnosis of "coagulopathy" or oozing from granulation tissue must be entertained. Because most clinical databases are not specific in codifying these problems (including our own), precise statistics are not available. We all look forward to a fully relational database which can address these infrequent but important events.

Rebleeding may not require reoperation, but the extent of this complication is difficult to quantify. In many patients with *mild to moderate* postoperative bleeding, the problem is not clearly recognized. Just the need for blood transfusion postoperatively is a serious concern, especially in this era of transfusion-related diseases (e.g., AIDS and hepatitis) for which there is no specific treatment. In this light, the use of heat-treated blood factor concentrates should be kept in mind as a possible alternative to blood transfusion in hemophiliacs or other patients who are experiencing some hemorrhagic phenomenon.[2,3]

There are many contributing and confounding factors in the need for postoperative transfusion. Before long, no doubt, there will be guidelines for acceptable rates of postoperative transfusion therapy in general surgical procedures, just as there are guidelines for the transfusion of blood and blood products after coronary bypass surgery.

INCIDENCE OF POSTOPERATIVE BLEEDING

The patients with postoperative bleeding whom we have information about are those who require reoperation for bleeding; the reported incidence is quite low. The fact that a postoperative hemorrhage has occurred may not be reflected in the postoperative problem list unless the precise cause of bleeding was apparent. As a result, these data may be incomplete. At Cook County Hospital, there were 15,600 operations on the General Surgery Service between July 1986 and July 1991; only eight patients (0.05%) required reoperation for bleeding during that period. If only bleeding from suture lines, persistent ulcers, or the gastric lumen are included, the number of reoperations falls to only two

(0.01%). These data do not include any of the patients operated on for nongastrointestinal disease; postoperative bleeding after vascular or cardiac operations is an entirely different problem. There is a higher incidence of gastrointestinal procedures needing aggressive anticoagulation intraoperatively or antithrombotic therapy in the postoperative period.[4-6]

During a 20-year period, the author's personal experience has included 36 patients whose recurrent bleeding required reoperation (Table 28.1). This series includes not only patients undergoing celiotomy for bleeding but also those with bleeding following an endoscopic treatment. This inclusion is based upon the fact that endoscopic treatments are analogous to surgical procedures and the complications must be considered in a similar manner.

The incidence of surgical interventions for gastrointestinal bleeding has shown a dramatic decrease in the past 10 years as the endoscopic techniques to control bleeding have become widespread, applied by a national cadre of well-trained physician and

TABLE 28.1. Source of Rebleeding (Requiring operation or endoscopic therapy)

1. Suture Line:7
   1—hand-sewn
   2—EEA anastomoses (gastrojejunostomy, jejunojejunostomy)
   *4—gastrojejunostomy (2 sewn),
   gastroduodenostomy (1 sewn),
   jejunojejunostomy (1 stapled)
2. Ulcer site: 3
   1—aortoesophageal fistula (monilia)
   1—penetrating duodenal ulcer (progressive ulcer after vagotomy (gastric pH always > 5.0)
   1—multiple superficial ulcers (cytomegalovirus?) throughout jejunum and ileum
3. Pseudoaneurysm—peripancreatic necrosis: 3
   1—gastroduodenal artery
   1—left gastric artery
   1—splenic artery (after splenectomy)
4. Unrecognized site: 4
   1—arteriovenous malformation of jejunum
   1—posterior pharynx/nasopharynx (facial trauma)
   1—esophageal ulcer after sclerotherapy
   1—jejunal ulcer
5. Acute gastric mucosal lesions: 3
6. Failure of endoscopic injection or thermal therapy: 14
   5—gastritis
   5—duodenal ulcer
   2—duodenal ulcer
   2—Mallory-Weiss tear
7. Bleeding from granulation tissue or small vessels: 3
   1—duodenal ulcer (reoperation, antrectomy)
   1—primary gastric resection for gastric ulcer
   1—left colon resection (cancer of splenic flexure)

*Endoscopic treatment.

surgeon-endoscopists. Rebleeding after endoscopic treatment is more common than after surgical treatment; for example, after surgical treatment, a rebleeding rate within seven days of more than 1–2% may be excessive, whereas the rate of rebleeding after endoscopic treatment (as reported) varies between 5% and 30%.[5-14] When reviewing these data, however, one should highlight the average 10% operative mortality observed during emergent operations for gastrointestinal bleeding. Therefore, most experienced physicians and surgeons are in favor of aggressive endoscopic attempts to control upper gastrointestinal bleeding as the initial treatment. Hopefully, future discussions of rebleeding after endoscopic procedures will be based upon more valid data derived from the fully integrated databases now coming on line.

The recognition of serious postoperative bleeding may be either difficult or self-evident, depending on the circumstances. For example, the patient who has bloody nasogastric secretions noted on the second postoperative day will be recognized promptly, whereas an individual with a sudden hematemesis on the morning of hospital discharge may have no premonitory symptoms. Similarly, the patient with low-volume intraperitoneal bleeding will be suspected only if serial postoperative hematocrits are being monitored for some reason. Fortunately, this type of bleeding is not usually a serious concern and seldom requires operative intervention.

At this point, one should note that postoperative bleeding is *not necessarily,* of itself, a quality-of-care issue; to be sure, patients with postoperative hemorrhage are a highly visible group who demand careful evaluation and treatment. Many (if not most instances) represent an inevitable progression of the underlying disease. Each requires individualized treatment based upon consideration of the global aspects of the patient's condition and response to treatment. While this fact is self-evident to experienced surgeons, it is important that it be stated clearly for the benefit of patients, their families, and their attorneys. If an occasional patient experiences a problem (an incidence of 0.01–0.001% of hospital admissions), corrective action plans are of dubious utility; on the other hand, awareness of the possible causes of this problem may help prevent future occurrences or help practitioners organize their approach to the bleeding patient.

MANAGEMENT OF BLEEDING FROM THE GASTROINTESTINAL TRACT

The individual with gastrointestinal bleeding after an operation on the gastrointestinal tract has a special type of gastrointestinal bleeding, but the overall approach to diagnosis and treatment is not unique. The site and cause of bleeding are variable, and each varies further in the severity of bleeding and the total morbidity (Table 28.2).

There is a major difference of opinion with respect to the management of these patients. While most instances of primary bleeding from the upper gastrointestinal tract can be managed endoscopically, the use of fiberoptic endoscopes has a more limited role in patients with postoperative bleeding. Further, individual gastroenterologists and surgeons may have different opinions about the utility/possibility of endoscopic control for these problems.

The timing of the rebleeding must be considered (Table 28.3). If there is substantial bleeding within the first 24–48 hours, there is a greater chance that the original site has continued to bleed or that some problem with the original suture line exists. Endoscopy

TABLE 28.2. Differential Diagnosis of Upper Gastrointestinal Hemorrhage

Location	*Lesion*	*Endoscopic Therapy*
Mouth	Arteriovenous malformations	+
	Telangiectasia	+
	Traumatic tears/lacerations	no
Oropharynx	Telangiectasia	+
Nose	Hypertension	no
	Telangiectasia	+
	Trauma	no
Nasopharynx	Trauma	
Esophagus	Esophagitis	+
	Esophageal varices	+
	Peptic ulceration	+
	Neoplasm	+
	Mallory-Weiss tear	+
Stomach	Acute gastric mucosal lesions	+
	Gastric ulcer	+
	Neoplasm	+
	Heterotopic tissue (pancreas)	+
	Gastric varices	+
	Dieulafoy lesions	+
	Arteriovenous malformations	+
	Thrombocytopenia (any cause)	±
	Rupture of retrogastric aneurysm	
	Hereditary hemorrhagic telangiectasia	+
	Anastomotic bleeding	+
	Visible vessels $\leq$1.5 mm in diameter	+
	Visible vessels >1.5 mm in diameter	±
	Nasogastric tube–induced lesions	+
Duodenum/jejunum	Duodenal ulcer	+
	Duodenitis	+
	Neoplasm (adenoma, carcinoma)	+
	Duodenal varices	+
	Aortoenteric fistula (atherosclerotic/graft-related)	
	Hemosuccus pancreaticus	
	Hemobilia	
	Telangiectasias	+
	Arteriovenous malformations	+
	Ulcerated diverticulum	
	Inflammatory bowel disease (Crohn's disease, etc.)	
	Visible vessels $\leq$1.5 mm in diameter	+
	Visible vessels >1.5 mm in diameter	±

Source: Reference 18.

TABLE 28.3. Differential Diagnosis of Postoperative Bleeding by Time and Site

- I. *Bleeding*—Postoperative time bleeding is noted
  - Suture line
    - Hand-sewn (1–72 hours; 7–12 days))
    - Stapled (immediately; 7–12 days)
  - Missed lesion (hours, days, or months)
  - Inappropriate operation (hours, days, or months)
  - Wrong operation (hours to days)
  - Persistence or recurrence of the primary problem
    - Technical failure of the operation
    - Progression of disease despite appropriate treatment
  - Nonspecific response to stress
    - Acute gastric mucosal lesion(s)
    - Acute duodenal ulcer or perforative intestinal lesion
- II. *Bleeding sites which may be difficult to find/control*
  - Esophagus
    - Atypical ulcers, diverticula, fistulas
    - Rebleeding varices
    - Coagulopathic diffuse bleeding
  - Stomach
    - Persistent arterial bleeding site
    - High gastric ulcers
    - Gastric varices with gastritis
    - Coagulopathic diffuse bleeding
  - Duodenum
    - Persistent artery in ulcer base
    - Bleeding from ampulla of Vater
    - Aortoenteric fistula
    - Atypical ulcer
    - Advanced cancer of pancreas or duodenum
  - Jejunum—ileum
    - Arteriovenous anomalies/malformations
    - Diverticula
    - Diffuse infectious ulcers (viral syndromes)
  - Colon
    - Arteriovenous malformations
    - Diverticula
    - Neoplastic lesions

in this setting is rarely indicated unless the amount of bleeding is considerable. If an endoscopic investigation is to be performed, the goals are limited (e.g., inspection of a suture line or exclusion of certain anatomical points as the source.). Angiography is rarely employed for this type of bleeding unless there is an unusual or compelling feature of the patient's history or clinical course, such as pancreatic necrosis or major surgical resections.

When the original site of bleeding was in the lower gastrointestinal tract and a postoperative bleeding episode ensues, the possibility of an incorrect diagnosis or therapy is paramount; parenthetically, lower gastrointestinal sources of bleeding still retain some of the mystery that upper gastrointestinal sources have lost since the advent of flexible endoscopic approaches for diagnosis. In the lower gastrointestinal tract, the inability to make an accurate diagnosis of midgut lesions by means of conventional endoscopes is occasionally a problem. When the site of bleeding is in the colon, the most common diagnostic entities are not associated with obvious craters or other visible clues to the source of the bleeding. In all cases, the diagnostic and therapeutic approaches need to be individualized.

At this point, it is important to consider the rebleeding episode with respect to the postoperative interval, the original site and treatment of bleeding, the common causes of rebleeding, and the author's treatment recommendations. The proposals for therapy are made with the full realization that the expertise and experience in different medical centers may indicate the use of alternatives in a different sequence. At times, it might be impossible to have a specific diagnosis prior to recommending reoperation. Another bias, which deserves additional emphasis is: *When a postoperative patient has unstable vital signs, with symptoms of postoperative bleeding, consistent with or accompanied by signs of postoperative bleeding, the most definitive diagnostic test is often the diagnostic laparotomy.*

THREE POTENTIAL CONCERNS IN POSTOPERATIVE BLEEDING

Wrong Diagnosis

For each part of the gastrointestinal tract, the first problem to be considered is whether the original diagnosis was correct. Since the advent of flexible endoscopes, however, the problem of incorrect diagnosis is less common. There are several explanations for an incorrect endoscopic diagnosis (Table 28.4). Of these, the most common is poor preparation of the stomach due to retained blood clots. Retained blood clot is not always due to poor preparation, since the rapidity of bleeding and the tenaciousness of the blood clot sometimes cause difficulty for the most skilled endoscopist. Good patient preparation is facilitated by vigorous lavage of the stomach through a wide-bore tube such as the Ewald tube; vigorous manual irrigation and suction of such tubes with a Toomey syringe is the best way to remove fresh clot from the stomach.

Rapidity of bleeding, a corollary problem to the one of excessive clot, is a common cause of difficulty in reaching a correct diagnosis. The mature surgical endoscopist will readily recognize when the rapidity of bleeding necessitates operative intervention. Retained clot lying in a dependent portion of the stomach can obscure the bleeding site,

TABLE 28.4. Causes of Incorrect Endoscopic Diagnosis

Poor preparation of stomach/patient
Rapidity of bleeding
Multiple potential bleeding sites
Anatomic deformity
Bleeding beyond the endoscopic field (Hemobilia, hemosuccus pancreaticus)
Inexperienced operator
Equipment failure

especially if the bleeding is not in the usual esophageal or lesser gastric curve sites. For example, gastric varices, gastric ulcers, or lesions on the greater curve of the stomach will not be discovered unless the patient is repositioned several times during the endoscopic examination. Repositioning is no mean feat in such individuals and must be accomplished with adequate assistance, attention to oxygenation by pulse oximetry, and extreme care.

The presence of multiple lesions that might account for the bleeding is a common problem in our institution. During a one-year period at Cook County Hospital, over 20% of 600 patients examined initially for acute bleeding had more than one lesion noted as a source of the bleeding. When one of multiple bleeding sites cannot be seen, subsequent decision making is compromised and the likelihood of late postoperative bleeding rises. Although the endoscopic approaches are discussed elsewhere, failure to identify a second bleeding lesion must be kept in mind as a potential cause of postoperative bleeding.

When two potential sites of massive hemorrhage are bleeding at the time of the original examination, the utmost diligence must be taken to determine which of the lesions is responsible for the major risks with respect to morbidity, rebleeding, and death. In general, both of the potential sites are managed as separate and potentially lethal problems until one or the other is shown to be the more dangerous and significant. Other sources of difficulty during endoscopic investigation are anatomical deformities which prevent direct visualization of the bleeding source. Stenosis of any visceral lumen may occur as a result of fibrosis, neoplasia, or postoperative changes. The experienced endoscopist will recognize when an examination is not complete, and should make that clear to the individual who is managing the patient.

For postoperative bleeding identified within the first 48 hours, the following questions need to be considered (Table 28.3):

1. Is there a suture/staple site (anastomosis)? Every suture line is at risk for bleeding, either in the first 48 hours or by five to seven days postoperatively. In the first case, unligated mucosal bleeders are the cause, while in the second case, a late reaction/ slough of the sutured mucosal vessels is thought to be the usual cause.
2. What is the potential for bleeding from the original site of pathology? This question addresses the potential for failure of the original attempt at hemostasis and must be viewed in the context of the natural history of the original bleeding lesion, with or without surgical therapy. Following porto-systemic shunting, varices rebleed at times, depending on the site, the portal pressure, and factors which control the integrity or healing potential of the mucosa. Since mucosal factors cannot be measured at present, we must expect and accept a failure rate for these operations, but a few of the failures will remain inexplicable.
3. How fast is the patient bleeding? If torrential bleeding is encountered, a return to the operating room might be the prudent or only way to establish the cause and treat it appropriately.
4. What resources are available in terms of endoscopic and radiographic intervention? One of the most difficult tasks is for the operating surgeon to remain objective about managing postoperative bleeding in his or her patient. Assuming that the primary operation identified the site of bleeding and dealt with it in an appropriate fashion, the presence of postoperative bleeding is quite demoralizing. The case must be managed on its own merits, without assuming that any of the previous care has or

has not been effective. Since every possible circumstance which can go wrong *does* go wrong occasionally, the mature surgeon will be prepared to react in a way which takes nothing for granted.

The most common bleeding problem I have encountered in the immediate postoperative period has been related to stapled anastomoses. Only one such patient required reoperation during the first 48 hours after operation; the bleeding site was a stapled anastomosis which was not visually inspected after completion of a Roux-en-Y limb constructed by passing the EEA stapler into the end of the defunctionalized limb. This type of bleeding can be prevented by visual inspection of stapled anastomoses and is viewed as a judgmental error rather than a technical failure of the stapler. Since stapled anastomoses preserve the blood supply distal to the staple line, occasional arterial bleeding occurs in the middle of a staple line. If the problem is noted immediately, a suture can be placed under direct vision or the bleeding point can be coagulated; however, if the bleeding point is not identified and bleeding continues, a massive hemorrhage can result. A bleeding rate of 1.0 cc/min which continues for 24 hours results in almost a 1,500 cc blood loss, an amount of bleeding which certainly qualifies as "massive."

A more common time for anastomotic hemorrhage after stapled anastomosis is the fifth to seventh day after the operation. Most such patients have been successfully managed with endoscopic thermal therapy. Why a stapled anastomosis should bleed at this point is unknown, but the potential for a slough of tissue included in anastomotic sites (stapled or sutured) at this time is well established.

Wrong Operation

Occasionally, there are situations in which the patient does so poorly after a first operation that the surgeon may wish that another operation had been employed the first time. Despite this, prospective judgments about the adequacy of operations for lesions of the stomach and intestines are extremely difficult. The only individuals who can make such clear-sighted distinctions, as a rule, are the plaintiff's attorneys and the "experts" whom they dredge up retrospectively to discuss bad-outcome situations.

Every well-known operation shows some evidence of having accomplished a stated goal. Variations in response to an operation, however, may reflect differences in tissue status, the presence or absence of previous or associated pathology, and many other factors. Clearly, no two people have the same background, the same medical history, and the same type of gastrointestinal bleeding.

Academic surgeons, as well as the community of surgeons, often disagree about the relative merits of different operations for specific diseases. When an experienced surgeon reviews the indications for a procedure, myriad considerations come to bear on the question. These include prior experience, work of teachers or respected colleagues, and previous complications of their own or those of colleagues. One surgical option may have little or no relevance in some settings but may be very useful for some surgeons in a different setting. One must remember that the precise operation employed is in many ways the prerogative of the operating surgeon. Although there are some real differences among surgical alternatives, depending on the primary pathology, a rigorous analysis of alternatives is not within the purview of this chapter.

Technical Problem

The technical problem of an unligated major vessel must always be a potential consideration in a patient with postoperative hemorrhage. The possibility of technical problems is sometimes hard for the operating surgeon to address objectively, since there is a natural tendency for the operator to assume that the initial problem was dealt with successfully.

Some circumstances, such as postoperative abscess or reoperations/resections in the presence of abscess, have a greater potential for postoperative hemorrhage. For example, a patient with a gastric resection for bleeding gastritis might have had a pancreatic abscess or peritonitis as a predisposing factor to the hemorrhage. Thus, persistent infection might cause a ligated vessel to bleed suddenly, with catastrophic results. We have had this problem in three patients who had exsanguinating hemorrhage as a late sequela to drainage of the pancreatic abscess; one individual bled from a ligated renal artery, another from the gastroduodenal artery, and another from the right gastric artery. Another group of patients with major risk factors for this type of hemorrhage are those in whom gastric resection was part of a Whipple procedure or a bypass for biliary obstruction; when a leak or abscess occurs in these individuals, hemorrhage can be a lethal event.

When treating the patient with unstable vital signs and a falling hematocrit, the team must consider a number of possibilities (see Table 28.5). However, when vital signs are unstable in the immediate postoperative period, there may be no way to ascertain that the intra-abdominal site is free of bleeding *except* by a second-look operation.

COAGULOPATHY

When a patient has postoperative bleeding, one should consider and search for a hematological problem as a contributing factor. The guide to effective management of these patients is a stepwise consideration of the possible causes of bleeding (Table 28.5).

TABLE 28.5. Types of Coagulopathy Associated with Postoperative Bleeding

Dilution of coagulation proteins from hemorrhage
Dilutional thrombocytopoenia
Hypothermia
Liver failure (liver resection, cirrhosis)
Factor VII or factor IX deficiency
Overheparinization
Aspirin or other nonsteroidal anti-inflammatory drugs
Disseminated intravascular coagulation
Fibrinolysis
Antibodies to heparin
Antithrombin 3 deficiency
Transfusion reaction
Previous streptokinase therapy
Antibiotic therapy (vitamin K deficiency)

A patient with recurrent gastrointestinal hemorrhage can be managed without serial platelet counts, prothrombin and partial thromboplastin times, bleeding time, and specific factor analysis[14-16] (see Chapter 8) but these studies are often useful.

Vitamin K deficiency must be considered in the patient who is jaundiced, in the patient in whom the gut has been sterilized, and in the patient who has been receiving antibiotics for long periods of time.

Specific management of the patient with gastrointestinal hemorrhage includes the correction of any identified clotting deficiency. If the patient is cold, then active warming measures are instituted. If there is a deficiency of special factors, fresh frozen plasma is indicated. If the platelet count is low, then platelet transfusions are appropriate; usually 1 unit of platelets is required for every unit of packed red blood cells employed, but a clinical need does not arise unless the hemorrhage is equal to or greater than 6 units.

In all cases, one must not become mesmerized by the postoperative clotting factor measurements and lose sight of the possibility of a less esoteric cause of postoperative bleeding, such as an unligated blood vessel.[17,18]

REFERENCES

1. Donahue PE, Nyhus LM: Massive upper gastrointestinal hemorrhage, Nyhus LM, Wastell C (eds): in *Surgery of the Stomach and Duodenum,* ed. 4. Boston, Little, Brown, 1986, pp 422–456.
2. Conlan MG, Hoots WK: Disseminated intravascular coagulation and hemorrhage in hemophilia B following elective surgery. *Am J Hematol* 35:203–207, 1990.
3. Scott TA, Jackler RK, Koerper MA: Management of hemophilia in otolaryngologic surgery. A contemporary protocol. *Arch Otolaryngol* 114:1445–1448, 1988.
4. Lee KF, Mandell J, Rankin JS, et al: Immediate versus delayed coronary grafting after streptokinase treatment. Postoperative blood loss and clinical results. *J Thorac Cardiovasc Surg* 95:216–222, 1988.
5. Chan KH, Mann KS, Lai EC, et al: Factors influencing the development of gastrointestinal complications after neurosurgery: results of multivariate analysis. *Neurosurgery* 25:378–382, 1989.
6. Donahue PE, Mobarhan S, Layden TJ, et al: Control of upper gastrointestinal bleeding with a bipolar coagulation device. *Surg Gynecol Obstet* 159:113–118, 1984.
7. Chung SCS, Leung JWC, Sung JY, et al: Injection or heat probe for bleeding ulcer. *Gastroenterology* 100:33–37, 1991.
8. Laine L: Determination of the optimal technique for bipolar electrocoagulation treatment. *Gastroenterology* 100:107–112, 1991.
9. Waring JP, Sanowski RA, Sawyer RL, et al: A randomized comparison of multipolar electrocoagulation and injection sclerosis for the treatment of bleeding peptic ulcer. *Gastrointest Endosc* 37:295–298, 1991.
10. Sugawa C, Fujita Y, Ikeda T, et al: Endoscopic hemostasis of bleeding of the upper gastrointestinal tract by local injection of 98% dehydrated alcohol. *Surg Gynecol Obstet* 162:159–163, 1986.
11. Sugawa C, Steffes CP, Nakamura R, et al: Upper GI bleeding in an urban hospital. Etiology, recurrence, and prognosis. *Ann Surg* 212:521–526, 1990.
12. Hui WM, Ng MMT, Lok ASF, et al: A randomized comparative study of laser photocoagulation, heater probe, and bipolar electrocoagulation in the treatment of actively bleeding ulcers. *Gastrointest Endosc* 137:299–304, 1991.

13. Lin HJ, Tsai YT, Lee SD, et al: A prospectively randomized trial of heat probe thermocoagulation versus pure alcohol injection in nonvariceal peptic ulcer hemorrhage. *Gut* 31:753–757, 1990.
14. Barak S, Shaked Y, Bar ZG, et al: Drug induced postsurgical haemorrhage resulting from trimethoprim sulfamethoxazole. A case report. *Int J Oral Maxillofacial Surg* 18:206–207, 1989.
15. Armstrong CP, Blower AL: Non-steroidal anti-inflammatory drugs and life threatening complications of peptic ulceration. *Gut* 28:527–532, 1987.
16. Kitler ME, Hays A, Enterline JP, et al: Preventing postoperative acute bleeding of the upper part of the gastrointestinal tract. *Surg Gynecol Obstet* 171:366–372, 1990.
17. Donahue PE: Acute and chronic duodenal ulcers, in Dent TL, Kukora JS, McCombs PR, et al (eds): *Surgical Tips*. Philadelphia, McGraw-Hill Book Co, 1988, pp 381–398.
18. Donahue PE: Gastroduodenal and non-variceal esophageal bleeding, in Madden RL (ed): *Problems in General Surgery*, ed 3, Vol 4. Philadelphia, JB Lippincott, 1987, pp 332–346.

VI

TREATMENT OF VARICEAL BLEEDING

29

VARICEAL BLEEDING: EMERGENCY TREATMENT, TAMPONADE, AND PHARMACOLOGICAL CONTROL

J. Loren Pitcher, M.D.

NATURAL HISTORY OF VARICEAL BLEEDING

Regardless of the cause of portal hypertension, variceal hemorrhage is unquestionably the most serious and potentially fatal complication of this condition. The most common cause of portal hypertension in Western countries is cirrhosis. The true natural history of patients with cirrhosis, portal hypertension, and variceal bleeding is, to a great extent, unknown and probably varies considerably depending upon the etiology of the cirrhosis. Much of our current knowledge of the natural history is based upon specific populations of patients, such as the control patients in prophylactic portal caval shunt trials, after the manifestations of their illness have led to a correct diagnosis.

Varices coexist with cirrhosis in about 60% of patients based upon autopsy series and in 33 to 98% of patients in endoscopic series. Approximately 25 to 40% of patients with varices will experience variceal bleeding. Of those patients who do have variceal bleeding, 70% will do so within two years of diagnosis.[1]

Following an index bleed from varices, 30 to 50% or more of such patients may die. Of those who survive their first bleed, 65 to 70% will rebleed and only 30% will survive for one year.

Almost 75% of the deaths associated with variceal hemorrhage occur during the first week after the onset of bleeding. From 30 to 60% of early deaths and 40% of late deaths are attributable to bleeding per se; many late deaths are due to hepatic failure.[2,3]

Early survival after an index bleed may be the best marker of later survival. However, at least one-third of cirrhotics with an index bleed may be in a terminal state of their liver disease, when no therapy will improve their survival. One should also realize that, on the average, 30 to 50% of patients with bleeding varices will spontaneously cease bleeding—albeit temporarily. These figures are important to remember when assessing the effectiveness of various therapeutic modalities in treating variceal bleeding.

PORTAL HYPERTENSION

Portal pressure results from an interaction of resistance and flow. This is reflected in Ohm's law: $\Delta P = Q \times R$, where ΔP is the change in pressure, Q is the flow, and R is the resistance in a vessel. Resistance depends on several factors expressed in Poiseuille's law: $R = 8nL/\pi r^4$, in which n is the coefficient of viscosity, L is the length of the vessel, and r is the radius of the vessel. Since length and viscosity do not usually change significantly, resistance is most influenced by the vessel radius. Small increases or decreases in r (taken to the fourth power) can cause significant increases or decreases in resistance and, hence, changes in pressure.[4]

Portal hypertension in most patients results primarily from increased resistance to portal flow to the liver secondary to increased intrahepatic resistance (the so-called backward flow theory).

Intrahepatic causes of increased resistance may include pressure from regenerative nodules on hepatic venules, collagenation of venules and sinusoids, capillarization of sinusoids, and hepatocyte enlargement. Evidence exists that some of the intrahepatic resistance may be lowered by vasodilators such as clonodine and isoproterenol, by the loss of hepatocyte swelling (as may occur after resolution of alcoholic hepatitis), or by other pharmacological manipulations of myofibroblasts around heptic sinusoids.[4,5]

Besides intrahepatic causes of increased resistance to flow, there are those conditions which inhibit hepatic venous outflow (i.e., constrictive pericarditis, severe right heart failure, vena cava obstruction, hepatic vein obstruction, etc.). Other causes of increased resistance to flow are presinusoidal obstruction (such as in schistosomiasis) and extrahepatic causes such as portal and splenic vein obstruction.

If resistance increases but flow decreases, increased portal pressure may not occur. However, despite the development of multiple venous collaterals, which should decrease portal pressure, the pressure actually increases, reflecting an increase in total splanchnic flow (a concept reflected in the traditional *forward flow* theory). The causes for this increased splanchnic flow are multiple and include increased cardiac output, expanded blood volume, a hyperdynamic splanchnic circulation, the vasodilatory effects of increased levels of circulating endogenous compounds (e.g., glucagon), and a decreased sensitivity to endogenous vasoconstrictors.

Thus, the portal hypertension syndrome is caused by multiple factors which cause both increased resistance and total portal flow. Some of these factors may be static, while others may be dynamic and subject to alteration.

VARICEAL BLEEDING

Esophagogastric varices (EGV) develop over time from preexisting embryonic venous channels in an attempt to decompress portal hypertension. They are the most vulnerable of the multiple collaterals which develop (intercostal, azygos, hemorrhoidal, paraumbilical, diaphragmatic, retroperitoneal, abdominal wall, and peri-ileostomy veins). A threshold hepatic venous pressure gradient, which correlates with portal pressure in alcoholic cirrhosis, of 12 mm Hg or more is usually required for the formation of EGV.

Elegant anatomical studies have helped to clarify the venous channels in the lower 4 or 5 cm of the esophagus (the so-called critical area) in both normal humans and those with portal hypertension.[6-10] Major varices primarily represent dilated deep intrinsic veins in the esophageal lamina propria which communicate outwardly with adventitial, periesophageal, and communicating (perforating) veins to the azygos system. In addition, there are smaller veins in the superficial esophageal mucosa overlying the deep intrinsic veins. These superficial veins may become compressed over the dilating deep intrinsic veins, may be the source of minimal or limited venous bleeding, and may be the source of various endoscopic signs, such as red spots, noted over varices. In this ''critical area'' of the distal 4 to 5 cm of the esophagus, the number and size of veins and venules are significantly increased, and this increase correlates with the location of the entrance of both the perforating veins from the periesophageal venous plexus and the venous channels which flow from across the esophagogastric junction. A bulbous enlargement on a variceal chain in this critical area is often the point of variceal bleeding and may overlay the location of a perforating vein.

Variceal bleeding usually results from a rupture at a point on one of the three to five chains of varices located in the critical area. Variceal bleeding solely due to erosions and esophagitis is unusual compared to the frequency of rupture. The factors leading to rupture most likely relate to pressure and varix wall tension.[11] Varix wall tension is best expressed by a modified form of Laplace's law, where $T = TP \times r/w$. T is tension, TP is transmural pressure (intravariceal pressure minus esophageal luminal pressure), r is the radius, and w is the wall thickness. Increases in TP or varix radius (r) or a decrease in wall thickness (w) results in an increase in variceal wall tension and an increased risk of varix rupture. Larger, and thinner-walled varices with thin overlying supportive mucosa have been correlated with a higher risk of variceal bleeding. However, absolute *portal* pressure levels above 12 mm Hg have not previously correlated well with predictions of which patients might bleed from their varices. This has been somewhat perplexing, as one might expect patients with higher portal pressures to bleed more often than those with lower pressures. Recent positive correlations between *intravariceal* pressures, but not *portal* pressures, in predicting variceal bleeding have been published.[12,13] Sarin et al.[12] found mean *intravariceal* pressures of 21.4 mm Hg in variceal bleeders versus 12.9 mm Hg in nonbleeders. Rigau et al.[13] also found that variceal bleeders had significantly higher variceal pressures than nonbleeders in spite of similar portal pressures in both groups. More than 60% of bleeders but only 22% of nonbleeders had *variceal* pressures greater than 15 mm Hg. These important findings expand the intravariceal pressure studies conducted by Palmer in the 1950s.[14,15] Once variceal rupture has occurred, however, other factors such as portal pressure levels, varix flow rates, size of the rent, the patient's coagulation status, blood viscosity, and intravariceal pressure may be important relative to the severity, continuation, duration, or recurrence of the variceal bleeding.

DIAGNOSIS

An accurate diagnosis of bleeding varices is critical for both immediate and future therapy and for the proper assessment of therapeutic trials. Panendoscopy is the best method to ensure an accurate diagnosis. Evidence of an actively bleeding varix or a fresh clot or fibrin plug on a varix reasonably confirms vericeal bleeding. The presence of nonbleeding varices, with or without variceal red spots or other endoscopic signs, and no evidence of another bleeding site identified during panendoscopy are often used as criteria for probable recent variceal hemorrhage. However, these are less reliable endoscopic findings unless there is bright red blood in the stomach and/or excessive time has not elapsed since the cessation of the bleeding. Some prospective randomized controlled therapeutic trials may be associated with the inclusion of a larger percentage of patients with these less reliable endoscopic criteria for variceal bleeding, and this could significantly influence the outcome and results unrelated to the treatment being studied.

The frequency of other bleeding causes, especially acute mucosal lesions or multiple lesions, in various patient populations with esophagogastric varices warrants early endoscopic diagnosis.[16]

Barium esophagograms or attempts at diagnosis through trials of balloon tamponade or pharmacological therapy to see if bleeding stops are unreliable for the confirmation of variceal bleeding. Transhepatic venography is rarely necessary or indicated for diagnostic purposes and rarely documents a venous leak to ensure variceal bleeding. Often, a second delayed endoscopic examination, especially if rebleeding occurs, will help to confirm the correct diagnosis in questionable cases.

GENERAL CARE

The general care of patients with suspected variceal bleeding incorporates many of the well-known tenets of managing patients with upper gastrointestinal bleeding. A relevant history and physical examination; resuscitation with packed red blood cells, platelets, and fresh frozen plasma; infusion of intravenous fluids while avoiding sodium overload; gastric lavage; and the establishment of an accurate diagnosis can be accomplished expeditiously and often simultaneously. Other measures include the reduction of tense ascites by judicious paracentesis; obtaining appropriate laboratory tests; monitoring major organ systems; necessary vitamin and electrolyte replacement; avoidance of excessive volume replacement with blood, colloid, or fluids; and assessment of both the etiology of the portal hypertension and the functional hepatic reserve of the patient. Hepatic encephalopathy and infections should be vigorously treated, harmful and unnecessary medications avoided, at least two major intravenous pipelines established, and meticulous medical record logs kept. The immediate goal of therapy—after appropriate resuscitation, general care measures, and the establishment of an accurate diagnosis—is to achieve rapid cessation and control of bleeding, even if the control is only temporary. The next goal should always be to plan the next therapeutic step should the initial or subsequent attempts to control variceal bleeding succeed or fail, rebleeding occur, or complications develop.

BALLOON TAMPONADE

Balloon tamponade was introduced by Westphal in 1930; significant tube design modifications by Sengstaken and Blakemore (1950), Linton and Nachlas (1953 and 1955), Boyce (1962), and Edlick, et al. (1968) followed. Numerous reports attest to the efficacy of balloon tamponade to stop variceal bleeding temporarily for at least 12 to 24 hours if utilized properly in patients proven to be bleeding from EGV and if instituted early in the bleeding episode.[17-25] Tamponade is potentially and actually very hazardous if careful attention is not paid to management protocols directed at the prevention of the many major and minor complications associated with this therapy.[17] Rebleeding after initial hemostasis is common. Therefore, tamponade should be regarded as temporary emergency therapy administered for bleeding control until more definitive therapy can be provided when necessary.

Worldwide, balloon tamponade is used by some as the initial therapy of choice. Many physicians, however, reserve the use of tamponade, with or without pharmacological therapy, as either a backup, second line of therapy after the failure of other treatments (i.e., sclerotherapy) or as a temporary measure before more definitive therapy is instituted. Most experts now prefer emergency sclerotherapy at the time of emergency endoscopy, despite active variceal bleeding, while others prefer to use tamponade to gain temporary control of bleeding and, hence, convert sclerotherapy to a more elective, less difficult procedure with fewer potential risks.

Balloon tamponade can be an unpleasant experience for both the patient and the health care team. The technique must be implemented in an intensive care unit staffed with highly trained and experienced personnel. Tamponade is neither a reliable diagnostic technique, as it was once thought to be, nor a safe and effective treatment during the transportation of patients from remote facilities to tertiary care centers.

Early reports on the safety and effectiveness of balloon tamponade were often confusing and conflicting due to such factors as poor endoscopic techniques, lack of endoscopic proof of variceal bleeding, poor techniques for tube placement and management, wide variation in tube design and quality, excessive time delays before initiating therapy, and a paucity of prospective, controlled therapeutic trials.

Table 29.1 presents prospective trials of balloon tamponade in which endoscopic proof of variceal bleeding was required, tamponade was initiated soon after the diagnosis, and patients were managed in an intensive care setting by experienced physicians and medical personnel.[17-25] The range of initial bleeding control for at least 12 to 24 hours was 76% to 98%. This exceeds the average 50% rate of spontaneous cessation of variceal bleeding noted among control patients in many trials.

The results of eight randomized controlled trials of tamponade with either pharmacological therapy or sclerotherapy are noted in Table 29.2.[26-33] It should be noted that the one unusually low bleeding control rate for tamponade in the report by Barsoum et al.[30] actually relates to definitive (no bleeding for up to four weeks) and not temporary control of bleeding. The low 70% bleeding control rate of Correia et al.[27] may be attributed to delayed inflation of the esophageal balloon, which was used only if initial gastric balloon inflation and traction failed. The remaining initial bleeding control rates range from 73% to 87%. Tamponade is as good as or better than vasopressin therapy, is equal to terlipressin plus nitroglycerine, and is generally less effective than endoscopic variceal sclerotherapy for the initial short-term control of variceal bleeding.

Tamponade alone does not ensure reduced blood transfusion requirements, reduce mortality, prevent early or late rebleeds, or reduce the length of the hospital stay. Most experts prefer the Linton-Nachlas tube for treating bleeding gastric varices,[19,28] and either the four-lumen Minnesota type Sengstaken-Blakemore (SB) tube or the Boyce modification of the standard SB tube for treating bleeding esophageal varices. The fourth lumen helps to prevent the accumulation of fluids and blood emanating from both above and below the esophageal balloon and, hence, reduces the frequency and severity of pulmo-

TABLE 29.1 Results of Selected Trials with *Balloon Tamponade* to Control Active Variceal Bleeding*

Author(s)	*Year*	*Number of Episodes*	*% Initial Bleeding Control***	*Type Balloon*
Pitcher (17)	1971	50	92	SBB
Novis et al (18)	1976	41	85	SBB
Terés et al (19)	1978	31	87	SB
		48	92	LN
Mitchell et al (20)	1980	14	78	Minn
		14	76	SBB
Hunt et al (21)	1982	103	94	SBB + Minn
Sarin et al (22)	1984	62	87	SB
Panés et al (23)	1988	118	92	SB
Feneyrou et al (24)	1988	82	95	SB
Haddock et al (25)	1986	126	98	Minn

Abbreviations: SB—Sengstaken-Blakemore Tube, SBB—Sengtaken-Blakemore Boyce Modification, LN—Linton-Nachlas Tube, Minn—Minnesota-Edlick Tube.

*Bleeding varices diagnosed by endoscopy.

**for 12–24 hours.

nary aspiration. For bleeding esophageal varices, the inflation of both the esophageal and gastric balloons is more effective than relying solely upon gastric balloon inflation and traction. Endotracheal intubation of obtunded patients or for mechanical ventilation may be indicated but is not necessary in most patients.

The complications of tamponade are legion and include esophageal rupture and laceration, aspiration, tube impaction, balloon deflation, tube migration with asphyxiation, chest pain, hiccups, and misplacement in the lung, chest, duodenum, and jejunum. Other complications are mucosal erosions and ulcerations, blockage of thoracic lymph flow or the innominate vein, nasopharyngeal bleeding, and patient self-extubation. Most, if not all, of these complications are preventable, or their frequency can be reduced to an acceptable level with minimal morbidity and mortality if a proper protocol, designed to minimize or prevent these complications, is followed by an experienced, knowledgeable team.[17] Guidelines or protocols without expertise in patient care management are not sufficient, and the absence of both should preclude the use of balloon tamponade.

A safe and effective method for the use of the modified SB tube has been previously reported[17] and is noted in Appendix I.

PHARMACOLOGICAL CONTROL

The pharmacological control of variceal bleeding is an appealing concept due to its potential ease of administration, wide availability, low cost, and patient acceptance if agents can be found which are proven to be relatively safe and effective. Ideally, the goal of rapid and definitive control of variceal bleeding is desired but, practically, the

TABLE 29.2 Results of Selected Randomized Controlled Trials with *Balloon Tamponade* to Control Active Variceal Bleeding*

Author(s)	*Year*	*Number of Episodes*	*Treatment*	*% Initial (12–24 hrs) Bleeding Control*
Hernomo et al (26)	1983	30	SB	87
		30	VP	83
		30	Ice Water	47
Correia et al (27)	1984	20	SB	70
		17	VP	65
Terés et al (28)	1990	52	SB + LN	87
		56	VP	66
Fort et al (29)	1990	24	SB	79
		23	GLY VP + Nitro	78
Barsoum et al (30)	1982	50	SB	42**
		50	EVS	74
Söderlund et al (31)	1985	50	SB	84
		57	EVS	95
Paquet et al (32)	1985	21	SB	73
		21	EVS	95
Moretó et al (33)	1988	20	SB	80
		23	EVS	100

Abbreviations: SB—Sengstaken-Blakemore, VP vasopressin, LN—Linton Nachlas, Nitro—nitroglycerin, Gly VP—glypressin or terlipressin, EVS—endoscopic variceal sclerotherapy

*Bleeding varices diagnosed by endoscopy.

**Required no bleeding in first four *weeks* post tube removal.

agents to date are best viewed as providing temporary control or adjunctive therapy to allow stabilization of the patient before more definitive therapy, such as sclerotherapy, long-term beta blocker therapy, surgical decompression, or other surgical procedures such as liver transplantation can be used.

Pharmacological agents used in the control of active variceal bleeding act primarily, but not exclusively, in one of two ways. Some reduce portal blood flow and pressure by causing vasoconstriction (vasopressin, terlipressin, somatostatin), while others cause vasodilatation (nitrates, pentagastrin, isoproterenol). A third group of agents, including agents such as metoclopramide and pentagastrin, which may act by constricting the lower esophageal sphincter area and thus inhibiting variceal flow, have not been adequately tested to date.

The major agents which have been subjected to even limited trials are discussed below. Although the various pharmacological agents and other therapeutic modalities are considered separately, they are often used sequentially or simultaneously despite the lack of controlled trials regarding combinations of therapy.

Propranalol and other beta blockers, although used to prevent bleeding or rebleeding, have not been shown to date to be effective, alone or as adjunctive therapy, in the direct control of active variceal bleeding. Therefore, they are not discussed further.

Vasopressin

Vasopressin increases mesenteric vascular resistance via vasoconstriction, leading to decreased portal flow and pressure. It temporarily decreases hepatic artery flow, which then returns toward normal. Venous collateral flow is decreased, along with the portasystemic pressure gradient and intravariceal pressure. Vasopressin may also cause increased esophageal muscle wall tone, which decreases flow and pressure in varices. Vasopressin decreases wedge hepatic venous pressure, increases free hepatic vein pressure, and, hence, decreases the hepatic venous pressure gradient.

Unfortunately, vasopressin causes hypertension, reflex bradycardia, coronary artery ischemia and myocardial infarction, decreased cardiac output, intestinal necrosis, antidiuresis, increased gastrointestinal motility and cramps, generalized vasoconstriction of skin and muscle, and the release of plasminogen activator and factor VIII, and is associated with a host of adverse side effects and possible complications.

Despite the unconvincing and limited number of placebo-controlled trials involving small numbers of patients, vasopressin, surprisingly, has been one of the most widely utilized pharmacological agents for the control of variceal bleeding for almost 30 years.[34,35]

Tables 29.2 through 29.5 include some of the selected randomized controlled trials comparing vasopressin to balloon tamponade, placebo, vasopressin plus nitroglycerin, terlipressin, and somatostatin relative to the immediate control of variceal bleeding.

Overall, vasopressin, as monotherapy, appears to have an efficacy of approximately 50 to 55%, although this figure is adversely affected by the study by Fogel et al.,[36] in

TABLE 29.3 Results of Selected Randomized Controlled Trials with Vasopressin to Control Active Variceal Bleeding

Author(s)	*Year*	*Number of Episodes*	*Treatment*	*% Initial Bleeding Control*
Merigan et al (36)	1962	23	VP	69
		16	P	0
Ramsby et al (37)	1975	17	VP	71
		16	P	25
Fogel et al (38)	1982	14	VP	29
		19	P	32
Tsai et al (40)	1986	19	VP	47
		20	VP + NG (Sub L)	55
Gimson et al (41)	1986	34	VP	44
		38	VP + NG (IV)	68
Bosch et al (42)	1989	30	VP + NG (T. DERM)	83
		35	VP + P (T. DERM)	74

Abbreviations: VP—vasopressin, P—placebo, NG—nitroglycerin, Sub L—Sublingual, I.V.—intravenous, T. DERM—transdermal patch

TABLE 29.4 Results of Selected Randomized Controlled Trials with Terlipressin to Control Active Variceal Bleeding

Author(s)	*Year*	*Number of Episodes*	*Treatment*	*% Initial Bleeding Control*
Freeman et al (43)	1982	10	TP	70
		11	VP	9
Freeman et al (44)	1989	15	TP	60
		16	P	37
Söderlund et al (45)	1990	31	TP	90
		29	P	59

Abbreviations: TP—Terlipressin (Glypressin®), VP—Vasopressin, P—Placebo

which the endoscopic criteria for bleeding varices are unclear. Vasopressin, usually given by continuous intravenous infusion, is relatively low in cost and readily available, and so is often used.[36-38] The usual doses consist of continuous intravenous infusion rates titrated from to 0.4 to 0.8 units/min (some advocate an initial bolus infusion of 15–20 units over 15 minutes). One trial using rates as high as 1.5 units/min has been reported.[39] Careful patient monitoring, including cardiac output, is usually recommended if vasopressin monotherapy is used.

Nitroglycerin

Nitroglycerin, a powerful venous and mild arterial dilator, enhances the reduction in portal pressure caused by vasopressin due to a reduction in portal venous resistance.

TABLE 29.5 Results of Selected Randomized Controlled Trials with Somatostatin to Control Active Variceal Bleeding

Author(s)	*Year*	*Number of Episodes*	*Treatment*	*% Initial Bleeding Control*
Valenzuela et al (47)	1989	48	ST	65
		36	P	83
Burroughs et al (48)	1990	61	ST	64
		59	P	41
Avgerinos et al (49)	1989	20	ST	90
		18	SBT	55
Kravetz et al (50)	1984	30	ST	87
		31	VP	74
Jenkins et al (51)	1985	10	ST	100
		12	VP	33
Saari et al (52)	1990	32	ST	84
		22	VP	57

Abbreviations: ST—Somatostatin, P—Placebo, SBT—Sengstaken-Blakemore Tube, VP—Vasopressin

The combination of vasopressin and nitroglycerin thus offers the possibility of achieving a further fall in portal pressure without additional reductions in portal blood flow.[35] At the same time, it may ameliorate many of the major and undesirable systemic side effects of vasopressin. The use of nitroglycerin, either intravenously or sublingually, presents a problem in maintaining stable drug concentrations.[40,41] This problem appears to be overcome with the transdermal slow release of approximately 5–10 mg of nitroglycerin per 24 hours.[42]

The report by Bosch et al.[42] indicates that when compared to vasopressin plus a placebo transdermal patch, vasopressin plus a transdermal nitroglycerin patch yields initial control of variceal bleeding in 83% vs. 74% of episodes and definitive control of 73% vs. 54%. Decreased transfusion requirements, lower doses of vasopressin, and less need for balloon tamponade and emergency surgery were observed, but with no significant differences in minor side effects and mortality.

The factors of cost, ease of administration, current availability, and the relative safety and effectiveness of vasopressin plus transdermal nitroglycerin make this combined therapy very attractive if the results of Bosch et al.[42] are confirmed by others. Such therapy, if confirmed to be both safe and effective, might be ideal for use in patients who must be transported from remote areas to tertiary centers or as temporary emergency therapy in hospitals until specialists can be mobilized.

Terlipressin

Terlipressin (Glypressin) is a vasopressin analog which has no significant activity on smooth muscle. After injection, its terminal amino acid residues are released in vivo, resulting in a slow release of vasopressin. Its actions are otherwise thought to be similar to those of vasopressin relative to its hemostatic effects on variceal bleeding. The slow release of vasopressin results in smooth muscle constriction for up to 10 hours compared to 20 to 40 minutes with equipotent doses of intravenous vasopressin. Terlipressin has less adverse systemic effects than vasopressin and is said not to alter clotting mechanisms. Table 29.4 presents limited trials comparing terlipressin to vasopressin[43] or to placebo.[44,45] More trials are needed to evaluate its effectiveness compared to vasopressin plus nitroglycerin, somatostatin, or other drugs. Terlipressin is not yet available in the United States for routine use.

Somatostatin

Somatostatin (Stilamin) is a peptide inhibitor which, in pharmacological doses, inhibits splanchnic blood flow without causing any significant effects on the systemic circulation or other serious side effects such as those observed with vasopressin.[46] A very short half-life (two to three minutes) requires continuous infusions at a dose of approximately 250 μg/hr. Somatostatin reduces effective hepatic blood flow, wedge hepatic venous pressure, and hepatic venous pressure gradient. The mechanism of action is thought to be direct and indirect vasoconstriction of venous collaterals in the portal circuit, thus reducing variceal blood flow. Unlike vasopressin, which decreases intravariceal pressure, somatostatin may produce either no change or a slight increase in intravariceal pressure, but its protective effect may be the associated reduction in venous flow to the varices.

Published clinical trials with somatostatin compared with placebo,[47,48] balloon tamponade,[49] or vasopressin[50-52] are noted in Table 29.5.

The multicenter trial reported by Valenzuela et al.,[47] as noted in Table 29.5, has been criticized relative to patient selection and exclusion criteria, the short duration of drug infusion (250 μg IV bolus × 30 hours), and especially a placebo response rate of 83%.[46] This latter rate far exceeds the expected 30 to 50% rate for spontaneous cessation of variceal bleeding in most trials. The well-designed and controlled clinical trial by Burroughs et al.[48] has confirmed that somatostatin (250 μg IV bolus, 250 μg/hr × five days) is safe and more effective than placebo for the control of bleeding. In addition, requirements for blood transfusions and balloon tamponade were reduced. There were no differences in 30-day mortality rates or general complication rates. However, none of the complications which occurred could be attributed to either the drug or the placebo. To be effective, somatostatin may need to be infused for longer than 30 hours.

Unfortunately, somatostatin is very expensive and not yet available in the United States for routine use for variceal bleeding. Based upon the preliminary trials, further trials comparing somatostatin with vasopressin plus dermal nitroglycerin are currently indicated and eagerly anticipated.

Octreotide

Preliminary reports on octreotide (Sandostatin; SMS201-995), an octapeptide somatostatin analog, are encouraging for the control of bleeding varices.[53] This drug is administered subcutaneously, has a 90- to 115-minute half-life and has clinical effects for up to 12 hours.[54] At a 25 μg/hr dose, its effects on variceal bleeding control have been compared with balloon tamponade using the Minnesota tube. Octreotide was found to provide less immediate bleeding control than tamponade (55% vs. 75%) but similar control at four hours (90% vs. 95%). These latter results remained similar at 24 hours.[53] Further trials are anticipated for this apparently well-tolerated analog of somatostatin.

CONCLUSION

Convincing evidence exists that balloon tamponade, when used under proper protocols by experienced and trained personnel, is relatively safe and effective in controlling well-documented variceal bleeding. However, its potential risks, personnel requirements, lack of suitability and safety during the transport of patients, unpleasant aspects for patients, and the superior effectiveness of sclerotherapy to control bleeding and early rebleeding appear to limit the use of balloon tamponade by many physicians.

It would be ideal to have a highly reliable pharmacological agent, or combination of agents, which are readily available, easy to administer without the need for specialists, relatively low in cost and side effects, safe, and highly effective—even if effective for only temporary control of bleeding. Vasopressin, as monotherapy, does not appear to fulfill all of these goals. Hopefully, however, the effectiveness of vasopressin-nitroglycerin or somatostatin, or analogs of either vasopressin or somatostatin, will be confirmed as fulfilling these goals in the near future.

Ironically, despite earlier and more effective control of variceal bleeding, mortality rates in most studies of balloon tamponade and pharmacological therapy have not been significantly decreased. However, it seems obvious that the optimal control of acute bleeding and the prevention of early rebleeding are the major factors which we can control by therapy. There must be patients for whom this will make a difference, and our future challenge is to attempt to better identify this group. If this is possible, effective therapy will probably be found in a regimen of therapies applied in the most appropriate sequence and not in a single therapy.

APPENDIX I: TECHNIQUE FOR THE SAFE AND EFFECTIVE USE OF THE MODIFIED SENGSTAKEN-BLAKEMORE (SB) TUBE*

1. Complete an accurate diagnosis with endoscopy to ensure that the acute bleeding is from gastric and/or esophageal varices.
2. Use a new 20 French (or smaller sizes, when appropriate) SB tube with the Boyce[17] modification [Accessory nagogastric (NG tube)] attached (or use the Minnesota tube.
   a. Always check balloons underwater just before use to ensure that there are no leaks.
3. Ensure that the stomach and esophagus are reasonably empty to prevent aspiration during SB tube passage. Use a large-bore tube for gastric lavage just before step 4.
4. Lubricate the modified SB tube, attach the accessory NG tube to constant suction, and then pass the SB tube through the mouth (not the nose) until the gastric lumen tip and balloon are well within the stomach.
   a. Tubes are easiest to introduce with the patient in the left lateral decubitus position.
   b. A guidewire or flexible wand in the gastric lumen channel may ease tube insertion; introduce the tube as if inserting a gastroscope.
5. Flush the gastric lumen channel with 25 to 50 ml of air, while auscultating over the epigastric area, to ensure that the gastric lumen tube tip and the gastric balloon are in the stomach, not the esophagus, before performing step 6.
6. Slowly inflate the gastric balloon, in 50-ml aliquots, to a total of 250 to 275 ml of air (no more or less) while auscultating over the epigastric area. Stop immediately if the patient develops sudden substernal pain and/or the insufflation of air is not audible in the epigastric area. (Waiting to check the position of the gastric balloon with x-rays taken after inflation is often too late to prevent serious complications.)
7. Double-clamp the gastric balloon inlet with two rubber-shod surgical clamps.
8. Apply firm but gentle traction on the SB tube at the mouth so that the gastric balloon is firmly snugged against the diaphragm at the cardia. Too much traction causes retching or hiccups.
9. Connect the gastric lumen tube inlet to intermittent suction.

*See Reference 17 for more details, discussion, and equipment setup relative to the use of the modified SB tube.

10. Position a keyholed, padded traction pad at a corner of the mouth and tape the SB tube securely to the pad.
    a. In dentulous patients, add a protective plastic mouthpiece around the SB tube.
11. Inflate the esophageal balloon to 25 to 45 mm Hg of pressure. Use the lowest pressure necessary to stop bleeding. Do not exceed 45 mm Hg of pressure.
12. Double-clamp the esophageal balloon inlet with two rubber-shod surgical clamps.
13. Switch the suction on the accessory NG tube (or the fourth channel of the Minnesota tube) from constant to low intermittent suction and tape the connections on this system shut to preclude inadvertent lavage.
14. Maintain elevation of the head of the bed on 6-inch blocks (to prevent aspiration and decrease hiccups or retching).
15. Tape scissors to the head of the bed within the clear view and quick reach of attendants should emergency transection and removal of the tube become necessary.
16. Reinstruct all aides, nurses, interns, residents, and others who will be attending the patient in the proper management of the SB tube.
17. Irrigate the gastric channel approximately every half-hour and record the appearance of the return fluid.
18. Recheck and readjust the tube traction and esophageal balloon pressure every two hours; this should be performed by informed physicians only.
19. An informed, trained attendant must be at or near the bedside of the patient at all times.
20. Give the patient nothing by mouth, and so advise all visitors.
    a. Once bleeding is stopped, certain necessary medications (i.e., lactulose, neomycin, etc.) may be given in small volumes via the gastric lumen channel.
21. Ensure proper oral hygiene, frequent deep breathing or coughing, and changes of body position.
22. Continue tamponade for 24 to 48 hours (or less if this is an adjunct to sclerotherapy or other definitive treatments).
23. Deflate the esophageal balloon only; relax the traction on the gastric balloon but leave the gastric balloon inflated.
    a. This is best done at a time of day when close observation for rebleeding is ensured.
24. Observe for rebleeding while the esophageal balloon is deflated, the gastric balloon is inflated, and the tube is in place for another 12 to 24 hours.
25. If rebleeding does not occur during step 24, pull the SB tube out after complete transection of the tube with scissors to ensure that:
    a. The tube is not reused.
    b. Balloons are deflated before removal.
26. Begin an appropriate liquid diet and institute appropriate therapy for possible gastroesophagitis and erosions.
27. Should rebleeding occur during step 24 or after step 25, tamponade may be resumed as a temporary measure until other therapy is initiated.
28. From the time of tube insertion (step 4) until tube removal (step 25), continuously reevaluate what will be the next and best course of action should tamponade fail or rebleeding occur.

REFERENCES

1. Sivak MV Jr: *Esophageal Varices. Gastrointestinal Endoscopy*. Philadelphia, WB Saunders, 1987, pp 342–372.
2. Graham DY, Smith JL: The course of patients after variceal hemorrhage. *Gastroenterology* 80:800–809, 1981.
3. Smith JL, Graham DY: Variceal hemorrhage: A critical evaluation of survival analysis. *Gastroenterology* 182:968–973, 1982.
4. Mahl TC, Groszmann RJ: Pathophysiology of portal hypertension and variceal bleeding. *Surg Clin North Am* 70:251–266, 1990.
5. MacMathuna P, Westaby D, Williams R: Taking the tension out of the portal system: An approach to the management of portal hypertension in the 1990s. *Scand J Gastroenterol* 175:131–145, 1990.
6. McCormack TT, Smith PM, Rose JD, et al: Perforating veins and blood flow in oesophageal varices. *Lancet* 2:1442–1444, 1983.
7. Spence RAJ: The venous anatomy of the lower oesophagus in normal subjects and in patients with varices: An image analysis study. *Br J Surg* 71:739–744 1984.
8. Kitano S, Terblanche J, Kahn D, et al: Venous anatomy of the lower oesophagus in portal hypertension: Practical implications. *Br J Surg* 73:525–531, 1986.
9. Vianna A, Hayes PC, Moscoso G, et al: Normal venous circulation of the gastroesophageal junction: A route to understanding varices. *Gastroenterology* 93:876–889, 1987.
10. Spence RAJ, Terblanche J: Venous anatomy of the lower oesophagus: A new perspective on varices. *Br J Surg* 74:659–660, 1987.
11. Polio J, Groszmann RJ: Bleeding esophageal varices. *Pract Gastroenterol* 13:41–73, 1989.
12. Sarin SK, Sundaram KR, Ahuju RK: Prediction of variceal bleeding: An analysis of clinical, endoscopic, and haemodynamic variables, with special reference to intravariceal pressure. *Gut* 30:1757–1764, 1989.
13. Rigau J, Bosch J, Bordas JM, et al: Endoscopic measurements of variceal pressure in cirrhosis: Correlation with portal pressure and variceal hemorrhage. *Gastroenterology* 96:873–880, 1989.
14. Palmer ED: On correlations between portal venous pressure and the size and extent of esophageal varices in portal cirrhosis. *Ann Surg* 138:741–744, 1953.
15. Palmer ED: Correlations between the severity of esophageal varices in portal cirrhosis and their propensity toward hemorrhage. *Gastroenterology* 30:85–90, 1956.
16. Pitcher JL: Variceal hemorrhage among patients with varices and upper gastrointestinal hemorrhage. *South Med J* 70:1183–1185, 1977.
17. Pitcher JL: Safety and effectiveness of the modified Sengstaken-Blakemore tube: A prospective study. *Gastroenterology* 61:291–298, 1971.
18. Novis BH, Duys P, Barbezat GO, et al: Fiberoptic endoscopy and the use of the Sengstaken tube in acute gastrointestinal haemorrhage in patients with portal hypertension and varices. *Gut* 17:258–263, 1976.
19. Teres J, Cecilia A, Bordas JM, et al: Esophageal tamponade for bleeding varices: Controlled trial between the Sengstaken-Blakemore tube and the Linton-Nachlas tube. *Gastroenterology* 75:566–569, 1978.
20. Mitchell K, Silk DBA, Williams R: Prospective comparison of two Sengstaken tubes in the management of patients with variceal haemorrhage. *Gut* 21:570–573, 1980.
21. Hunt PS, Fracs MS, Korman MG, et al: An 8-year prospective experience with balloon tamponade in emergency control of bleeding esophageal varices. *Dig Dis Sci* 27:413–416, 1982.

22. Sarin SK, Nundy S: Balloon tamponade in the management of bleeding oesophageal varices. *Ann R Coll Surg* 66:30–32, 1984.
23. Panes J, Teres J, Bosch J, et al: Efficacy of balloon tamponade in treatment of bleeding gastric and esophageal varices: Results in 151 consecutive episodes. *Dig Dis Sci* 33:454–459, 1988.
24. Feneyrou B, Hanana J, Daures JP, et al: Initial control of bleeding from esophageal varices with the Sengstaken-Blakemore tube: experience in 82 patients. *Am J Surg* 155:509–511, 1988.
25. Haddock G, Garden OJ, McKee RF, et al: Esophageal tamponade in the management of acute variceal hemorrhage. *Dig Dis Sci* 34:913–918, 1989.
26. Hernomo K, Boedhi-Darmojo R, Oesman N, et al: Vasopressin vs. Sengstaken tube for bleeding varices. A prospective randomized controlled clinical trial. *Hepatology* 3:1058–1062, 1983.
27. Correia JP, Alves MM, Alexandrino P, et al: Controlled trial of vasopressin and balloon tamponade in bleeding esophageal varices. *Hepatology* 4:885–888, 1984.
28. Teres J, Planas R, Panes J, et al: Vasopressin/nitroglycerine infusion vs. esophageal tamponade in the treatment of acute variceal bleeding. A randomized controlled trial. *Hepatology* 11:964–968, 1990.
29. Fort E, Sautereau D, Silvain C, et al: A randomized trial of terlipressin plus nitroglycerin vs. balloon tamponade in the control of acute variceal hemorrhage. *Hepatology* 11:678–681, 1990.
30. Barsoum MS, Bolous FI, El-Rooby AA, et al: Tamponade and injection sclerotherapy in the management of bleeding oesophageal varices. *Br J Surg* 69:76–78, 1982.
31. Soderlund C, Ihre T: Endoscopic sclerotherapy v. conservative management of bleeding oesophageal varices. *Acta Chir Scand* 151:449–456, 1985.
32. Paquet KJ, Feussner H: Endoscopic sclerosis and esophageal balloon tamponade in acute hemorrhage from esophagogastric varices: A prospective controlled randomized trial. *Hepatology* 5:580–583, 1985.
33. Moreto M, Zaballa M, Bernal A, et al: A randomized trial of tamponade or sclerotherapy as immediate treatment for bleeding esophageal varices. *Surg Gynecol Obstet* 167:331–334, 1988.
34. Hussey KP: Vasopressin therapy for upper gastrointestinal tract hemorrhage. Has its efficacy been proven? *Arch Intern Med* 145:1263–1267, 1985.
35. Conn HO: Vasopressin and nitroglycerin in the treatment of bleeding varices: The bottom line. *Hepatology* 6:523–525, 1986.
36. Fogel MR, Knauer CM, Andres LL, et al: Continuous intravenous vasopressin in active upper gastrointestinal bleeding: A placebo-controlled trial. *Ann Intern Med* 96:565–569, 1982.
37. Merigan TC, Poltkin GR, Davidson CS: Effect of intravenously administered posterior pituitary extract on hemorrhage from bleeding esophageal varices. *N Engl J Med* 266:134–135, 1962.
38. Ramsby GR, Storer EH, Mutchnick MG, et al: Intraarterial vasopressin in the treatment of upper gastrointestinal hemorrhage: A prospective, controlled clinical trial. *Gastroenterology* 68:211–221, 1975.
39. Sirinek KR, Levine BA: High-dose vasopressin for acute variceal hemorrhage: Clinical advantages without adverse effects. *Arch Surg* 123:876–880, 1988.
40. Tsai YT, Lay CS, Lai KH, et al: Controlled trial of vasopressin plus nitroglycerin vs. vasopressin alone in the treatment of bleeding esophageal varices. *Hepatology* 6:406–409, 1986.
41. Gimson AES, Westaby D, Hegarty J, et al: A randomized trial of vasopressin and vasopressin plus nitroglycerin in the control of acute variceal hemorrhage. *Hepatology* 6:410–413, 1986.
42. Bosch J, Groszmann RJ, Garcia-Pagan JC, et al: Association of transdermal nitroglycerin to

vasopressin infusion in the treatment of variceal hemorrhage: A placebo-controlled clinical trial. *Hepatology* 10:962–968, 1989.

43. Freeman JG, Lishman AH, Cobden I, et al: Controlled trial of terlipressin ('Glypressin') versus vasopressin in the early treatment of oesophageal varices. *Lancet* 2:66–68, 1982.
44. Freeman JG, Cobden I, Record CO: Placebo-controlled trial of terlipressin (Glypressin) in the management of acute variceal bleeding. *J Clin Gastroenterol* 11:58–60, 1989.
45. Soderlund C, Magnusson I, Torngren S, et al: Terlipressin (triglycyl-lysine vasopressin) controls acute bleeding oesophageal varices. A double-blind, randomized, placebo-controlled trial. *Scand J Gastroenterol* 25:622–630, 1990.
46. Resnick RH: Somatostatin for variceal bleeders. *Gastroenterology* 99:1524–1526, 1990.
47. Valenzuela JE, Schubert T, Fogel MR, et al: A multicenter, randomized, double-blind trial of somatostatin in the management of acute hemorrhage from esophageal varices. *Hepatology* 10:958–961, 1989.
48. Burroughs AK, McCormick PA, Hughes MD, et al: Randomized, double-blind, placebo-controlled trial of somatostatin for variceal bleeding: Emergency control and prevention of early variceal rebleeding. *Gastroenterology* 99:1388–1395, 1990.
49. Avgerinos A, Klonis CH, Rekoumis G, et al: Controlled trial of somatostatin and balloon tamponade in bleeding esophageal varices. *Gastroenterology* 96:A18, 1989.
50. Kravetz D, Bosch J, Teres J, et al: Comparison of intravenous somatostatin and vasopressin infusions in treatment of acute variceal hemorrhage. *Hepatology* 4:442–446, 1984.
51. Jenkins SA, Baxter JN, Corbett W, et al: A prospective randomized controlled clinical trial comparing somatostatin and vasopressin in controlling acute variceal haemorrhage. *Br Med J* 290:275–278, 1985.
52. Saari A, Klvilaakso E, Inberg M, et al: Comparison of somatostatin and vasopressin in bleeding esophageal varices. *J Gastroenterol* 85:804–807, 1990.
53. McKee RF, Garden OJ, Anderson JR, et al: A long acting somatostatin analogue in the management of bleeding from oesophageal varices. (communication to the Assoc of Surg. of Great Britain and Ireland) referenced in *Lancet* 2:1276, 1989.
54. Editorial: Octreotide. *Lancet* 2:541–542, 1989.

30

ENDOSCOPIC SCLEROTHERAPY OF ESOPHAGOGASTRIC VARICES

John J. Vargo II, M.D.
Michael V. Sivak, Jr., M.D.

Endoscopic injection sclerotherapy remains the principal method for the nonsurgical management of bleeding esophageal varices despite the current technological renaissance in gastrointestinal endoscopy and pharmacological attempts to control variceal hemorrhage. The injection of a sclerosing solution into esophageal varices was suggested in 1933 by Pemberton and also Walters,[1] and the first procedure was performed by Crafoord and Frenckner[2] in 1939. Soon thereafter, Moersch[3] duplicated the procedure using sodium morrhuate in 10 patients, and larger series of cases began to appear in the 1970s.[4,5] However, the relative scarcity of such reports is no doubt related to the use of rigid endoscopes and general anesthesia for the injection procedure, as well as a greater interest in portal decompressive surgery. In the late 1970s, the use of the rigid endoscope was largely abandoned as sclerotherapy by means of a fiberoptic endoscope was shown to be technically feasible, safe, and effective.

PATHOGENESIS AND NATURAL HISTORY OF VARICEAL BLEEDING

Variceal Anatomy

The effects produced by injection of a chemical agent into a varix relate in part to the venous anatomy of the esophagus, which undergoes a significant transformation in response to portal hypertension. Vianna et al.[6] studied the venous circulation in specimens obtained from patients without portal hypertension using the techniques of corrosion casting and x-rays obtained after injection of a gelatin-barium mixture. This work should be contrasted with that of Butler[7] and Kitano et al.,[8] who studied specimens from patients with varices.

A detailed discussion of esophageal venous and variceal anatomy, including differences among the several studies of these veins, is beyond the scope of this chapter. However, the important components of the endoscopic treatment of variceal bleeding are three: an extrinsic (paraesophageal) system of veins, an intrinsic system (that seen at endoscopy), and a system of perforating channels which connect the intrinsic with the extrinsic veins. This simplified description conveys a useful concept, albeit not a precise anatomical description. Anastomoses between the intrinsic veins of the esophagus and corresponding veins in the stomach were considered rudimentary or even nonexistent by Butler,[7] although more recent studies demonstrate substantial connections at the mucosal and submucosal levels.[6,8]

The intrinsic and extrinsic venous systems have numerous interconnections along the length of the esophagus via the perforating veins. Since the extrinsic veins represent the primary collateral channel, the perforating veins are therefore of major importance with respect to the development of the intrinsic veins. Butler[7] found that the perforating veins have one-way valves that prevent blood flow from the extrinsic system to the intrinsic plexuses. This finding was not confirmed by Kitano et al.[8] Nevertheless, differences in venous anatomy may explain the fact that some patients with significant portal hypertension do not have varices.

Blood Flow in Esophageal Varices

Esophageal varices are usually regarded simply as conduits that direct portal blood to the systemic circulation as a consequence of portal hypertension. The actual blood flow dynamics are more complex than this. McCormack et al.[9] studied variceal blood flow by means of a 10-MHz Doppler probe placed against varices under endoscopic guidance. They demonstrated instances of caudad and bidirectional blood flow with respiratory variations. In some patients, the direction of flow changed at 1 to 4 cm proximal to the gastroesophageal junction; these investigators related the change of flow to the presence of perforating vessels. McCormack et al.[9] further suggested that the perforating veins are crucial in the pathogenesis of esophageal varices. With primary shunting of blood through the extrinsic system in portal hypertension, valvular incompetence of the perforating veins leads to retrograde flow from the extrinsic to the intrinsic veins.

Pathogenesis of Variceal Hemorrhage

The pathogenesis of portal hypertension and the ensuing development of the portosystemic collateral circulation are well established. However, very little is known about the events that lead to variceal hemorrhage.

Portal Pressure

Elevated portal venous pressure is required for the establishment of esophageal varices and the potential for variceal hemorrhage. However, a relation between increasing levels of portal pressure and the level of risk for variceal bleeding has proved to be more problematic.

Wedged hepatic-free hepatic venous pressure, which accurately reflects portal pressure, has been utilized to predict the occurrence of variceal hemorrhage. A gradient of 10–12 mm Hg appears to be necessary for the development of esophageal varices,[10] but an elevated gradient is not always predictive of the presence of varices. Most studies have not found a correlation between the degree of portal hypertension and the risk of variceal bleeding.[11,12] Other studies, such as that of Gluud et al.,[13] have found the venous pressure gradient, among other variables, to be prognostic of variceal bleeding and death.

The work of Dagradi[14] and other investigators[15,16] supports a relationship between portal hypertension and the diameter and extent of variceal vessels. However, these studies included patients with normal or slightly elevated portal pressure. Lebrec et al.[10] suggested that in patients with significant increases in portal pressure, there is no relationship between portal pressure and variceal size. In fact, there are substantial data to indicate that there is no relationship between variceal size and portal pressure.[17-20] McCormack et al.[9] have postulated that the absence of such a relationship may be due to differences in perforating vein competence.

Intravariceal Pressure

Intravariceal pressure appears to be a factor in variceal bleeding despite the fact that variceal bleeding cannot be correlated with the degree of portal hypertension. Rigau et al.[21] recorded intravariceal pressure by means of an endoscopically directed pressure gauge in 70 patients with cirrhosis and portal hypertension, including 47 with prior endoscopically proven variceal bleeding and 23 with varices but no prior bleeding. These pressure determinations were compared to wedged and free hepatic venous pressures. Variceal pressure was significantly higher in the group with prior variceal hemorrhage compared to those with no prior bleeding. The intravariceal pressure in both groups was less than the portal pressure. Variceal pressure and tension were also significantly higher in patients with large varices. The hepatic venous pressure gradient was elevated in patients with and without prior hemorrhage, but there was no significant difference in the degree of elevation for the two groups.

Red Color Signs

Dagradi[22] described the presence of "cherry red spots" or "varices on varices" on the surface of large varices. Collectively, these surface features are usually termed *red color signs*. Beppu et al.[23] regard them as microtelangiectasias or small, dilated vessels.

Spence et al.[24] examined rings of esophageal tissue obtained from 27 patients undergoing esophageal transection for varices and 17 patients without cirrhosis or portal hypertension. Those from patients with varices exhibited dilated intraepithelial blood channels immediately beneath the mucosa. These channels were lined with flattened cells with an incomplete basement membrane which proved to be squamous epithelial cells by electron microscopy. In some cases, visual inspection of the surgical specimens confirmed that the aforementioned histomorphometric abnormalities corresponded to "hemorrhagic petechiae" or "blood-filled blisters." Spence et al.[24] suggested that these findings correspond to the cherry red spots seen endoscopically and that they are important in the pathogenesis of variceal hemorrhage.

Kleber et al.[25] performed fine needle variceal punctures in 40 patients with cirrhosis and found intravariceal pressure to be significantly higher in varices with red color signs. There was no relationship between the transmural variceal pressure and the number and diameter of esophageal varices or the degree of liver dysfunction.

Precipitating Factors

The precipitating factor or factors in variceal bleeding are largely a matter of conjecture. Gastroesophageal reflux has been considered a prime candidate by virtue of mucosal erosions on the thin-walled surfaces of large varices. Earlier studies revealed esophageal ulcerations in 43 to 56% of patients who succumbed to acute variceal bleeding.[26,27] However, later studies which controlled for prior sclerotherapy and variceal tamponade disclosed no histological evidence of esophagitis.[28,29] Esophageal function in patients with cirrhosis and esophageal varices has also been found to be normal.[30] The degree of liver dysfunction has been found to represent an independent albeit additive risk factor in the occurrence of the first variceal hemorrhage.[31] However, once variceal bleeding has occurred, there is no clear relationship between the severity of liver disease and the risk of subsequent bleeding.

Natural History of Esophageal Varices

Hemorrhage is the only clinical symptom of esophageal varices. Since bleeding from esophageal varices is not invariable, an accurate assessment of the prevalence of esophageal varices is probably not possible. Autopsy series suggest that about two-thirds of patients with cirrhosis have varices. Between 35% and 84% of such patients have varices when studied by endoscopy. The reported incidence of bleeding among patients with varices is also highly variable. This relates in part to differences in the design of studies of these patients. In a prospective study of 321 patients with esophageal varices without prior bleeding, 26.5% eventually bled during the study period (median, 23 months).[31] Of the patients who bled, 67% did so within the first year and 90% by the second year of follow-up. By comparison, Paquet et al.[32] noted a 66% incidence of variceal bleeding. However, patients in this series had large varices and other endoscopic signs associated with an increased risk of bleeding.

The mortality from variceal bleeding was over 30% in the survey conducted by the American Society for Gastrointestinal Endoscopy (ASGE).[33] The mortality following an index variceal hemorrhage may be as high as 42% six weeks after the onset of bleeding.[34] Most of these deaths were related to hemorrhage. After six weeks, however, the mortality rate decreases and deaths occur equally from hepatic failure, bleeding, and other causes. Without intervention, over 60% of patients who survive an index hemorrhage will have recurrent bleeding.[35,36]

Thus, the natural course of esophageal varices is unpredictable, with the index hemorrhage being associated with a high mortality and a risk of further bleeding, although the rate of recurrent bleeding decreases over time.[31,37] Management may therefore be directed at prevention of variceal bleeding, control of the acute episode, and/or reduction of the risk of recurrent bleeding. Although current methods of therapy have led to some improvements in each of these circumstances, dramatic improvements in survival have not been shown for any type of treatment.

PREDICTION OF VARICEAL HEMORRHAGE

Stratification of patients with varices into risk categories is useful in the selection of patients for prophylactic therapy, but "high risk" doesn't necessarily mean impending

TABLE 30.1. General Rules for Recording Endoscopic Findings of Esophageal Varices

1. Red color signs (RCS)*
   a. Red wale marking (RWM)
   b. Cherry red spot (CRS)
   c. Hematocystic spot (HCS)
   d. Diffuse redness (DR)
2. Fundamental color
   a. White (Cw)
   b. Blue (Cb)
3. Form
   a. Small, straight varices (F1)
   b. Enlarged, tortuous, occupy less than one third of lumen (F2)
   c. Largest, coil-shaped, occupy more than one third of lumen (F3)
4. Location (longitudinal extent)
   a. Lower one third (Li)
   b. Middle one third below tracheal bifurcation (Lm)
   c. Upper one third above tracheal bifurcation (Ls)
5. Adjunctive Finding
   a. Erosion (E+)

*RWM and CRS are graded from 1+ to 3+, depending on number and length.
Source: The Japanese Research Society for Portal Hypertension.

hemorrhage, nor does a ''low-risk'' classification insure the patient against potentially fatal bleeding. Most methods for defining the risk of variceal hemorrhage have utilized variceal size (diameter and length) and certain aspects of variceal appearance. The Japanese Research Society for Portal Hypertension has proposed a classification based on certain aspects of endoscopic appearance of varices.[23,38] This classification, ''General Rules for Recording Endoscopic Findings on Esophageal Varices,'' is outlined in Table 30.1.

Variceal Size

Various studies have demonstrated a rough correlation between variceal size and the risk of bleeding.[10,22,31,39,40] Variceal size is not static, and changes to higher or lower grades as well as the disappearance of varices have been described.[39,40] Furthermore, endoscopic grading of esophageal varices is by no means standardized. Although similar terms (e.g., grade 1, grade 2) are used by many authors, their meaning can be different.

Variceal Appearance

Certain features of the endoscopic appearance of esophageal varices have been used to predict hemorrhage.[13,23,31,40] Beppu et al.[23] retrospectively analyzed the endoscopic appearance of varices with regard to color, morphology, and the presence of red color signs. Variceal hemorrhage had occurred in 58.7% of patients with red color signs versus only 9.1% of those without such signs. Column length did not correlate with the diameter of the varices or the risk of bleeding. Red color signs were subclassified into several types, and the authors concluded that the relative risk of bleeding was higher with certain varieties. We believe, however, that the risk of bleeding may simply be related to the presence of these markings, without reference to subtype.

Cales et al.[41] studied interobserver variability in the endoscopic assessment of variceal features in 100 consecutive patients with cirrhosis. Four independent observers assessed variceal size, color, extent, and the presence of red color signs. Agreement was good for variceal size and the presence of red color signs and poor for variceal extent and color. This study suggests that only certain endoscopic features of esophageal varices are recognized consistently by experienced clinicians.

In a multicenter study, 321 patients with cirrhosis and no history of variceal bleeding were followed for a median of 23 months in order to determine parameters that predict variceal bleeding.[31] During the study, 26.5% of the patients bled, esophageal varices being the source in over 90%. Large varices, the presence of red color signs, and the degree of liver dysfunction were found to be independent, additive risk factors for variceal bleeding. These parameters were then used in an index equation which determined the risk of bleeding during a one-year period in another group of 75 patients with cirrhosis and varices but no history of bleeding. No statistically significant difference between the predicted and observed incidence of bleeding was found.

Cutaneous Stigmata of Liver Disease

The presence, number, appearance, and distribution of the cutaneous vascular spiders characteristic of cirrhosis may be of value in predicting the risk of variceal hemorrhage. Foutch et al.[42] examined 92 men with cirrhosis and found the incidence of cutaneous spiders and varices to be similar (90%). There was a significantly higher incidence of variceal bleeding in patients with cutaneous spiders. Larger numbers (more than 20) of the cutaneous lesions and atypical location appeared to be risk factors for hemorrhage. Large spiders (i.e., those over 15 mm in diameter) correlated best with the presence of large varices and had the strongest association with variceal bleeding.

TECHNIQUE OF SCLEROTHERAPY

Comparing the results of sclerotherapy is difficult, since virtually all methods employed are empiric and no two regimens are precisely the same. The numerous permutations in technique make it difficult to ascertain whether a lower complication rate or better results are possible with one method as opposed to another. The list of variables includes choice of endoscope, use of various compression methods, schedule of procedures, types of resuscitative modalities employed, selection of sclerosing agent(s), injection volume, pattern of injection, intravariceal versus paravariceal injections, experience of the endoscopist, and the effect of randomization criteria.

Instruments

Certain attributes of the rigid endoscope are said by some authors to provide technical advantages during injection sclerotherapy.[4,5,43,44] These include variceal compression, vigorous suction of blood and clots, and the prevention of aspiration. However, the rigid esophagoscope also has disadvantages, including the risks associated with general anesthesia, added cost, and restrictions on the ability to perform emergency sclerotherapy in a timely manner. Bornman et al.[45] randomized 70 patients with variceal bleeding to receive sclerotherapy with a fiberoptic endoscope or with a rigid instrument under general anesthesia. There was no significant difference in outcome between the two groups with regard to control of acute bleeding, mortality, and eventual variceal eradication. However, sclerotherapy with the rigid instrument was associated with a significantly higher complication rate per injection. Based on the large number of techniques described in the literature, the flexible endoscopes are clearly the preferred instruments for sclerotherapy.

Variceal Compression

Variceal compression has several theoretic advantages, including tamponade of active bleeding vessels prior to sclerotherapy and a reduction in back bleeding following injection of the sclerosant. Compression is thought to retard the flow of the sclerosant and thereby to increase the duration of its contact with the varix endothelium, an effect which is thought to promote sclerosis of the vessel. The various methods and maneuvers that have been employed to achieve this effect include the use of a rigid endoscope, placement of a Sengstaken-Blakemore tube after the procedure, utilization of an overtube during the procedure, attachment of a balloon cuff to the endoscope, and placement of a balloon fixed in the cardia of the stomach during the procedure.

Inflation of a balloon in the gastric cardia has been used during sclerotherapy to stop or decrease active bleeding.[46,47] In one report, this type of compression was said to retard the fluoroscopically monitored clearance of a mixture of sclerosant and radiographic contrast medium.[47]

Williams and Dawson[48] introduced the use of a semiflexible overtube in conjunction with a fiberoptic endoscope for variceal compression and control of bleeding. Most versions of this device have a slot in the distal end by means of which a single variceal channel can be isolated. After injection of a varix, the tube is rotated until another varix protrudes into the slot.

Kitano et al.[49] randomized 102 consecutive patients to receive intravariceal sclerotherapy by a free-hand or overtube technique. Variceal obliteration and two-year mortality rates were similar for both groups. However, control of acute bleeding was significantly better with the overtube technique (100% versus 77%). In the free-hand injection group, ulcers appeared earlier, recurrent bleeding was earlier in onset, and the blood loss during the first two sclerotherapy sessions was significantly greater. The overtube method was compared to free-hand injection in another prospective randomized study of 40 patients with variceal bleeding.[50] Recurrent bleeding occurred with equal frequency in the two groups, but free-hand injection was associated with a higher mortality rate.

The theoretical value of variceal compression can be challenged on the basis of anatomical and physiological studies[6,7,9] which demonstrate the bidirectional nature of variceal blood flow with free communication between the intrinsic and extrinsic systems of veins. Rapid clearance of injected substances from the point of injection, with or without compression, has been clearly demonstrated. Radiographic contrast agents have been added to sclerosant solutions in order to study the movement of the injected material. Despite perceived intravariceal injections, local accumulation at the puncture site is a frequent occurrence.[51,52] Grobe et al.[51] observed that 42% of the injections resulted in a rapid clearance in a cephalad direction; in 14% there was clearance toward the gastric veins. Compression with a balloon proximal to the injection sites did not impede the cephalad clearance of the contrast agent. Similar observations have been reported by Barsuom et al.[52]

Free-hand injection is highly effective and clearly less complicated than sclerotherapy with compression, although it requires quickness and skill for both elective and emergent procedures. The aforementioned methods of variceal compression have not gained widespread acceptance.

Sclerosing Agents

There is little information to guide the selection of a sclerosing agent or agents. This problem is compounded by the wide variety of available sclerosing agents, the limited applicability of animal studies to humans, and a lack of controlled clinical trials. The variables that must be taken into account in any definitive comparative trial include the type and concentration of sclerosant(s), the volume of sclerosant per injection, the use of intravariceal versus paravariceal injection, emergency versus elective sclerotherapy, and the frequency of follow-up sessions. Combinations of agents, presumably with different modes of action, have also been used.

Some of the agents that have been employed for sclerotherapy are listed in Table 30.2. The precise mechanism(s) of action of the sclerosing agents currently employed is poorly understood. Kang et al.[53] studied the action of ethanolamine oleate in vivo by measuring specific fibrinopeptide levels. The sclerosant was found to cause transient activation of both clotting and fibrinolytic cascades. However, in vitro studies demonstrated an inhibition of fibrin clot formation, which was attributed to the calcium chelating effect of the ethanolamine constituent. Kang et al.[53] concluded that the predominant effect of ethanolamine in vivo is the local activation of the coagulation cascade. This may be enhanced by an oleate-induced inflammatory process. In another study, platelet aggregation, as well as the coagulative and fibrinolytic cascades, were evaluated in 45 patients who underwent sclerotherapy with 5% ethanolamine oleate.[54] Platelet aggregation was significantly decreased for as long as 48 hours following sclerotherapy and

TABLE 30.2. Agents Used for Variceal Sclerotherapy

Sodium morrhuate
Sodium tetradecyl sulfate
Cefazolin
Thrombin (bovine)
Hypertonic glucose
Ethanolamine oleate
Polidocanol
Linoleic acid
Sterile paraffin
Urea
Quinine
Phenol-almond oil
Bucrylate (tissue glue)
Ethanol

returned toward baseline values six days after treatment. Transient activation of both the coagulation and fibrinolytic systems occurred 1 hour after sclerotherapy and normalized 48 hours later.

McClave et al.[55] randomized 42 patients to receive sclerotherapy with either sodium tetradecyl sulfate or sodium morrhuate in a study designed to evaluate efficacy and complications. There was no difference between the groups with respect to control of acute bleeding, mortality, variceal obliteration, transfusion requirements, or complications. Recurrent bleeding was more frequent in the group treated with sodium tetradecyl sulfate (81% versus 51%), but this difference did not reach statistical significance.

It would be difficult to recommend a specific sclerosing agent on the basis of currently available data. A wide variety of substances appear to be effective. Experience with a specific agent probably plays a large role in determining its efficacy as the sclerosant volume and concentration are adjusted to achieve optimal effects.

Paravariceal versus Intravariceal Injections

A sclerosing solution may be injected into or adjacent to a varix. A combination of intravariceal and paravariceal injection sites have also been utilized. Based on the number of reports, it appears that intravariceal injection is the preferred method, although this varies from region to region.

Local accumulations of contrast have been demonstrated at intravariceal injection sites in studies of variceal blood flow using solutions of sclerosant and a radiographic contrast agent.[51,52] This suggests that perivascular leakage of sclerosant occurs with intravascular injections, probably by leakage along the needle tract, and/or that it is not always possible to position the needle precisely in a varix. In a study of the accuracy of placement of intravariceal injections, the overall success rate was 75%, with that for large varices being somewhat higher (82%).[56] The addition of methylene blue to the sclerosant in an attempt to improve the accuracy of intravariceal injection was studied by Waring et al.[57] Intravariceal injections were confirmed fluoroscopically in 60.7% of the injections with methylene blue and 69% without it; the authors concluded that the addition of the dye did not improve the accuracy of intravariceal sclerotherapy.

Rose et al.[56] found intravariceal injections to be more thrombogenic than paravariceal injections. Their follow-up period was relatively short, so that the long-term effect of intravariceal versus paravariceal injections could not be assessed. In a randomized trial of intravariceal versus paravariceal sclerotherapy in 54 patients, Sarin et al.[58] found the former technique to be more effective for control of variceal bleeding (91% versus 19%). In this study, intravariceal injections of 50% ethanol shortened the time required for eradication of varices and reduced the number of treatment sessions. Other investigators have found paravariceal injections to be efficacious.[59,60]

Schedule of Procedures

The most effective and safe schedule of sclerotherapy has not been established. Most likely, the optimal interval between procedures will vary with other elements of technique, including the selection of an agent, its concentration, the pattern for placement of injections, and the number of injection points. In theory, a relatively large number of sessions over a short time interval leads to rapid variceal eradication at the risk of an increased frequency of sclerotherapy-induced complications. Early eradication might influence the prognosis by rapidly reducing the risk of recurrent bleeding. Sclerotherapy sessions at longer intervals might minimize sclerosant-induced complications at the risk of further bleeding and a longer interval until variceal eradication is achieved.

Sarin et al.[61] randomized 96 patients with recent esophageal hemorrhage to undergo sclerotherapy with absolute alcohol at one-week and three-week intervals. The weekly sessions resulted in earlier variceal eradication and a reduction in recurrent bleeding (8.5% versus 26.5%). The volume of sclerosant, number of sessions required for eradication, and mortality were the same for both groups. However, 23% of the patients undergoing treatment on a weekly basis had procedures postponed because of the presence of diffuse ulceration. In a similar study by Westaby et al.,[62] 55 patients with recent variceal bleeding were randomized to undergo sclerotherapy with 5% ethanolamine according to a one-week or three-week schedule. Weekly sessions significantly shortened the time required for variceal eradication but had no advantage with respect to recurrent bleeding and mortality. Weekly sclerotherapy led to the postponement of 19 sessions due to the presence of extensive ulceration. Although the group treated weekly had an increased incidence of significant ulceration, this observation may be biased, as weekly surveillance endoscopies were not performed in patients undergoing sclerotherapy every three weeks.

Injection Pattern and Volume of Sclerosant

The pattern for placement of injections is another important element in sclerotherapy technique. Injections can be restricted to the distal few centimeters of the esophagus,[63,64] or they may be made over longer segments. The distance between puncture sites may also be important to the overall outcome. This should be related to the strength of the sclerosing agent, which is a function of its inherent chemical properties and concentration. Close approximation of injection points with a relatively potent sclerosant solution may increase the chance of significant ulceration. The volume per injection and the total volume used per procedure are other variables that must be considered in relation to the strength of the agent.

Outpatient Sclerotherapy

Sclerotherapy can be performed safely on an ambulatory basis. Korula[65] reported a trial of outpatient sclerotherapy in 34 patients who underwent a total of 117 sclerotherapy sessions. Only five patients (15%) were classified as having Child's C liver disease. Each session was completed without hospitalization. Although 24% of the procedures resulted in a complication, all were considered minor. These included chest pain (14% of sessions), dysphagia (6%), fever (2%), and bleeding (2%).

Drell et al.[66] performed sclerotherapy in 14 hospitalized patients (30 sessions) and in 34 nonhospitalized patients (133 sessions). In each group, sclerotherapy was considered elective and was performed at least one week after an index hemorrhage. In contrast to the study of Korula, 79% of the ambulatory patients and 57% of the hospitalized patients were classified as Child's C. Major complications occurred in 14% and 2.9% of the hospitalized and ambulatory patients, respectively. There were no deaths among outpatients versus a 7% mortality for hospitalized patients. Minor complications were noted in 26% of the ambulatory patients; apparently, none occurred in the hospitalized group. The cost of sclerotherapy was markedly reduced in the outpatient setting.

Variceal Ligation

Variceal ligation is a new form of endoscopic treatment for esophageal varices.[67] The ligation device, consisting of an inner and an outer cylinder, fits over the distal end of the endoscope. Round elastic rings are stretched over the inner cylinder, which is connected to a trip wire that runs retrograde through the accessory channel of the endoscope. A varix is drawn by suction into the cylinder, whereupon the endoscopist pulls the trip wire, which retracts the inner cylinder and thereby releases the rubber ring over the varix.

Stiegmann et al.[67] have reported the results of variceal band ligation in 100 consecutive patients with variceal hemorrhage. Bleeding was active in 21% at the time of band ligation and was eventually controlled in 86% of these patients. The remaining 79 patients had ceased bleeding prior to the index ligation. Mortality during the initial hospitalization was 12%, with recurrent bleeding leading to death in only one patient. Variceal ligation procedures were continued in the survivors (mean, 15 months), and variceal eradication was achieved in 60 patients after an average of five ligation sessions. The rate of recurrent bleeding was 47% over the course of therapy. The source of recurrent hemorrhage in five patients was presumed to be shallow ulcers observed at most sites after sloughing of the ligated varix. Three complications of a nonbleeding nature occurred (stricture in two patients and meat impaction in another). There were no pulmonary, mediastinal, or systemic complications. Most patients described transient dysphagia or chest pain.

Preliminary results from a prospective randomized study comparing endoscopic variceal ligation with intravariceal sclerotherapy in 70 patients with active or recent variceal bleeding suggest that variceal ligation might have advantages over conventional therapy with regard to recurrent bleeding, complications, variceal eradication, and survival.[68] However, statistical significance was not achieved for any of these parameters. Larger randomized controlled trials comparing variceal ligation with sclerotherapy are needed to determine the value of this new technique.

Endoscopic variceal ligation may be appropriate as a salvage procedure for patients who fail conventional endoscopic sclerotherapy. Saeed et al.[69] prospectively evaluated 12 patients who were considered failures on the basis of recurrent bleeding, transfusion requirements, persistent large variceal channels, or complications including deep ulceration, severe chest pain, and intramural hematoma formation. Initial hemostasis was achieved in all 10 patients who were bleeding acutely. Eradication of varices was achieved in five patients, who required a total of 19 ligation sessions. Bleeding recurred in 58%, although this was attributed in part to poor patient compliance.

COMPLICATIONS OF SCLEROTHERAPY

The esophageal varices seen at endoscopy are merely one component of a more extensive venous plexus that develops in response to portal hypertension.[7] Complications of sclerotherapy may occur not only at the site of injection but also as a result of systemic dissemination in areas removed from the esophagus. Sukigara et al.[70] have demonstrated widespread systemic distribution of a technetium-labeled sclerosant mixture following intravariceal sclerotherapy. Certain minor complications such as fever, chest pain, and dysphagia occur so frequently that they are regarded as side effects by some authors.[71]

Complication Rate

Determining an overall complication rate for sclerotherapy is difficult. Variations in technique, differences in the action of various sclerosants, and varying levels of experience among endoscopists are just a few of the factors that may affect the outcome of the procedure. A complication occurs in 2 to 20% of patients.[3,4,72-76] A complication occurred in 20% of 107 patients who underwent 240 procedures in the report of Macdougall et al.[77] If minor, transient complications such as esophageal ulceration and chest pain are included, complication rates as high as 78% have been reported.[78] Schuman et al.[79] reported an overall complication rate of 52% in a series of 42 patients.

Side Effects

Chest Pain

Substernal chest pain occurs after sclerotherapy in 25 to 50% of patients. The discomfort is usually mild but sometimes can be severe. Characteristically, the pain persists for 12 to 24 hours and is occasionally associated with odynophagia.[80] Pain or discomfort has been reported following paravariceal injections, intravariceal injections,[47,71,80,81] and combinations of the two.[82] Pain that occurs immediately after sclerotherapy usually does not indicate necrosis or perforation, although the latter complication can sometimes present with chest pain during or immediately after sclerotherapy. However, necrosis and perforation usually develop insidiously, requiring several days to become clinically apparent. Although Harris et al.[83] indicated that chest pain is more likely to occur with ethanolamine than with tetradecyl sulfate, it is not established that the type or concentration of sclerosant or the pattern of injection has any bearing on the pathogenesis of chest pain.

Gebhard et al.[84] studied the relationship between sclerotherapy-induced chest pain and abnormalities found on barium esophograms obtained immediately after sclerotherapy in 11 patients. A positive correlation between the degree of spasm seen radiographically and the severity of chest pain was established. However, balloon tamponade used during sclerotherapy may have had a confounding effect by precipitating both chest pain and esophageal spasm. Shoenut and Micflikier[85] performed esophageal manometry before and immediately after upper endoscopy in a trial involving seven patients undergoing sclerotherapy and seven control subjects undergoing upper endoscopy for other reasons. Transient diffuse esophageal spasm was demonstrated in the patients who had sclerotherapy. Failure of relaxation of the lower esophageal sphincter was also noted in five of the sclerotherapy patients.

Fever

Low-grade fever occurs in almost half of the patients undergoing sclerotherapy[75,78] and lasts for 24 to 48 hours. It appears that this mild temperature elevation is not the result of bacteremia in the great majority of cases.[86] The cryptic etiology of this fever may be a chemical phlebitis or an acute inflammatory response.[87] Antibiotic therapy should not be instituted for this fever. When fever persists for more than 48 hours or significant temperature spikes occur, a source of sepsis should be sought.

Local Complications

Esophageal Ulceration

Esophageal ulceration is extremely common following sclerotherapy. The incidence varies with the endoscopic technique and, more important, with the frequency of endoscopic surveillance. Sarles et al.[78] noted a 78% incidence of ulceration in a trial of sclerotherapy that included follow-up sessions every five to seven days. Erosions or exudate were present over the varices in all patients. Sarin et al.[88] performed serial endoscopic examinations in 48 patients over a three-week period following intravariceal sclerotherapy with absolute alcohol. Ulcers were present in 94% of the patients 24 hours after sclerotherapy. The incidence of ulceration decreased to 69% at one week and to 12.5% at three weeks. Sarin et al. concluded that the development of esophageal ulceration probably represented a ''necessary accompaniment'' of sclerotherapy and should not be considered a complication.

The pathogenesis of esophageal ulceration is uncertain. Since ulcers have been noted with all agents, the sclerotherapy technique and the concentration of the sclerosant likely play major roles in their occurrence. In theory, a large number of injections in a localized area or a single injection with a large volume of sclerosant could result in ulceration. There was a strong correlation between the volume of sclerosant and the incidence of ulceration in the study by Sarin et al.[88] However, the pathogenesis of esophageal ulceration is probably more complex than localized irritation and necrosis at the injection site. Castro-Fernandez et al.[89] reported a case in which ulceration developed in the gastric fundus following a fourth session of intravariceal esophageal sclerotherapy. This site of ulceration was some distance from any injection site and was not present during previous sclerotherapy sessions.

Significant ulceration, whether gauged by the surface area of esophageal mucosa involved or the depth of penetration into the esophageal wall, can lead to serious complications. Ayres et al.[90] reported two patients in whom postsclerotherapy ulceration may have resulted in recurrent hemorrhage. In one patient, a visible vessel was identified endoscopically and histologically. In the other patient, there was bleeding from the border of an ulcer which may have eroded into an adjacent varix. Bleeding from a sclerotherapy-induced ulcer can be difficult to treat, since further sclerotherapy or other methods of endoscopically detected hemostasis may result in further tissue damage. Balloon tamponade and surgery would most likely be hazardous in areas of necrosis. Chronic postsclerotherapy ulceration has been reported by Subramanyam and Patterson.[91] Their patient had a large esophageal ulceration for 23 months, and this caused gastrointestinal blood loss on two occasions.

Postsclerotherapy ulceration appears in about one to seven days[92] and usually heals in three weeks.[88] Most ulcers leave small, clinically insignificant mucosal defects in the esophageal wall or, more rarely, result in the formation of pseudodiverticula.[93]

Various methods of treatment have been proposed for sclerotherapy-induced ulcers, none of which have been evaulated in prospective randomized trials. Treatment of sclerotherapy-induced bleeding ulcers with a sucralfate suspension led to a cessation of hemorrhage in three of four patients in one report.[94] Endoscopy revealed satisfactory adherence of the sucralfate to the ulcer bases. An eight-week course of omeprazole resulted in endoscopically documented healing of chronic esophageal ulcers that were resistant to treatment with sucralfate and high-dose H2 receptor antagonists.[95] In each of the 10 patients treated, a complication of chronic ulceration was present, including severe chest pain, stricture formation, or bleeding. Two patients relapsed but responded to a further course of therapy.

Esophageal Perforation

Perforation of the esophagus, both traumatic and postnecrotic, occurs in 1 to 6% of patients undergoing sclerotherapy.[96,97] Traumatic perforation is less frequent now that rigid esophagoscopes have been largely replaced by flexible endoscopes. A period of five to seven days is usually required for the development of a sclerotherapy-induced esophageal perforation. Signs and symptoms of perforation can be minimal. Soderlund and Wiechel[98] reported four cases in which the diagnosis was clinically evident prior to death in only one patient. In another report, the clinical diagnosis of esophageal perforation became apparent three weeks after sclerotherapy, during which time the patient was relatively asymptomatic.[99] Conservative treatment with broad-spectrum antibiotics and occasional chest tube drainage is indicated. Shemesh and Bat[100] described successful management by conservative measures alone in two patients with esophageal perforations and localized extravasation of radiocontrast. Oral antibiotics and nasoduodenal tube feedings were successful in the treatment of a patient who had developed an esophagobronchial fistula six weeks after sclerotherapy.[101]

Esophageal Stricture

The incidence of esophageal stricture is estimated at 3%,[96] although rates as high as 31% have been reported.[102] Acid-induced injury as a result of transient dysfunction of the normal acid clearance mechanism of the esophagus has been postulated as a mechanism of stricture formation.[103] However, the lack of significant lower esophageal sphincter (LES) abnormalities[104] or increases in the duration of reflux episodes following sclerotherapy[105] have cast some doubt on this hypothesis. More likely, the strictures form in response to the local action of the sclerosant. Paravariceal injections should logically result in a higher rate of stricture formation than would be expected with the intravariceal technique. However, stricture formation has been reported with every agent and sclerosing technique. Intermittent dysphagia without evidence of stricture formation is usually due to esophageal spasm, which resolves without treatment. Fortunately, stricture formation even in the presence of residual varices can be managed by bougienage.

Sorenson et al.[106] noted a 59% incidence of dysphagia and/or stricture formation in 34 patients undergoing long-term paravariceal sclerotherapy with 3% polidocanol. The sclerotherapy sessions were performed every three days until obliteration occurred. Sessions were postponed if ulcers or necrosis were found on follow-up examination. Of the 18 patients with strictures, 14 described concomitant dysphagia but the remaining 4 patients were asymptomatic. The number of treatment sessions and the volume of sclerosant injected were significantly greater in patients who developed strictures. Mucosal necrosis was frequently noted prior to the development of a stricture. Recurrence of bleeding and variceal eradication were similar in patients with and without stricture formation. Eder-Puestow bougienage was performed in 11 patients and led to the development of a transdiaphragmatic fistula in one patient.

Haynes et al.[107] studied the clinical characteristics of a group of 24 patients in whom variceal eradication was achieved by repeated sclerotherapy. The incidence of stricture formation was 42%. Stricture formation occurred an average of 55 days after initiation of sclerotherapy. All patients with strictures had a one- to two-week history of dysphagia for solid foods, and two of these patients also experienced difficulty in swallowing liquids. Haynes et al.[107] reported that patients with strictures did not undergo more sclerotherapy sessions or receive a greater volume of sclerosant than patients who did not develop strictures. Treatment by Maloney bougienage was successsful and without complication in all patients.

Esophageal Manometry and Acid Clearance

Disruption of normal esophageal motility and acid-clearing mechanisms may result, theoretically, from damage to the esophageal musculature and neurovascular structures by the sclerosing agents. The results of studies of sclerotherapy on acid clearance and esophageal motility are conflicting. A decline in the LES pressure was described in one study,[108] but other studies found no significant changes in motility.[109,110]

Sauerbruch et al.[105] studied the effects of repeated sclerotherapy on gastroesophageal reflux by means of long-term pH monitoring in 19 patients who underwent a mean of 10.3 sclerotherapy sessions. Fifteen cirrhotic patients with untreated varices served as controls. No significant differences were found with respect to the percentage of time during which the esophageal pH was less than 4 on the mean duration of reflux episodes. However, Snady and Korsten[103] found a marked increase in the number of swallows needed for the clearance of a standard acid load following sclerotherapy in a study comparing the results of esophageal manometry and acid clearance before and 24 hours after sclerotherapy. An increase in swallow-induced simultaneous contractions in the distal esophagus was observed following sclerotherapy. Both the manometric and acid clearance abnormalities resolved within one week.

Esophageal manometry and 24-hour pH monitoring were performed in five children undergoing intravariceal sclerotherapy for extrahepatic portal vein obstruction before and five months after the procedure.[104] A decrease in the mean amplitude of peristaltic contractions was demonstrated following sclerotherapy. There was no significant effect on the resting LES pressure.

Reilly et al.[111] obtained esophageal pH determinations and manometry in 22 patients undergoing sclerotherapy. However, only 60% of the patients were studied before and after sclerotherapy. After a mean of 2.9 sclerotherapy sessions, there was no significant change in LES pressure. However, there was a significant increase in peristaltic abnormalities consisting of broad-based, double-peaked waveforms and aperistalsis of the distal 5 cm of the esophagus. Although gastroesophageal reflux was more common following sclerotherapy, this finding failed to reach statistical significance.

The manometric findings in 14 patients with prior variceal hemorrhage were compared to those in 19 patients who had undergone ablative sclerotherapy a median of seven months prior to manometry.[112] There was no significant difference between the two groups except for a subgroup of patients with dysphagia after sclerotherapy. These eight patients exhibited a significant decrease in the percentage of deglutitive peristaltic contractions in the distal esophagus. The dysphagia and manometric abnormalities improved over time.

Systemic Complications

Pulmonary Complications

Pleural and mediastinal changes are common after sclerotherapy, occurring in up to 79% of patients.[113] Hughes et al.[75] found that 60% of patients developed pulmonary infiltrates or effusions within 48 hours of sclerotherapy. Saks et al.[113] studied chest radiographs in 15 patients undergoing a total of 38 sclerotherapy sessions. One-half of the patients had pleural effusions. These were bilateral or on the right side with equal frequency, while left-sided effusions were less common. The effusions resolved in all cases. A 48% incidence of pleural effusions was found by Bacon et al.[114] in 30 patients after 65 sclerotherapy sessions; right, left, and bilateral effusions occurred with equal frequency. Patients who developed pleural effusions were more likely to have chest pain and received a significantly greater sclerosant volume. The pleural fluid was exudative in 11 of 12 patients who underwent thoracentesis.

Computerized axial tomography was used to study anatomic changes in the esophagus, mediastinum, and lungs following intravariceal sclerotherapy in nine patients.[115] Although esophageal wall thickness was normal in seven of these patients prior to sclerotherapy, all nine exhibited an increase in thickness after sclerotherapy. Homogeneous or heterogeneous effusions with obliteration of the paraesophageal fat planes were noted in the paraesophageal mediastinum of all patients. In six patients, the effusion was mass-like and caused flattening of the right atrial wall.

A mixture of sodium morrhuate and a technetium-labeled radiopharmaceutical was used to study the embolization of sclerosant in 18 patients undergoing a total of 25 intravariceal sclerotherapy sessions.[116] Embolization was documented in 15 procedures (60%). There was no correlation between embolization to the pulmonary circulation and chest x-ray abnormalities. Patients with embolization tended to have low-grade fever following sclerotherapy.

Monroe et al.[117] reported the occurrence of the adult respiratory distress syndrome (ARDS) in two patients following intravariceal sclerotherapy with sodium morrhuate. Both patients developed dyspnea, bilateral pulmonary infiltrates, and hypoxemia. Administration of sodium morrhuate in an animal model produced profound transient hemodynamic changes including a marked increase in baseline pulmonary artery pressure, but there was no histological equivalent of ARDS or alterations in lung permeability. Using invasive hemodynamic monitoring in eight patients undergoing intravariceal sclerotherapy with sodium morrhuate, Bailey-Newton et al.[118] failed to show any clinically significant changes in pulmonary or systemic hemodynamics. Korula et al.[119] were unable to detect any significant short- or long-term differences in gas exchange or lung function in 11 patients undergoing sclerotherapy.

Cardiac Complications

Bradyarrhythmias have been reported in two patients undergoing sclerotherapy with sodium morrhuate;[120] both were known to have conduction abnormalities. The electrocardiographic abnormalities included periods of sinus bradycardia, sinus arrest, asystole, and second-degree atrioventricular block. In one patient the arrhythmia recurred during a sclerotherapy session.

Chest pain and electrocardiographic abnormalities consistent with transient coronary spasm were detected in a patient by Charng et al.[121] The authors felt that the stress of the procedure rather than the direct effect of ethanolamine oleate on the myocardium was the precipitating factor.

Knauer and Fogel[122] reported the occurrence of acute pericarditis in three patients following sclerotherapy with sodium morrhuate. One patient required a pericardiocentesis, which yielded 1,550 ml of a bloody, nonclotting fluid. In the other two patients with small and large pericardial effusions, respectively, there was gradual resolution without hemodynamic embarrassment. The authors concluded that this complication should be considered in the differential diagnosis of postsclerotherapy chest pain.

Central Nervous System Injury

Seidman et al.[123] reported a patient with irreversible paraplegia within eight hours of a third session of sclerotherapy using 5% sodium morrhuate. This four-year-old girl with cryptogenic cirrhosis, diagnosed at the age of one year, had been undergoing sclerotherapy sessions with a rigid endoscope under general anesthesia. During the third session, three injections were performed using a total of 6 ml of sclerosant. Blood loss, estimated at 150 ml, was noted following withdrawal of the needle from the third injection site. The child died two years later, and an autopsy revealed evidence of an old spinal cord infarction and occlusion of the anterior spinal artery by organized thrombi.

Hemorrhage from Other Collateral Vessels

Bleeding from duodenal varices is uncommon.[124,125] In a patient undergoing esophageal variceal sclerotherapy, Sauerbruch et al.[124] were able to control hemorrhage from a duodenal varix by means of intravariceal injections of polidocanol. The mechanism for the development of duodenal varices remains speculative but may involve obliteration of the coronary-azygous system, which could lead to increased portal flow through the intestinal venous system.[126] Arst and Reynolds[127] reported a patient with ileal variceal hemorrhage occurring six hours after an initial sclerotherapy procedure. The development of bleeding ileal varices within an adhesion between the small intestine and a surgical scar in a patient undergoing sclerotherapy was reported by Fry et al.[128] Foutch and Sivak[126] described bleeding rectosigmoid varices in three patients who were undergoing sclerotherapy. All three patients were managed conservatively, without subsequent recurrence of bleeding. In another report, balloon tamponade of bleeding rectal varices was unsuccessful, but ligation with elastic bands proved to be an effective temporizing measure.[129]

Vascular Complications

Extraesophageal vascular disorders are an uncommon group of complications following sclerotherapy. These are regarded as complications of sclerotherapy by association and usually involve obliteration of blood flow in a branch of the portal venous system, with the ensuing risk of ischemia or infarction over the compromised watershed. The pathogenesis of these complications is poorly understood. Sluggish portal blood flow secondary to cirrhosis coupled with localized activation of the clotting cascade as a result of disseminated sclerosant could theoretically lead to thrombosis. Ng and Chan[130] reported the development of digital ischemia and subsequent gangrene following intraoperative sclerotherapy with intravariceal ethanolamine. Following partial amputation, the lumina of the digital arteries were found to be completely obliterated by organized thrombi. There was no evidence of a vasoculopathy or an obvious thromboembolic source. This phenomenon could have been due to systemic dissemination of ethanolamine oleate or to embolization of clots formed in the injected esophageal varices.

At least four cases of portal vein thrombosis following sclerotherapy have been reported.[80,87,131] Barsuom et al.[87] treated a patient in whom a fresh thrombus was found extending from the submucosal and subepithelial veins of the esophagus into the left gastric vein and ultimately into the portal vein.

Thatcher et al.[132] reported two patients with mesenteric venous thrombosis after sclerotherapy with a mixture of 0.75% sodium tetradecyl sulfate and 50% glucose. Extension of a portal vein thrombus into the superior mesenteric vein, which was successfully treated with a distal splenorenal shunt, has also been described.[131] Sauerbruch and Moser,[133] using the technique of hepatosplenic radionuclide angiography, failed to demonstrate any change in the portal venous blood flow in eight patients six months after initiation of chronic sclerotherapy.

Bacteremia/Infectious Complications

The incidence of bacteremia following sclerotherapy has not been clearly established. Camara et al.[134] documented transient bacteremia in 5% of sclerotherapy procedures performed on 18 patients. Cohen et al.[86] found 14 episodes of bacteremia in 11 patients. Most positive blood cultures were obtained in the first five minutes following sclerotherapy. Oropharyngeal flora were the most common organisms isolated. The occurrence of bacteremia may be a function of the length of the injector needle. Snady et al.[135] found that the incidence of bacteremia increased by a factor of 3.5 with use of a 6- to 8-mm needle compared to that for a needle 3–4 mm long.

Low et al.[136] obtained blood cultures prior to sclerotherapy and at 5 minutes and 10 minutes after injection in 38 patients who underwent 104 procedures. Surveillance cultures were obtained from the pharynx and the accessory channel of the endoscope. There was no significant difference between the rates of bacteremia before injection (1.9%) and after sclerotherapy (4.3%). Positive bacterial cultures were obtained from the endoscope in 4% of the procedures, although none of these organisms were subsequently found in the blood cultures. In only one procedure was the same organism isolated in blood cultures and at both 5 and 10 minutes.

Hegnhj et al.[137] studied 30 consecutive patients with cirrhosis and esophageal varices who underwent either sclerotherapy or a diagnostic upper endoscopy. Although bacteremia was documented in 19% of patients undergoing sclerotherapy versus 6% of patients undergoing diagnostic endoscopy, this difference did not achieve statistical significance. The microorganisms recovered were either oropharyngeal or normal skin flora. The bacteremia was transient, and no patient developed clinical evidence of sepsis.

Serious infections as a result of sclerotherapy have been reported. Van Zaanen et al.[138] reported the development of meningococcal septicemia and peritonitis in a diabetic patient with alcoholic cirrhosis who received intra- and paravariceal polidocanol. The type of meningococcus isolated can be found in the nasopharynx and is almost never pathogenic. Contamination of the accessory channel of the endoscope by oropharyngeal flora was considered to be the source of the infection. Acute bacterial meningitis with *Klebsiella pneumoniae,* another gram-negative organism known to inhabit the oropharynx, occurred in a patient one day after intravariceal sclerotherapy with a mixture of 50% glucose and 3% sodium tetradecyl sulfate.[139] The occurrence of a solitary brain abscess following sclerotherapy has also been reported.[140]

Barthel et al.[141] described the development of a candidal esophageal abscess in a patient who was undergoing intravariceal injections of sodium morrhuate. The patient eventually died as a result of overwhelming candidal sepsis.

Ritchie et al.[142] reported a case of bilateral perinephric abscesses that developed three weeks after a fifth sclerotherapy session using sodium morrhuate. Despite an intensive search, the only source that could be implicated was the sclerotherapy procedure itself. *Streptococcus pneumoniae,* an organism commonly found in the nasopharynx, was the infectious organism.

Baskin[143] described a 66-year-old man with a prior mitral valve replacement for endocarditis who developed fever, a new mitral regurgitant murmur, and multiple positive blood cultures for *Streptococcus viridans.* A careful search for other sources of bacteremia was unsuccessful. The patient had been given an intramuscular antibiotic as a prophylactic measure, but it was determined retrospectively that this provided suboptimal bactericidal concentrations. The author concluded that there was a strong association between the infection and prior sclerotherapy sessions. Antibiotic prophylaxis was recommended for patients with prosthetic heart valves who are to undergo sclerotherapy. These reports on sclerotherapy-related sepsis are clouded by the frequent occurrence of spontaneous bacteremia of cryptic origin in cirrhotic patients.

Based upon the low incidence of bacteremia following sclerotherapy and the infrequent nature of significant sequelae to transient bacteremia, it is not clear at present that routine antibiotic prophylaxis should be administered prior to sclerotherapy. Prudence, however, favors prophylaxis in patients with a history of rheumatic valvular heart disease, valve replacement, or prior episode(s) of endocarditis. Given the low incidence of bacteremia, a relatively large controlled study would be needed to determine the efficacy of routine antibiotic prophylaxis.

Miscellaneous Complications

At least eight patients with esophageal carcinoma following sclerotherapy with a variety of agents have been reported.[144-146] Seven had squamous cell carcinomas and one an adenocarcinoma. The interval between the last sclerotherapy session and the onset of esophageal carcinoma ranged from 6 to 30 months. In theory, a sclerosant could be carcinogenic, although there are no data to support this supposition. A causal relationship between sclerotherapy and esophageal cancer seems dubious given the small number of patients in whom the two diseases occurred in the same patient. Furthermore, other risk factors including the use of tobacco and alcohol often coexist.

One patient with chylous ascites and pleural effusion[147] and one with isolated right chylothorax[148] after sclerotherapy have been reported. These unusual complications have been attributed to inadvertent puncture of the thoracic duct with the sclerotherapy needle.

Rasbridge et al.[149] described three patients with intestinal pseudo-obstruction after sclerotherapy. The patients developed abdominal distention, high-pitched bowel sounds, and radiographic evidence of small and large bowel distention which resolved spontaneously after 48 hours.

Gastric bezoars developed in five patients with alcoholic cirrhosis who underwent sclerotherapy.[150] The bezoar was transient in most patients, but persistent and recurrent episodes were also documented. Davion et al.[150] suggested that the development of a bezoar could be due to delayed gastric emptying as a result of sclerotherapy-induced vagal injury.

The formation of large splenorenal shunts has been noted after variceal eradication by sclerotherapy in three patients with extrahepatic portal hypertension.[151] These collateral vessels were clinically insignificant in all cases.

Intramural hematomas have led to perforation in one patient and to bacteremia and death in another.[71,83] Transient complete obstruction of the esophagus as a result of a large intramural hematoma has been reported following intravariceal sclerotherapy with sodium tetradecyl sulfate.[152] This patient eventually recovered with conservative management. Transient bacteremia was thought to have led to significant intravascular hemolysis in a patient with glucose-6-phosphate dehydrogenase deficiency after a third sclerotherapy session.[153] Alcohol, the sclerosant used, could not be incriminated, as it is a reducing substance.

SCLEROTHERAPY OF GASTRIC VARICES

Gastric varices are an important sequela of portal hypertension of any etiology. Splenic vein obstruction or occlusion by an inflammatory process or, more rarely, pancreatic malignancy can result in isolated gastric varices. Uncommon causes of splenic vein occlusion include polycythemia rubra vera, retroperitoneal fibrosis or bleeding, lymphadenopathy, and splenic artery aneurysm.

The incidence of gastric varices varies widely in different groups of patients. Mathur et al.[154] found that 48% of a group of 104 patients with portal hypertension had gastric varices. A further 31 patients subsequently developed gastric varices, presumably as a result of esophageal sclerotherapy. Sarin et al.[155] found a 16% incidence of gastric varices in 309 patients with portal hypertension. Concomitant esophageal varices were noted in 88% of these patients. Isolated gastric varices were present in only six patients. It is difficult to estimate the incidence of bleeding from gastric varices, since relatively few series with small numbers of patients have been published. In the two largest series, the incidence of hemorrhage from gastric varices ranged from 11% to 23%.[154,155]

The role of sclerotherapy for the treatment of gastric varices remains uncertain. The little information available is derived from relatively small and uncontrolled series. Eradication of esophageal varices resulted in the disappearance of gastric varices in 28% of patients with esophagogastric varices in the series of Sarin et al.[155]

A canine model of bleeding gastric varices was used to compare the efficacy of endoscopic variceal ligation to that of high-volume sclerotherapy.[156] Both methods achieved controlled bleeding in all instances, but variceal ligation led to significantly larger ulcers and was considered the more difficult procedure.

Trudeau and Prindiville[157] performed intravariceal injections of 1.5% sodium tetradecyl in nine patients with advanced liver disease and bleeding gastric varices who were not considered surgical candidates and then compared the results in these patients to those in 47 patients with bleeding esophageal varices and similarly advanced liver disease. The initial level of hemostasis was equivalent for both groups. However, the rate of recurrent bleeding was significantly higher in patients with gastric varices (89% versus 51%). Sclerotherapy to control recurrent bleeding was also less effective in patients with gastric varices (44% versus 94%). Mortality, transfusion requirements, average length of hospitalization, and average hospital costs were all significantly higher in the patients with gastric varices.

Elective intravariceal sclerotherapy for gastric varices was followed by immediate or delayed bleeding in four of five patients reported by Sarin et al.[155] Two of these patients exsanguinated despite balloon tamponade. Combined paravariceal and intravariceal injections controlled bleeding in four of six patients. Combination sclerotherapy was employed electively in 32 patients. Variceal obliteration was achieved in 12 patients (38%), and reduction in variceal size was seen in an additional 7 patients (12%) after a minimum of four sessions. Bleeding recurred in 16%. Complications included retrosternal pain (36%), fever (28%), dysphagia (14%), and ulceration (38%). At a mean follow-up period of 9.7 months, there was no recurrence or increase in variceal size in the 19 patients who responded to sclerotherapy.

Recently, Lee et al.[158] reported the results of a trial in which 28 patients with actively bleeding gastric varices were treated by intravariceal sclerotherapy. High-volume injections (average, 6.8 ml) were performed in 13 patients with isolated fundic varices. Fifteen patients with esophagogastric varices received injections 1 cm above the esophagogastric junction. High-volume sclerotherapy of isolated fundic varices resulted in hemostasis in all cases. Subsequent bleeding and mortality rates were 15% for this group. Treatment of patients with esophagogastric varices led to a lower rate of hemostasis (86%), a similar number of complications, and a higher mortality rate (26%).

The tissue adhesive butyl cyanoacrylate has been used to obliterate large and/or actively bleeding gastric varices in a series of 27 patients.[159] The procedure was performed for active bleeding in only six patients in whom the blood loss was termed "moderate," although immediate hemostasis was achieved in all cases. Recurrent bleeding was controlled in one of two patients in this group. It was difficult to distinguish patent from occluded varices at endoscopy, and occlusion of the accessory channel of the endoscope or the injection needle occurred with 8% of injection attempts. Rauws et al.[160] treated 39 consecutive patients with actively bleeding gastric varices or signs of a recent hemorrhage (a fibrin plug or an adherent clot) by injection of the cyanoacrylate adhesive. Hemostasis was achieved in the 27 patients with active bleeding. During the follow-up period, which ranged from three months to three years, there were 40 episodes of recurrent bleeding from gastric varices and 23 episodes of esophageal variceal bleeding. Death due to recurrent hemorrhage or liver failure occurred in five patients. No major complications related to the tissue adhesive were noted.

Optimal treatment of gastric varices, whether by sclerotherapy, endoscopic ligation, or injection of a tissue adhesive, is uncertain at present. Until more data are available, these methods should generally be considered investigative. When the options for treatment are limited by other clinical circumstances, sclerotherapy may be performed. However, it should be recognized that sclerotherapy for this condition is probably less effective and is associated with a higher complication rate compared to sclerotherapy for esophageal varices.

REFERENCES

1. Walters W: Discussion. *Proc Staff Meet Mayo Clin* 8:163–165, 1932.
2. Crafoord C, Frenckner P: New surgical treatment of varicose veins of the oesophagus. *Acta Otolaryngol* 27:422–429, 1939.
3. Moersch HJ: Further studies on the treatment of esophageal varices by injection of a sclerosing solution. *Ann Otol Rhinol Laryngol* 50:1233–1244, 1941.
4. Johnston GW, Rodgers HW: A review of 15 years' experience in the use of sclerotherapy in the control of acute haemorrhage for oesophageal varices. *Br J Surg* 60:797–800, 1973.
5. Paquet KJ, Oberhammer E: Sclerotherapy of bleeding oesophageal varices by means of endoscopy. *Endoscopy* 10:7–12, 1978.
6. Vianna A, Hayes PC, Moscoso G, et al: Normal venous circulation of the gastroesophageal junction. A route to understanding varices. *Gastroenterology* 93:876–889, 1987.
7. Butler H: The veins of the oesophagus. *Thorax* 6:276–296, 1951.
8. Kitano S, Terblanche J, Kahn D, et al: Venous anatomy of the lower oesophagus in portal hypertension: Practical implications. *Br J Surg* 73:525–531, 1986.
9. McCormack TT, Rose JD, Smith PM, et al: Perforating veins and blood flow in esophageal varices. *Lancet* 2:1442–1444, 1983.
10. Lebrec D, DeFleury P, Rueff B, et al: Portal hypertension, size of esophageal varices, and risk of gastrointestinal bleeding in alcoholic cirrhosis. *Gastroenterology* 79:1139–1144, 1980.
11. Reynolds TB, Ito S, Iwatsuki S: Measurement of portal pressure and its clinical application. *Am J Med* 49:649–657, 1970.
12. Garcia-tsao G, Groszmann RJ, Fisher R, et al: Portal pressure, presence of gastroesophageal varices and variceal bleeding. *Hepatology* 5:419–424, 1985.
13. Gluud C, Henriksen JH, Nielsen G: Prognostic indicators in alcoholic cirrhotic men. *Hepatology* 8:222–227, 1988.
14. Dagradi AE: Esophageal varices, splenic pulp pressure and "directional" flow patterns in alcoholic liver cirrhosis. A correlation study. *Am J Gastroenterol* 59:15–22, 1973.
15. Joly JG, Marleau D, Legare A, et al: Bleeding from esophageal varices in cirrhosis of the liver: Hemodynamic and radiological criteria for the selection of potential bleeders through hepatic and umbilicoportal catheterization studies. *Can Med Assoc J* 104:576–580, 1971.
16. Willoughby EO, David D, Smith CW, et al: The significance of small esophageal varices in portal cirrhosis. *Gastroenterology* 47:375–381, 1964.
17. Greene L, Weisberg H, Rosenthal WS, et al: Evaluation of esophageal varices in liver disease by splenic-pulp manometry, splenoportography, and esophagogastroscopy. Diagnostic discrepancies. *Am J Dig Dis* 10:284–292, 1965.
18. Westaby S, Wilkinson SP, Warren R, et al: Spleen size and portal hypertension in cirrhosis. *Digestion* 17:63–68, 1978.
19. Simert G, Lunderquist A, Tylen U, et al: Correlation between percutaneous transhepatic portography and clinical findings in 56 patients with portal hypertension. *Acta Chir Scand* 144:27–34, 1978.
20. Smith-Laing G, Camilo ME, Dick R, et al: Percutaneous transhepatic portography in the assessment of portal hypertension. Clinical correlations and comparison of radiographic techniques. *Gastroenterology* 78:197–205, 1980.
21. Rigau J, Bosch J, Bordas JM, et al: Endoscopic measurement of variceal pressure in cirrhosis: Correlation with portal pressure and variceal hemorrhage. *Gastroenterology* 96:873–880, 1989.

22. Dagradi AE: The natural history of esophageal varices in patients with alcoholic liver cirrhosis: An endoscopic and clinical study. *Am J Gastroenterol* 57:520–540, 1972.
23. Beppu K, Inokuchi K, Koyanagi N, et al: Prediction of variceal hemorrhage by esophageal endoscopy. *Gastrointest Endosc* 27:213–218, 1981.
24. Spence RAJ, Sloan JM, Johnston GW, et al: Oesophageal mucosal changes in patients with varices. *Gut* 24:1024–1029, 1983.
25. Kleber G, Sauerbruch T, Fisher G, et al: Endoscopic markers of impending variceal hemorrhage: Correlation with the pressure in the varices. *Gut* 30:228–232, 1989.
26. Chiles NH, Baggenstoss AH, Butt HR, et al: Oesophageal varices: Comparative incidence of ulceration and spontaneous rupture as a cause of fatal hemorrhage. *Gastroenterology* 25:565–573, 1953.
27. Wagenknecht TW, Noble JF, Barnofsky ID: Nature of bleeding in esophageal varices. *Surgery* 33:869–874, 1953.
28. Ponce J, Froufe A, de la Morena E, et al: Morphometric study of the esophageal mucosa in cirrhotic patients with variceal bleeding. *Hepatology* 1:641–646, 1981.
29. Spence RA, Anderson JR, Johnston GW: Twenty-five years of injection sclerotherapy for bleeding varices. *Br J Surg* 72:195–198, 1985.
30. Eckardt VF, Grace ND: Gastroesophageal reflux and bleeding esophageal varices. *Gastroenterology* 76:39–42, 1979.
31. The North Italian Endoscopic Club for the Study and Treatment of Esophageal Varices: Prediction of the first variceal hemorrhage in patients with cirrhosis of the liver and esophageal varices. A prospective multicenter study. *N Engl J Med* 319:983–989, 1988.
32. Paquet KJ: Prophylactic endoscopic sclerosing treatment of the esophageal wall in varices—a prospective controlled randomized trial. *Endoscopy* 14:4–5, 1982.
33. Silverstein FE, Gilbert DA, Tedesco FJ, et al: The national ASGE survey on upper gastrointestinal bleeding. II. Clinical prognostic factors. *Gastrointest Endosc* 27:80–93, 1981.
34. Graham DY, Smith JL: The course of patients after variceal hemorrhage. *Gastroenterology* 80:800–809, 1981.
35. Jackson FC, Perrin EB, Degradi AE, et al: Clinical investigation of the portacaval shunt. I. Study design and preliminary survival analysis. *Arch Surg* 91:43–54, 1965.
36. Christensen E, Fauerholdt L, Schlichting P, et al: Aspects of the natural history of gastrointestinal bleeding in cirrhosis and the effect of prednisone. *Gastroenterology* 81:944–952, 1981.
37. Resnick RH, Iber FL, Ishihara AM, et al: A controlled study of the therapeutic portacaval shunt. *Gastroenterology* 67:843–857, 1974.
38. Fujita R: Endoscopic diagnosis and classification of esophageal varices in Japan, in Sivak MV Jr (ed): *Sclerotherapy of Esophageal Varices*. New York, Praeger, 1984, pp 35–42.
39. Baker LA, Smith C, Lieberman G: The natural history of esophageal varices. A study of 115 cirrhotic patients in whom varices were diagnosed prior to bleeding. *Am J Med* 26:228–237, 1959.
40. Palmer ED, Brick IB: Correlation between the severity of esophageal varices in portal cirrhosis and their propensity toward hemorrhage. *Gastroenterology* 30:85–90, 1956.
41. Cales P, Zabotto B, Meskens C, et al: Gastroesophageal endoscopic features in cirrhosis. Observer variability, interassociations, and relationship to hepatic dysfunction. *Gastroenterology* 98:156–162, 1990.
42. Foutch PG, Sullivan JA, Gaines JA, et al: Cutaneous vascular spiders in cirrhotic patients: Correlation with hemorrhage from esophageal varices. *Am J Gastroenterol* 83:723–726, 1988.

43. Hennessy TPJ, Stephens RB, Keane FB: Acute and chronic management of esophageal varices by injection sclerotherapy. *Surg Gynecol Obstet* 154:375–377, 1982.
44. Terblanche J, Yakoob HI, Bornman PC, et al: Acute bleeding varices. A five-year prospective evaluation of tamponade and sclerotherapy. *Ann Surg* 194:521–530, 1981.
45. Bornman PC, Kahn D, Terblanche J, et al: Rigid versus fiberoptic endoscopic injection sclerotherapy. *Ann Surg* 208:175–178, 1988.
46. Lewis J, Chung RS, Allison J: Sclerotherapy of esophageal varices. *Arch Surg* 115:476–480, 1980.
47. Kirkman JS, Quayle JB: Oesophageal varices: Evaluation of injection sclerotherapy without general anesthesia using the flexible fiberoptic gastroscope. *Ann R Coll Surg Engl* 64:401–405, 1982.
48. Williams KGD, Dawson JL: Fiberoptic injection of oesophageal varices. *Br Med J* 2:766–767, 1979.
49. Kitano S, Koyanagi N, Iso Y, et al: Prospective randomized trial comparing two injection techniques for sclerosing oesophageal varices: over-tube and free-hand. *Br J Surg* 74:603–606, 1987.
50. Westaby D, Macdougall BRD, Melia W, et al: A prospective randomized study of two sclerotherapy techniques for esophageal varices. *Hepatology* 3:681–684, 1983.
51. Grobe JL, Kozarek RA, Sanowski RA, et al: Venography during endoscopic injection sclerotherapy of esophageal varices. *Gastrointest Endosc* 30:6–8, 1984.
52. Barsoum MS, Khattar NY, Risk-Allah MA: Technical aspects of injunction sclerotherapy of acute oesophageal variceal haemorrhage as seen by radiography. *Br J Surg* 65:588–589, 1978.
53. Kang JH, Kambayashi J, Sakon M, et al: Mechanism of the haemostatic effect of ethanolamine oleate in the injection sclerotherapy for oesophageal varices. *Br J Surg* 74:50–53, 1987.
54. Yamaga H, Hashizume M, Kitano S, et al: Platelet aggregability after endoscopic variceal injection of 5 percent ethanolamine oleate into esophageal varices. *Br J Surg* 76:939–942, 1989.
55. McClave SA, Kaiser SC, Wright RA, et al: Prospective randomized comparison of esophageal sclerotherapy agents: Sodium tetradecyl sulfate versus sodium morrhuate. *Gastrointest Endosc* 36:567–571, 1990.
56. Rose JDR, Crane MD, Smith PM: Factors affecting successful endoscopic sclerotherapy for oesophageal varices. *Gut* 24:946–949, 1983.
57. Waring JP, Sanowski RA, Pardy K, et al: Does the addition of methylene blue to the sclerosant improve the accuracy of injections during sclerotherapy? *Gastrointest Endosc* 57:159–160, 1991.
58. Sarin SK, Nanda R, Sachdev G, et al: Intravariceal versus paravariceal sclerotherapy: A prospective, controlled, randomized trial. *Gut* 28:657–662, 1987.
59. Stray N, Jacobsen CD, Rosseland A: Injection sclerotherapy of bleeding oesophageal and gastric varices using a flexible endoscope. *Acta Med Scand* 211:125–129, 1982.
60. Paquet KJ, Feussner H: Endoscopic sclerosis and esophageal balloon tamponade in acute hemorrhage from esophagogastric varices: A prospective controlled randomized trial. *Hepatology* 5:580–583, 1985.
61. Sarin SK, Sachdev G, Nanda S, et al: Comparison of the two time schedules for endoscopic sclerotherapy: A prospective randomised controlled study. *Gut* 27:710–713, 1986.
62. Westaby D, Melia WM, Macdougall BRD, et al: Injection sclerotherapy for oesophageal varices: A prospective randomised trial of different treatment schedules. *Gut* 25:129–132, 1984.

63. Smith PM, Jones DB, Rose JDR: Simplified fibre endoscopic sclerotherapy for oesophageal varices. *J R Col Physicians Lond* 16:236–238, 1982.

64. Soehendra N, de Heer K, Kempeneers I, et al: Sclerotherapy of esophageal varices: Acute arrest of gastrointestinal hemorrhage of long-term therapy? *Endoscopy* 15:136–140, 1983.

65. Korula J: Outpatient esophageal variceal sclerotherapy: Safe and cost-effective. A prospective study. *Gastrointest Endosc* 32:1–3, 1986.

66. Drell E, Prindiville T, Trudeau W: Outpatient endoscopic injection sclerosis of esophageal varices. *Gastrointest Endosc* 32:4–6, 1986.

67. Stiegmann G, Goff JS, Sun JH, et al: Endoscopic ligation of esophageal varices. *Am J Surg* 159:21–25, 1990.

68. Stiegmann G, Goff JS, Michaletz P, et al: Endoscopic variceal ligation vs. sclerotherapy for bleeding esophageal varices: Early results from a prospective randomized trial (abstract). *Gastrointest Endosc* 36:188, 1990.

69. Saeed ZA, Michaletz PA, Winchester CB, et al: Endoscopic variceal ligation after failed endoscopic sclerotherapy. *Gastrointest Endosc* 36:572–574, 1990.

70. Sukigara M, Omoto R, Miyamae T: Systemic dissemination of ethanolamine oleate after injection sclerotherapy for esophageal varices. *Arch Surg* 120:833–836, 1985.

71. Palani CK, Abuabara S, Kraft AR, et al: Endoscopic sclerotherapy in acute variceal hemorrhage. *Am J Surg* 141:164–168, 1981.

72. Cello JP, Grendell JH, Crass RA, et al: Endoscopic sclerotherapy versus portacaval shunt in patients with severe cirrhosis and variceal hemorrhage. *N Engl J Med* 311:1589–1594, 1984.

73. Sivak MV Jr, Stout DJ, Skipper G: Endoscopic injection sclerosis (EIS) of esophageal varices. *Gastrointest Endosc* 27:52–57, 1981.

74. Clark AW, Westaby D, Silk DBA, et al: Prospective controlled trial of injection sclerotherapy in patients with cirrhosis and recent variceal hemorrhage. *Lancet* 2:552–554, 1980.

75. Hughes RW Jr, Larson DE, Viggiano TR, et al: Endoscopic variceal sclerosis: A one-year experience. *Gastrointest Endosc* 28:62–66, 1982.

76. Patterson CO, Rouse MO: The sclerosing therapy of esophageal varices. *Gastroenterology* 9:391–395, 1947.

77. Macdougall BRD, Westaby D, Theodossi A, et al: Increased long-term survival in variceal haemorrhage using injection sclerotherapy. Results of a controlled trial. *Lancet* 1:124–127, 1982.

78. Sarles HE, Sanowski RA, Talbert G: Course and complications of endoscopic variceal sclerotherapy: A prospective study of 50 patients. *Am J Gastroenterol* 80:595–599, 1985.

79. Schuman BM, Beckman JW, Tedesco FJ, et al: Complications of endoscopic injection sclerotherapy: A review. *Am J Gastroenterol* 82:823–830, 1987.

80. Goodale RL, Silvis SE, O'Leary JF, et al: Early survival after sclerotherapy for bleeding esophageal varices. *Surg Gynecol Obstet* 155:523–538, 1982.

81. Ayres SJ, Goff JS, Warren GH: Endoscopic sclerotherapy for bleeding esophageal varices: Effects and complications. *Ann Intern Med* 98:900–903, 1983.

82. Barsoum MS, Bolous FI, El-Rooby AA, et al: Tamponade and injection sclerotherapy in the management of bleeding oesophageal varices. *Br J Surg* 69:76–78, 1982.

83. Harris OD, Dickey JD, Stephenson PM: Simple endoscopic injection sclerotherapy of oesophageal varices. *Aust NZ J Med* 12:131–135, 1982.

84. Gebhard RL, Ansel HJ, Silvis SE: Origin of pain during variceal sclerotherapy (abstract). *Gastrointest Endosc* 28:131, 1982.

85. Shoenut JP, Micflikier AB: Retrosternal pain subsequent to sclerotherapy. *Gastrointest Endosc* 32:84–87, 1986.

86. Cohen LB, Korsten MA, Scherl EJ, et al: Bacteremia after endoscopic injection sclerosis. *Gastrointest Endosc* 29:198–200, 1983.
87. Barsoum MS, Mooro HAW, Bolous FI, et al: The complications of injection sclerotherapy of bleeding oesophageal varices. *Br J Surg* 69:79–81, 1982.
88. Sarin SK, Nanda R, Vij JC, et al: Oesophageal ulceration after sclerotherapy—a complication or an accompaniment? *Endoscopy* 18:44–45, 1986.
89. Castro-Fernandez M, Guerrero-Jimenez P, Herrera-Justiniano JM, et al: Ulcer of the gastric fundus associated with sclerosis of esophageal varices. *Endoscopy* 19:143–144, 1987.
90. Ayres SJ, Goff JS, Warren GH, et al: Esophageal ulceration and bleeding after flexible fiberoptic esophageal vein sclerosis. *Gastroenterology* 83:131–136, 1982.
91. Subramanyam K, Patterson M: Chronic esophageal ulceration after endoscopic sclerotherapy. *J Clin Gastroenterol* 8:58–60, 1986.
92. Novis, B, Bat L, Pomerantz I, et al: Endoscopic sclerotherapy of esophageal varices. *Isr J Med Sci* 19:40–44, 1983.
93. Scherl EJ, Fabry TL: Pseudodiverticula secondary to injection sclerotherapy. *J Clin Gastroenterol* 5:401–403, 1983.
94. Roark G: Treatment of postsclerotherapy esophageal ulcers with sucralfate. *Gastrointest Endosc* 30:9–10, 1984.
95. Gimson A, Potson R, Westaby D, et al: Omeprazole in the management of intractable ulceration following injection sclerotherapy. *Gastroenterology* 99:1829–1831, 1990.
96. Sivak MV Jr: Endoscopic injection sclerosis of esophageal varices: ASGE survey (letter). *Gastrointest Endosc* 28:41, 1982.
97. Perino LE, Gholson CF, Goff JS: Esophageal perforation after fiberoptic variceal sclerotherapy. *J Clin Gastroenterol* 9:286–289, 1987.
98. Soderlund C, Wiechel K-L: Oesophageal perforation after sclerotherapy for variceal haemorrhage. *Acta Chir Scand* 149:491–495, 1983.
99. Carr-Locke DL, Sidky K: Broncho-oesophageal fistula: A late complication of endoscopic variceal sclerotherapy. *Gut* 23:1005–1007, 1982.
100. Shemesh E, Bat L: Esophageal perforation after fiberoptic endoscopic injection sclerotherapy for esophageal varices. *Arch Surg* 121:243–245, 1986.
101. Wilborn SL, Rector WG, Schaefer JW: An esophagobronchial fistula after endoscopic variceal sclerotherapy. Development and successful nonsurgical management. *J Clin Gastroenterol* 10:81–83, 1988.
102. Kjaergaard J, Fischer A, Miskowiak J, et al: Sclerotherapy of bleeding esophageal varices. Long-term results. *Scand J Gastroenterol* 17:363–367, 1982.
103. Snady H, Korsten MA: Esophageal acid-clearance and motility after endoscopic sclerotherapy of esophageal varices. *Am J Gastroenterol* 81:419–422, 1986.
104. Greenholz SK, Hall RJ, Sondheimer JM, et al: Manometric and pH consequences of esophageal endosclerosis in children. *J Pediatr Surg* 23:38–41, 1988.
105. Sauerbruch T, Wirsching R, Holl J, et al: Effects of repeated injection sclerotherapy on acid gastroesophageal reflux. *Gastrointest Endosc* 32:81–83, 1986.
106. Sorensen T, Burcharth F, Pedersen ML, et al: Oesophageal stricture and dysphagia after endoscopic sclerotherapy for bleeding varices. *Gut* 25:473–477, 1984.
107. Haynes WC, Sanowski RA, Foutch PG, et al: Esophageal strictures following endoscopic variceal sclerotherapy: Clinical course and response to dilation therapy. *Gastrointest Endosc* 32:202–205, 1986.
108. Ogle SJ, Kirk CJC, Bailey RJ, et al: Oesophageal function in cirrhotic patients undergoing injection sclerotherapy for oesophageal varices. *Digestion* 18:178–185, 1978.

109. Larson GM: Esophageal motility after injection sclerotherapy (abstract). *Gastrointest Endosc* 29:164, 1983.

110. Simon C, Cohen L, Scherl E, et al: Esophageal motility and symptoms after endoscopic injection sclerotherapy (abstract). *Gastrointest Endosc* 29:192, 1983.

111. Reilly JJ Jr, Schade RR, Van Thiel DS: Esophageal function after injection sclerotherapy: Pathogenesis of esophageal stricture. *Am J Surg* 147:85–88, 1984.

112. Soderlund C, Thor K, Wiechel KL: Oesophageal motility after sclerotherapy for bleeding varices. *Acta Chir Scand* 151:249–253, 1985.

113. Saks BJ, Kilby AE, Dietrich PA, et al: Pleural and mediastinal changes following endoscopic injection sclerotherapy of esophageal varices. *Radiology* 149:639–642, 1983.

114. Bacon BR, Bailey-Newton RS, Connors AF Jr: Pleural effusions after endoscopic variceal sclerotherapy. *Gastroenterology* 88:1910–1914, 1985.

115. Mauro MA, Jaques PF, Swantkowski TM, et al: CT after uncomplicated esophageal sclerotherapy. *AJR* 147:57–60, 1986.

116. DePuey EG, Richards WO, Millikan WJ, et al: Scintigraphic detection of pulmonary embolization of esophageal variceal sclerosant. *Endoscopy* 20:91–94, 1988.

117. Monroe P, Morrow CF Jr, Millen JE, et al: Acute respiratory failure after sodium morrhuate esophageal sclerotherapy. *Gastroenterology* 85:693–699, 1983.

118. Bailey-Newton RS, Connors AF Jr, Bacon BR: Effect of endoscopic variceal sclerotherapy on gas exchange in humans. *Gastroenterology* 89:368–373, 1985.

119. Korula J, Baydur A, Sassoon C, et al: Effect of esophageal variceal sclerotherapy (EVS) on lung function. *Arch Intern Med* 146:1517–1520, 1986.

120. Perakos PG, Cirbus JJ, Camara DS: Persistent bradyarrhythmia after sclerotherapy for esophageal varices. *South Med J* 77:531–532, 1984.

121. Charng MJ, Wang SP, Chang MS, et al: Coronary spasm complicating sclerotherapy of esophageal varices. *Chest* 93:204–205, 1988.

122. Knauer CM, Fogel MR: Pericarditis: Complication of esophageal sclerotherapy. A report of three cases. *Gastroenterology* 93:287–290, 1987.

123. Seidman E, Weber AM, Morin CL, et al: Spinal cord paralysis following sclerotherapy for esophageal varices. *Hepatology* 4:950–954, 1984.

124. Sauerbruch T, Weinzierl M, Dietrich HP, et al: Sclerotherapy of a bleeding duodenal varix. *Endoscopy* 14:187–189, 1982.

125. Eleftheriadis E: Duodenal varices after sclerotherapy for esophageal varices. *Am J Gastroenterol* 83:439–441, 1988.

126. Foutch PG, Sivak MV Jr: Colonic variceal hemorrhage after endoscopic injection sclerosis of esophageal varices: A report of three cases. *Am J Gastroenterol* 79:756–760, 1984.

127. Arst HF, Reynolds JD: Acute ileal variceal hemorrhage secondary to esophageal sclerotherapy. *J Clin Gastroenterol* 8:603–604, 1986.

128. Fry RD, Fischer KC, Susman N, et al: Adhesion related variceal hemorrhage following sclerosis of esophageal varices. *Arch Surg* 94–95, 1988.

129. Keane RM, Britton DC: Massive bleeding from rectal varices following repeated injection sclerotherapy of oesophageal varices. *Br J Surg* 73:120, 1986.

130. Ng WD, Chan YT: Digital gangrene complicating intraoperative injection sclerotherapy. *Gastrointest Endosc* 34:151–153, 1988.

131. Ashida H, Yoshinao K, Nishioka A, et al: Portal and mesenteric vein thrombosis as a complication of endoscopic sclerotherapy. *Am J Gastroenterol* 84:306–310, 1989.

132. Thatcher BS, Sivak MV Jr, Ferguson DR, et al: Mesenteric venous thrombosis as a possible

complication of endoscopic sclerotherapy: A report of two cases. *Am J Gastroenterol* 81:126–129, 1986.

133. Sauerbruch T, Moser E: Influence of long-term injection sclerotherapy on portal venous component of total liver perfusion measured by hepatosplenic radionuclide angiography. *Hepatogastroenterology* 33:17–19, 1986.
134. Camara DS, Gruber M, Barde CJ, et al: Transient bacteremia following endoscopic injection sclerotherapy of esophageal varices. *Arch Intern Med* 143:1350–1352, 1983.
135. Snady H, Korsten MA, Waye JD: The relationship of bacteremia to the length of the injection needle in endoscopic variceal sclerotherapy. *Gastrointest Endosc* 31:243–246, 1985.
136. Low DE, Shoenut JP, Kennedy JK, et al: Infectious complications of endoscopic injection sclerotherapy. *Arch Intern Med* 146:569–571, 1986.
137. Hegnhj J, Andersen JR, Jarlv JO, et al: Bacteriaemia after injection sclerotherapy of oesophageal varices. *Liver* 8:167–171, 1988.
138. Van Zaanen HCT, Shotborgh RH, Chamuleau RAFM: Meningococcus septicemia: A complication of endoscopic injection sclerotherapy (letter). *Am J Gastroenterol* 85:631–632, 1990.
139. Wang W, Chen C, Jan C, et al: Central nervous system infection after endoscopic injection sclerotherapy. *Am J Gastroenterol* 85:865–867, 1990.
140. Cohen FL, Koerner RS, Taub SJ: Solitary brain abscess following endoscopic injection sclerosis of esophageal varices. *Gastrointest Endosc* 31:331–333, 1985.
141. Barthel JS, Sprouse RF, Dix JD, et al: Fatal *Candida* esophageal abscess and sepsis complicating endoscopic variceal sclerosis. *Gastrointest Endosc* 33:107–110, 1987.
142. Ritchie MT, Lightdale CJ, Botet JF: Bilateral perinephric abscesses: A complication of endoscopic injection sclerotherapy. *Am J Gastroenterol* 82:670–673, 1987.
143. Baskin G: Prosthetic endocarditis after endoscopic variceal sclerotherapy: A failure of antibiotic prophylaxis. *Am J Gastroenterol* 84:311–312, 1989.
144. Bochna GS, Harty RF, Harned RK, et al: Development of squamous cell carcinoma of the esophagus after endoscopic variceal sclerotherapy. *Am J Gastroenterol* 83:564–568, 1988.
145. Kokudo N, Sanjok S, Nebutaka V, et al: Squamous cell carcinoma after variceal injection sclerotherapy for esophageal varices. *Am J Gastroenterol* 85:861–864, 1990.
146. Guillemot F, Bonniere P, Bretagne JF, et al: Cancer esophagien et sclerose endoscopique des varices oesophaiennes: une association forfuite? *Gastroenterol Clin Biol* 12:858–861, 1988.
147. Barritt AS: Chylous ascites and esophageal sclerotherapy. *Gastroenterology* 94:1109–1110, 1988.
148. Gertsch P, Mosimann R: Chylothorax complicating sclerotherapy for bleeding oesophageal varices. *Br J Surg* 70:562, 1983.
149. Rasbridge S, Sheldon C, Hardman SM, et al: Intestinal pseudo-obstruction: A new complication of oesophageal sclerotherapy. *Br Med J* 292:991, 1986.
150. Davion T, Delamarre J, Reix A, et al: Gastric bezoar: Another side effect of endoscopic variceal sclerotherapy. *Scand J Gastroenterol* 24:818–820, 1989.
151. Dilawari JB, Chawla DM, Chakraborty MD: Development of splenoadrenal shunts after obliteration of esophageal varices by endoscopic sclerotherapy. *Am J Gastroenterol* 84:304–305, 1989.
152. Low DE, Patterson DJ: Complete esophageal obstruction secondary to dissecting intramural hematoma after endoscopic variceal sclerotherapy. *Am J Gastroenterol* 83:435–438, 1988.
153. Bhatia V, Goenka MK, Kochhar R, et al: Intravascular hemolysis following endoscopic variceal sclerotherapy (letter). *Am J Gastroenterol* 85:1435–1436, 1990.

154. Mathur SK, Dalvi AN, Somesthwar V, et al: Endoscopic and radiological appraisal of gastric varices. *Br J Surg* 77:432–435, 1990.

155. Sarin SK, Sachdev G, Nanda R, et al: Endoscopic sclerotherapy in the treatment of gastric varices. *Br J Surg* 75:747–750, 1988.

156. Egan J, Jensen DM, Jensen K, et al: Randomized, controlled study of endoscopic rubber band ligation and high volume sclerotherapy for actively bleeding gastric varices in dogs (abstract). *Gastrointest Endosc* 37:239, 1991.

157. Trudeau W, Prindiville T: Endoscopic injection sclerosis in bleeding esophageal varices. *Gastrointest Endosc* 32:264–268, 1986.

158. Lee RE, Prindiville TP, Trudeau WL: Endoscopic injection sclerotherapy for bleeding esophageal varices (abstract). *Gastrointest Endosc* 37:237, 1991.

159. Ramond JM, Valla D, Mosner JF, et al: Successful endoscopic obturation of gastric varices with butyl cyanoacylate. *Hepatology* 10:488–493, 1989.

160. Rauws EAJ, Jansen PLM, Tytgat GNJ: Endoscopic sclerotherapy of gastric varices with bucrylate (abstract). *Gastrointest Endosc* 37:242, 1991.

31

OUTCOME AFTER SCLEROTHERAPY OF ESOPHAGOGASTRIC VARICES: A COMPARISON WITH OTHER THERAPIES

John J. Vargo II, M.D.
Michael V. Sivak, Jr., M.D.

EVALUATING METHODS OF TREATMENT

Most therapy for variceal hemorrhage is initiated after the fact because the bleeding is essentially unpredictable. This makes it difficult to evaluate different methods of treatment in relation to the natural history of esophageal varices. Moreover, the time of intervention can affect the outcome.[1] Delayed therapy can seemingly improve survival, irrespective of other variables. This is because many high-risk patients are ''excluded'' in the period following hemorrhage due to a lethal bleed.[1]

POSTMORTEM STUDIES

The effects of sclerosants on esophageal tissue have been the subject of several postmortem studies.[2-7] By arranging autopsy material according to interval after the initiation of sclerotherapy, one can define the sequence of microscopic and gross changes in the variceal channels and esophageal wall.

The initial histological changes appear to include thrombus formation, endothelial damage of the variceal wall, and an intense inflammatory cell response that is initially composed of polymorphonuclear leukocytes.[2,5,8] After 24 hours, a lymphocytic infiltration develops which includes activated macrophages and fibroblasts.[2] The onset of fibrosis may begin as early as two weeks[2] or as late as several months.[5] Matsumoto[7] analyzed autopsy specimens from 26 patients obtained at various intervals after the initiation of sclerotherapy with intravariceal ethanolamine. Thrombotic obliteration of variceal channels was observed within 20 days. Organization and shrinkage of thrombi were seen at one month. Development of edema and necrosis paralleled the appearance of thrombi and tended to decrease over time. At 10 days, the first foci of granulation tissue were recognized, with subsequent transformation of fibroblasts into fibrocytes. By 10 weeks after initiation of sclerotherapy, a fibrotic, virtually acellular stroma was present.

CONTROL OF ACUTE VARICEAL HEMORRHGE

Sclerotherapy by means of a wide variety of sclerosing agents is reported to control at least 75% of acute bleeding episodes.[9-17] In most series, intravenous vasopressin and/or tamponade were used to stabilize the patients prior to sclerotherapy.[9,11,13,14,18] Sclerotherapy was also performed serially following the initial control of bleeding.

EFFECT ON BLEEDING

Sclerotherapy reduces the severity of variceal bleeding, decreases transfusion requirements,[19,20] and lowers the number and frequency of rebleeding episodes.[19,21] Clark et al.[14] compared the efficacy of medical management in 28 patients versus that of sclerotherapy in 36 patients. Recurrent bleeding was seen in one-third of the sclerotherapy patients versus two-thirds of the control patients. Differences in the rate of recurrent bleeding remained statistically significant throughout the course of the study.

A randomized controlled trial of sclerotherapy for acute variceal bleeding was reported by Larson et al.[20]; 44 patients underwent sclerotherapy and 38 patients received conventional medical therapy. By two weeks, the rate of recurrent bleeding in the control group was 53% compared to only 23% for the sclerotherapy group, a statistically significant difference. The mean transfusion requirement for acutely bleeding patients who received conventional therapy was significantly higher than that for the sclerotherapy group (8.5 versus 2.5 units).

This study by Larson et al.[20] contained 58 patients who were not actively bleeding at randomization; 31 underwent sclerotherapy and 27 were managed by conventional means. There was no significant difference in the number of transfusions in each group. However, 52% of the patients in the control group had recurrent bleeding versus 19% of those receiving sclerotherapy; this difference was statistically significant. Four deaths occurred in the medically managed patients; three were related to recurrent bleeding. There were no deaths in the sclerotherapy group.

CONTROL OF RECURRENT VARICEAL HEMORRHAGE

Although sclerotherapy appears to be effective for the control of acute variceal bleeding, the efficacy of long-term sclerotherapy for the prevention of recurrent bleeding or for the reduction of the severity of such episodes is more difficult to establish. A reduction in recurrent bleeding and transfusion requirements has been emphasized by some[19-24] but not all authors.[25] Terblanche et al.[10] found that acute injection plus long-term sclerotherapy was superior to acute sclerotherapy alone with regard to the number and severity of rebleeding episodes.

Soderlund and Ihre[26] compared conservative treatment with tamponade and/or vasopressin infusion with conservative therapy plus sclerotherapy in 107 randomized patients. No significant difference with respect to control of the index bleeding episode or hospital mortality was found. During follow-up (median, 28 months), patients receiving conservative therapy alone had an almost fourfold higher rate of recurrent bleeding than those who also had sclerotherapy. Although the overall mortality was the same for both groups, there were significantly more deaths attributable to variceal hemorrhage in the control patients.

Terblanche et al.[27] randomized 75 patients to receive long-term sclerotherapy or medical management. Recurrent bleeding in either group was managed by sclerotherapy. Varices were eradicated in 95% of the patients in the sclerotherapy group, but the rate of recurrent bleeding was 66% during follow-up (mean, 21.5 months). The cumulative percentage chance of remaining free of variceal bleeding was slightly higher in the sclerotherapy group after six months, but this was not statistically significant. The number of episodes of recurrent bleeding in the control group was significantly higher than for the group receiving sclerotherapy. This may be due in part to the fact that the control group had a significantly worse Child-Pugh score. There was no difference in survival between the two groups.

A multicenter study from Copenhagen involved 187 patients who were randomized to receive medical therapy including tamponade or medical therapy plus paravariceal sclerotherapy with polidocanol.[28] Sclerotherapy had no effect in terms of recurrent bleeding during the 40-day period following the index hemorrhage. After 40 days, the patients receiving sclerotherapy bled significantly less and had fewer recurrent bleeding episodes.

Despite evidence supporting long-term sclerotherapy as a prophylaxis against variceal bleeding, recurrent hemorrhage remains a major problem. The exact frequency of recurrent bleeding during long-term therapy is difficult to establish, but controlled trials comparing medical treatment and long-term sclerotherapy suggest that the rate of recurrent bleeding ranges from 28 to 58%.[26,27] One may assume that the immediate control of variceal bleeding by sclerotherapy results from thrombus formation within the variceal channels.[2,5,29,30] However, long-term prevention of variceal bleeding most likely hinges upon eventual obliteration of variceal channels.[7] Therefore, a "window" period may exist during the series of sclerotherapy sessions when variceal channels have not been completely replaced by fibrotic stroma. Until this process is complete, there is a risk of variceal bleeding. Other factors such as recanalization of fibrosed varices, nonuniformity of the fibrotic process with the esophageal wall, and variceal recurrence may also add to the risk of bleeding even in patients with endoscopic evidence of variceal eradication.

Based on available data, repeated sclerotherapy procedures have a favorable influence on recurrent bleeding once initial hemostasis has been achieved. The objective of serial procedures is the eradication of all variceal channels in the esophagus.

VARICEAL ERADICATION

Variceal eradication does not occur in a predictable fashion. Small varices may require only a few injections, while numerous injections in a long series of procedures may be needed to eliminate larger variceal channels.[30] Moreover, the endoscopic definition of variceal eradication may vary from complete obliteration to the presence of small residual varices.[31] In controlled series addressing the efficacy of chronic sclerotherapy, obliteration rates varied from 62% in a group of patients undergoing treatment for three months[19] to 95% in patients treated for up to five years.[27]

De Franchis et al.[31] performed sclerotherapy procedures in patients until there was either complete variceal obliteration, partial obliteration with residual small white varices, or partial obliteration with small blue varices. After at least six months of endoscopic surveillance, there was no statistical difference among the groups with any of these three endpoints with regard to variceal recurrence, further episodes of bleeding, or hemorrhage-related deaths.

The endoscopic assessment of variceal patency or thrombosis is inexact. Hosking et al.[32] studied variceal patency via intravariceal pressure recordings with a manometric device connected to the injection needle. Thirty-five control patients had maintenance sclerotherapy based on endoscopic appearance alone, and 33 patients received sclerotherapy only if the varices were patent by manometry. Sclerotherapy was performed every three weeks until variceal obliteration occurred. The sensitivities for recognition of thrombosis and variceal patency by visual assessment alone were 86% and 45%, respectively. The predictive value for visual diagnosis of thrombosis was 80% and 56% for variceal patency when compared to the manometric method of assessing these parameters. During follow-up (mean, 13 months), 20% of the patients treated on the basis of visual assessment alone had recurrent bleeding compared to 3% of the group in which treatment was guided by manometry, a significant difference. Eradication of esophageal varices (absent varices in the distal 2 cm of the esophagus) was achieved in a significantly higher number of patients in the manometry group. Episodes of esophageal sloughing were more common in the group treated according to visual assessment. The results of this study suggest that the failure to inject all patent vessels may be an important factor in the recurrence of variceal bleeding. The injection of channels that appear patent but are actually thrombosed (as determined by manometric assessment) may also be a significant factor in the development of severe esophageal ulceration or slough.

Takase et al.[33] utilized percutaneous transhepatic portography to study the anatomy of esophageal varices and their feeder vessels in 26 patients in whom obliteration of esophageal varices was achieved with sclerotherapy. Embolization of the feeder vessels was complete in 16 patients and incomplete in 10. Over a two-year period, varices recurred in 70% of the patients with incomplete embolization compared to only one patient with complete embolization. Takase et al. concluded that sclerosis of both the esophageal varices and their feeding vessels is essential for prevention of recurrent bleeding.

There are relatively few data regarding the recurrence of varices after eradication. In controlled studies of the efficacy of long-term sclerotherapy, recurrence rates vary from 15 to 62% over median follow-up intervals of 13 to 21.5 months, respectively.[26,27]

De Franchis et al.[31] reported a 41.6% recurrence rate in patients followed for a minimum of six months after variceal eradication. Sarin et al.[34] performed endoscopic surveillance in 101 patients at monthly intervals after variceal eradication. There were 54 patients with cirrhosis, 31 with noncirrhotic portal fibrosis, and 16 with extrahepatic portal venous obstruction. The recurrence rate at six months for patients with cirrhosis and those with noncirrhotic portal fibrosis was the same: 22%. These patients (2.9%) had recurrent variceal bleeding. Variceal recurrence was not observed in any patient with extrahepatic portal venous obstruction.

Westaby and Williams[35] followed 147 patients prospectively after variceal eradication for periods that ranged from six months to six years. Varices recurred in 99 (67%) patients, and in 28 (19%) there was also recurrent variceal bleeding. The majority of the recurrences, as well as recurrent episodes of bleeding, were observed during the first six months after eradication. The mortality associated with recurrent bleeding was only 3%. Recurrent varices were easily obliterated in most cases by further sclerotherapy (median, two sessions). Van Hootegem et al.[36] noted a 35% recurrence rate in a group of 68 patients followed for up to four years after variceal eradication. As in other studies, the recurrence of varices and further bleeding were most frequent during the first year following eradication.

SURVIVAL

Based upon the available data, it is difficult to ascertain whether sclerotherapy has a favorable effect on the survival of patients with variceal bleeding. The randomized controlled trials of long-term sclerotherapy differ with respect to important factors such as sample size, entry criteria, the point of randomization in relation to the index variceal hemorrhage, treatment intervals, and surveillance. With such variability in study design, the survival results of such trials, not surprisingly, are mixed.

A randomized Copenhagen trial of sclerotherapy versus medical therapy illustrates the problematic nature of assessing survival in patients undergoing sclerotherapy.[28] Overall, survival of patients receiving sclerotherapy was no better than that of the medically treated group. However, when other factors such as the presence of ascites and/or encephalopathy were taken into account, the overall mortality of the sclerotherapy group was significantly less than that of the control group. Survival curves revealed that mortality was somewhat lower in the sclerotherapy group during the first 10 days following randomization. Between 10 and 40 days, mortality was higher in the sclerotherapy group. Both of these differences failed to achieve statistical significance. On the whole, the Kaplan-Meier curves did not disclose an overall difference in mortality but late survival was significantly better in the sclerotherapy group.

The study of Macdougall et al.,[21] which is an extension of the report of Clark et al.,[14] found that the rate of recurrent bleeding for patients undergoing sclerotherapy was 43% versus 75% for a control group. One-year survival in the sclerotherapy group (75%) was significantly better than that of patients managed medically (58%). Variceal obliteration was thought to lead to improved survival. In a third report from this group,[37] 56 patients were randomized to undergo sclerotherapy and 60 patients to receive medical management. After a median follow-up of 37 months, a significant reduction in mortality was seen in the sclerotherapy group compared to controls (18% versus 32%). Death due to bleeding was significantly higher in the control (25%) versus the sclerotherapy patients (5%). Other reports also indicate a favorable effect of sclerotherapy on survival.[38-40]

In one prospective randomized trial, 63 patients were treated in sclerotherapy and 57 patients by conservative means.[19] Mean follow-up was 12.5 and 14.9 months for the sclerotherapy and control groups, respectively. A significant improvement in regard to transfusion requirements, recurrence of bleeding, and the length of the bleeding-free interval were noted in the sclerotherapy patients. However, no significant difference in survival was found between the groups.

Terblanche et al.[27] reported a trial of long-term sclerotherapy in 37 patients versus medical management plus emergency sclerotherapy as needed for recurrent bleeding in 38 patients. Although the number of episodes of recurrent bleeding was significantly reduced in the patients receiving chronic sclerotherapy, there was no improvement in survival. There was a relatively high and unexplained rate of recurrence of varices after eradication.

In an uncontrolled study, Sauerbruch et al.[41] prospectively followed 96 patients undergoing long-term sclerotherapy for a mean period of 25 months. A highly significant difference in survival in relation to the Child's classification was found. One-year survival for patients initially classified as Child's class A was 100% versus only 38% of those in Child's class C.

In an attempt to evaluate the effect of repeated sclerotherapy on long-term survival, Infant-Rivard et al.[42] performed a meta-analysis involving seven randomized clinical trials.[19,26-28,37,43,44] This analysis indicated that repeated sclerotherapy reduced the number of deaths by 25%.

PROPHYLACTIC SCLEROTHERAPY

Since the first episode of hemorrhage from esophageal varices is associated with significant morbidity and mortality, the concept of prophylactic treatment of esophageal varices has theoretical merit. However, this should be considered in light of the fact that several trials of portasystemic shunt surgery in patients with varices but no prior bleeding have failed to show improvement in survival despite virtual elimination of variceal hemorrhage.[45,46]

Prophylactic sclerotherapy has been found superior to conservative management in certain studies[47-49] and of some benefit in selected patients in other studies.[50,51] However, prophylactic sclerotherapy may also represent a source of increased morbidity and mortality.[52]

Witzel et al.[47] reported a randomized trial of prophylactic sclerotherapy in which patients were stratified according to Child classification and variceal size. Intravariceal sclerotherapy was performed on a monthly basis with polidocanol over a mean follow-up period of 25 months. Variceal bleeding occurred in 5 of 56 sclerotherapy patients (9%) versus 30 of 53 control patients (57%). There was a correlation between the frequency of variceal bleeding and variceal size in the control group. A significant difference was noted in overall mortality rates between the sclerotherapy group (21%) and patients who were treated conservatively (55%). This difference was generally attributed to a significantly higher mortality from variceal bleeding in the control group (36%) compared to those who received sclerotherapy (4%).

Paquet et al.[48,49] performed two randomized controlled trials of prophylactic sclerotherapy. In the first, entry criteria included large varices with erosions or the presence of large varices with sufficiently abnormal clotting characteristics.[48] There was a significant difference between the incidence of variceal bleeding in the control group (66%) and the sclerotherapy group (6%). The mortality for the control group was 42% versus 6% for patients undergoing sclerotherapy. In the second trial of Paquet et al.,[49] entry criteria were changed to include patients with large varices that exhibited *surface telangiectasia* (a term that is probably equivalent to *red color signs*) or abnormal clotting characteristics.

In the group randomized to conservative management, there was a high rate of variceal bleeding (66%) and death (42%), while the sclerotherapy-treated patients had a significantly lower incidence of variceal bleeding (6%) and death (6%).

In another controlled trial, patients were randomized according to variceal size and the Pugh-modified Child classification to receive conservative management or combined peri- and intravariceal polidocanol.[51] Although the rate of bleeding was lower in the sclerotherapy group (13% versus 30%), mortality rates were similar for both groups. Child-Pugh class A patients undergoing sclerotherapy had a significantly lower mortality rate than their conservatively managed counterparts. The most frequent cause of death was liver failure in the treatment group and variceal bleeding in the controls.

Patients with a Child-Pugh score less than 12 and at least two esophageal varices 5 mm or more in diameter were randomized to receive sclerotherapy with polidocanol or expectant management with periodic endoscopic surveillance in the trial of Sauerbruch et al.[50] No statistical differences were found in mortality or the incidence of variceal bleeding. Surivival in patients with alcoholic cirrhosis and Child-Pugh class B liver dysfunction was significantly better in those receiving sclerotherapy. However the risk of bleeding from esophageal varices was only marginally decreased in the sclerotherapy group. This suggests that the survival benefit in this study was due to a factor(s) other than sclerotherapy.

Santangelo et al.[52] randomized 95 patients with large varices to undergo treatment with intravariceal 1% tetradecyl sulfate or to serve as controls. After a mean follow-up period of 13 months, bleeding had occurred in 17 of 49 sclerotherapy patients (35%) compared to 7 of 46 control patients (15%). Although there was no difference in the overall mortality rates (24% in both groups), there were significantly more episodes of variceal bleeding in the sclerotherapy group. In fact, 75% of the deaths in the treatment group were attributed to bleeding compared to 18% for the control patients.

The collective data on the efficacy of prophylactic sclerotherapy should be regarded as inconclusive. More recent studies have shown no clinical benefit and also an increased risk of hemorrhage and death with treatment. The incidence of first variceal bleeding episodes was extremely high in earlier studies compared to later series or to the control arms of studies of prophylactic portasystemic shunt surgery in a similar population.[45,46] In the three negative studies,[50-52] patients were not stratified according to variceal appearance, specifically the presence of red color signs, a finding that is known to be an independent risk factor for variceal bleeding.[53,54] Sclerotherapy technique is another variable that is difficult to account for in these studies. The development of esophageal ulcers in response to the injection procedure may contribute to the incidence of variceal bleeding. Abstinence from alcohol is another variable that may influence the outcome but is difficult to assess in these trials. Based on current information and reports, sclerotherapy cannot be recommended as routine prophylactic treatment for esophageal varices that have not bled. Further controlled trials are needed that incorporate patient stratification according to current endoscopic and clinical methods of risk assessment.[53-55]

SCLEROTHERAPY VERSUS DRUG THERAPY

Modern pharmacotherapy for hemorrhage as a result of portal hypertension began with the observation of Lebrec et al.[56,57] that the administration of propranolol significantly reduced the rate of recurrent variceal bleeding in low-risk patients with cirrhosis.

However, subsequent studies have questioned the efficacy of beta blockade in such patients. Villeneuve et al.[58] found that this form of treatment had no significant effect on recurrent bleeding or survival. Similar results were reported by Burroughs et al.[59] Garden et al.[60] found that modified Child class C patients had a significantly lower incidence of recurrent variceal hemorrhage after 60 days of therapy with propranolol but no improvement in survival.

One controlled trial of sclerotherapy versus oral metoprolol showed that the risk of recurrent bleeding per patient-month of follow-up was three times higher in those receiving the drug than in the cohort undergoing sclerotherapy.[61] O'Connor et al.[62] randomized cirrhotic patients with Child's class C liver dysfunction and recent hemorrhage to receive propranolol alone or beta blockade with sclerotherapy. After three to six years of observation, the rate of recurrent bleeding was 84% in the propranolol group and 65% in the propranolol plus sclerotherapy group. Mortality was 81% in the former versus 55% in the latter group. O'Connor et al.[63] then compared oral propranolol, sclerotherapy plus propranolol, and transhepatic sclerotherapy plus propranolol. Patients treated with propranolol alone had a significantly higher mortality rate and tended to have more episodes of serious bleeding. Those receiving endoscopic sclerotherapy and beta blockade tended to have a lower mortality rate and a lower incidence of variceal bleeding.

Fleig et al.[64] randomized 70 patients with at least one episode of variceal bleeding to treatment with propranolol or sclerotherapy with 1% polidocanol to the point of variceal eradication. Recurrent bleeding from esophageal varices occurred in 28% of the sclerotherapy group (mean follow-up period, 14 months) and 29% of the propranolol group (mean follow-up period, 9.2 months). The mortality rate was 8% and 14% in the sclerotherapy with propranolol and propranolol alone groups, respectively. These differences were not statistically significant.

Another trial of 108 patients with Childs-Pugh class A or B liver dysfunction randomized patients after the spontaneous cessation of an index hemorrhage to receive long-term sclerotherapy or oral propranolol.[65] Patients receiving propranolol underwent one session of sclerotherapy if active variceal bleeding ensued. If the recurrent episode of hemorrhage was major (i.e., required transfusion of more than 10 units of blood) or if more than three episodes of recurrent bleeding took place while receiving propranolol, a series of sclerotherapy procedures was instituted. Data were analyzed on an intention-to-treat basis. There was no significant difference between the sclerotherapy and propranolol-treated groups with respect to recurrent bleeding (45% versus 54%) or mortality (42% versus 38%) during follow-up periods that ranged from 12 to 64 months. For propranolol-treated patients, 31% required at least one session of sclerotherapy, and in 26%, a series of procedures was performed.

SCLEROTHERAPY VERSUS SURGERY

A randomized controlled trial of sclerotherapy compared to portacaval shunt surgery was reported by Cello et al.[12,66] Sixty-four Child's class C patients with acute variceal hemorrhage requiring 6 or more units of blood were randomized. Treatment was initiated one to six hours after randomization. A portacaval shunt was performed in 32 patients, while the other 32 patients underwent intravariceal sclerotherapy with 5% sodium morrhuate. During the initial hospitalization, the transfusion requirement was significantly lower and the length of hospitalization significantly shorter for the sclerotherapy patients, but the rate of recurrent bleeding was higher. The 30-day survival was similar for both groups. After the index hospitalization, the advantages of sclerotherapy noted in the early phase of the trial were less evident. Patients undergoing sclerotherapy had significantly higher rates of rehospitalization, total days of hospitalization, and units of blood transfused. Long-term survival (mean follow-up period, 530 days) was the same in both groups. Although the total cost of care was significantly lower for the sclerotherapy patients during the initial hospitalization, rehospitalization for recurrent variceal bleeding and the cost of elective sclerotherapy during long-term follow-up equalized the overall costs of the two treatment programs. Of the 14 sclerotherapy patients discharged from the index hospitalization, 7 were eventually considered treatment failures due to severe and/or repeated bleeding. All seven underwent surgery and one died within 30 days. The authors concluded that sclerotherapy was as effective as the portacaval shunt in high-risk patients with massive bleeding and the patients who fail sclerotherapy should be considered for elective shunt surgery.

Planas et al.[67] carried out a randomized trial involving 82 patients with Child-Campbell class A and B dysfunction; all received either sclerotherapy with 1% polidocanol or an end-to-side portacaval shunt. Hemodynamic stability for three days after the index hemorrhage was required for randomization, and 31 patients were excluded because of uncontrollable bleeding or recurrent hemorrhage. The sclerotherapy group had a significantly higher incidence of recurrent bleeding (40% versus 2.9%) but the incidence of hepatic encephalopathy was significantly higher in the shunted group (40% versus 12%). Disabling encephalopathy, however, was present in only 8.8% of the surgically treated patients. Long-term mortality, hospitalization period, complication rates, and medical costs were similar.

Teres et al.[68] randomized 112 patients to receive sclerotherapy or distal splenorenal shunt. They were either Child's class A or B patients, were stable at randomization, and were randomized 10 to 15 days after the index variceal hemorrhage. Of the 57 patients randomized to surgery, 14 were excluded because of venous thrombosis, inadequate splenic vein size, or medical contraindications to surgery. Four of 55 patients initially randomized to sclerotherapy were excluded because of bleeding gastric varices or massive esophageal hemorrhage. Survival at two years was similar for the surgical (71%) and sclerotherapy (68%) groups. A significantly higher rate of recurrent bleeding was noted in patients treated with sclerotherapy (37.5% versus 14.3%). However, hepatic encephalopathy was significantly more frequent in the surgical group (24% versus 8%). As in other studies, sclerotherapy-treated patients spent significantly fewer days in the hospital for the index hemorrhage, but the higher rates of recurrent bleeding and complications for this group eventually resulted in an equal number of hospital days for both groups. Based on the number of patients excluded from both treatment arms, the authors concluded that sclerotherapy had wider applicability.

Henderson et al.[69] recently reported the final results of a randomized controlled trial comparing sclerotherapy and the distal splenorenal shunt. Preliminary results of this trial were reported by Warren et al.[70] In contrast to the study of Teres et al.,[68] Child's class C patients were included and 90% of the patients were randomized within two weeks of the index hemorrhage. After a median follow-up period of 61 months, the estimated four-year survival was significantly better for the sclerotherapy group. This survival advantage remained significant for low-risk as well as high-risk patients. However, seven patients, classified as treatment failures in the sclerotherapy group, underwent surgery. No increase in operative mortality was noted for these patients. Survival in patients with alcoholic cirrhosis receiving sclerotherapy was significantly better than in those who underwent surgery. No survival advantage was found for either modality if the etiology of the liver disease was nonalcoholic. As in previous studies, the rate of recurrent bleeding remained significantly higher in the sclerotherapy group (39% versus 3%). The authors noted that successful surgical therapy in patients deemed treatment failures in the sclerotherapy group was an important factor in the survival advantage.

Huizinga et al.[71] reported a prospective randomized trial of sclerotherapy versus esophageal transection in which 37 patients received sclerotherapy and 39 patients underwent surgery. Recurrent bleeding early in the course of treatment was noted in 48.6% of those receiving sclerotherapy as opposed to 2.5% of the operated patients, a highly significant difference. Recurrent variceal hemorrhage led to six deaths in the sclerotherapy group and none in the surgical group. During the later phases of the trial, 13 of the sclerotherapy patients experienced 22 episodes of bleeding versus no bleeding in the surgically treated patients. The 30-day mortality rate was 33.3% in the group that underwent transection compared to 24.3% for the patients who received sclerotherapy; this difference was not statistically significant. There were no operative deaths among 15 Child's class B patients who underwent transection, but 13 of 24 patients with Child's class C liver disease died.

A total of 101 patients were randomized to receive sclerotherapy or staple transection of the esophagus in a study by Burroughs et al.[72] Patients were enrolled if treatment with drugs, transfusion, and colloid infusion failed to control the index hemorrhage within five days. There was no significant difference in survival at six weeks or at 12 months of follow-up. Proportional hazards analysis revealed that the severity of ascites and encephalopathy, a prolonged prothrombin time, and balloon tamponade were independently associated with death at six weeks. As in other studies, surgical intervention resulted in a significantly larger number of patients who remained free of bleeding for five days after initiation of therapy. In nine patients, three sessions of sclerotherapy failed to control bleeding. Five of these patients underwent esophageal transection, which controlled bleeding in all cases, but only one patient survived. The authors felt that esophageal transection was as safe as sclerotherapy and was superior to a single sclerotherapy session with respect to prevention of recurrent bleeding. Due to the poor outcome of patients after three sclerotherapy sessions, an attempt at surgical salvage was recommended after the second episode of recurrent bleeding.

Sclerotherapy and surgery are the primary methods for management of acute or recurrent variceal hemorrhage. However, the exact role of each in relation to the other remains a matter of conjecture. Comparing the various studies of sclerotherapy and surgery is difficult because the surgical procedures, sclerotherapy technique, entry criteria, and time of randomization in relation to the index variceal hemorrhage differ substantially from study to study. Nevertheless, some general conclusions are possible.

The survival of patients with Child's class C liver disease and variceal bleeding is poor regardless of the type of therapeutic intervention. Burroughs et al.[72] noted that three of the four independent predictors of death within six weeks following endoscopic or surgical intervention are components of the Child's classification. The only operative deaths in the series of Huizinga et al.[71] occurred in patients with Child's class C liver dysfunction. Therefore, endoscopic sclerotherapy is the treatment of choice for variceal hemorrhage in patients with severe liver disease. One has difficulty recommending surgery in such patients, even when sclerotherapy fails, given the risk of encephalopathy and death.

Sclerotherapy was associated with a significantly higher rate of recurrent variceal bleeding in all of the studies of sclerotherapy versus surgical therapy. In several of these trials, however, documentation of variceal eradication was not defined. Possibly a more aggressive plan of sclerotherapy or a more effective technique could have altered the outcome of these studies.

Surgery and sclerotherapy appear to be equivalent with regard to survival and the overall cost of treatment. The choice of therapy may be influenced by patient preference, hospital resources, technical expertise, and an assessment of the patient as a candidate for orthotopic liver transplantation. The last factor is important, because sclerotherapy does not entail the marked surgical alterations that may make transplantation more difficult. Henderson et al.[69] demonstrated that surgery may be used to "rescue" or "salvage" patients in whom sclerotherapy fails to control recurrent bleeding. The operative mortality for these patients was the same as that for those who underwent primary surgical treatment. Thus, a strong argument can be made for endoscopic sclerotherapy as the initial method of treatment of variceal bleeding. If this fails to prevent life-threatening recurrent bleeding or if the frequency of recurrent bleeding becomes unacceptable, surgical intervention should be considered.

PREHEPATIC PORTAL HYPERTENSION

Extrahepatic portal vein thrombosis, fibrosis, and congenital malformation are the most common causes of portal hypertension and subsequent variceal bleeding in the pediatric population. However, many patients with extrahepatic portal vein obstruction may present with major variceal bleeding for the first time as adults.[73,74] Attempts at surgical treatment of this condition have met with only limited success. In children, small vessel size often precludes a shunting procedure. Fonkalsrud et al.[75] found that over half of their 164 operations were done to correct problems created by a previous operation.

Stellan and Lilly[76] performed endoscopic sclerotherapy in 11 children with portal vein thrombosis. The mean number of sessions needed for variceal eradication was 7.3, which, on average, required two years. No deaths or recurrent variceal bleeds occurred during follow-up (mean, 2.6 years). Thatcher et al.[73] performed sclerotherapy in eight patients with extrahepatic portal vein obstruction and variceal bleeding. All but one were adults when sclerotherapy was initiated; six had sustained episodes of recurrent bleeding after a variety of surgical procedures. Five patients had no further bleeding during a mean follow-up period of 26 months. Three patients had episodes of bleeding prior to variceal eradication. There was one death, which was attributable to cardiac disease.

Howard et al.[77] performed sclerotherapy in 152 children with portal hypertension (extrahepatic, 42; intrahepatic, 110). Variceal eradication was achieved in all patients with extrahepatic portal hypertension and in 84% of those with intrahepatic portal hypertension. Prior to variceal eradication, the rate of recurrent bleeding was 39%, with 20% of these episodes being attributed to sclerotherapy-induced ulceration. During a mean follow-up period of 2.9 years after variceal obliteration, bleeding recurred in 9% of the patients, with only one death.

Kahn et al.[74] performed sclerotherapy in 39 adults and in teenage patients with extrahepatic portal venous obstruction and variceal hemorrhage. Variceal eradication was accomplished in 33 patients, with a median of seven injection sessions over an average of 14.5 months. Fewer sessions were needed for eradication of varices in patients over the age of 20 (four sessions) than for younger patients (eight sessions). Four patients bled from recurrent varices over an average surveillance interval of 45.5 months. There were no deaths. Sixteen patients with extrahepatic obstruction underwent endoscopy monthly for an average of 17.9 months following variceal eradication in a study by Sarin et al.[34] There was no variceal recurrence in these patients, whereas a cohort with either cirrhosis or noncirrhotic portal fibrosis had a 22% recurrence rate over the same surveillance interval.

The results of virtually all studies of sclerotherapy for variceal bleeding due to extrahepatic portal vein obstruction have been good, probably superior to those in patients with portal hypertension due to hepatic parenchymal disease. The complication rate for sclerotherapy in this circumstance is low, and variceal recurrence is relatively infrequent. The normal liver function of these patients undoubtedly contributes to this favorable outcome.

REFERENCES

1. Smith JL, Graham DY: Variceal hemorrhage: A critical evaluation of survival analysis. *Gastroenterology* 82:968–973, 1982.
2. Helpap B, Bollweg L: Morphologic changes in the terminal oesophagus with varices, following sclerosis of the wall. *Endoscopy* 13:229–233, 1981.
3. Evans DMD, Jones DB, Cleary BK, et al: Oesophageal varices treated by sclerotherapy: A histopathological study. *Gut* 23:615–620, 1982.
4. Novis B, Bat L, Pomerantz I, et al: Endoscopic sclerotherapy of esophageal varices. *Isr J Med Sci* 19:40–44, 1983.
5. Hunt BL, Mitros FA, Lewis JW: Histologic changes in esophagus after injection sclerotherapy (abstract). *Gastrointest Endosc* 28:137, 1982.
6. Pushpanathan C, Idikio H: Pathological findings in the esophagus after endoscopic sclerotherapy for variceal bleeding. *Am J Gastroenterol* 81:9–13, 1986.
7. Matsumoto S: Clinicopathological study of sclerotherapy of esophageal varices. I. A review of 26 autopsy cases. *Gastroenterol Jpn* 21:99–105, 1986.
8. Sarin SK, Kumar A: Sclerosants for variceal sclerotherapy: A critical appraisal. *Am J Gastroenterol* 85:641–649, 1990.
9. Terblanche J, Northover JMA, Bornman P, et al: A prospective evaluation of injection sclerotherapy in treatment of acute bleeding from esophageal varices. *Surgery* 85:239–245, 1979.
10. Terblanche J, Northover JMA, Bornman P, et al: A prospective controlled trial of sclerotherapy in the long term management of patients after esophageal variceal bleeding. *Surg Gynecol Obstet* 148:323–333, 1979.
11. Sivak MV Jr, Stout DJ, Skipper G: Endoscopic injection sclerosis (EIS) of esophageal varices. *Gastrointest Endosc* 27:52–57, 1981.
12. Cello JP, Grendell JH, Crass RA, et al: Endoscopic sclerotherapy versus portacaval shunt in patient with severe cirrhosis and acute variceal hemorrhage. Long-term follow-up. *N Engl J Med* 316:11–15, 1987.
13. Palani CK, Abuabara S, Kraft AR, et al: Endoscopic sclerotherapy in acute variceal hemorrhage. *Am J Surg* 141:164–168, 1981.
14. Clark AW, Westaby D, Silk DBA, et al: Prospective controlled trial of injection sclerotherapy in patients with cirrhosis and recent variceal hemorrhage. *Lancet* 2:552–554, 1980.

15. von Ryll-Gryska P, Hedberg SE: Injection thrombosclerosis of esophageal varices. *Surg Gynecol Obstet* 161:438–444, 1985.
16. Spence RA, Anderson JR, Johnston GW: Twenty-five years of injection sclerotherapy for bleeding varices. *Br J Surg* 72:195–198, 1985.
17. Lewis J, Chung RS, Allison J: Sclerotherapy of esophageal varices. *Arch Surg* 115:476–480, 1980.
18. Stray N, Jacobsen CD, Rosseland A: Injection sclerotherapy of bleeding oesophageal and gastric varices using a flexible endoscope. *Acta Med Scand* 211:125–129, 1982.
19. Korula J, Balart LA, Radvan G, et al: A prospective, randomized controlled trial of chronic esophageal variceal sclerotherapy. *Hepatology* 5:584–589, 1985.
20. Larson AW, Cohen H, Zweiban B, et al: Acute esopahgeal variceal sclerotherapy. Results of a prospective randomized controlled trial. *JAMA* 255:497–500, 1986.
21. Macdougall BRD, Westaby D, Theodossi A, et al: Increased long-term survival in variceal haemorrhage using injection sclerotherapy. Results of a controlled trial. Lancet 1:124–127, 1982.
22. Hughes RW Jr, Larson DE, Viggiano TR, et al: Endoscopic variceal sclerosis: A one-year experience. *Gastrointest Endosc* 28:62–66, 1982.
23. Ayres SJ, Goff JS, Warren GH: Endoscopic sclerotherapy for bleeding esophageal varices: Effects and complications. *Ann Intern Med* 98:900–903, 1983.
24. Sivak MV Jr, Williams GW: Endoscopic injection sclerosis (EIS) of esophageal varices: Analysis of survival and transfusion requirement (abstract). *Gastrointest Endosc* 27:129, 1981.
25. Hennessy TPJ, Stephens RB, Keane FB: Acute and chronic management of esophageal varices by injection sclerotherapy. *Surg Gynecol Obstet* 154:375–377, 1982.
26. Soderlund C, Ihre T: Episodic sclerotherapy. V. Conservative management of bleeding oesophageal varices. A 5 year prospective controlled trial of emergency and long-term treatment. *Acta Chir Scand* 151:449–456, 1985.
27. Terblanche J, Bornman PC, Kahn D, et al: Failure of repeated injection sclerotherapy to improve long-term survival after oesophageal variceal bleeding. A five-year prospective controlled clinical trial. *Lancet* 2:1328–1332, 1983.
28. Copenhagen esophageal varices sclerotherapy project: Sclerotherapy after first variceal hemorrhage in cirrhosis. *N Engl J Med* 311:1594–1600, 1984.
29. Kang JH, Kambayashi J, Sakon M, et al: Mechanism of the haemostatic effect of ethanolamine oleate in the injection sclerotherapy for oesophageal varices. *Br J Surg* 74:50–53, 1987.
30. Rose JDR, Crane MD, Smith PM: Factors affecting successful endoscopic sclerotherapy for oesophageal varices. *Gut* 24:946–949, 1983.
31. de Franchis R, Vitagliano P, Agape D, et al: Eradication of esophageal varices by endoscopic sclerotherapy: How much is enough? *Gastrointest Endosc* 34:395–399, 1988.
32. Hosking SW, Robinson P, Johnson AG: Usefulness of manometric assessment of varices in maintenance sclerotherapy. A controlled trial. *Gastroenterology* 93:846–851, 1987.
33. Takase Y, Susumu S, Chikamori F, et al: Recurrence factors studied by transhepatic portography before and after sclerotherapy for esophageal varices. *Hepatology* 11:348–352, 1990.
34. Sarin SK, Sachdev G, Nada R: Follow-up of patients after variceal eradication. A comparison of patients with cirrhosis, noncirrhotic portal fibrosis, and extrahepatic obstruction. *Ann Surg* 204:78–82, 1986.
35. Westaby D, Williams R: Elective sclerotherapy—technique and results. *Endoscopy* 18 (Suppl 2):28–31, 1986.
36. Van Hootegem P, Besian K, Broekaert L, et al: Endoscopic sclerotherapy of esophageal varices. Long term follow-up, recurrence, and survival. *J Clin Gastroenterol* 10:368–372, 1988.

37. Westaby D, Macdougall BR, Williams R: Improved survival following injection sclerotherapy for esophageal varices: Final analysis of a controlled trial. *Hepatology* 5:827–830, 1985.
38. Goodale RL, Silvis SE, O'Leary JF, et al: Early survival after sclerotherapy for bleeding esophageal varices. *Surg Gynecol Obstet* 155:523–538, 1982.
39. Hedberg SE, Fowler DL, Ryan RLR: Injection sclerotherapy of esophageal varices using ethanolamine oleate. A pilot study. *Am J Surg* 143:426–431, 1982.
40. Trudeau W, Prindiville T, Gibbert V, et al: Endoscopic injection sclerosis in Child's C patients with bleeding gastroesophageal varices (abstract). *Gastrointest Endosc* 29:168, 1983.
41. Sauerbruch T, Weinzierl M, Kopcke W, et al: Long term sclerotherapy of bleeding esophageal varices in patients with liver cirrhosis. An evaluation of mortality and rebleeding risk factors. *Scand J Gastroenterol* 20:51–58, 1985.
42. Infante-Rivard C, Esnaola S, Villeneuve J-P: Role of endoscopic variceal sclerotherapy in the long-term management of variceal bleeding: A meta-analysis. *Gastroenterology* 96:1087–1092, 1989.
43. Barsoum MS, Bolous FI, El-Rooby AA, et al: Tamponade and injection sclerotherapy in the management of bleeding oesophageal varices. *Br J Surg* 69:76–78, 1982.
44. Paquet KJ, Feussner H: Endoscopic sclerosis and esophageal balloon tamponade in acute hemorrhage from esophagogastric varices: A prospective controlled randomized trial. *Hepatology* 5:580–583, 1985.
45. Resnick RH, Iber FL, Ishihara AM, et al: A controlled study of the therapeutic portacaval shunt. *Gastroenterology* 67:843–857, 1974.
46. Conn HO, Lindenmuth WW, May CJ, et al. Prophylactic portacaval anastomosis. A tale of two studies. *Medicine* 51:27–40, 1972.
47. Witzel L, Wolbergs E, Merki H: Prophylactic endoscopic sclerotherapy of oesophageal varices. A prospective controlled study. *Lancet* 1:773–775, 1985.
48. Paquet KJ: Prophylactic endoscopic sclerosing treatment of the esophageal wall in varices—a prospective controlled randomized trial. *Endoscopy* 14:4–5, 1982.
49. Paquet KJ, Koussouris P: Is there an indication for prophylactic endoscopic paravariceal injection sclerotherapy in patients with liver cirrhosis and portal hypertension? *Endoscopy* 18(Suppl 2):32–35, 1986.
50. Sauerbruch T, Wotzka R, Wolfgang K, et al: Prophylactic sclerotherapy before the first episode of variceal hemorrhage in patients with cirrhosis. *N Engl J Med* 319:8–15, 1988.
51. Koch H, Henning H, Grimm H, et al: Prophylactic sclerosing of esophageal varices—results of a prospective controlled study. *Endoscopy* 18:40–43, 1986.
52. Santangelo WC, Dueno MI, Estes BL, et al: Prophylactic sclerotherapy of large esophageal varices. *N Engl J Med* 318:814–818, 1988.
53. Beppu K, Inokuchi K, Koyanagi N, et al: Prediction of variceal hemorrhage by esophageal endoscopy. *Gastrointest Endosc* 27:213–218, 1981.
54. The North Italian Endoscopic Club for the Study and Treatment of Esophageal Varices: Prediction of the first variceal hemorrhage in patients with cirrhosis of the liver and esophageal varices. A prospective multicenter study. *N Engl J Med* 319:983–989, 1988.
55. Sarin SK, Sundarm KR, Ahuja RK: Predictors of variceal bleeding: An analysis of endoscopic, and haemodynamic variables with special reference to intravariceal pressure. *Gut* 30:1757–1764, 1989.
56. Lebrec D, Poynard T, Hillon P, et al: Propranolol for prevention of recurrent gastrointestinal bleeding in patients with cirrhosis, a controlled study. *N Engl J Med* 305:1371–1374, 1981.
57. Lebrec D, Poynard T, Bernuau J, et al: A randomized controlled study of propranolol for prevention of recurrent gastrointestinal bleeding in patients with cirrhosis: A final report. *Hepatology* 4:355–358, 1984.

58. Villeneuve JP, Promier-Layrargues G, Infante-Rivard C, et al: Propranolol for the prevention of recurrent variceal hemorrhage: A controlled trial. *Hepatology* 6:1239–1243, 1986.
59. Burroughs AK, Jenkins WJ, Sherlock S, et al: Controlled trial of propranolol for the prevention of recurrent variceal hemorrhage in patients with cirrhosis. *N Engl J Med* 309:1539–1542, 1983.
60. Garden OJ, Mills PR, Birnie GC, et al: Propranolol in the prevention of variceal hemorrhage in cirrhotic patients. A controlled trial. *Gastroenterology* 98:185–190, 1990.
61. Westaby D, Melia WM, Macdougall BR, et al: B1 selective adrenoreceptor blockade for the long term management of variceal bleeding. A prospective randomised trial to compare oral metoprolol with injection sclerotherapy in cirrhosis. *Gut* 26:421–425, 1985.
62. O'Connor K, Benage D, Lehman G, et al: A comparison between propranolol, propranolol plus endoscopic sclerotherapy, and propranolol plus transhepatic sclerotherapy in preventing major rebleeding and death from esophageal varices. *Gastrointest Endosc* 34:A180, 1988.
63. O'Connor KW, Lehman G, Yune H, et al: Comparison of three non-surgical treatments for esophageal varices. *Gastroenterology* 96:899–906, 1989.
64. Fleig WE, Stange EF, Hunecke R, et al: Prevention of recurrent bleeding in cirrhotics with recent variceal hemorrhage: Prospective, randomized comparison of propranolol and sclerotherapy. *Hepatology* 7:355–361, 1987.
65. Westaby D, Polson RJ, Gimson AES, et al: A controlled trial of oral propranolol compared with injection sclerotherapy in the long-term management of variceal bleeding. *Hepatology* 11:353–359, 1990.
66. Cello JP, Grendell JH, Crass RA, et al: Endoscopic sclerotherapy versus portacaval shunt in patients with severe cirrhosis and variceal hemorrhage. *N Engl J Med* 311:1589–1594, 1984.
67. Planas R, Boix J, Broggi M, et al: Portacaval shunt versus endoscopic sclerotherapy in the elective treatment of variceal hemorrhage. *Gastroenterology* 100:1078–1086, 1991.
68. Teres J, Bordas JM, Bravo D, et al: Sclerotherapy vs. distal splenorenal shunt in the elective treatment of variceal hemorrhage: A randomized controlled trial. *Hepatology* 7:430–436, 1987.
69. Henderson JM, Kutner MH, Millikan WJ, et al: Endoscopic variceal sclerosis compared with distal splenorenal shunt to prevent recurrent variceal bleeding. *Ann Intern Med* 112:267–269, 1990.
70. Warren WD, Henderson JM, Millikan WJ, et al: Distal splenorenal shunt versus endoscopic sclerotherapy for long-term management of variceal bleeding. Preliminary report of a prospective, randomized trial. *Ann Surg* 203:454–462, 1986.
71. Huizinga WK, Angorn IB, Baker LW: Esophageal transection versus injection sclerotherapy in the management of bleeding esophageal varices in patients at high risk. *Surg Gynecol Obstet* 160:539–546, 1985.
72. Burroughs AK, Hamilton G, Phillips A, et al: A comparison of sclerotherapy with staple transection of the esophagus for the emergency control of bleeding from esophageal varices. *N Engl J Med* 321:857–862, 1989.
73. Thatcher BS, Sivak MV, Petrini JL: Endoscopic sclerotherapy for bleeding esophageal varices secondary to extrahepatic portal vein obstruction. *Gastrointest Endosc* 33:214–219, 1987.
74. Kahn D, Terblanche J, Kitano S, et al: Injection sclerotherapy in adult patients with extrahepatic portal venous obstruction. *Br J Surg* 74:600–602, 1987.
75. Fonkalsrud EW, Myers NA, Robinson MJ: Management of extrahepatic portal hypertension in children. *Ann Surg* 180:487–493, 1974.
76. Stellen GP, Lilly JR: Esophageal endosclerosis in children. *Surgery* 98:970–975, 1985.
77. Howard ER, Stringer MD, Mowat AP: Assessment of injection sclerotherapy in the management of 152 children with oesophageal varices. *Br J Surg* 75:404–408, 1988.

32

RADIOLOGIC THERAPY FOR ESOPHAGEAL VARICES

Ernest J. Ring, M.D.

Since selective angiography was first developed in the late 1950s and early 1960s, radiological techniques have played an important role in the evaluation and management of patients with portal hypertension and variceal bleeding. Visualization of the portal vein and its tributaries by splenoportography, arterial portography, and transhepatic catheterization has provided the details of venous anatomy and patterns of portal flow that are necessary to plan shunt operations. More recently, noninvasive imaging methods including Doppler ultrasound, computed tomography (CT), and magnetic resonance imaging (MRI) have been used to evaluate the patency of the major portal venous structures and increasingly are being used as an alternative to angiography to demonstrate portal vein patency and follow shunts after surgery. Along with the diagnostic role of selective angiography, there have been several attempts to modify catheterization techniques and develop transcatheter procedures which treat variceal hemorrhage. This chapter reviews the status of these transcatheter interventional therapies and discusses their current role in the management of patients with portal hypertension and bleeding varices.

SELECTIVE MESENTERIC ARTERY INFUSIONS OF VASOPRESSIN

In 1967, Nusbaum and colleagues first showed that continuous infusion of vasopressin directly into the superior mesenteric artery (SMA) at a dose rate of 0.2 ug/min reduced portal pressure by approximately 50%, with few systemic side effects.[1] In their initial clinical experience, they found that SMA vasopressin at this dose rate resulted in cessation of variceal bleeding in 95% of cases.[2] Subsequent investigators confirmed the effectiveness of low-dose SMA vasopressin in reducing portal pressure but had less success in controlling bleeding in patients with severe liver disease. Most series showed that overall only about 50% of patients bleeding from esophageal varices responded to SMA vasopressin.[3] Throughout the late 1960s and early 1970s, selective SMA catheterization and low-dose vasopressin infusion became a popular treatment for acute variceal hemorrhage. When Nusbaum et al. reported in 1968 that intraoperative vasopressin could reduce blood loss during shunt surgery, mesenteric artery catheterization became widely employed as an adjunct to surgery.[4]

In 1975, Barr and his colleagues were investigating the effect of vasopressin on the hepatic artery and incidentally noted that systemically administered vasopressin caused a reduction in portal pressure that was comparable to the effect obtained with SMA infusion at similar doses.[5] Subsequently, Johnson et al. confirmed that continuous low-dose intravenous vasopressin was just as effective in controlling variceal bleeding as SMA infusions.[6] Since that time, low-dose systemic vasopressin has continued to be an important first-line therapy for variceal bleeding, and the use of selective catheterization of the mesenteric artery to deliver the drug has been abandoned.

PERCUTANEOUS CATHETERIZATION OF THE PORTAL VEIN AND SELECTIVE EMBOLIZATION OF GASTRIC AND ESOPHAGEAL VARICES

In 1974, Lunderquist and Vang developed a technique for percutaneous access to the portal vein which permitted selective catheterization of any of the major portal venous tributaries.[7] They employed this method to perform transcatheter embolization of the coronary vein and esophageal varices as a new way of treating variceal hemorrhage. Numerous subsequent reports have evaluated the efficacy of this therapy and found varying results.[8-10] In 1989 L'Hermine et al. reported the largest experience with this procedure. They used hepatic embolization with ethanol and stainless steel coils to obliterate varices in 400 consecutive patients and were able to control variceal bleeding in 83% of cases.[11]

As more experience was gained with transhepatic variceal obliteration, two important problems became evident. First, recurrent variceal bleeding is extremely common. Even after successful embolization of the coronary vein and all other angiographically visible gastric veins, new collaterals to the varices rapidly develop (Figure 32.1). In L'Hermine's series, bleeding recurred in 55% of surviving patients at six months and in 66% at one year.[11] Second, there is a high incidence of portal vein thrombosis after the procedure because patients with severe liver disease have very high resistance to portal flow, and in many cases the coronary and gastric veins provide the only significant outflow for the entire portal venous system. Portography in these patients generally shows greatly enlarged coronary and gastric veins which not only flow into the submucosal esophageal varices that cause bleeding but also supply much larger collateral veins in the mediastinum around the esophagus (Figure 32.1B,C). If these mediastinal collateral veins are occluded, flow in the portal vein stagnates and thrombus begins to form. By the early 1980s, most radiologists and surgeons believed that these problems severely limited the application of the procedure. Moreover, as endoscopic sclerotherapy became more widely used, it became clear that the endoscopic method of treatment was not only effective in controlling variceal bleeding but also caused fewer complications, so that most centers stopped routinely performing transhepatic variceal embolization.

There are a few clinical settings where transhepatic variceal embolization may still be indicated. High-risk patients who are bleeding from endoscopically inaccessible duodenal or intestinal varices can be successfully treated by the transhepatic approach. Transcatheter embolization can also be very effective after distal splenorenal shunt surgery when persistent venous connections between the portal vein and the distal splenic vein become large enough to cause bleeding or encephalopathy. Although the coronary vein and other proximal venous communications to the stomach are usually ligated during distal splenorenal shunt surgery, accessory venous connections are sometimes overlooked. Alternatively, veins that are too small to be identified intraoperatively can enlarge as they become collateral pathways decompressing the high-pressure portal side of the shunt. Transhepatic portal vein catheterization and portal venography can identify these venous connections, and selective embolization can be used as an alternative to reoperation to occlude this new collateral flow (Figure 32.2).

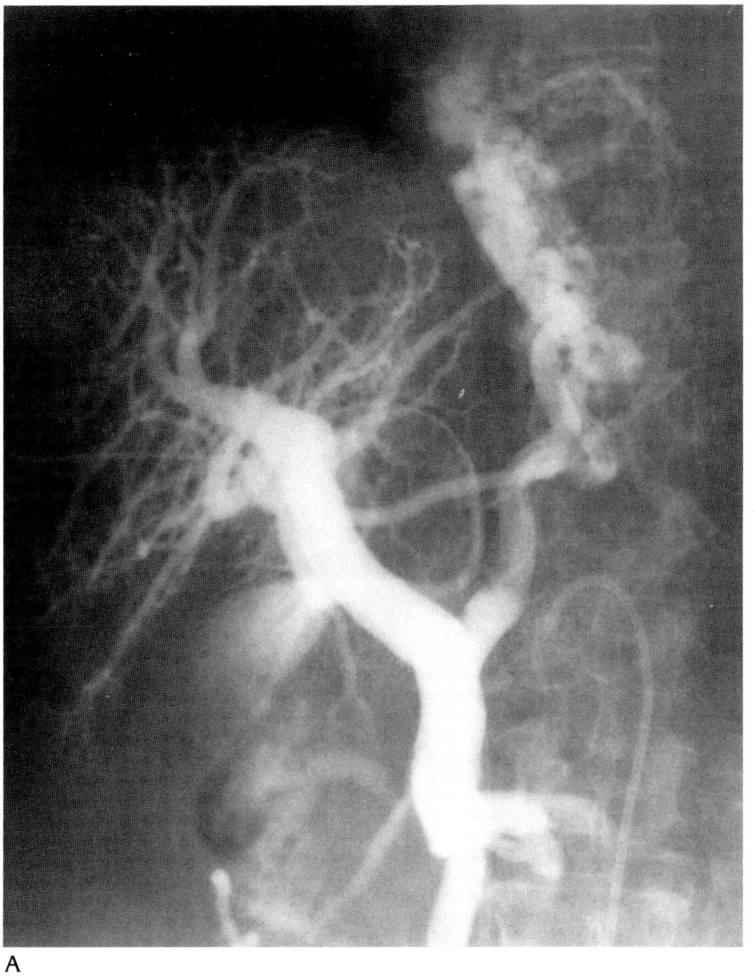

A

Figure 32.1. Transhepatic embolization for acute hemorrhage. (*A*) A transhepatic mesenteric venogram demonstrates hepatofugal flow into a large coronary vein.

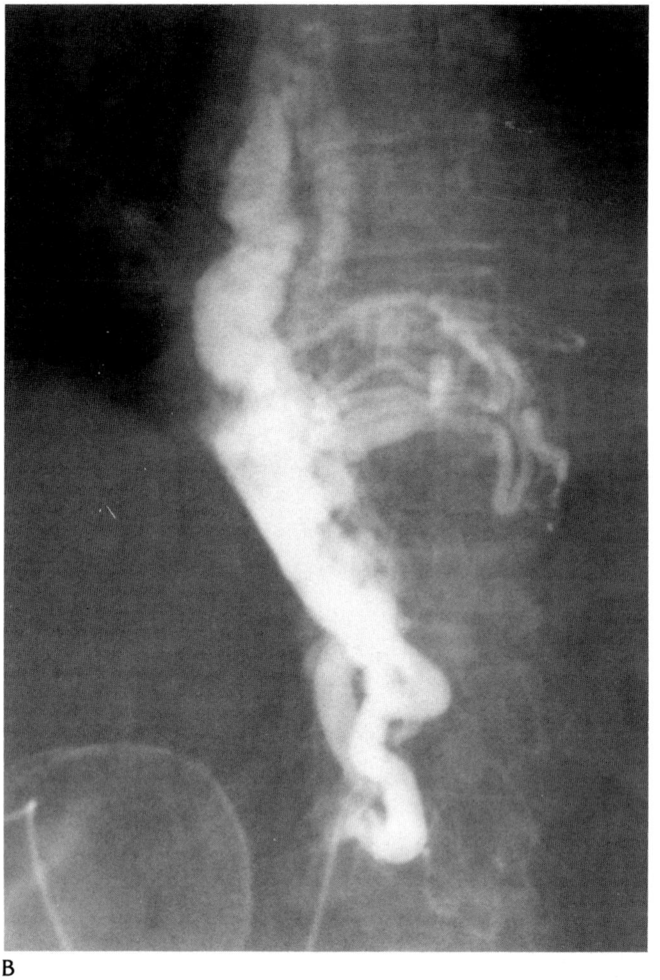

B

Figure 32.1. (*B*) The coronary vein was selectively catheterized and embolized with Gelfoam pledgets. Note that the veins filled during the selective coronary venogram appear to course in the mediastinum to the right of the location of the esophagus. (*C*) A vein that joined the distal splenic vein was catheterized, and an injection of contrast appears to fill the esophageal varices. After this vein was embolized, the patient stopped bleeding. (*D*) Twenty-four hours later there was recurrence of the variceal hemorrhage. A repeat transhepatic portogram showed that the two veins previously embolized remained occluded (*arrows*), but new collaterals to the esophageal varices had already formed.

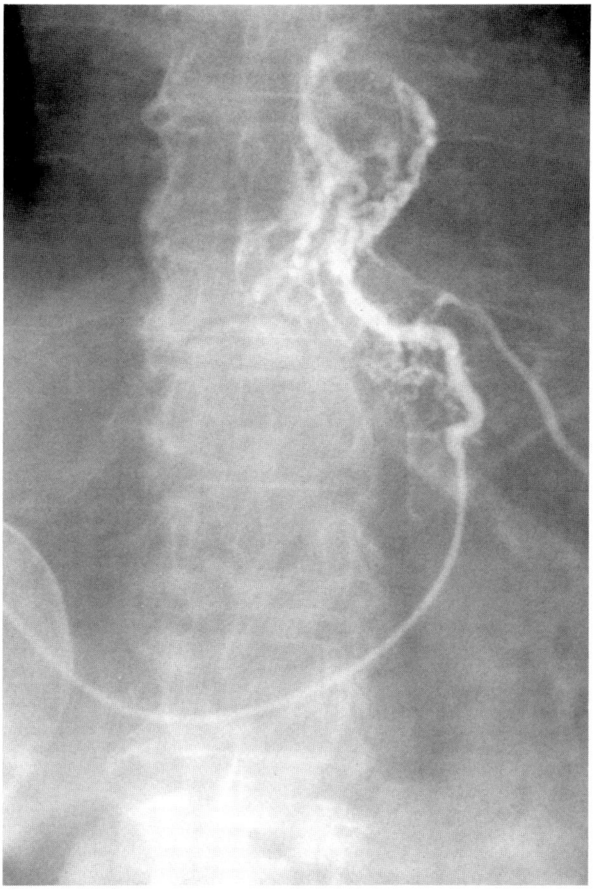

C

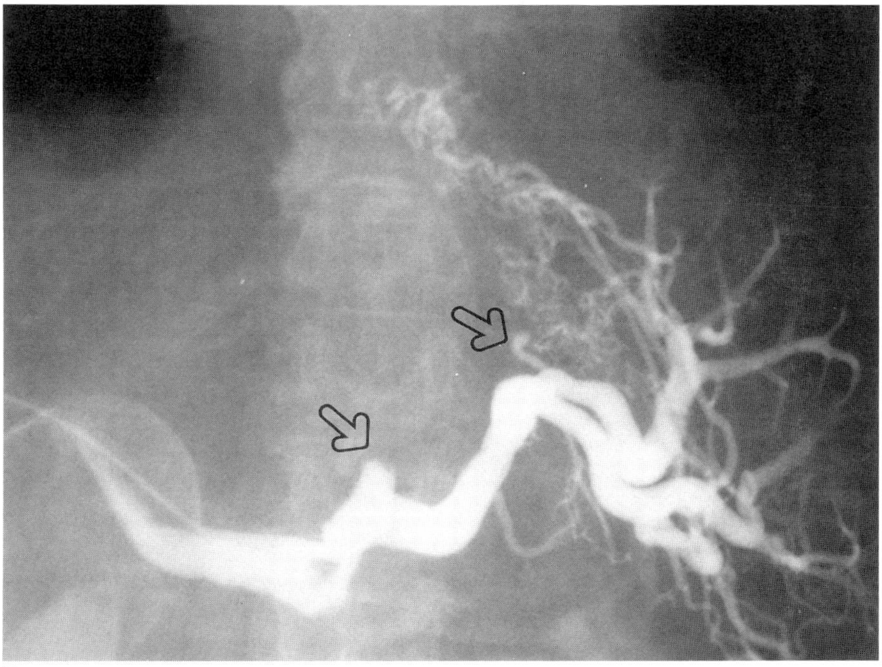

D

Figure 32.1. *(continued)*

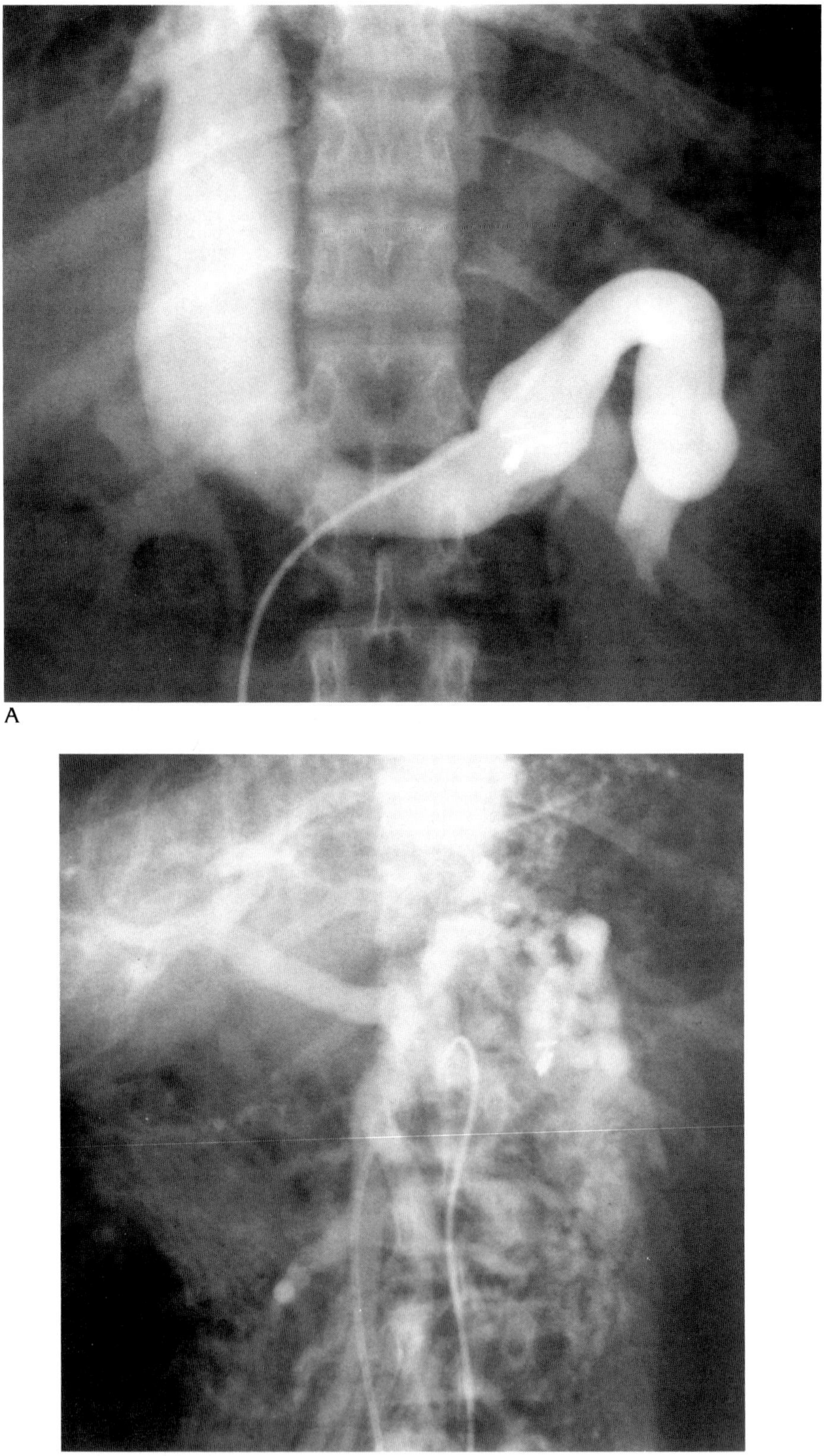

A

B

Figure 32.2.

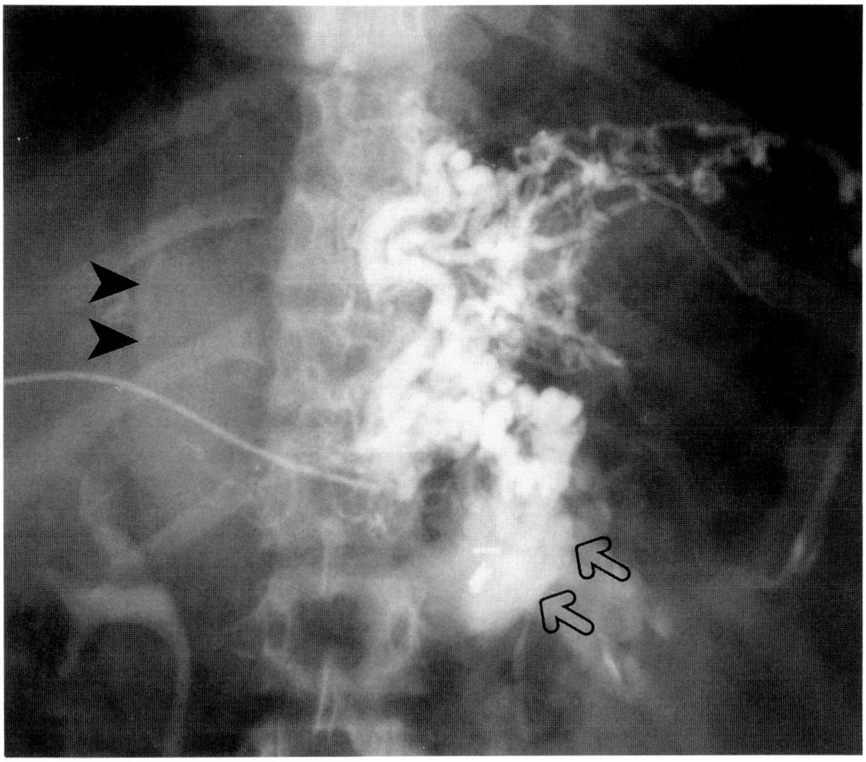

C

Figure 32.2. Recurrent variceal bleeding following placement of a distal splenorenal shunt. (*A*) A 14-year-old girl was bleeding from gastric varices three years after placement of a distal splenorenal shunt. The shunt was catheterized through the renal vein and was found to be widely patent. (*B*) The venous phase of a superior mesenteric arteriogram showed gastric varices between the shunt and the portal vein. (*C*) The portal vein was catheterized transhepatically. A selective injection into an accessory left gastric vein shows large gastric varices flowing toward the shunt (*arrows*) and filling of the inferior vena cava (*arrowheads*).

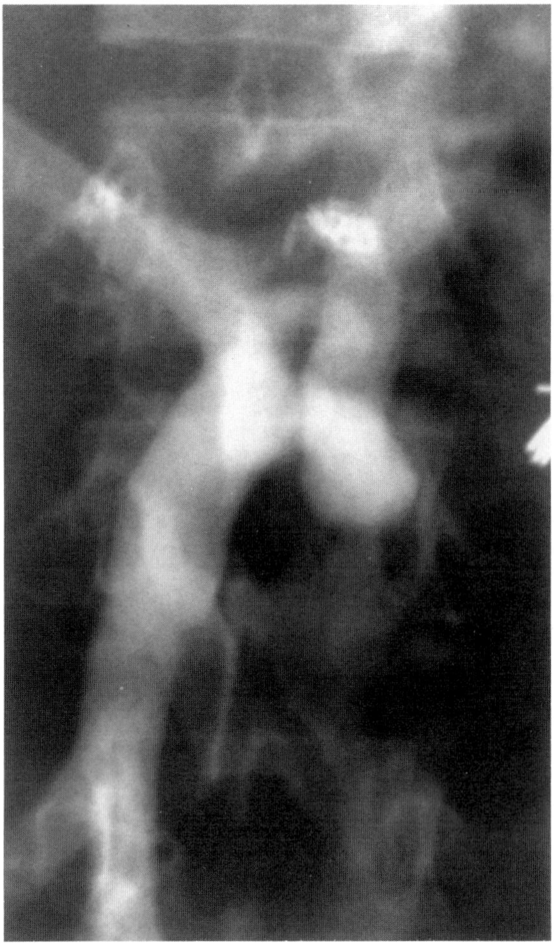

D

Figure 32.2. (*D*) A superior mesenteric venogram performed after the coronary vein had been occluded with stainless steel coils shows no further connection to the gastric varices.

TRANSSHUNT INTERVENTIONS

Patent portosystemic shunts can usually be readily catheterized from the inferior vena caval side of the shunt through a femoral vein approach. Once across the shunt, the catheter can be manipulated throughout the portal venous system to perform a variety of therapeutic interventions. For example, there have been numerous reports describing the use of this approach to perform balloon dilatation of stenotic mesocaval and portacaval shunts (Figure 32.3). Transshunt catheterization can also be used postoperatively to embolize persistent varices. Recently, there has been a trend in the surgical literature to recommend smaller-diameter portosystemic shunts to preserve hepatic perfusion and lower the incidence of postoperative encephalopathy. With the more modest reduction in portal pressure that is achieved using shunts as small as 8 mm, significant esophageal varices can persist. Although Johansen reported recurrent bleeding from persistent varices in only 1 of 50 patients who underwent small-caliber portacaval shunting,[12] Coldwell et al. recently catheterized 33 consecutive small-caliber portacaval shunts and embolized the residual varices that were present in 13 patients.[13]

Completely occluded portosystemic shunts are generally difficult to catheterize from the vena caval side. This is especially true for occluded portacaval shunts, since there is usually nothing angiographically visible to help identify the site of the anastomosis. On the other hand, one can advance a catheter with relative ease through an occluded mesocaval or splenorenal shunt. The success of shunt catheterization is much greater if the procedure is attempted soon after the occlusion, when the clot is still soft enough to readily permit passage of a guidewire; a clip or other metal marker left at surgery helps fluoroscopic identification of the anastomosis. In some patients, it may be technically easier to catheterize an occluded shunt from the portal vein side, since there is usually some deformity at the anastomosis to guide the catheterization. Transhepatic catheteriza-

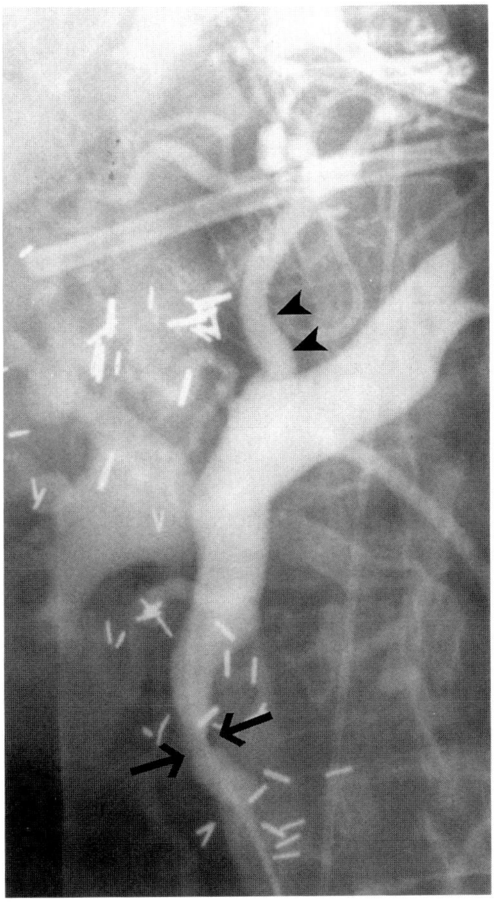

A

Figure 32.3. Embolization of residual varices and balloon angioplasty of a stenotic mesocaval shunt. (*A*) Because of recurrent variceal bleeding seven months after placement of a mesocaval shunt, the portal venous system was catheterized through the shunt. A splenic venogram demonstrates filling of the coronary vein (*arrowheads*) and persistent esophageal varices. Narrowing is present in the graft (*arrows*), and there is relatively little flow into the IVC. Corrected portal pressure was 21 cm H_2O.

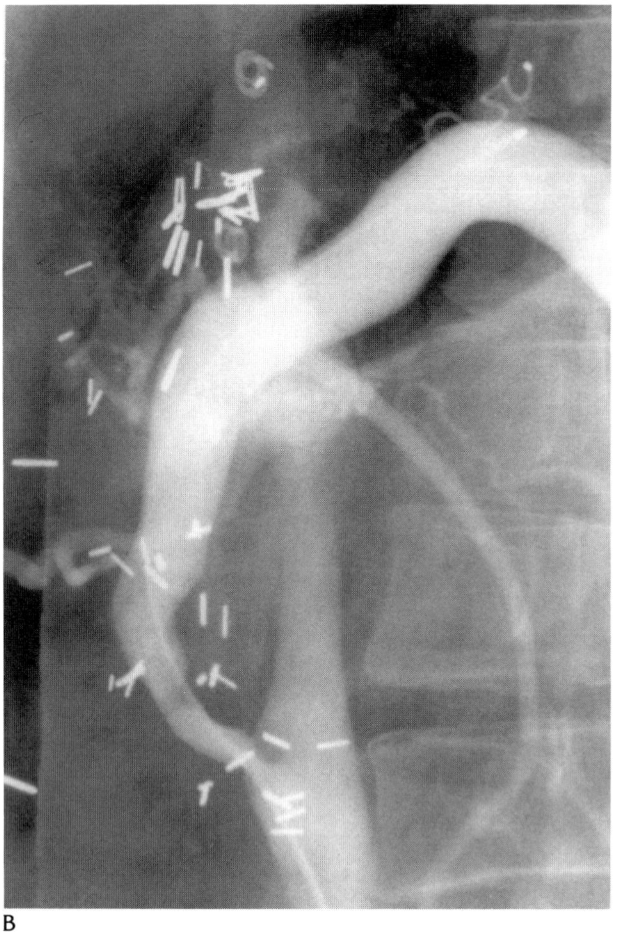

B

Figure 32.3. (*B*) The coronary vein was selectively catheterized and occluded with ethanol and coils (*arrows*). Repeat splenic venography shows no flow to the varices and improved opacification of the IVC. Corrected portal pressure was 23 cm H_2O.

tion is particularly useful for occluded proximal splenorenal shunts, since the angle between the veins at the anastomosis does not favor catheterization from the renal vein.

Once a catheter has been advanced across an occluded shunt, it can be used to reestablish shunt patency. Cope reported the use of fibrinolytic infusions to dissolve clotted mesocaval shunts.[14] When one wishes to avoid the risk of induced or increased bleeding from fibrinolytic therapy, balloon catheters can be used to fragment and then push the clot into the portal venous system. The clot can then flow into either an intrahepatic portal branch or, more likely, into a vein flowing away from the liver, such as the coronary vein. If the situation is urgent enough and the amount of thrombus is relatively small, the clot can be pulled into the inferior vena cava (IVC) with the balloon catheter. The resulting pulmonary embolus is not without risk, but we have used this approach as emergency therapy for six patients and have found that iatrogenic emboli are surprisingly well tolerated. None of our patients had pulmonary sequela or even evidence that pulmonary embolization had occurred.

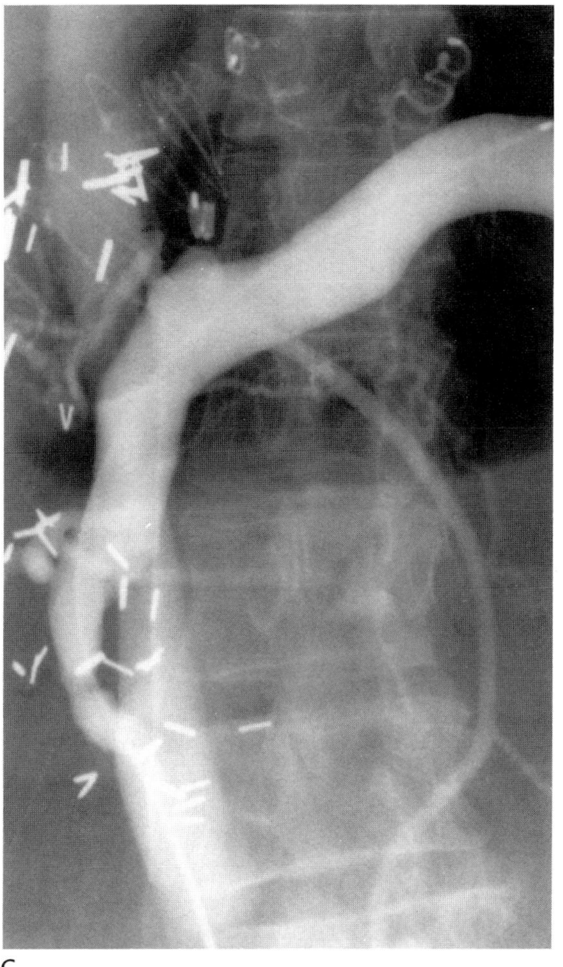

C

Figure 32.3. (*C*) An 8-mm angioplasty balloon was inflated across the shunt, and the splenic venogram was again repeated. The stenosis was reduced, and there was rapid flow into the IVC. Corrected portal pressure fell to 14 cm H_2O.

RECANALIZATION OF PORTAL VENOUS OCCLUSIONS

Since the technique of transhepatic portal vein catheterization was first popularized, it has been known that catheters can be manipulated across occlusions of the portal vein or its tributaries. Originally, this technique was used mainly to embolize varices associated with portal vein occlusions. However, the recent introduction of expandable metallic stents has made it possible to extend the therapeutic potential of this approach and reestablish flow through venous occlusions. The Wallstent, which is the thinnest of these devices, can be placed through a relatively small-diameter percutaneous puncture hole (7-F), which makes introduction using the transhepatic approach feasible. It enlarges up to a full 10-mm luminal diameter, so that when deployed across an occluded segment of vein, a large conduit is provided for blood to flow in. After just a few weeks in the vascular system, metallic stents become incorporated in a neointima that is histologically similar to the lining of a porous vascular graft. We have had the opportunity to use expandable metallic stents to treat occlusions of the main portal vein, as well as the splenic and mesenteric veins, and have been successful in controlling bleeding from varices caused by these extrahepatic venous obstructions (Figure 32.4).

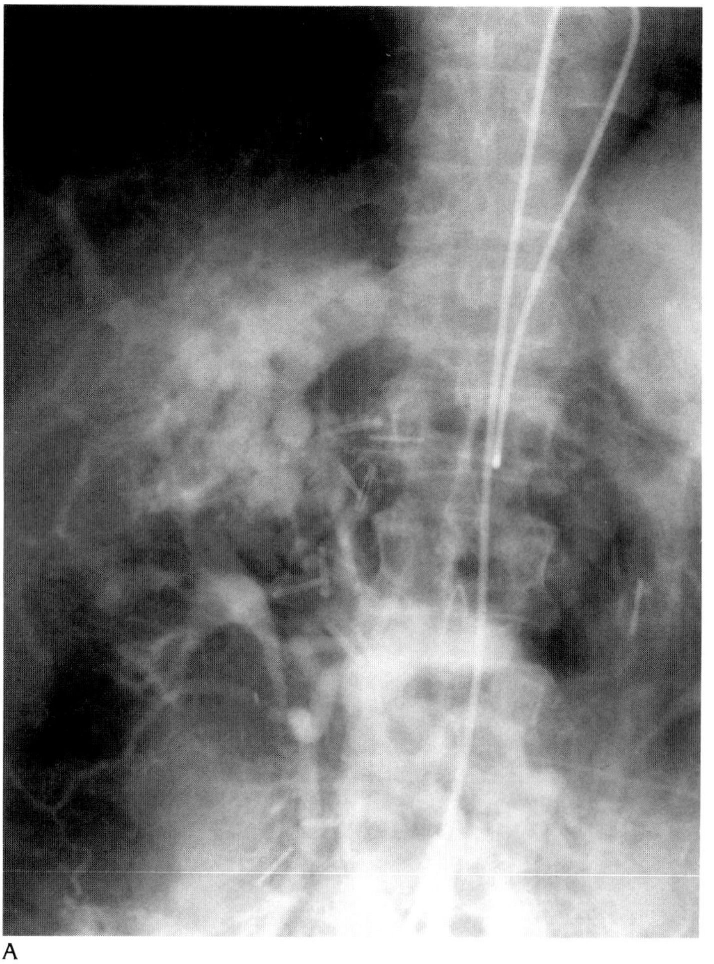

A

Figure 32.4. Percutaneous transhepatic recanalization of an occluded superior mesenteric vein. (*A*) Five months following pancreaticoduodenectomy for chronic pancreatitis, this 56-year-old woman began to bleed from the lower gastrointestinal tract. The venous phase of a superior mesenteric arteriogram showed occlusion of the superior mesenteric vein. Large subhepatic varices fill the intrahepatic branches of the portal vein. (*B*) A catheter was placed transhepatically into a peripheral portal vein branch and advanced to the point of obstruction. (*C*) A catheter was manipulated through the obstructed segment of the superior mesenteric vein. An injection in the distal superior mesenteric vein shows large jejunal varices that are probably related to the Roux-en-Y jejunal loop anastomosed to the biliary tree.

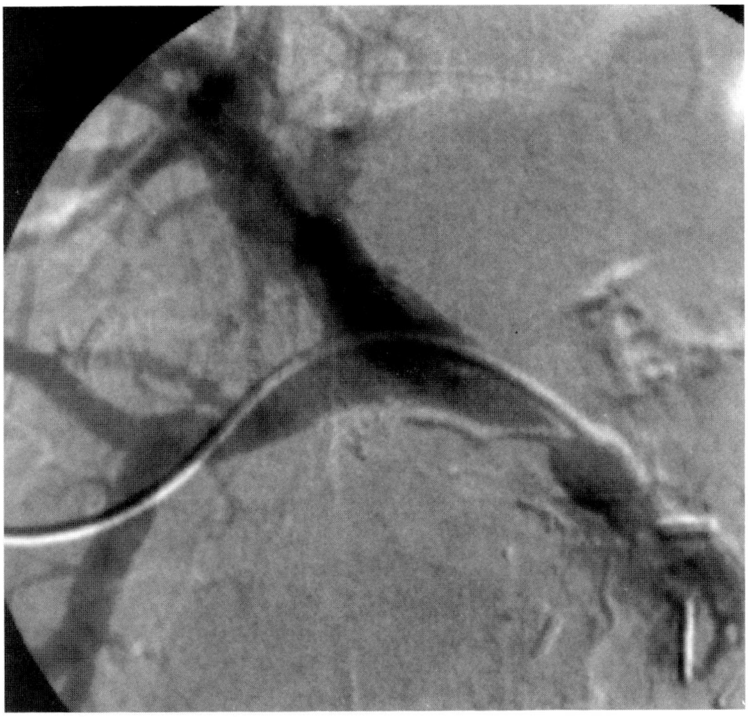

B

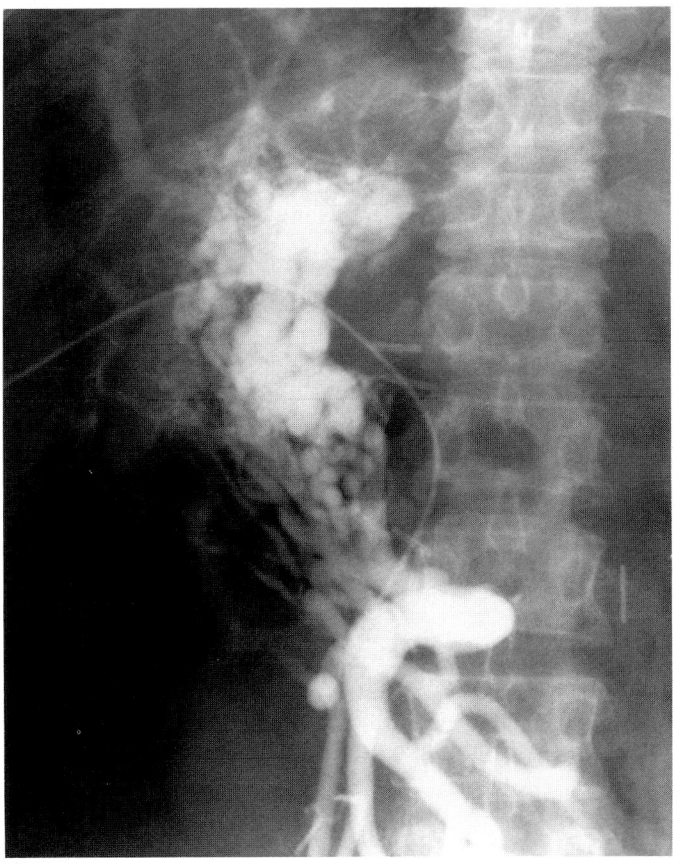

C

Figure 32.4.

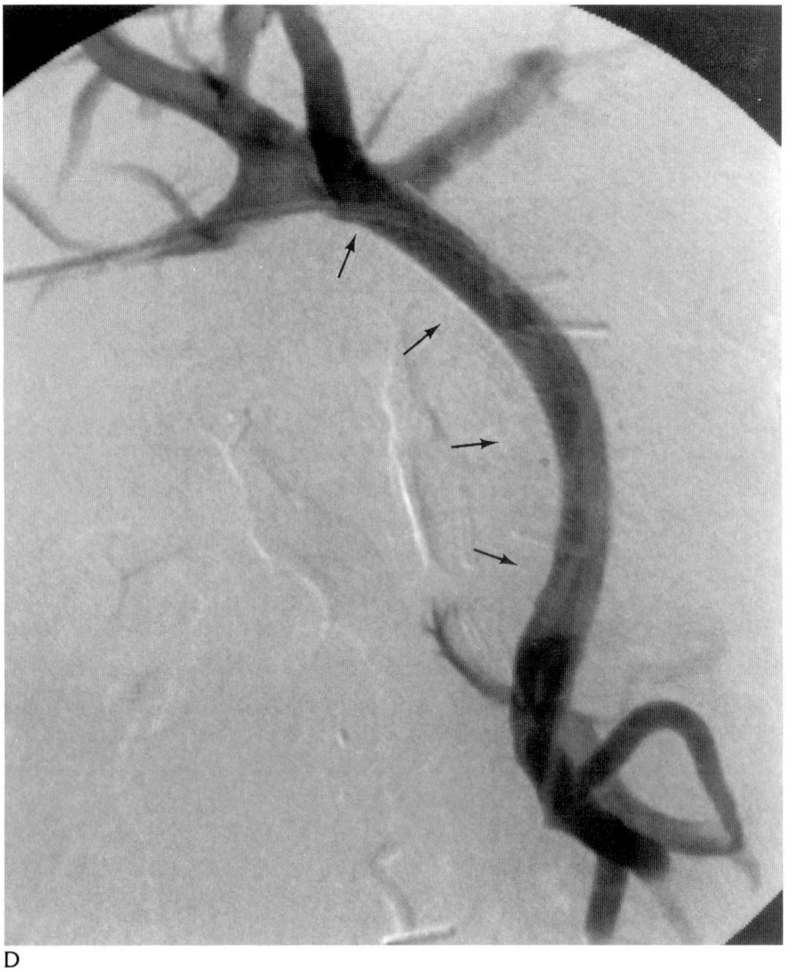

D

Figure 32.4. (*D*) A 10-mm expandable metallic stent was deployed across the obstructed segment of vein (*arrows*). The mesenteric venogram was repeated and showed freeflow through the stent into the portal vein. There was no longer filling of the jejunal varices.

HEPATIC VEIN INTERVENTIONS FOR BUDD-CHIARI SYNDROME

Typically, patients with Budd-Chiari syndrome present with a triad of ascites, hepatomegaly, and abdominal pain; associated portal hypertension can occasionally lead to variceal hemorrhage. The syndrome has numerous causes: In Asians there is almost always an obstructing web at the outflow of the hepatic veins or the intrahepatic vena cava. Diffuse thrombosis of the intrahepatic veins is commonly associated with toxins or hypercoagulable conditions such as polycythemia rubra vera or the use of birth control drugs. Webs obstructing the hepatic vein or inferior vena cava have been fractured intraoperatively.[15] Alternatively, numerous reports have described successful use of balloon angioplasty to disrupt hepatic vein and caval webs[16,17] (Figure 32.5). Recurrences of these venous obstructions appear to be common after angioplasty, and expandable stents have been used to treat recurrent stenoses.[18]

When the intrahepatic veins are diffusely filled with thrombus, very little can be done to improve hepatic venous flow. Surgical therapy is directed to diversion of portal flow into either the vena cava or the right atrium. We have recently begun to use percutaneous transhepatic catheterization of peripheral hepatic vein branches to evaluate the anatomy of the obstruction and, when feasible, to recanalize venous occlusions (Figure 32.6). Though experience with this method is still preliminary, the results thus far in three patients suggest that transhepatic recanalization may become a useful approach to the management of this difficult clinical problem.

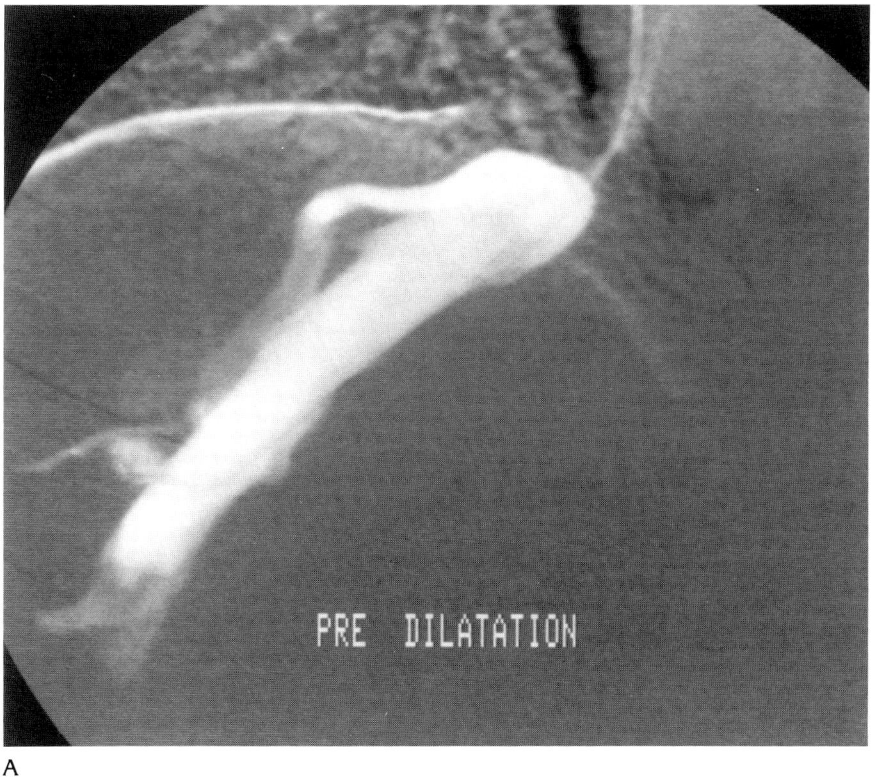

A

Figure 32.5. Budd-Chiari syndrome, caused by a web at the junction of the hepatic vein with the inferior vena cava, treated by balloon angioplasty. (*A*) A hepatic venogram performed on a 29-year-old man with ascites and portal hypertension shows only retrograde opacification of the hepatic vein. A web at the hepatic vein caval junction did not allow flow into the IVC.

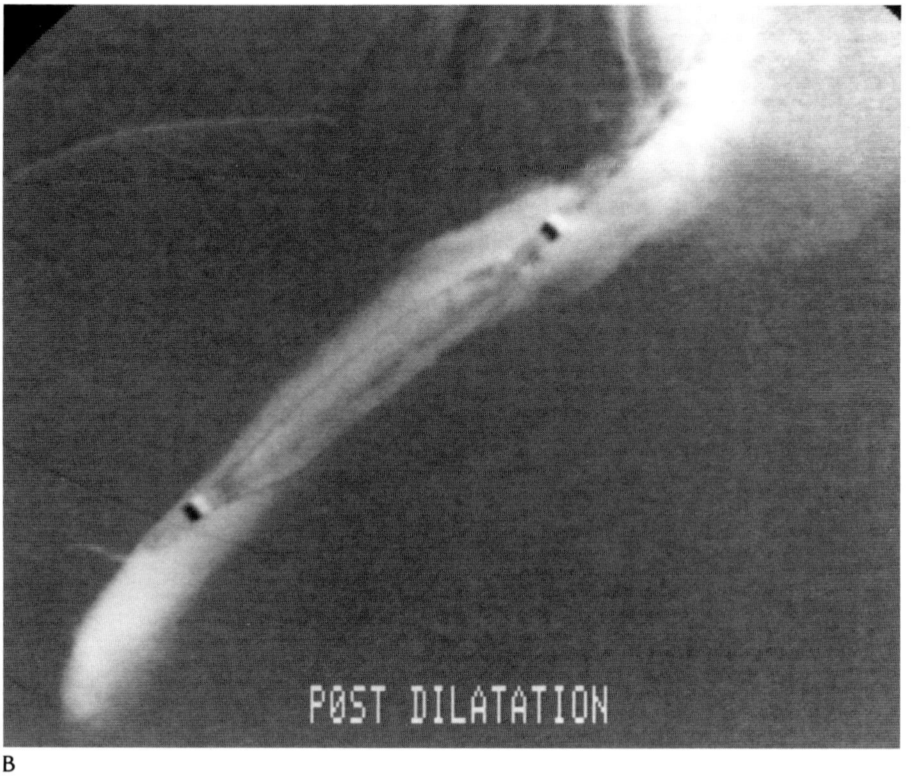

B

Figure 32.5. (*B*) The web was disrupted with a 20-mm angioplasty balloon. A repeat venogram shows free flow to the IVC.

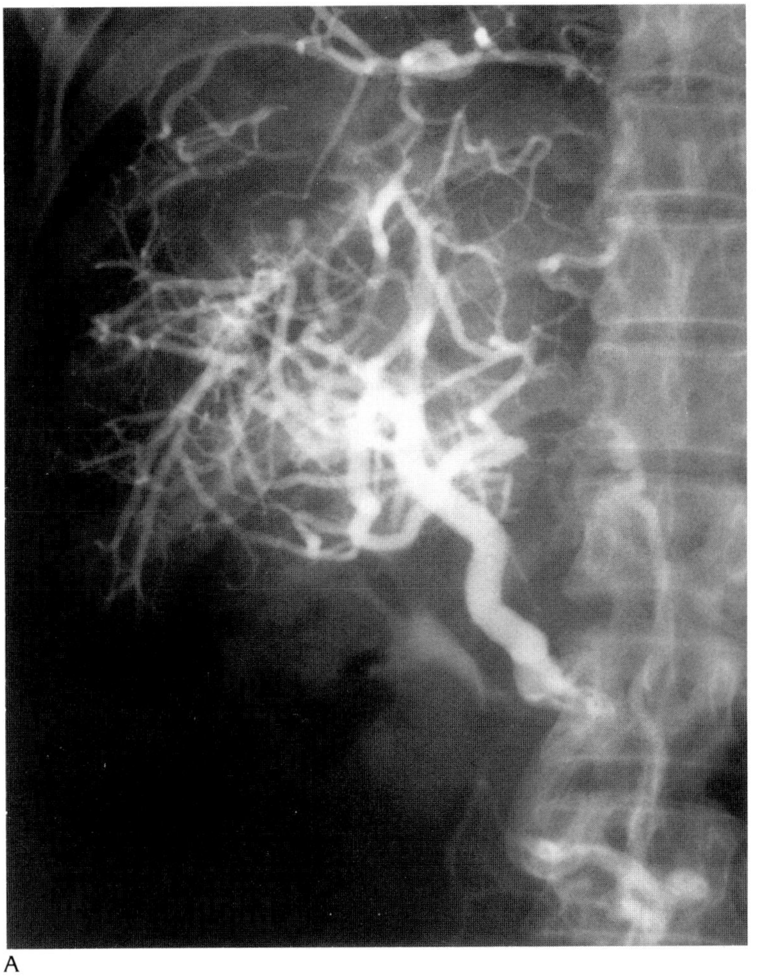

A

Figure 32.6. Budd-Chiari syndrome, caused by diffuse hepatic vein occlusion, treated by transhepatic recanalization stenting. (*A*) A transhepatic catheter was introduced into a peripheral right hepatic vein. Hepatic venography demonstrates numerous intrahepatic collaterals.

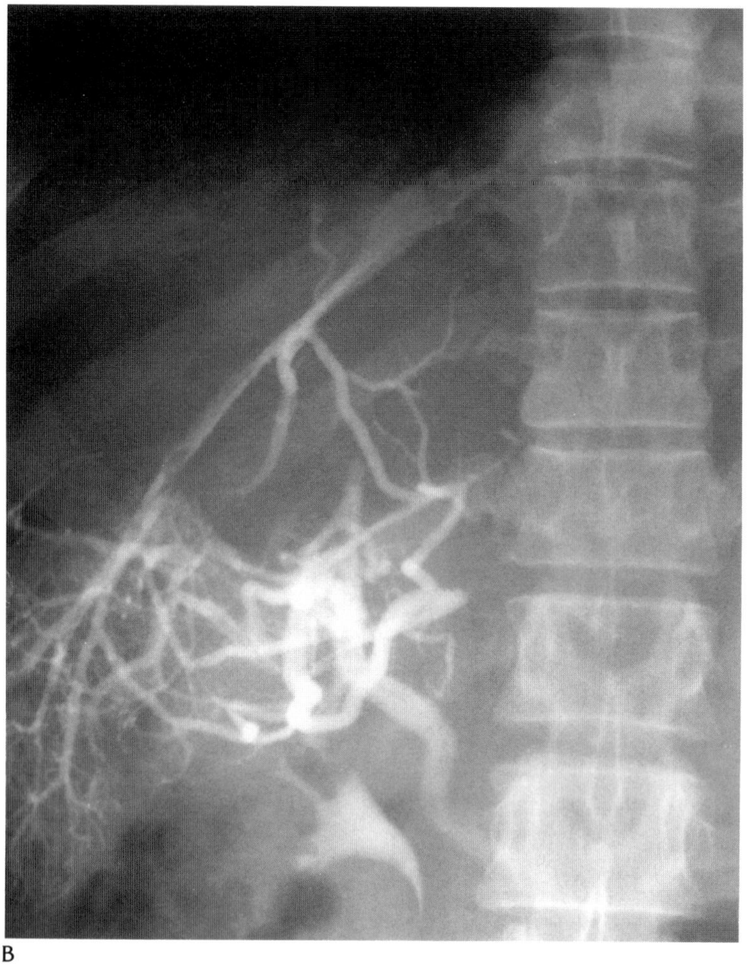

B

Figure 32.6. (*B*) A transhepatic catheter was manipulated through the occlusion into the IVC. The occluded segment was dilated with a 6-mm angioplasty balloon. (*C*) The transhepatic catheter was removed, and a catheter was introduced through a femoral approach into the hepatic vein. The vein was then dilated to 8 mm with an angioplasty balloon catheter. A repeat venogram shows a widely patent lumen, with the exception of a linear lucency at the junction of the hepatic vein with the IVC. The pressure gradient from the hepatic vein to the IVC was 26 cm H_2O. (*D*) An expandable metallic stent was placed across the web. This completely eliminated the gradient. A repeat venogram shows free flow into the IVC.

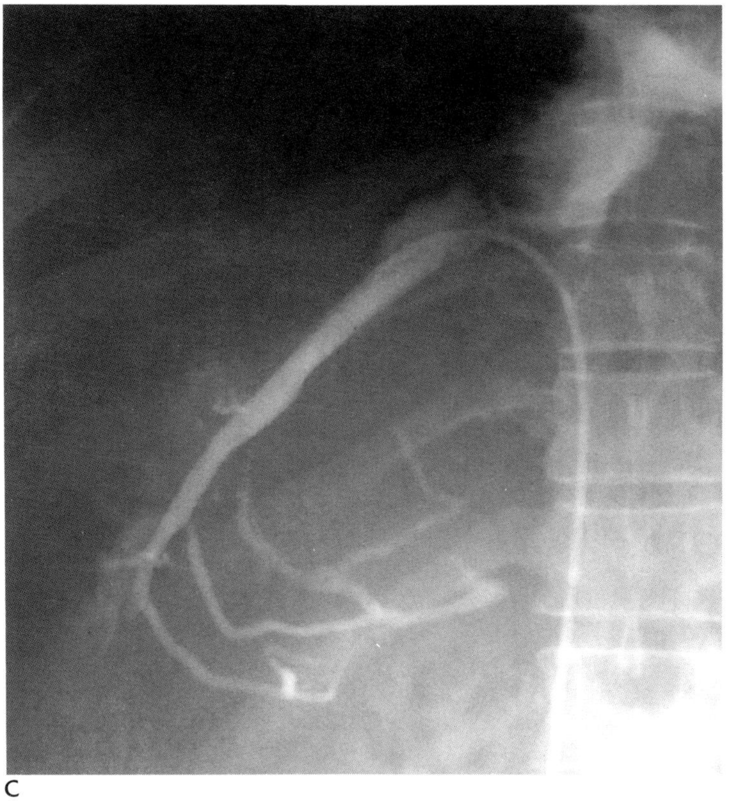

C

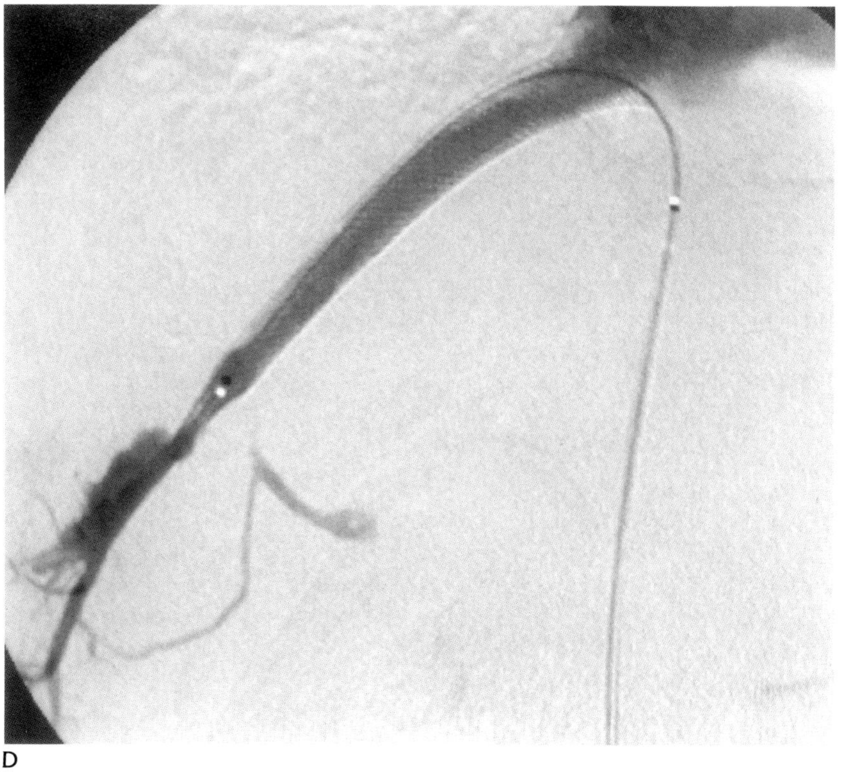

D

Figure 32.6.

TRANSJUGULAR INTRAHEPATIC PORTOSYSTEMIC SHUNTS (TIPS)

Portal decompression through a percutaneously established communication between the hepatic and portal veins was first conceived of by Rosch et al. in 1969.[19] Subsequently, several experimental methods have been developed to expand the venous connection up to a diameter that would be adequate for portal decompression. In 1982, Colapinto et al. first reported performing percutaneous intrahepatic shunts in humans.[20] They used angioplasty balloon catheters and repeated dilatation to try to establish a large transparenchymal track. While these shunts were effective in lowering portal pressure, they tended to occlude rapidly because of elastic recoil in the adjacent hepatic parenchyma.

Palmaz et al. in 1985[21] and Rosch et al. in 1987[22] used expandable metallic vascular stents to create TIPs in animals and showed that a neointimal lining formed on the stent within just a few weeks. Palmaz et al. in 1986[23] found that expandable metallic intrahepatic shunts placed in dogs with experimentally induced portal hypertension remained patent for 48 weeks. Richter et al. in 1990 successfully created intrahepatic shunts in 10

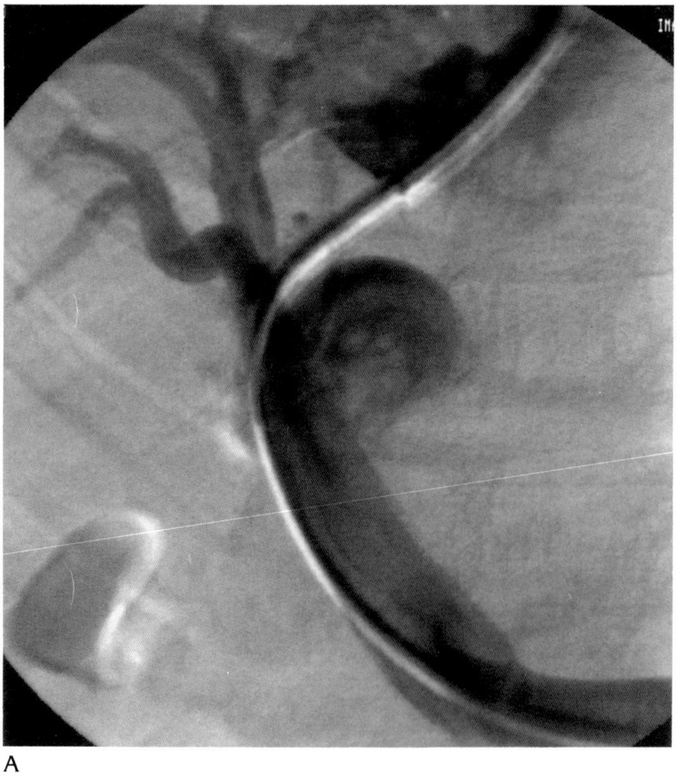

A

Figure 32.7. Transjugular intrahepatic portosystemic shunt. (*A*) A transjugular catheter was advanced into the right hepatic vein, and then a needle was passed through the catheter into the right portal vein. A guidewire was advanced into the mesenteric vein followed by a 5-F catheter. A portal venogram performed through the 5-F catheter demonstrates hepatofugal flow in the coronary vein. The flow in the intrahepatic portal vein branches is hepatopedal.

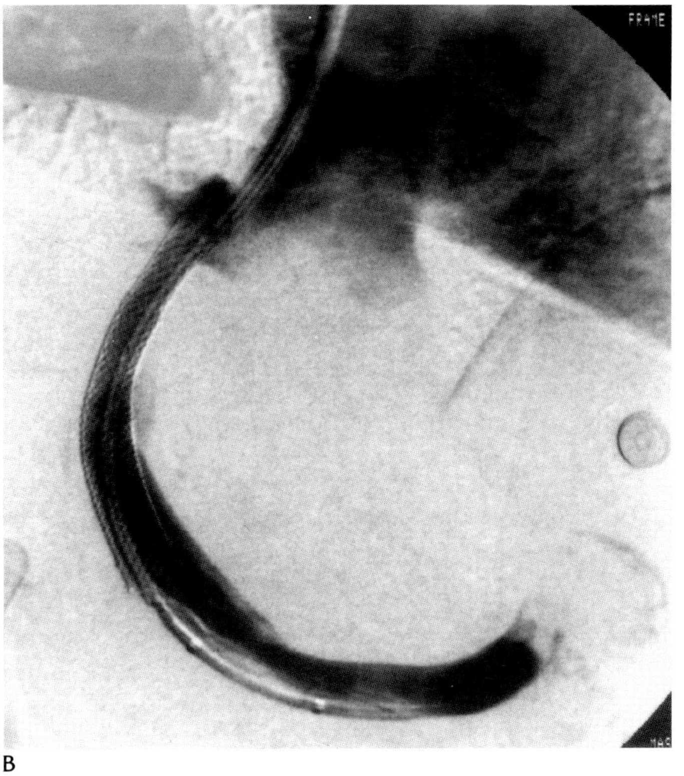

B

Figure 32.7. (*B*) After dilating the track between the hepatic vein and the portal vein with an 8-mm balloon, an expandable metallic Wallstent was positioned across the parenchymal tract. A repeat portal venogram shows total diversion of portal flow through the shunt.

of 14 patients using the Palmaz balloon-expandable stent.[24] The procedures were performed using a combination of transjugular hepatic vein catheterization and transhepatic portal vein catheterization; a transjugular needle advanced out of the hepatic vein was directed toward a Dormia basket that had been placed transhepatically in the portal vein. Once the communication between the veins was established, the track was dilated, and a Palmaz* expandable stent was positioned to connect the hepatic and portal venous systems.

Over the past year, we have performed TIPS on 23 patients and are mainly using this procedure as a bridge to transplantation in patients who continue to bleed from varices despite multiple endoscopic sclerotherapies. TIPS is an attractive alternative in these high-risk patients because it is effective in controlling bleeding without surgery or general anesthesia. In addition, the shunt's intrahepatic location avoids the technical problems that are commonly associated with liver transplantation after conventional portacaval shunts.

Our approach is a modification of the technique described by Richter et al.[24] A 9-F angiographic sheath is advanced from the right internal jugular vein into the right or

*Johnson & Johnson Interventional Systems, Warren, New Jersey.

middle hepatic vein. A Colapinto transjugular needle (16-gauge needle within a 7.5-F catheter) is then advanced through the sheath and directed anteriorly under ultrasound guidance through the liver parenchyma into a right portal vein branch. A guidewire is then passed into the portal vein, and the needle is removed. The parenchymal tract is then dilated to 8 mm with an angioplasty balloon. An expandable metallic Wallstent is placed across the connection between the portal and hepatic veins, and the angioplasty balloon is used to distend the parenchymal segment of the stent to 8 mm (Figure 32.7). If subsequent portography demonstrates continued flow into the varices, the stent is further expanded to its maximum 10-mm diameter (Figure 32.8). The portogram is repeated, and if there is still filling of varices with the stent fully expanded, the coronary vein is selectively catheterized and occluded with stainless steel coils (Figure 32.9).

Using these methods, we have been successful in establishing effective shunts in all the patients in whom this procedure was attempted, and there were no procedural complications. Portal pressure was reduced from an initial 34.5 ± 3.5 cm H_2O to 20.5 ± 3.9 cm H_2O. Embolization of the coronary vein was necessary in only one patient. Histological examination of the shunts taken from the livers removed at transplantation revealed that by three weeks the stent's wires had become incorporated in a smooth

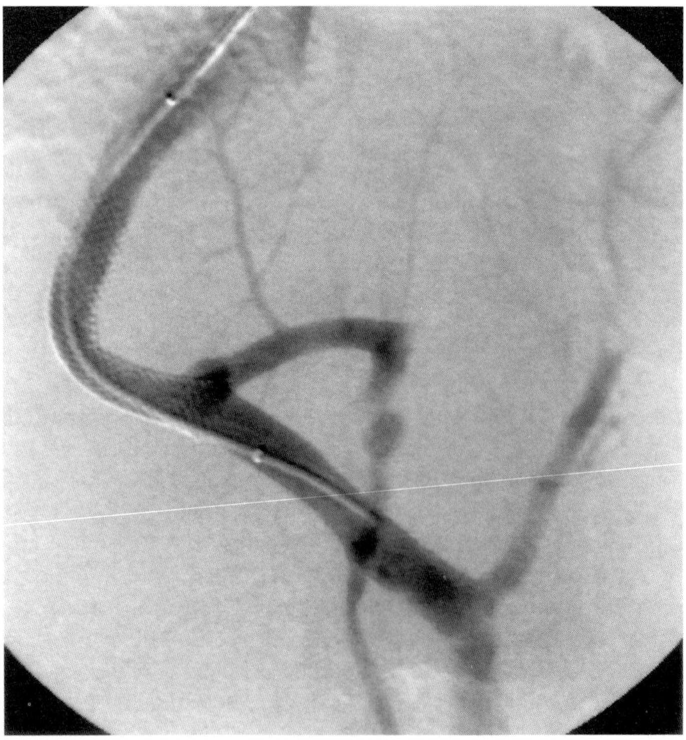

A

Figure 32.8. Transjugular intrahepatic portosystemic shunt requiring dilatation to 10 mm in order to eliminate hepatofugal flow. (*A*) Portal venography performed after a TIPS had been opened to 8mm shows persistent filling of the coronary vein. There is also flow to the umbilical vein through the left portal vein.

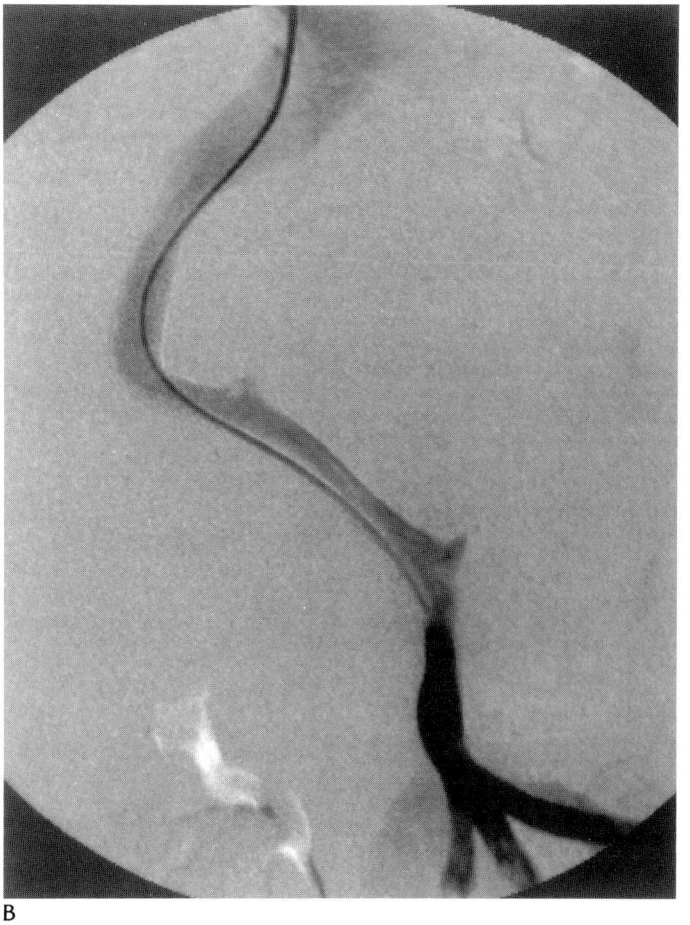

B

Figure 32.8. (*B*) The stent was further expanded using a 10-mm angioplasty balloon. This resulted in total diversion of portal flow through the stent.

neointima similar in appearance to the lining of an intra-arterial vascular graft (Figure 32.10).

There appear to be few potential complications from intrahepatic portal vein shunts using this approach. The procedure is accomplished through a jugular venipuncture alone, so there is little risk of hemorrhage even if the patient has a significant coagulopathy. Traversing a hepatic artery branch or biliary radical during the parenchymal puncture could conceivably cause hemobilia or arteriovenous fistula, but these complications have not yet occurred. Moreover, arterial injury is very unlikely because, when expanded, the metallic stent compresses and tamponades vessels within the parenchymal tract. Hemobilia should also be unlikely unless there is associated biliary obstruction and dilated intrahepatic ducts. Since the puncture is entirely within the liver, ascites poses no additional risks.

Because most of our TIPS procedures were performed in patients who subsequently went on to liver transplantation (4–106 days), there is insufficient long-term follow-up to compare this method with the surgical and endoscopic therapies that are currently being used for variceal bleeding. However, since less than half of Child's class C patients who bleed from varices survive for 30 days, regardless of whether they undergo portosystemic shunt surgery or sclerotherapy, and since only a few are alive at one year,[25] there clearly is a need to explore new treatment options if the dismal prognosis for these patients is ever to bc improved. TIPS represents the latest in a long line of percutaneous interventions for portal hypertension and bleeding varices that have been developed and evaluated by radiologists. As more experience is obtained, it is likely that new devices will be developed to improve these methods further, and that other percutaneous alternatives will evolve for the treatment of patients with variceal hemorrhage.

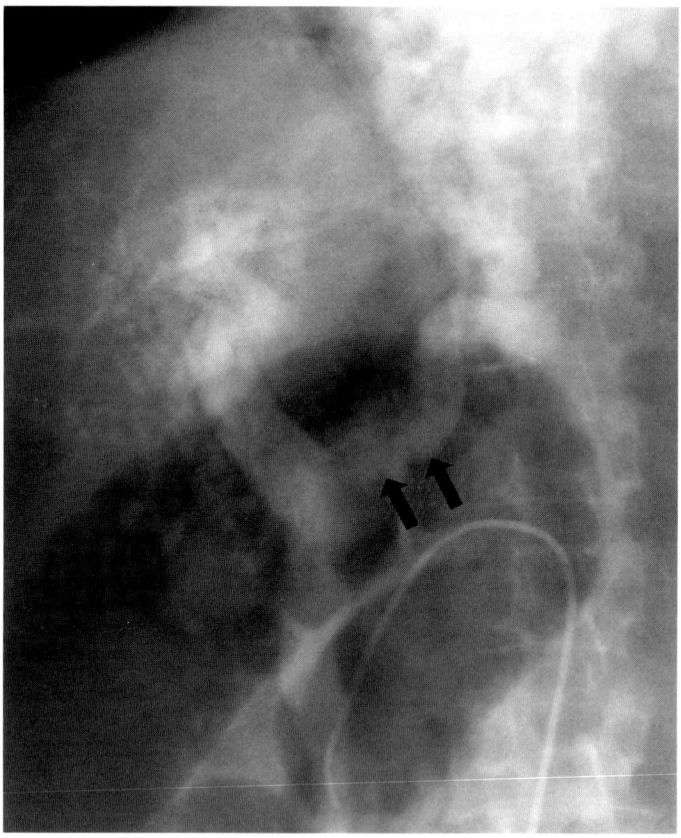

A

Figure 32.9. Combined TIPS and variceal embolization in a patient with portal vein occlusion. (*A*) The venous phase of a superior mesenteric arteriogram shows occlusion of the intrahepatic portal vein. There is hepatofugal flow into a greatly enlarged coronary vein (*arrows*). (*B*) A catheter was placed transhepatically into a peripheral portal vein branch and injected. There are numerous intrahepatic collateral veins. (*C*) The catheter was manipulated through the occlusion into the main portal vein. (*D*) TIPS was performed and the metallic stent was distended to 8 mm. Portal venography shows continued hepatofugal flow into the coronary vein. (*E*) The TIPS was further distended with a 10-mm balloon. There is still some flow into the coronary vein (*arrow*). (*F*) The coronary vein was selectively catheterized, and flow to the varices was occluded with stainless steel coils.

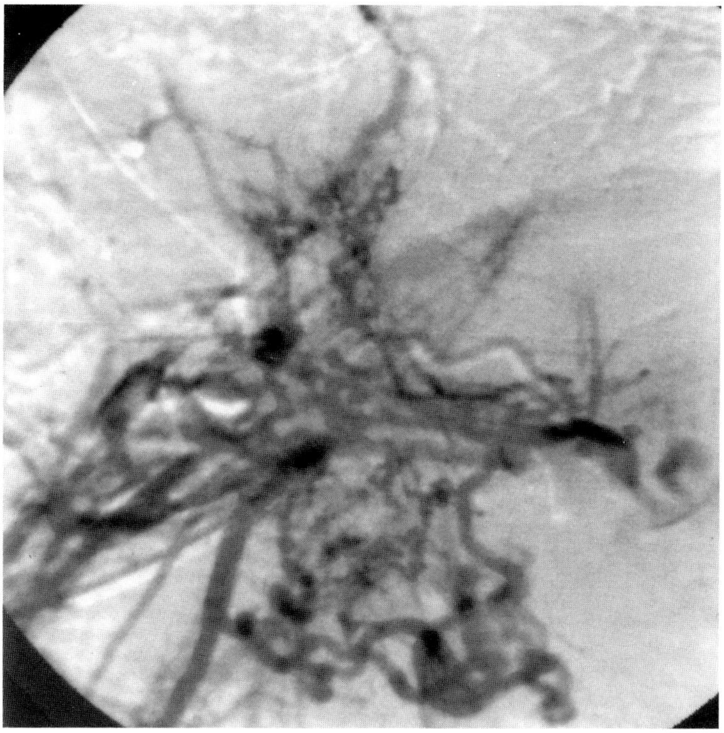

B

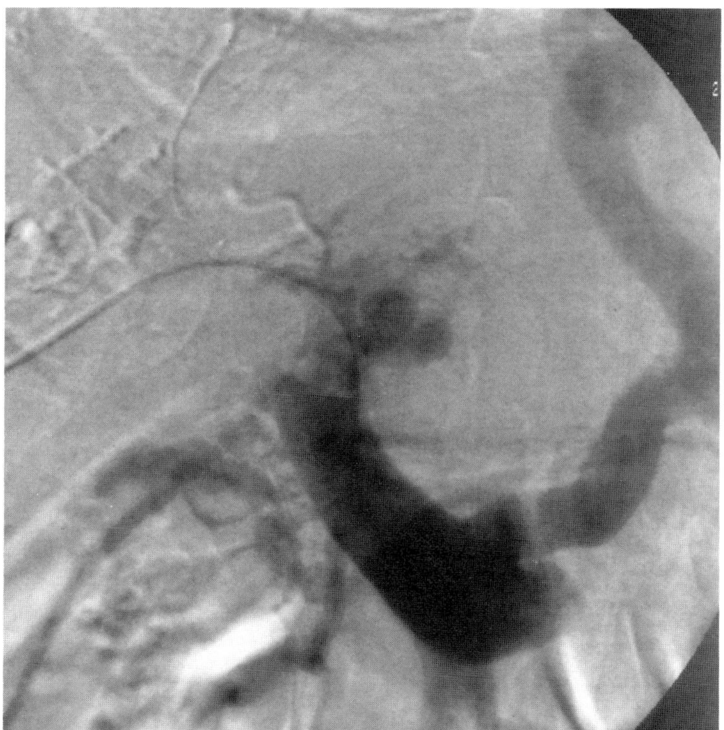

C

Figure 32.9.

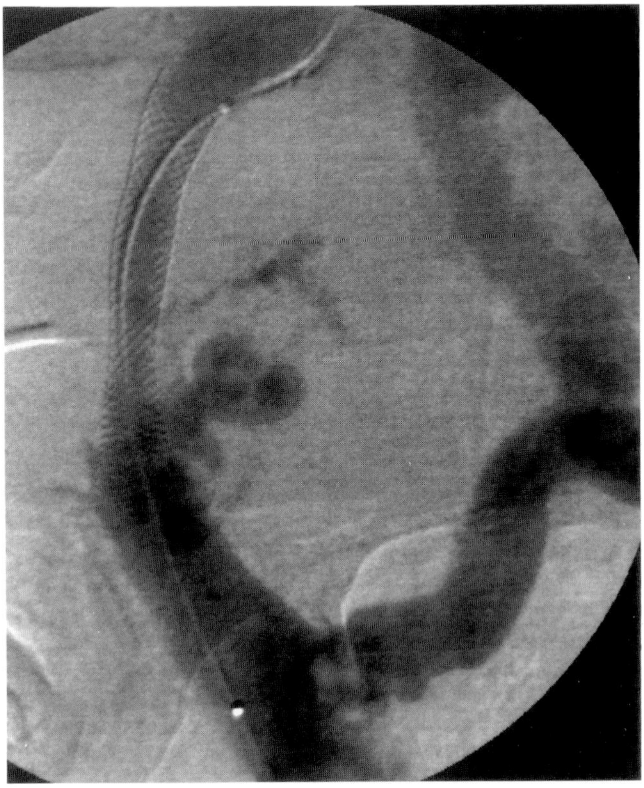

D

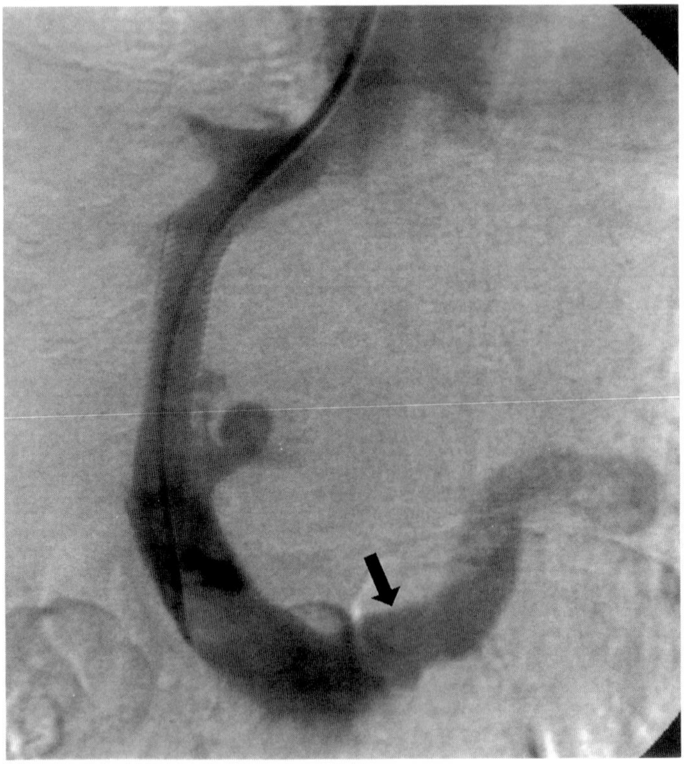

E

Figure 32.9. *(continued)*

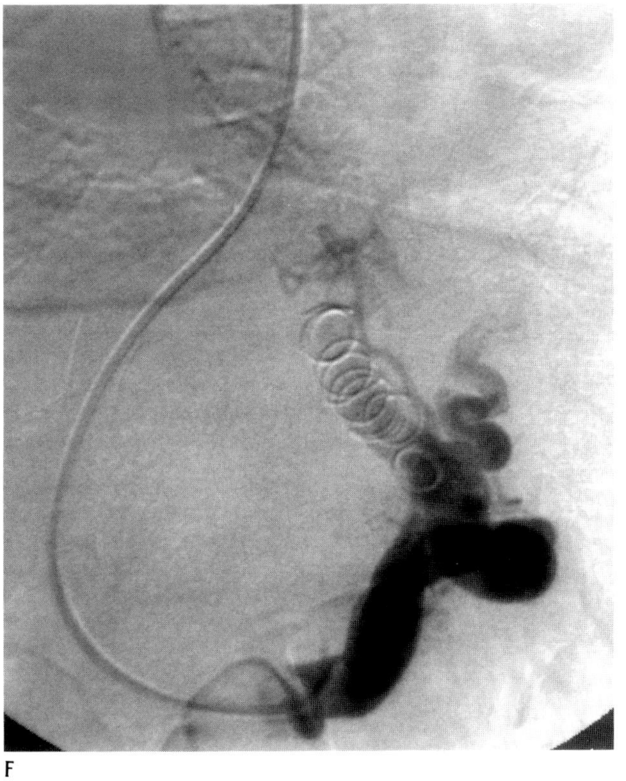

F

Figure 32.9. (*continued*)

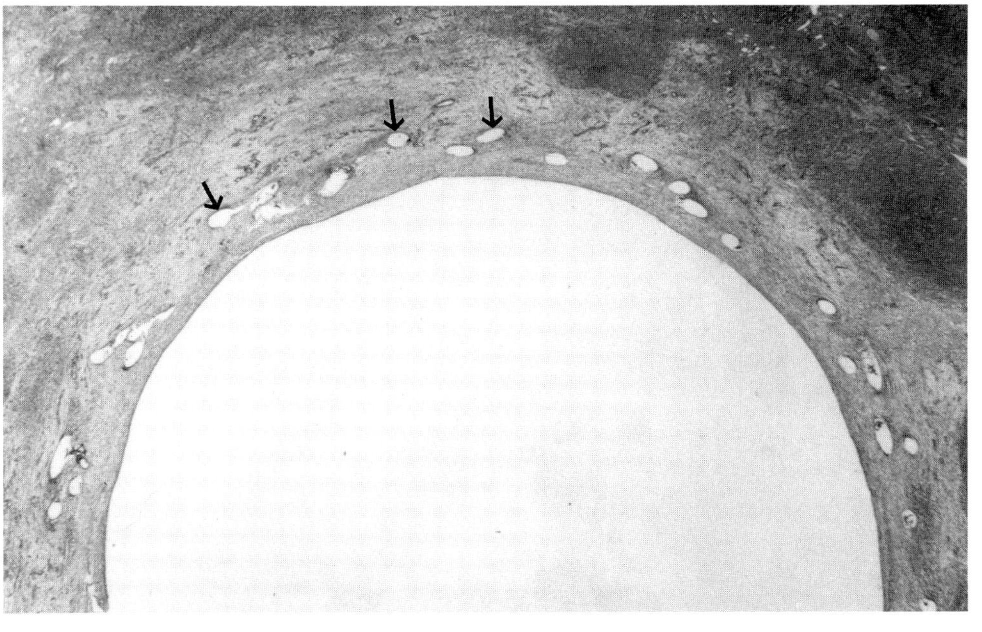

Figure 32.10. Histological section of TIPS 20 days after insertion. The lumen of the TIPS is round and smooth. The wires (*arrows*) are incorporated in a developing neointima.

REFERENCES

1. Nusbaum M, Baum S, Sakiyalak P, et al: Pharmacologic control of portal hypertension. *Surgery* 62:299–310, 1967.
2. Baum S, Nusbaum M, Tumen HJ: The control of gastrointestinal hemorrhage by selective mesenteric arterial infusion of pitressin (abstract). *Gastroenterology* 58:926, 1970.
3. Conn H, Ramsey GR, Storer EH, et al: Intraarterial vasopressin in the treatment of upper gastrointestinal hemorrhage: A prospective controlled clinical trial. *Gastroenterology* 68:211–221, 1975.
4. Nusbaum M, Baum S, Kuroda K, et al: Control of portal hypertension by selective mesenteric arterial drug infusion. *Arch Surg* 97:1005–1013, 1968.
5. Barr JW, Lakin RC, Rosch J: Similarity of arterial and intravenous vasopressin on portal and systemic hemodynamics. *Gastroenterology* 69:13–19, 1975.
6. Johnson WC, Widrich WC, Ansell JE, et al: Control of bleeding varices by vasopressin: A prospective randomized study. *Ann Surg* 186:369–376, 1977.
7. Lunderquist A, Vang J: Transhepatic catheterization and obliteration of the coronary vein in patients with portal hypertension and esophageal varices. *N Engl J Med* 291:646–649, 1974.
8. Viamonte M, Pereiras R, Russell E, et al: Transhepatic obliteration of gastroesophageal varices: Results in acute and nonacute bleeders. *AJR* 129:237–241, 1977.
9. Funaro AH, Ring EJ, Freiman DB, et al: Transhepatic obliteration of esophageal varices using the stainless steel coil. *AJR* 133:1123–1125, 1979.
10. Menu Y, Gayet B, Nahum H: Bleeding duodenal varices: Diagnosis and treatment by percutaneous portography and transcatheter embolization. *Gastrointest Radiol* 12:111–113, 1987.
11. L'Hermine CL, Chastanet P, Delemazure O, et al: Percutaneous transhepatic embolization of gastroesophageal varices: Results in 400 patients. *AJR* 152:755–760, 1989.
12. Johansen K: Partial portal decompression for variceal hemorrhage. *Am J Surg* 157:479–482, 1989.
13. Coldwell DM, Moore ADA, Ben-Menachem Y, et al: Bleeding gastroesophageal varices: Gastric vein embolization after partial portal decompression. *Radiology* 178:249–251, 1991.
14. Cope C: Angioplasty and thrombolytic therapy for portosystemic shunt obstruction, in Kadir (ed): *Current Practice of Interventional Radiology*. Philadelphia, B C Decker, 1990, pp 476–480.
15. Eguchi S, Takeuchi Y, Asano K: Successful balloon membranotomy for obstruction of the hepatic portion of the inferior vena cava. *Surgery* 76:837–840, 1974.
16. Uflacker R, Francisconi CF, Rodriguez MP, et al: Percutaneous transluminal angioplasty of the hepatic veins for treatment of Budd-Chiari syndrome. *Radiology* 153: 641–642, 1984.
17. Furui S, Yamauchi T, Ohtomo K, et al: Hepatic inferior vena cava obstructions: Clinical results of treatment with percutaneous transluminal laser-assisted angioplasty. *Radiology* 166:673–677, 1988.
18. Walker WS, Rholl KS, Register TE, et al: Percutaneous placement of a hepatic vein stent in the treatment of Budd-Chiari syndrome. *JVIR* 1:23–27, 1990.
19. Rosch J, Hanafee WN, Snow H: Transjugular portal venography and radiologic portacaval shunt: An experimental study. *Radiology* 92:1112–1114, 1969.
20. Colapinto RF, Stronell RD, Birch SJ, et al: Creation of an intrahepatic portosystemic shunt with a Gruntzig balloon catheter. *CMA* 126:267–268, 1982.
21. Palmaz JC, Sibbitt RR, Reuter SR, et al: Expandable intrahepatic portacaval shunt stents: Early experience in the dog. *AJR* 145:821–825, 1985.

22. Rosch J, Uchida BT, Putnam JS, et al: Experimental intrahepatic portacaval anastomosis: Use of expandable Gianturco stents. *Radiology* 162:481–485, 1987.

23. Palmaz JC, Garcia F, Sibbitt RR, et al: Expandable portacaval shunt stents in dogs with chronic portal hypertension. *AJR* 147:1251–1254, 1986.

24. Richter GM, Noeldge G, Palmaz JC, et al: Transjugular intrahepatic portacaval stent shunt: Preliminary clinical results. *Radiology* 174:1027–1030, 1990.

25. Cello JP, Grendell JH, Crass RA, et al: Endoscopic sclerotherapy versus portacaval shunt in patients with severe cirrhosis and variceal hemorrhage. *N Engl J Med* 311:1589–1594, 1984.

33

SURGICAL SHUNTS FOR BLEEDING ESOPHAGEAL VARICES

Jeremiah G. Turcotte, M.D.

HISTORY

In 1877 Nicolai Eck, a Russian military surgeon, performed a portosystemic shunt in eight dogs.[1] He anastomosed the side of the portal vein to the side of the vena cava and ligated the hepatic limb of the portal vein, thus constructing a functional end-to-side portacaval shunt. Only one dog survived, and this dog ran away after three weeks. Nevertheless, this landmark experiment was the first demonstration that an animal could survive after all portal blood was diverted around the liver. This observation motivated surgeons to attempt shunt operations in patients with portal hypertension. To this day, an end-to-side portacaval shunt is frequently referred to as an *Eck fistula*.

In the early twentieth century, European surgeons attempted portacaval shunts in humans but, not surprisingly, the operative mortality was excessive. Interest in constructing portacaval shunts remained dormant until the 1945 presentation by Whipple to the American Surgical Association, in which he reviewed the early experience with the end-to-side portacaval shunts at the Columbia Presbyterian Hospital[2] Spleen Clinic in New York City where balloon tamponade to control acute variceal hemorrhage was also introduced.

Much of the next 25 years was devoted to defining the indications for shunt operations, describing and evaluating different types of shunts, and determining the prognosis for patients undergoing portal decompressive operations. In 1959 C. Gardner Child 3rd joined the faculty at the University of Michigan. His interest in portal hypertension began while he was at New York Hospital. The team he developed at Michigan placed the evaluation of various portosystemic shunt procedures on a more rational basis by emphasizing the need to categorize patients according to hepatic reserve and the etiology of their liver disease.[3-5] This work resulted in the widespread use of the Child-Turcotte classification system of hepatic reserve to estimate operative mortality and long-term prognosis following shunt operations. The reports from Michigan utilized actuarial statistical methods for estimating survival. This was one of the first uses of this now common place statistical technique to estimate postoperative survival.[3] During the 1960s and 1970s, Dean Warren promulgated the concept of selective shunts and introduced the distal splenorenal shunt. Sarfeh et al., in the 1980s, extended the concept of the selective shunt with their description of the small-caliber interposition portacaval shunt.[6] In 1973 Johnston and Rodgers reintroduced sclerotherapy as a method to control variceal hemorrhage.[7] Today, an initial trial of serial sclerotherapy is the usual treatment for prevention of recurrent variceal bleeding for most patients.

Sir Roy Calne, in 1979, reported that the new immunosuppressive drug cyclosporine was effective in preventing rejection in human recipients of kidneys, pancreases, and livers.[8] This finding provided the impetus for the widespread application of liver transplantation in patients with end-stage liver disease. Liver transplantation is now used commonly for patients with bleeding varices who have poor liver function. Currently, the insertion of stented intrahepatic shunts introduced percutaneously via the jugular or femoral vein is under evaluation[9,10] (Figure 33.1). This minimally invasive procedure has been demonstrated to halt acute variceal hemorrhage effectively. Stented intrahepatic shunts have also been demonstrated to remain patent for at least several months, but more follow-up will be needed to determine the long-term patency rate.

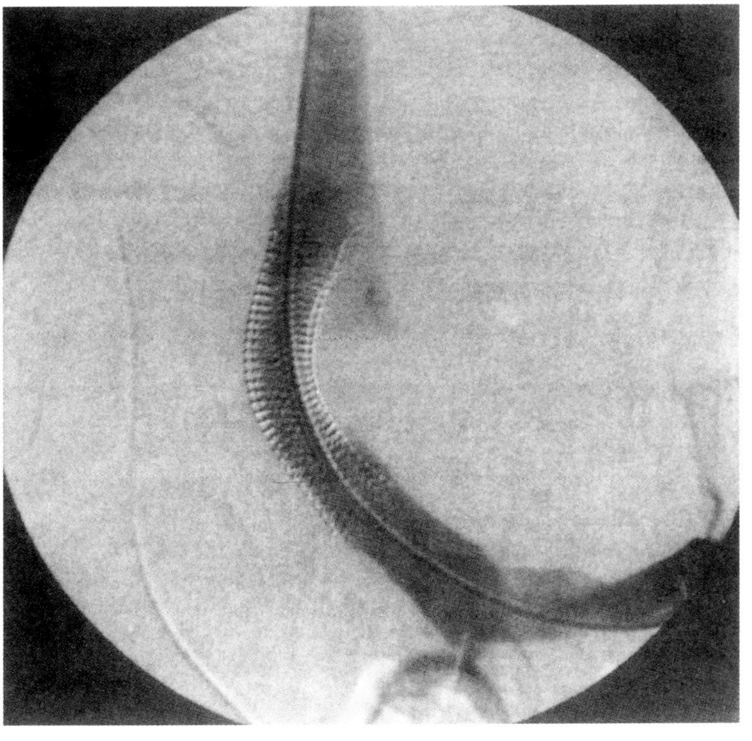

Figure 33.1. Intrahepatic stented portacaval shunt. This portal angiogram demonstrates portal flow into the vena cava across the shunt. A 10-mm-diameter stainless steel stent is in place. (Reproduced with permission from Ring E, Lake J, Sterneck M, et al: Intrahepatic portacaval shunt for variceal hemorrhage prior to liver transplantation. *Transplantation* 2:160–163, 1991.)

PATHOPHYSIOLOGY OF PORTAL HYPERTENSION AND BLEEDING VARICES

An understanding of the pathophysiology associated with cirrhosis and bleeding varices is necessary for the proper management of these patients during an acute variceal hemorrhage and in the perioperative period should the patient require a portosystemic shunt. The pathogenesis of portal hypertension involves more than simple obstruction of portal blood flow.[11] If the portal vein is obstructed in primates or humans, collateral flow will develop around the site of obstruction and portal hypertension will diminish or disappear in approximately one month. With so-called idiopathic portal hypertension, the histology of the liver appears normal with standard histological stains, and no obvious intrahepatic obstruction can be demonstrated. Most investigators believe that persistence of portal hypertension in this disease requires the development of a so-called hyperdynamic state. Typically, with liver disease a hyperdynamic state with increased splanchnic blood flow evolves. Permanent elevation of portal pressure usually requires an increase in portal flow, an increase in resistance to portal flow, and maintenance of tension in the walls of the portosystemic venous system. Obstruction to portal flow may be the major initiating etiologic factor in diseases such as the Budd-Chiari syndrome, whereas increased splanchnic blood flow may be the most important factor in the pathogenesis of portal hypertension in diseases such as idiopathic portal hypertension.

A number of neurohumoral mechanisms are implicated in the pathogenesis of portal hypertension.[12] For instance, neurotensin and some prostaglandins increase splanchnic flow, while neuroepinephrine, somatostatin, other prostaglandins, and thromboxane B2 may decrease it. This hyperdynamic state, together with other pathophysiological changes induced by liver disease, results in very significant changes in cardiorespiratory hemodynamics (Table 33.1). Alterations in neurohumoral mechanisms also account for the profound fluid and electrolyte abnormalities found in patients with advanced cirrhosis and

TABLE 33.1. Cardiorespiratory Pathophysiology Associated with Hepatic Cirrhosis and Portal Hypertension

Abnormality	*Pathophysiology*	*Physical Signs**
pO_2 and oxyhemoglobin saturation decreased	Portopulmonary and intrapulmonary shunts	Cyanosis, clubbing of fingers
Arteriovenous oxygen difference decreased	Arteriolar or capillary shunts	Palmer erythema, spider telangiectasia
Peripheral resistance decreased	Systemic and splanchnic arteriovenous shunts	Tendency to hypotension; hypertension unusual; widened pulse pressure
Cardiac output increased	Low peripheral resistance, expanded plasma volume	Systolic ejection murmur, rapid pulse
Plasma volume increased	Increased total body sodium and water, secondary aldosteronism	Edema, ascites, high output cardiac failure if severe

*The pathogenesis of the abdominal physical signs listed in this third column is related to the pathophysiology listed in the second column. Awareness of this pathophysiology is important for interpretation of cardiorespiratory studies and the treatment of patients with cirrhosis.

portal hypertension. Secondary hyperaldosteronism, an overactive sympathetic nervous system, and the presence of an as yet unidentified antinatiuretic factor are important mechanisms that decrease the ability of the kidney to excrete sodium. Hyperaldosteronism and the inability of the kidney to excrete sodium lead to a high total body sodium load, expanded plasma and the interstitial fluid volumes, and low total body exchangeable potassium.

When sodium retention is severe, ascites may result. Important factors in the development of ascites and peripheral edema are increased capillary hydrostatic pressure in the splanchnic system caused by the portal hypertension and decreased colloid osmotic pressure because of a low serum albumin concentration. Recently, a unitary hypothesis to explain the pathogenesis of ascites has been proposed.[13] In the first stage, increased hepatic sinusoidal resistance leads to splanchnic pooling and a reduced effective intravascular volume. A reduced intravascular volume triggers the retention of sodium and water by the kidney. In the next stage (the overflow phase), the rate of lymph production increases, with overflow into the peritoneal cavity and the peripheral interstitial space. The maximum amount of fluid that can be reabsorbed from the peritoneal cavity in 24 hours has been estimated to be 900 ml. In the advanced stage, tense ascites occurs. This increases abdominal pressure, interferes with lymph resorption, reduces venous return, and leads to compromised cardiac function.

DIAGNOSIS OF PORTAL HYPERTENSION AND BLEEDING VARICES

In the United States, the most common cause of portal hypertension in adults is alcoholic cirrhosis of the liver. There are multiple physical signs suggesting the diagnosis of advanced cirrhosis. These include muscle wasting, ascites, encephalopathy, cyanosis of the lips, earlobes and nail beds, and liver palms. The presence of portal hypertension may be indicated by splenomegaly and the appearance of venous collaterals over the abdomen and chest. When patients present with massive upper gastrointestinal bleeding, these physical signs, plus a history compatible with variceal bleeding, should immediately lead the clinician to suspect bleeding varices.

Not infrequently, standard liver function tests are normal in the patient with bleeding varices. One should keep in mind that only 15–20% of the liver is needed to maintain normal function. Coagulation tests such as prothrombin time are the most sensitive in detecting the presence of liver disease. Portal hypertension is by far the most common cause of splenomegaly, and the presence of an enlarged spleen requires that portal hypertension be suspected. The presence of portal hypertension can be confirmed by measuring the wedged hepatic vein pressure. This is usually measured while obtaining a mesenteric angiogram. However, wedged hepatic vein pressure does not reflect portal hypertension if the site of obstruction to portal flow is presinusoidal or infrahepatic (extrahepatic). A mesenteric arteriogram will often demonstrate intra-abdominal portosystemic collaterals, such as paraesophageal varices or splenorenal collateral vessels, in addition to confirming the presence of splenomegaly and corkscrew arteries within the liver typical of hepatic cirrhosis.

The definitive diagnosis of gastroesophageal varices as a source of upper gastrointestinal bleeding is usually made by esophagogastroduodenal endoscopy. Endoscopy can also visualize portal hypertensive gastropathy.[14,15] This rather recently recognized form of gastritis is caused by portal hypertension and can be a nonvariceal source of upper gastrointestinal bleeding. The presence of gastroesophageal varices does not, in itself, prove that the varices are the source of bleeding. Only about 50% of patients with cirrhosis develop gastroesophageal varices. Furthermore, only 30–50% of patients with varices actually bleed from their varices. When endoscopy is performed during a bleeding episode, one may see continued oozing or a clot on the varix. These findings confirm the diagnosis of bleeding varices. More commonly, however, the varices have stopped bleeding by the time endoscopy is performed. Usually the presence of varices, together with a history typical of variceal bleeding and the absence of other sources of upper gastrointestinal bleeding, is sufficient to make a diagnosis of bleeding varices.

At times, patients bleed slowly from their varices and present with anemia or melena, and only small varices are seen on endoscopy. After a thorough evaluation to rule out other sources of gastrointestinal bleeding, these small varices usually prove to be the source of the cryptogenic hemorrhage. Varices can also form at unusual sites and be a source of gastrointestinal bleeding.[16,17] Unusual sites include the duodenum, the sites of adhesions from previous operations to the bowel and abdominal wall, pericolostomy and peri-ileostomy regions, and, rarely, the ileum, rectum, or bladder. Often, bleeding from varices at unusual sites can be controlled with nonshunt procedures.[16,17]

CHOICE OF THERAPY

The major selection criteria for a specific type of therapy are the patient's hepatic reserve, the presence or absence of active bleeding, the location of the varices, and the patient's response to previous therapeutic interventions. Tables 33.2 and 33.3 list emergent and elective options available for treatment of patients with active or quiescent variceal bleeding. Pertinent current references are included with the tables. Surgical portosystemic shunts are indicated in the following circumstances: (1) failure of sclerotherapy, (2) inability of the patient to cooperate with the follow-up necessary for serial sclerotherapy, (3) bleeding gastric varices that cannot be adequately treated with sclerotherapy, (4) portal hypertensive gastropathy, and (5) unusual sites of bleeding varices which cannot be treated with sclerotherapy or transhepatic embolization. To be candidates for a shunt, patients must have sufficient liver function to tolerate a major operation. Shunts are usually performed in Child-Turcotte class A and B patients and are contraindi-

TABLE 33.2. Acute Variceal Hemorrhage: Options for Treatment

Intravenous pitressin ± nitroglycerin[18]
Intravenous somatostatin[19]
Sclerotherapy[20]
Balloon tamponade[20]
Beta blockers—Propranalol[21]
Percutaneous embolization[22]
Esophageal stapling/transection[23]
Percutaneous intrahepatic shunt[24]
Portosystemic shunts[25]
Liver transplantation[26]

Note: These options are not necessarily listed in order of preference or in the order in which they would be employed. Additional discussion is included in the text and in the listed references.

TABLE 33.3. Elective Treatment of Variceal Bleeding: Options for Treatment

Serial sclerotherapy[27]
Beta blockers—propranalol[21]
Endoscopic ligation of varices[28]
Portosystemic shunt[29]
Percutaneous intrahepatic shunt[24]
Transection procedure (Sugiura)[30]
Devascularization procedure (Tanner)[31]
Splenic transposition[32]
Splenopneumopexy[33]
Liver transplantation[26]

Note: Sugiura and Tanner are the eponyms for the more common types of transection and devascularization operations. Both the text and the listed references provide additional discussion of these options for treatment.

cated for most class C patients. Liver transplantation may be preferable for a few class A and some class B patients if the patient's liver disease is progressive of if such symptoms as pruritis, severe fatigue, or disabling encephalopathy are present. A patent portal, splenic, or superior mesenteric vein of sufficient diameter must be present to perform one of the standard shunts.

A number of nonshunt operations have been utilized to control or prevent recurrent variceal hemorrhage (Tables 33.2, 33.3). The indications for most of these operations are not fully clarified or the results of the procedures have varied so widely that the use of the procedures remains controversial. This is the status of most transection and devascularization procedures, such as the Sugiura and Tanner operations. Recently, there has been a renewed interest in splenic transposition and splenopneumopexy. These two procedures are designed to divert portal blood and thus relieve portal hypertension through the spleen after transposing it into the chest above the diaphragm and, in the case of splenopneumopexy, also suturing the spleen to the lung. Percutaneous embolization of the coronary vein has not been effective in halting hemorrhage permanently, but more recent reports utilizing more extensive embolization in combination with splenectomy have been more encouraging. Several groups are investigating the effectiveness of the percutaneously placed intrahepatic shunt. The shunt is placed percutaneously through either the jugular vein or the femoral vein. An opening is made within the liver between a branch of the portal vein and a branch of the hepatic vein. An 8- to 10-mm stent is placed across the opening to maintain the patency of the shunt. These shunts have been used successfully to halt acute variceal hemorrhage, both as a bridge to transplantation and as definitive treatment to prevent recurrent hemorrhage. The stented shunt has been demonstrated to remain patent reliably for several months, but obviously long-term follow-up is needed to determine if these shunts should be utilized as a definitive permanent treatment for bleeding varices.

EMERGENT, URGENT, AND ELECTIVE SHUNTS

There is an important distinction between an emergent shunt and an urgent shunt. A true *emergent* shunt is one that is performed promptly after the patient presents with acute variceal bleeding. If emergent shunts are routinely performed, the treatment group will include Child-Turcotte class A, B, and C patients. The class A and B patients will do well, but the class C patients will have a high mortality. Today, acute variceal hemorrhage is controlled in most of these patients with a combination of intravenous vasopressin, sclerotherapy, and balloon tamponade. An *urgent* shunt is one that is performed after an initial attempt to stop hemorrhage by nonoperative means. Usually several days will have elapsed before deciding to perform an urgent decompressive procedure, and the patient's general condition may have deteriorated. In general, nonoperative attempts to halt hemorrhage will be more successful in patients with better residual liver function. Thus, the process of attempting to halt hemorrhage selects those patients with the poorest liver function who eventually require an urgent shunt. Operative mortalities of up to 70% are reported in this group. Elective shunts are those performed after acute variceal hemorrhage has been halted and recurrent hemorrhage prevented for a sufficient length of time for the patient to have recovered from the insult of the acute hemorrhage. These patients are also self-selected, since many of those who initially entered the hospital with variceal hemorrhage will have died. Modern therapy, with the possible exception of liver transplantation, has not significantly changed the prognosis for patients entering the hospital with acute variceal hemorrhage. From 40 to 60% of these patients will die during hospitalization after the hemorrhage. Thus, those who survive are self-selected, probably because of their better liver function, and may also tolerate operations and other interventions with less mortality and morbidity compared to the entire group initially admitted to the hospital with acute variceal hemorrhage. Patients who survive a portosystemic shunt operation are also self-selected (Figure 33.2). Usually those with poorer liver function are the ones who die in the early postoperative period. Those who survive the operation have a reasonable long-term prognosis regardless of their Child-Turcotte preoperative risk classification. Some clinicians have recommended that all patients with bleeding varices uncontrolled by nonoperative methods undergo an emergent or urgent portacaval shunt, since some of these patients will be salvaged. These distinctions are important both in selecting the type of therapy for an individual patient and in evaluating the results of the therapy reported in the literature.

CATEGORIES OF SHUNTS

Shunts can be categorized according to their hemodynamic characteristics (Table 33.4). End-to-side portacaval shunts, (category I shunts), divert all blood around the liver and prevent blood from leaving the liver through the hepatic limb of the portal vein. Most surgeons active in this field believe that this type of shunt is the least desirable of those available because the liver is deprived of all portal blood and the risk of accelerating progressive hepatic insufficiency is increased. Ligating the hepatic limb of the portal vein during the construction of an end-to-side shunt may decrease the incremental hepatic artery blood flow which frequently occurs after construction of a shunt. The magnitude of incremental hepatic artery blood flow after construction of a portosystemic shunt has been demonstrated to correlate with survival. The blood exiting the liver through the hepatic limb of the portal vein also has a lower pO_2 and lower concentrations of other metabolites than the hepatic artery blood. This indicates that blood exiting via the portal vein has been used as a nutrient by hepatic cells. Side-to-side shunts or modifications thereof (category II lateral shunts) all have an anastomosis or conduit interposed between the splanchnic and systemic venous systems while maintaining a patent hepatic limb of

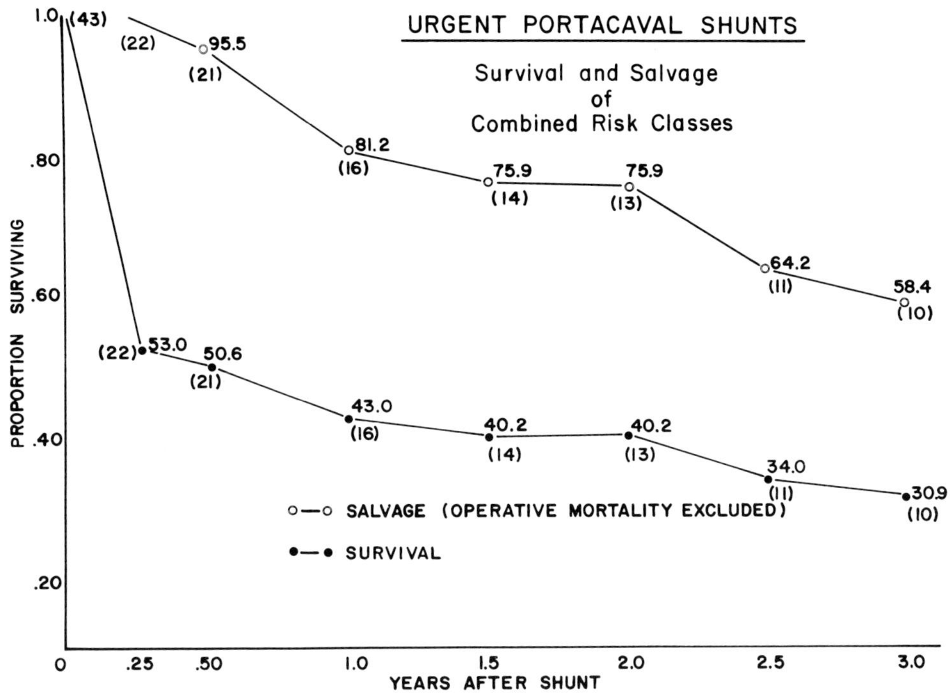

Figure 33.2. Actuarial survival of patients after construction of emergent and urgent portacaval shunts. Child-Turcotte A, B and C risk classes have been combined. Most were class C. The lower curve includes operative mortality and the upper curve excludes operative mortality. Those patients who are alive three months after the operation have a relatively good long-term prognosis, with a three-year actuarial survival of 58.4% regardless of their preoperative risk classification. See text for explanation.

TABLE 33.4. Hemodynamic Categories of Shunts

I. End-to-side portacaval[34]

II. Side-to-side and interposition portacaval[34]
- Portarenal[35]
- Interposition mesocaval[36]
- Marion-Clatworthy cavomesal[37]
- Central splenorenal[38]

III. Distal splenorenal[39]
- With splenopancreatic disconnection[40]
- Splenocaval modification[41]

Small-diameter shunts
- Interposition portacaval[42]
- Small diameter side-to-side portacaval[43]
- Small diameter mesocaval[44]
- Coronary-caval (Inokuchi)[45]

Note: See text for explanation. Pertinent current references are listed. Other types of shunts have also been described, but these are not employed with any frequency and most have a tendency to thrombose.

the portal vein. All lateral shunts are constructed within a few centimeters of the confluens of the splenic, superior mesenteric, and portal veins. Most of these shunts are totally diverting. These shunts may not be totally diverting if the anastomosis or conduit has a small diameter, if the veins used for the anastomosis are small in diameter or become kinked in the process of constructing a shunt, or if the shunts are performed more peripherally in the splanchnic venous system. For instance, a mesocaval shunt which interposes a conduit between the vena cava and a branch of the superior mesenteric vein, rather than of the main superior mesenteric vein, may not be totally diverting, but also may not prevent variceal hemorrhage as reliably.

The Category III shunts are the so-called selective shunts. These include the distal splenorenal shunt and its modifications, and the small-diameter side-to-side portacaval, interposition portacaval, and mesocaval shunts (Table 33.4). Selective shunts are preferred by many surgeons because gastroesophageal varices are selectively decompressed, while portal blood flow to the liver is maintained. Most prospective randomized studies have demonstrated that less encephalopathy occurs after a selective distal splenorenal shunt compared to a totally diverting shunt. Two recent prospectively randomized studies, however, did not show a difference in encephalopathy.[46,47] All studies show no significant differences in postoperative mortality or long-term survival when comparing selective and nonselective shunts. The major determinant of long-term survival is the natural history of the underlying liver disease, not the type of shunt unless the shunt itself accelerates the progression of hepatic decompensation. There are little data available to suggest that one type of selective shunt is preferable to another. Warren and colleagues have claimed that patients with alcoholic cirrhosis do better with the distal splenorenal shunt combined with splenopancreatic disconnection, but their patients have not been randomized and this observation has not been confirmed by others.

SELECTION OF SHUNTS

When operating in emergent or urgent circumstances, the surgeon should select a shunt which can be constructed expeditiously. Interposition mesocaval or side-to-side portacaval shunts are commonly selected, but some who have become very proficient at performing distal splenorenal shunts recommend this shunt even for emergent portal decompression.[25] The distal splenorenal shunt operation has the potential disadvantage of requiring more time to perform, and this shunt is not as reliable for immediately halting variceal hemorrhage.

A selective shunt is preferred in elective circumstances, provided that no contraindication is present. The distal splenorenal shunt is an "ascitogenic" operation, that is, it induces the formation of ascites in many patients. This can be a serious problem in the early postoperative period. For this reason, this shunt is contraindicated unless ascites can easily be controlled preoperatively. If the ascites disappears on a 40- to 70-mEq sodium per day diet and no more than 50 mg of spironolactone tid is required, a distal splenorenal shunt is recommended. If a more intense diuretic regimen is required, one of the lateral shunts, such as the side-to-side portacaval, portarenal, or mesocaval shunt, is advocated. We have also had good results with the small-diameter interposition portacaval shunt when used electively and when ascites it is not a major problem.[6] The presence of hepatofugal flow preoperatively is usually also considered a contraindication to performing a selective shunt. The reasoning is that one of the major rationales for performing a selective shunt is to preserve hepatopetal flow. Thus, although no comparative data have been published, it does not seem logical to choose this particular type of shunt when portal blood already flows away from the liver. Good results have been reported with the distal splenorenal shunt in the presence of a thrombosed portal vein.

Another important consideration in shunt selection is the likelihood that a patient may require a liver transplant in the future.[26] The major consideration is to avoid dissection in the area of the hepatic trinity and subhepatic space. Although previous right upper quadrant surgery is no longer considered a contraindication to liver transplantation, the presence of adhesions and an accompanying venous collateral in the area of the porta hepatis considerably complicates the performance of a transplant. The usual recommendation is to construct a distal splenorenal shunt in elective circumstances and a mesocaval shunt in emergent or urgent circumstances when there is a significant probability that a liver transplant may be required in the future. Usually these shunts are dismantled at the time of the liver transplant in order to maximize hepatopetal portal flow to the new liver.

ANATOMICAL CONSIDERATIONS

Standard hepatic arterial anatomy is present in only approximately 55% of patients. Total or partial replacement of the right hepatic artery to the superior mesenteric artery occurs in 18% of patients. This artery courses beneath the head of the pancreas and behind the common bile duct (Figure 33.3). The portal vein usually crosses anterior to the artery. Because of its location, the artery may be easily damaged when skeletonizing the portal vein to construct a portacaval shunt. In addition, if an end-to-side or side-to-side portacaval shunt is fashioned, the portal vein may be kinked as it passes over the replaced right hepatic artery when the portal vein is displaced for anastomosis to the vena cava.[48] Thus effective portal decompression is not achieved even though the anastomosis itself may appear technically very adequate. We usually avoid performing a portacaval shunt when a replaced right hepatic artery is demonstrated on a preoperative mesenteric angiogram. In 25% of patients there is total or partial replacement of the left hepatic artery to the left gastric artery. If the left gastric artery is ligated as part of a devascularization procedure or when performing a distal splenorenal shunt, the arterial supply to an already diseased liver may be compromised. This could be detrimental to the patient, especially if liver function is already marginal or flow in the portal vein is already reversed.

There is also considerable anatomical variation of the splanchnic venous system. Some patients do not have a single superior mesenteric vein trunk but have several mesenteric branches, which the splenic vein joins to form a portal vein. These patients are usually not good candidates for any shunt utilizing the mesenteric vein. If one uses a branch of the mesenteric vein, portal decompression may not be sufficient to prevent variceal hemorrhage and the shunt is more prone to thrombosis.

There are several other important anatomical considerations pertinent to shunt selection. The patient must have an adequate portal, splenic, or superior mesenteric vein. In 10–20% of patients with cirrhosis, one or more of these veins is thrombosed preoperatively. In other patients, one of these veins may be absent or of inadequate diameter. A splenic vein at least 7 mm and optimally 10 mm in diameter is preferred to perform an adequate distal splenorenal shunt. Likewise, the left renal vein should be visualized preoperatively if one is planning to shunt blood through the renal vein to the vena cava. Renal veins may be small, aberrant, retroaortic, or of the H type; usually such veins are

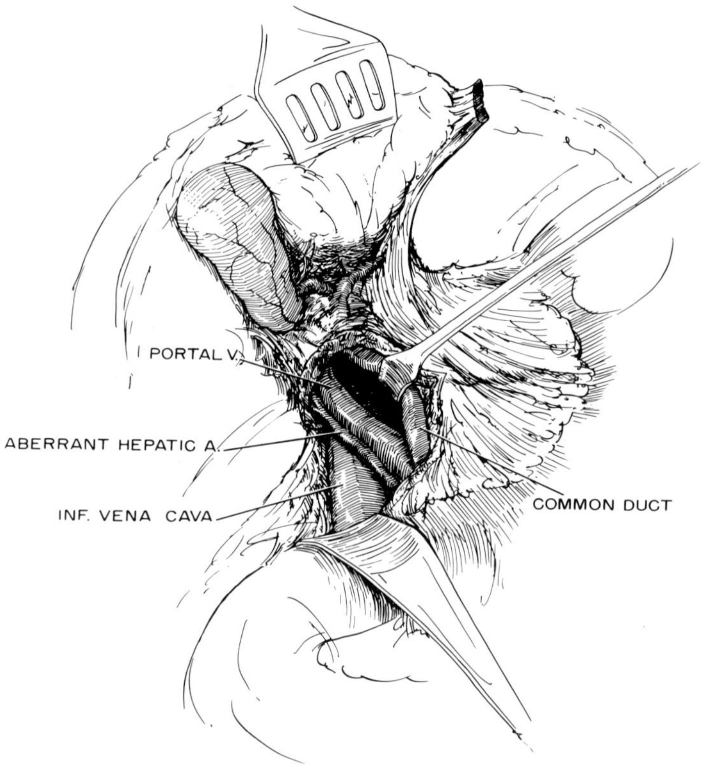

Figure 33.3. Replaced right hepatic artery. The replaced artery originates from the side of the superior mesenteric artery, courses behind the head of the pancreas, and then courses behind the common bile duct. This artery may be injured while dissecting within the hepatic trinity. When attempting to construct an end-to-side or side-to-side portacaval shunt, the portal vein may be kinked by the aberrant hepatic artery when the vein is displaced toward the vena cava to construct the shunt and adequate portal decompression may not be achieved.

not suitable for anastomosis. Rarely, the portal vein courses anterior to the pancreas and, in this circumstance, precludes construction of a portacaval shunt. Side-to-side portacaval shunts are very difficult or sometimes impossible to perform in the presence of an enlarged caudate lobe of the liver. Usually, one should select another type of shunt and avoid the blood loss associated with resection of this lobe to facilitate construction of a portacaval shunt. Because of the frequent variations and anomalies of hepatic arteries, splanchnic veins, and renal veins, a mesenteric angiogram is a very important preoperative study that assists in the selection of the appropriate type of shunt for an individual patient.

SPECIFIC TYPES OF SHUNTS AND TECHNICAL CONSIDERATIONS

Most of the dissection and anastomoses for the major types of shunts are performed in the central portion of the upper abdomen. An incision which gives generous exposure to this area is appropriate. For thin individuals with an acutely angled costal margin, a midline incision gives good exposure if a strong upper abdominal retractor is used to spread the margins of the incision. The retractor converts the vertical incision into a transverse exposure. In heavy-set individuals or those with a broad costal margin angle, either a generous right subcostal or a bilateral subcostal incision should be used. A fixed upper abdominal retractor such as an upper hand, Rochard, or Buckwalter retractor greatly facilitates exposure. With the availability of strong fixed retractors, a thoracoabdominal incision is not necessary even when performing a central splenorenal shunt.

We have found certain maneuvers helpful when isolating the portal vein to construct a portacaval shunt. Usually a patent portal vein can be palpated within the trinity. The peritoneum on the inferior or posterior margin of the trinity is incised and the surface of the vein exposed. We avoid skeletonizing the common bile duct. In patients with cirrhosis the wall of the bile duct may be very thin. Patients with cirrhosis also produce large quantities of bile. With this combination, even a small needle hole in the common duct may produce a persistent leak that may require insertion of a T tube for control. A maximum length of portal vein can be exposed by dividing the peritoneum and sometimes a thin tongue of pancreas which overlies the portal vein as it disappears behind the pancreas. The hepatic end of the portal vein should also be mobilized to above the bifurcation. When constructing a side-to-side portacaval shunt the clamp on the vena cava should be placed parallel to the portal vein. No margins from the posterior portion of the anastomosis should be excised from either the cava or portal vein, but a fairly generous margin of tissue should be trimmed from the anterior side of the anastomosis to provide for an adequately sized anastomosis (Figure 33.4). In adults the incision in the portal vein and cava should be 2 to 2.5 cm long. Recently, a small-diameter anastomosis has been advocated, with the goal of maintaining perfusion of the liver with portal blood.[43]

When constructing an interposition mesocaval shunt, the second and third portions of the duodenum and often at least a portion of the right colon should be fully mobilized medially. The third portion of the duodenum must also be mobilized superiorly to provide a generous exposure of the vena cava. Usually a C-type shunt, as described by Lillemoe and Cameron,[36] is necessary to anastomose the graft to the main trunk of the superior mesenteric vein (Figure 33.5). Depending upon the anatomy present, we fashion this anastomosis on the anterior or lateral border of the main trunk of the superior mesenteric vein. The mesenteric vein must be mobilized as it passes over the anterior surface of the uncinate process of the pancreas to the point where it disappears behind the neck of the pancreas to expose sufficient main trunk of superior mesenteric vein. Originally, 18- to 20-mm-diameter grafts were recommended. Recently, smaller ringed grafts measuring 12–14 mm in diameter have been used. With the smaller grafts, the mesocaval shunt may be partially selective and may allow some portal blood to continue to perfuse the liver.[44]

Sclerotherapy is very effective in most infants and children for preventing variceal bleeding.[49] Successful prophylaxis against recurrent hemorrhage has been reported in over 90% of patients in some series. If a shunt is needed, consideration should be given to constructing an interposition mesocaval shunt utilizing the internal jugular vein.[50] In children the jugular vein is relatively large compared to that of adults. In addition, the distance between the superior mesenteric vein and the vena cava is less. Use of a plastic prosthesis and the necessity of dividing the vena cava, an essential step in the construction of a Marion-Clatworthy mesocaval shunt, are thus avoided. Several European centers have reported excellent results with the jugular vein interposition mesocaval shunt.

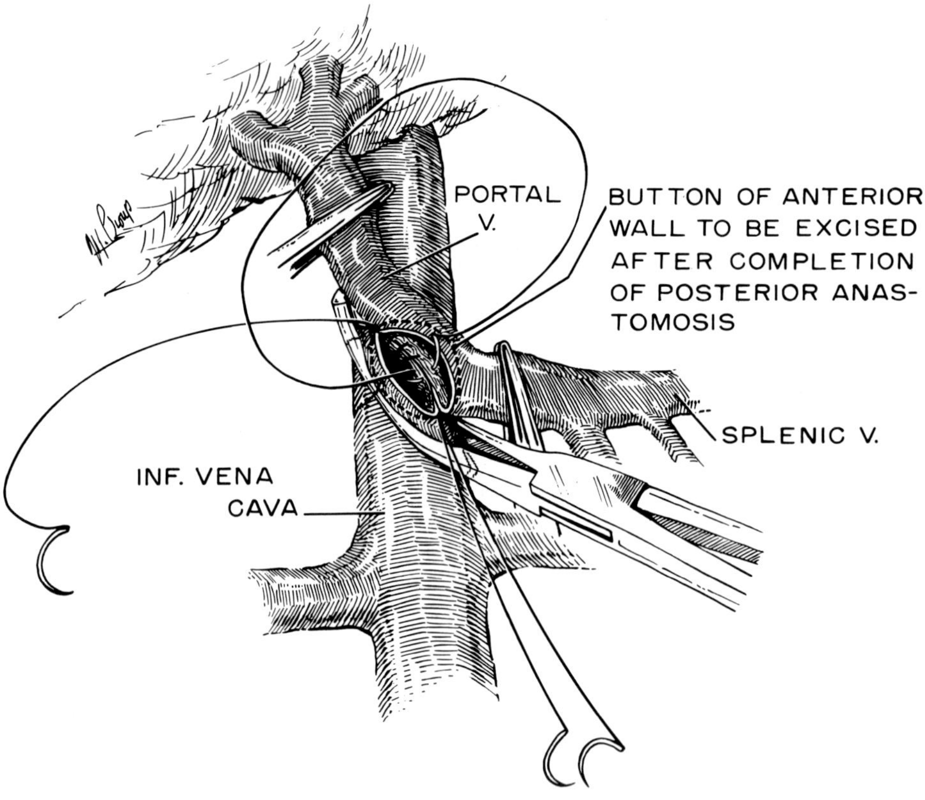

Figure 33.4. Construction of a side-to-side portacaval shunt. The vascular clamp on the vena cava has been placed parallel to the portal vein. No vein wall is excised from the posterior rim of the anastomosis. Excising a crescent of vein wall from the anterior rim of the anastomosis helps provide for a generous anastomotic ostium.

A distal splenorenal shunt can be fashioned with minimal blood loss if the dissection is precise. There are usually fewer collateral veins in the retropancreatic area than are encountered when constructing a portacaval or mesocaval shunt. The splenic artery may be encircled as it passes along the superior margin of the pancreas and temporarily occluded with a Rummel sling. This decreases the pressure in the splenic vein and facilitates dissection of this vein. An effort should be made to separate the portal-superior mesenteric vein side of the splanchnic system completely from the left side of the system (splenic and short gastric veins). This is accomplished by devascularizing the greater curve of the stomach from the pylorus to the first short gastric vein. The branches of the gastroepiploic vessels are divided adjacent to the greater curve of the stomach, leaving the gastroepiploic artery and vein intact to vascularize the omentum. The left side of the omentum is divided vertically from the area of the first short gastric vein on the stomach down to the superior surface of the left transverse colon. The splenic vein is mobilized from the junction of the superior mesenteric vein until it disappears behind the tail of the pancreas. We do not routinely perform a complete splenopancreatic dissection as described. The left renal vein is most easily located as it crosses anteriorly over the aorta.

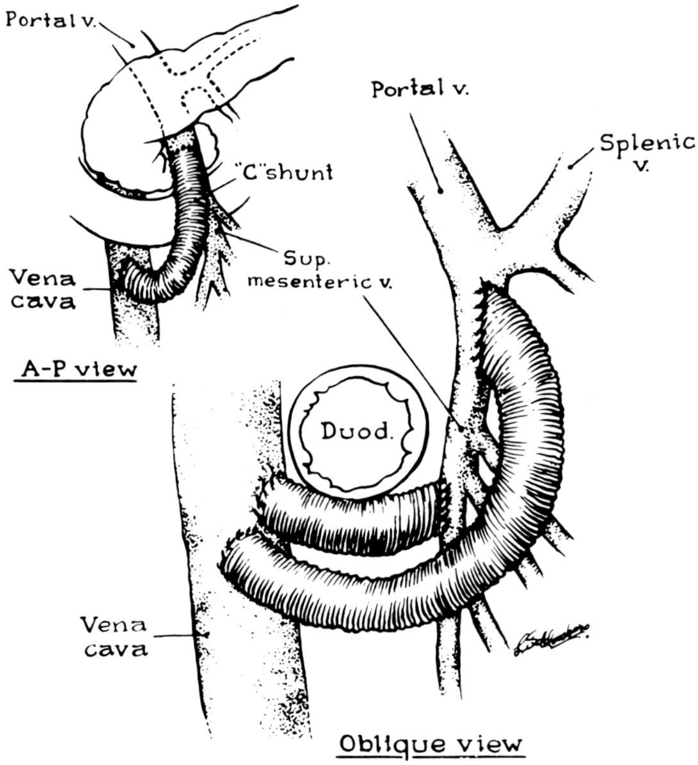

Figure 33.5. Relative positions of the interposed prosthesis with the mesocaval H-shunt and the mesocaval C-shunt. The C-shunt is usually preferable because it allows anastomosis to the main trunk of the superior mesenteric vein. (Reprinted with permission from Lillemoe KD, Cameron JL: The interposition mesocaval shunt. *Surg Clin North Am* 70:379–393, 1990.)

The left renal vein is completely mobilized from the cava to near the hilum of the kidney; this usually requires division of both the left gonadal and adrenal veins. The lymphatic tissue comprising the roof of the tunnel behind the superior mesenteric artery through which the left renal vein courses should be divided to ensure that the renal vein will not kink on the tunnel roof after the shunt is fashioned. The devascularization of the stomach is completed by bluntly mobilizing the left gastric pedicle behind the stomach. This pedicle contains both the coronary vein, the left gastric artery, and their branches. The pedicle is doubly ligated but not divided. If the coronary vein has joined the splenic vein, it should also be ligated in the course of mobilizing the splenic vein. If the devascularization of the stomach has been adequate, usually the upper third or half of the stomach appears gray and somewhat ischemic, but this has not led to ischemic ulcers, gastritis, or other problems.

The portarenal shunt is a technically convenient type of shunt to perform as an alternative to a side-to-side portacaval or interposition portacaval shunt[35] (Figure 33.6). The vena cava and left renal vein can be mobilized from the right side of the abdomen after performing a Kocher maneuver. A thin retractor, such as a Dever retractor, can be inserted anterior to the left renal vein to elevate the superior mesenteric vessels and help

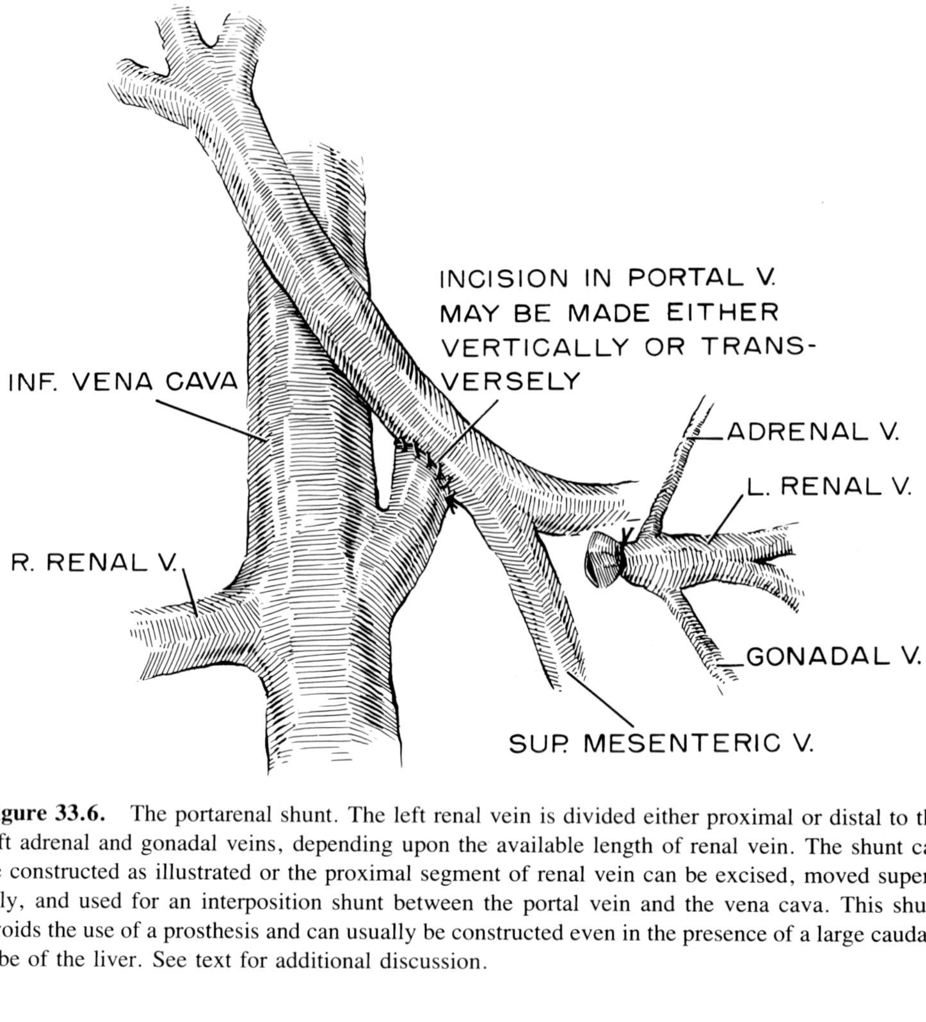

Figure 33.6. The portarenal shunt. The left renal vein is divided either proximal or distal to the left adrenal and gonadal veins, depending upon the available length of renal vein. The shunt can be constructed as illustrated or the proximal segment of renal vein can be excised, moved superiorly, and used for an interposition shunt between the portal vein and the vena cava. This shunt avoids the use of a prosthesis and can usually be constructed even in the presence of a large caudate lobe of the liver. See text for additional discussion.

visualize the left gonadal and adrenal veins. Usually it is best to divide one or both of these tributaries to obtain a sufficient length of renal vein. The left vein can then simply be turned superiorly and anastomosed to the underside of the portal vein, or the entire segment of vein can be excised and used as an interposition graft between the cava and the portal vein. Division of the left renal vein, especially in a patient with portal hypertension, does not have any lasting detrimental effect on kidney function. Serial intravenous pyelograms suggest some diminution in the function of the left kidney for approximately one week. The right renal vein cannot be divided without serious consequence to the right kidney.

As discussed previously, there are few indications for an end-to-side portacaval shunt. There are also few indications for a central splenorenal shunt.[38] This shunt may be chosen if a concomitant splenectomy is necessary. It can also be constructed without removing the spleen. In children, sclerotherapy and the jugular vein interposition mesocaval shunt have largely supplanted the use of the Marion-Clatworthy shunt.

We recommend measuring the pressure gradient across the newly constructed portosystemic shunt before closing the abdomen. The splanchnic venous system is a low-pressure system, so that even small kinks or technical problems with the anastomosis can significantly compromise portal decompression. The simplest technique for measuring pressure is to place a purse-string suture in a convenient area of vein adjacent to the shunt. A small polyethylene catheter can then be placed through the purse string across the shunt anastomosis. With a water manometer, pressures can be measured on either side of the shunt. If necessary, an operative venogram can be obtained through the catheter.

COMPLICATIONS

The usual complications associated with any major abdominal operation occur after constructing a portosystemic shunt. Patients with cirrhosis have compromised immune systems and are more prone to develop all types of infections. Other complications which tend to occur in patients requiring portosystemic shunts are continued variceal or intra-abdominal bleeding, excessive ascites formation, progressive hepatic insufficiency and encephalopathy, and shunt stenosis or thrombosis.

The two most important measures to avoid intra-abdominal bleeding are adequate hemostasis during the operation and generous replacement of coagulation factors. Electrocoagulation of bleeding points is not as reliable in patients with cirrhosis and portal hypertension as in patients with normal portal pressures and normal livers. Fresh frozen plasma, cryoprecipitate, and platelets should be administered during the operation in a prophylactic manner. If one attempts to correct coagulation deficiencies after they have become severe, usually more blood products are needed than if the deficiency was prevented. Likewise, coagulation factors should be monitored and replaced generously for the first 24–48 hours postoperatively. The levels of factor V or VII are better indicators of the need for fresh frozen plasma than the prothrombin time or partial thromboplastin time. Intraoperatively, most significant bleeding points should be ligated.

Fluid and electrolyte administration must be carefully monitored and the administration of sodium and potassium modified when cirrhosis is present. Estimated third space losses should be replaced conservatively so as not to administer excessive sodium. We often replace third space losses with half-strength saline, containing 77 mEq of sodium per liter, rather than lactated Ringer's or normal saline, which contains 130 and 154 mEq of sodium, respectively. After third space losses have been replaced, nonsodium-containing glucose solutions, such as 10% dextrose, are administered. These patients receive significant quantities of sodium from other sources. Most drugs are provided in the sodium salt form, and all blood products contain significant quantities of sodium. Potassium should be monitored and replaced generously if renal function is adequate because patients with cirrhosis frequently have a total body deficit of potassium that may induce or aggravate encephalopathy. Because of the hyperaldosteronism associated with cirrhosis, spironolactone is the diuretic of first choice. Furosemide or other loop diuretics should be used in conjunction with spironolactone and only when spironolactone alone is not sufficient. These measures, as well as attempts to ligate major lymphatic leaks during the operation, usually avoid excessive ascites formation in the early postoperative period. Continuous arteriovenous hemoperfusion, with or without dialysis, is an effective method of managing renal failure, should this occur, and is effective in removing excess fluid. With this treatment, patients can continue to receive blood products and intravenous hyperalimentation as needed.

There is no reliable therapy to treat progressive postoperative hepatic failure except transplantation. Careful attention to fluid and electrolyte balance, and prevention of infection and hemorrhage, are important prophylactic measures to avoid liver failure. Many surgeons administer a glucose-insulin-potassium solution postoperatively to help support the liver, but there is little evidence that this is helpful. Oral lactulose is the most effective drug to treat encephalopathy should it occur. Neomycin should be used with caution because some patients will absorb significant amounts from the gastrointestinal tract, causing nephrotoxicity. Patients with severe hepatic failure are potential candidates for a liver transplant.

Early postoperative shunt thrombosis or significant stenosis usually results in recurrent variceal hemorrhage in the early postoperative period.[51,52] In most series this occurs in only 1 or 2% of patients, especially if adequacy of the shunt has been tested by obtaining intraoperative pressures or portograms. Usually the problem is technical, and an operation should be performed promptly to revise the shunt. In some cases, the shunt can be dilated percutaneously. The late thrombosis rate for distal splenorenal shunts is 2–13% (Table 33.5). Mesocaval shunts, especially if a plastic prosthesis is used, have a late thrombosis rate of 9–20%[6] (Table 33.5). Fortunately not all of these patients develop recurrent bleeding varices, but those who do may require another portosystemic shunt or a liver transplant.

RESULTS

The results of portosystemic shunts can be assessed in terms of recurrent hemorrhage, patient survival, and quality of life measures including the incidence of spontaneous encephalopathy (Table 33.5). Most series report recurrent gastrointestinal hemorrhage rates in the range of 15–35%. This incidence includes variceal hemorrhage, as well as gastritis, ulcer, and other sources of gastrointestinal hemorrhage. Survival of patients varies directly with the etiology and natural history of the primary liver disease and with the hepatic reserve at the time of operation. With class A patients three-year survival rates of 80–90%, and with class B patients 70–75% survival rates, are commonly reported. Survival of class C patients is poor. Given the low operative mortality and good long-term prognosis for class A and B patients, portosystemic shunts are a good choice of therapy for patients in whom sclerotherapy is not feasible or fails, provided that their liver disease is not rapidly progressive and that the symptoms of hepatic insufficiency do not interfere significantly with their quality of life. In most liver transplant series, the two-year patient survival rate approximates 65–70%. For class C patients, survival is clearly superior with liver transplantation compared to any other form of therapy.

CONCLUSIONS

Portosystemic shunt surgery continues to have an important role in the control and prevention of variceal hemorrhage despite the fact that several alternative modes of therapy have evolved in recent years. When feasible, selective shunts are preferred, since

TABLE 33.5. Results of Portosystemic Shunt Surgery

Series	*Type of Shunt*	N	% *Operative Mortality*	% *Actuarial Survival 2 yr*	% *Actuarial Survival 5 yr*	% *Incidence Spontaneous Encephalopathy*	% *Incidence GI Bleeding*	% *Incidence Shunt Thrombosis*
U. of Nebraska[53]	DSRS	23	0	65		16	19	13
Barcelona[54]	DSRS	42	2 to 3	71		24	26	10.5
U. of Southern California[47]	DSRS	26	11.5		46	39	47	7
U. of Southern California[47]	End-to-side porta-caval	27	6.4		31	32	36	3
Emory[40]	DSRS + splenopancreatic disconnection	78	6.4				14	2
	Child A	32		90				
	Child B	25		70				
	Child C	21		50				
Germany[55]	Mesocaval 14–16 mm graft	86	8		70	10		9
	Child A				90			
	Child B				65			
	Child C				60			
U. of South Florida[50]	Small-diameter Interposition	36	11	83 (6–12 month estimate)		11	10	11

Note: All but the study from Emory are the results taken from prospective randomized studies. These studies were selected because the data tend to be more accurate in a prospective study. In a few instances, the numbers were estimated from graphic illustrations and may only be approximate.

DSRS = distal splenorenal shunt

they are associated with a lesser incidence of encephalopathy than totally diverting shunts. In addition to the distal splenorenal shunt, small-diameter side-to-side portacaval, interposition portacaval, and interposition mesocaval shunts also appear to maintain portal perfusion and are associated with less postoperative encephalopathy. If liver transplantation is anticipated in the future, right upper quadrant dissections should be avoided and either a distal splenorenal or a mesocaval shunt constructed. The internal jugular vein interposition mesocaval shunt has proved to be very effective in small children. Currently, there are few circumstances in which a central splenorenal or Marion-Clatworthy mesocaval would be preferred. Although the data are not definitive, most surgeons active in the field of portal hypertension avoid end-to-side portacaval shunts because of concern for a possibly increased incidence of progressive hepatic insufficiency and encephalopathy. Initial results with stented intrahepatic shunts are encouraging, at least for short-term control of variceal hemorrhage. A promising area of investigation is the development of drugs that will reduce portal pressure and thus prevent variceal hemorrhage.

REFERENCES

1. Donovan AJ, Covey PC: Early history of the portacaval shunt in humans. *SGO* 147:423–430, 1978.
2. Whipple AO: Problem of portal hypertension in relation to hepatosplenopathics. *Ann Surg* 122:449–475, 1945.
3. Child CG III: *The Liver and Portal Hypertension*. Philadelphia, WB Saunders Co, 1964.
4. Turcotte JG: Portal hypertension as I see it, in Child CG III (ed): *Portal Hypertension*. Philadelphia, WB Saunders Co, 1974, p 78.
5. Conn HO: A peek at the Child-Turcotte classification. *Hepatology* 1:673–676, 1981.
6. Sarfeh IJ, Rypins EB, Mason GR: A systemic appraisal of portacaval H-graft diameters: Clinical and hemodynamic perspectives. *Ann Surg* 204:356–363, 1986.
7. Johnston GW, Rodgers HW: A review of 15 years' experience in the use of sclerotherapy in the control of acute haemorrhage from oesophageal varices. *Br J Surg* 60:797–800, 1973.
8. Calne RY, Rolles K, White DGJ, et al: Cyclosporin A initially as the only immunosuppressant in 34 recipients of cadaveric organs: 32 kidneys, 2 pancreases, and 2 livers. *Lancet* 2:1033–1036, 1979.
9. Richter GM, Noeldge G, Palmaz JC, et al: The transjugular intrahepatic portosystemic stent-shunt (TIPSS): Results of a pilot study. *Cardiovasc Intervent Radiol* 13:200–207, 1990.
10. Zemel G, Katzen BT, Becker GJ, et al: Percutaneous transjugular portosystemic shunt. *JAMA* 266:390–393, 1991.
11. Benoit JN, Granger DN: Splanchnic hemodynamics in chronic portal hypertension. *Semin Liver Dis* 6:287, 1986.
12. Reichen J: Liver function and pharmacological considerations in pathogenesis and treatment of portal hypertension. *Hepatology* 11:1066–1078, 1990.
13. Stanley MM: Pathogenesis of ascites in cirrhosis: A unitary hypothesis. *ASAIO Trans* 35:161–163, 1989.
14. McCormack TT, Sims J, Eyre-Brook I, et al: Gastric lesions in portal hypertension: Inflammatory gastritis or congestive gastropathy? *Gut* 26:1226–1232, 1985.
15. Sarfeh IJ, Juler GL, Stemmer EA, et al: Results of surgical management of hemorrhagic gastritis in patients with gastroesophageal varices. *SGO* 155:167–170, 1982.

16. Osaki CK, Hansen M, Kadir S: Transhepatic embolization of superior mesenteric varices in portal hypertension. *Surgery* 105:446–448, 1989.
17. Mosquera DA, Walker SJ, McFarland JB: Bleeding stomal varices treated by sclerotherapy. *J R Coll Surg Edinb* 33:337, 1988.
18. Sirinek KR, Adcock DK, Levine BA: Simultaneous infusion of nitroglycerin and nitroprusside to offset adverse effects of vasopressin during portosystemic shunting. *Am J Surg* 157:33–37, 1989.
19. Morgan JS, Groszmann RJ: Somatostatin in portal hypertension. *Dig Dis Sci* 34(Suppl):40S–47S, 1989.
20. Moreto M, Zaballa M, Bernal A, et al: A randomized trial of tamponade or sclerotherapy as immediate treatment for bleeding esophageal varices. *SGO* 167:331–334, 1988.
21. Hayes PC, Davis JM, Lewis JA: Meta-analysis of value of propranolol in prevention of variceal hemorrhage. *Lancet* 336:153–156, 1990.
22. Durham JD, Van Stiegmann G: Direct catheterization of the mesenteric vein: Combined surgical and radiologic approach to the treatment of variceal hemorrhage. *Radiology* 177:229–233, 1990.
23. Wexler MJ, Stein BL: Nonshunting operations for variceal hemorrhage. *Surg Clin North Am* 70:425–448, 1990.
24. Richter GM, Noeldge G, Palmaz JC: Transjugular intrahepatic portacaval stent shunt: Preliminary clinical results. *Radiology* 174:1027–1030, 1990.
25. Mitchell RL, Ignatius JA: Distal splenorenal shunt: Standard procedure for elective and emergency treatment of bleeding esophageal varices. *Am J Surg* 156:169–172, 1988.
26. Wood RP, Shaw BW Jr, Rikkers LF: Liver transplantation for variceal hemorrhage. *Surg Clin North Am* 70:449–461, 1990.
27. Terblanche J, Kahn D, Bornman PC: Long-term injection sclerotherapy treatment for esophageal varices: A 10-year prospective evaluation. *Ann Surg* 210:725–731, 1989.
28. Saeed ZA, Michaletz PA, Winchester CB, et al: Endoscopic variceal ligation in patients who have failed endoscopic sclerotherapy. *Gastrointest Endosc* 36:572–574, 1990.
29. Rikkers LF: Definitive therapy for variceal bleeding: A personal view. *Am J Surg* 160:80–85, 1990.
30. Idezuki Y, Sanjyo K: Twenty-five-year experiences with esophageal transection for esophageal varices. *J Thorac Cardiovasc Surg* 98:876–883, 1989.
31. Bardot DJ, Rosato EF: Experience with the esophagogastric devascularization procedure. *Surgery* 101:685–690, 1987.
32. Turcotte JG, O'Neal RM, Zuidema GD, et al: The effect of splenic transposition on portal circulation. *J Surg Res* 1:299–306, 1961.
33. Akita H, Sakoda K: Portopulmonary shunt by splenopneumopexy as a surgical treatment of Budd-Chiari syndrome. *Surgery* 87:85–94, 1980.
34. Levine BA, Sirinek KR: The portacaval shunt: Is it still indicated? *Surg Clin North Am* 70:361–378, 1990.
35. Simeone FA, Hopkins RW: Portarenal shunt for hepatic cirrhosis and portal hypertension. *Surgery* 61:153–168, 1967.
36. Lillemoe KD, Cameron JL: The interposition mesocaval shunt. *Surg Clin North Am* 70:379–393, 1990.
37. Lambert MJ, Tank ES, Turcotte JG: Late sequela of mesocaval shunts in children. *Am J Surg* 127:19–24, 1974.
38. Fischer JE, Bower RH, Atamian S, et al: Comparison of distal and proximal splenorenal shunts: A randomized prospective trial. *Ann Surg* 194:531–544, 1981.

39. Henderson JM, Millikan WJ Jr, Galloway JR: The Emory perspective of the distal splenorenal shunt in 1990. *Am J Surg* 160:54–59, 1990.

40. Henderson JM, Millikan WJ, Galloway JR: Distal splenorenal shunt with splenopancreatic disconnection: A 4-year assessment. *Ann Surg* 210:332–341, 1989.

41. Atta HM, Henderson JM, Galloway JR: Selective splenocaval shunt: Report of 26 cases and review of the literature. *Arch Surg* 126:582–585, 1991.

42. Rypins EB, Sarfeh IJ: Small-diameter portacaval H-graft for variceal hemorrhage. *Surg Clin North Am* 70:395–404, 1990.

43. Chabert M, Page Y, Cadi F, et al: Calibrated side-to-side portacaval anastomosis in the treatment of bleeding from ruptured esophageal varices. Results in 38 cirrhotic patients. *Gastroenterol Clin Biol* 14:698–704, 1990.

44. Mercado MA, Paquet KJ, Klingele H, et al: Portal perfusion following selective and non-selective diversions in portal hypertension. *Rev Gastroenterol Mex* 56:3–6, 1991.

45. Inokuchi K, Sugimachi K: The selective shunt for variceal bleeding: A personal perspective. *Am J Surg* 160:48–53, 1990.

46. Grace ND, Conn HO, Resnick RH: Distal splenorenal vs portal-systemic shunts after hemorrhage from varices: A randomized controlled trial. *Hepatology* 8:1475–1481, 1988.

47. Harley HAJ, Morgan T, Redeker AC: Results of a randomized trial of end-to-side portacaval shunt and distal splenorenal shunt in alcoholic liver disease and variceal bleeding. *Gastroenterology* 91:802–809, 1986.

48. Eckhauser FE, Strodel WE, Thompson NW, et al: Technical dilemmas in portacaval shunt operations as a consequence of replaced right hepatic artery. *Surg Gynecol Obstet* 151:533–537, 1980.

49. Fonkalsrud EW: Treatment of variceal hemorrhage in children. *Surg Clin North Am* 70:475–487, 1990.

50. Gauthier F, De Dreuzy O, Valayer J, et al: H-type shunt with an autologous venous graft for treatment of portal hypertension in children. *J Pediatr Surg* 24:1041–1043, 1989.

51. Eckhauser FE, Pomerantz RA, Knol JA: Early variceal rebleeding after successful distal splenorenal shunt. *Arch Surg* 121:547–552, 1986.

52. Levine BA, Sirinek KR: Variceal rebleeding after portosystemic shunting. *Surg Clin North Am* 71:117–129, 1991.

53. Rikkers LF, Burnett DA, Volentine GD: Shunt surgery versus endoscopic sclerotherapy for long-term treatment of variceal bleeding. *Ann Surg* 206:261–271, 1987.

54. Teres J, Bordas JM, Bravo D: Sclerotherapy vs. distal splenorenal shunt in the elective treatment of variceal hemorrhage: A randomized controlled trial. *Hepatology* 7:430–436, 1987.

55. Paquet K-J, Kalk J-F, Koussouris P: Prospective evaluation and long-term results of mesocaval interposition shunts. *Acta Chir Scand* 153:423–429, 1987.

56. Rosemurgy AS, McAllister EW, Kearney RE: Prospective study of a prosthetic H-graft portacaval shunt. *Am J Surg* 161:159–164, 1991.

34

STAPLER ESOPHAGEAL TRANSECTION

Yasuo Idezuki, M.D.

CONCEPT OF TRANSECTION AND DEVASCULARIZATION PROCEDURES

The concept of direct nonshunting operations for controlling acute bleeding from esophagogastric varices is not new. Blain, in 1918, proposed splenic artery ligation for portal hypertension and bleeding varices.[1] Pemberton and Kiernan, in 1945, suggested that this procedure was ineffective because 53% of their patients developed rebleeding after splenic artery ligation.[2] Walters et al., in 1927,[3] proposed ligation of coronary veins for bleeding esophageal varices. Since that time, many direct procedures have been proposed and performed. Womack and Peters first proposed a more extensive devascularization procedure consisting of splenectomy; ligation of the splenic, left and right gastroepiploic, and right gastric vasculature; omentectomy; and resection of the greater gastric curvature.[4] They noted an excellent short-term benefit but were frustrated by later collateralization and rebleeding. The frequent incidence of recurrent bleeding from varices after devascularization procedures, and the introduction of portal decompression procedures in the 1940s, discouraged the use of these direct operations, which were only sporadically performed as emergency operations in acute bleeders. Dumont and coworkers in 1972, however, noted that patients with splenic arteries measuring more than 9 mm in diameter stopped bleeding from esophageal varices acutely after percutaneous balloon occlusion of the splenic artery, thereby avoiding general anesthesia during the acute bleed.[5]

Indeed, a more recent follow-up on the Womack and Peters devascularization procedure questions the value of this procedure, since most patients develop collaterals and rebleed.[6]

In the early 1960s, Walker[7,8] reported the results of transthoracic esophageal transection. Although he seriously questioned the long-term efficacy of this procedure, the preliminary results were encouraging enough to stimulate further study. Subsequently, the techniques of direct operations for esophageal varices have matured and the extent of devascularization has increased.

The original concept of the direct approach to esophagogastric varices was to block all blood flow to the varices in the esophagocardiac region. As the knowledge of collateral circulation in portal hypertension accumulated, it became apparent that much wider devascularization was necessary and essential in order to effectively block the blood inflow to the varices. Also, prevention of cephalad blood flow within the wall of the cardiac region of the stomach mandates transection of the esophagus just above the esophagocardiac junction. Following animal experimentation to confirm the safety of extensive devascularization of the upper gastric and lower esophageal regions in conjunction with transection of the esophagus, this procedure was applied to patients.[9] This combined approach to esophageal varices became widely known as the *University of Tokyo method* or the *Sugiura procedure*.[10]

The objective of the Sugiura procedure is to block all blood inflow to the varices in the esophagocardiac region. Multiple studies have shown that this is best achieved by complete devascularization of the upper half of the stomach and the lower esophagus up to the level of the left pulmonary vein. Since complete devascularization of the lower esophagus up to the left pulmonary level may be achieved only by a transthoracic approach, the thoracoabdominal approach was used originally in the Sugiura procedure.[10] In low-risk patients (Child's A category), one-stage thoracoabdominal transection and devascularization are well tolerated; in many higher-risk patients (Child's B and C categories), it is necessary to perform these procedures in two stages (staged operations). When employing the two-stage approach, the thoracic procedure with devascularization of the lower esophagus and transection of the esophagus is done first. The second-stage abdominal procedure with splenectomy, devascularization of the stomach, and pyloroplasty is performed approximately one month later.

Avoiding the additive hazards of staged operations may be accomplished by the one-stage abdominal transection using an (EEA) stapler together with the devascularization procedure.[11] By necessity, this transabdominal approach results in some compromise in the extent of devascularization of the lower esophagus. Only 8 to 10 cm of the esophagus can be devascularized from the abdomen, whereas the transthoracic approach permits a more extensive devascularization of the esophagus from the esophagocardiac junction to the midesophagus 15 cm cephalad to this junction. This more complete devascularization of the esophagus yields about a 10 to 20% decrease in postoperative recurrence of esophageal varices. Long-term follow-up after these procedures, however, reveals that bleeding had not been observed in 80% of the patients following stapler transection and devascularization.[12] Patients with recurrent varices can easily be treated with adjuvant endoscopic sclerotherapy. A recent nationwide survey on the treatment of esophagogastric varices in Japan showed that the transabdominal stapler transection with devascularization was by far the most popular operative procedure for esophagogastric varices.[13]

INDICATIONS

There are many options for the treatment of esophagogastric varices, and one must select the most appropriate modality for each particular patient. Previously, emergency operations have often been performed in patients with massive bleeding; more recently, endoscopic sclerotherapy has become the treatment of choice in many institutions, thereby circumventing the prohibitive risk of emergency operation in acutely bleeding patients. In Japan, transabdominal stapler transection and esophagogastric devascularization were performed in most patients with esophagogastric varices until the mid-1980s. However, the more recent development and trials of sclerotherapy have changed the indications for this Sugiura procedure, which is now limited to lower-risk patients (Child's A and B) and is seldom performed as an emergency operation.[14]

Factors which should be considered when selecting the method of treatment are age of the patient, severity of hepatic dysfunction, clinical findings, location of varices, distribution and dynamics of portal collaterals, presence or absence of hypersplenism, history of abdominal or thoracic operations, associated diseases of other organs, and the technical hazards of the operative procedures.

Based on extensive experience with nonshunting operations for over 25 years,[13] the indications for transabdominal esophageal transection and devascularization procedures have become established (Table 34.1). The operative mortality from this procedure is very low when liver function is preserved, as judged by the indocyanine green (ICG) retention (15 minutes) and the ICG disappearance constant. ICG retention (15 minutes) is the plasma retention of ICG 15 minutes after bolus intravenous injection. This is expressed as the ratio of its plasma concentration measured 15 minutes after intravenous administration to that at 0 minutes (C_0). C_0 is assumed to be 10 μg/ml plasma when 0.5 mg/kg of ICG is administered intravenously. It has the same significance as the ICG disappearance constant in terms of the assumption about the plasma content. The plasma disappearance rate constant of ICG is calculated from its plasma concentrations during the brief period (usually within 15 minutes) after intravenous administration. The analysis is performed by supposing that ICG plasma concentrations decline monoexponentially after intravenous administration. We have experienced no operative mortality when the ICG retention (15 minutes) is over 40% and the ICG disappearance constant is over 0.06 min^{-1}. When the patient's risk, as judged from other liver function tests, is in question, the ICG retention (15 minutes) and ICG disappearance constant values are used to define

TABLE 34.1. Indications for Stapler Esophageal Transection

Age	<65 years old
History	History of bleeding
Endoscopic findings	R-C sign (+), F_2, F_3, C_B
Clinical symptoms	Encephalopathy (−) Ascites (−) Cachexia (−)
Liver Function Tests	
Albumin	<3.0 g/dl
Bilirubin	>2.0 mg/dl
SGOT	>100 units
SGPT	>100 units
Antipyrin clearance	<0.10 ml/min/kg
Prothrombin time	<50%
Hepaplastin test	<50%
ICG retention (15 min)	>40%
ICG disappearance constant	<0.06 min^{-1}
	No severe complications in other organs

the indication for operation. Unfortunately, ICG retention (15 minutes) and ICG disappearance constant values may be erroneous when a large extrahepatic shunt is present; therefore, this should be taken into consideration when planning the Sugiura procedure.

This procedure is seldom performed as an emergency operation, since most acute bleeding can now be controlled, at least tentatively, by balloon tamponade or sclerotherapy. In Child's A patients, however, surgery may still be performed immediately following balloon tamponade. In Child's B and C patients, surgery is usually carried out electively. Prophylactic operations have been performed when the patients have had varices at increased risk for recurrent bleeding,[15,16] but since the development of sclerotherapy, prophylactic operation is limited to patients in Child's A category with severe hypersplenism and high-risk varices. High-risk varices can be identified by their large (F_2, F_3) size and red (R-C sign +) or blue (C_B) coloration (Table 34.1), according to a classification of esophageal varices, based on size and appearance, which has been proposed by the Japanese Research Society for Portal Hypertension.[15,16]

TECHNIQUES OF THE SUGIURA PROCEDURE

The transabdominal esophageal transection and devascularization procedures consist of six components: (1) splenectomy; (2) devascularization of the greater curvature of the stomach; (3) devascularization of the lesser curvature of the stomach; (4) devascularization of the lower esophagus; (5) transection of the esophagus using the stapler (EEA); and (6) pyloroplasty (Table 34.2).

Usually, the abdominal cavity is entered by a long midline incision extending from the xiphoid process of the sternum to a point halfway between the umbilicus and pubis. A long transverse incision across the upper hypogastric region may be used, but the vertical midline incision avoids severance of many collaterals developing in the abdominal wall.

Devascularization of the greater curvature of the stomach is started at a point opposite to the incisura angularis on the lesser curve so that approximately three arterial and venous arcades of the right gastroepiploic vessels are doubly ligated and divided close to the gastric wall. Devascularization is continued cephalad until all the vascular arcades of the left gastroepiploic vessels and the short gastric vessels are also doubly ligated and divided.

The splenic artery is then located along the superior border of the pancreas, dissected free, and suture-ligated. This interrupts the main splenic inflow, thereby causing the enlarged spleen to shrink considerably. This facilitates safer dissection of the upper pole

TABLE 34.2. Steps of Operative Procedures

1. Devascularization of the greater curvature of the stomach
2. Splenectomy
3. Devascularization of the lesser curvature of the stomach
4. Devascularization of the lower esophagus
5. Esophageal transection using EEA
6. Pyloroplasty

of the spleen, devascularization of the cardia of the stomach, and splenectomy. Often, the most cephalad short gastric vessels, the most proximal arcades of the left gastroepiploic vessels, and the posterior gastric artery and vein are dissected, ligated, and divided after the splenic inflow has been interrupted. When these vessels have been divided, the proximal gastric fundus with its apical fat pad can safely be severed from small diaphragmatic attachments as hemostasis is achieved by ligature or electrocoagulation. Care should be taken not to tear the capsule of the spleen, which may bleed massively, despite hemostatic efforts, until the spleen is removed.

Other ligaments attached to the spleen are carefully ligated and divided. These ligaments (splenocolic, lienorenal, lienogastric, and phrenicolienal) often house abundant portal collaterals. These collaterals should be carefully ligated before division. After mobilizing the spleen, the splenic artery and vein are ligated by transfixing sutures, and the spleen is removed.

Once the spleen, which is usually very large due to portal hypertension, is removed, access to the left upper quadrant and esophagus is enhanced as sufficient working space becomes available. The remaining operative procedures may then be carried out, usually without much difficulty or significant bleeding.

Devascularization of the lesser curvature is also performed very close to the gastric wall, starting from a point just inferior to the incisura angularis and extending cephalad to the esophagus. The collaterals behind the stomach (innominate or retrogastric veins) should also be completely devascularized, since these minute veins communicate with the gastroesophageal varices.

After completely devascularizing the upper half of the stomach, devascularization is continued cephalad along the lower esophagus. Opening the esophageal hilum facilitates devascularization of the esophagus. Usually 8 to 10 cm of esophageal devascularization is possible by pulling the esophagus out into the abdomen (Figure 34.1). The fundic portion of the stomach may become ischemic after complete devascularization.

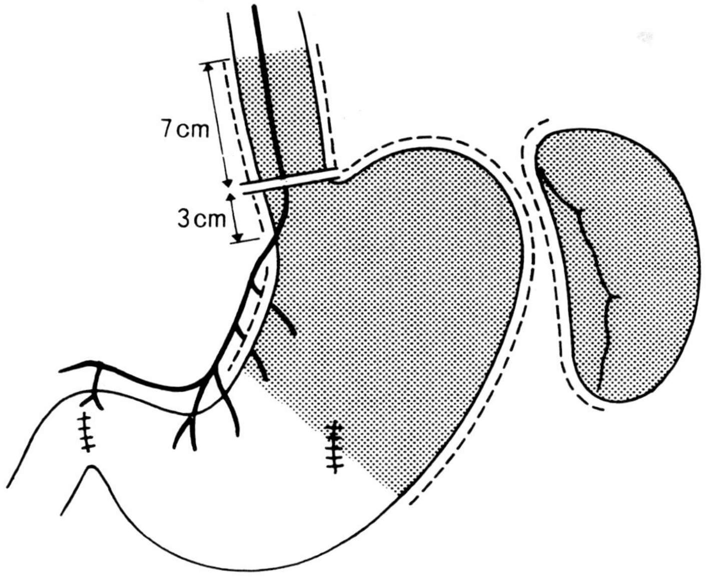

Figure 34.1. Extent of devascularization using the transabdominal approach (shaded area).

After devascularization of both the stomach and the esophagus, a 2-cm incision is made in the anterior stomach for insertion of the EEA (Figures 34.2, 34.3). This small gastrotomy should be made in the lower portion of the gastric body, where circulation is least altered by the devascularization.

The EEA stapler is introduced into the esophagus through this gastrotomy, and transection is carried out at a level 2 to 3 cm above the esophagogastric junction (Figures 34.4, 34.5). Usually, a 25- to 28-mm disposable cartridge is used in esophageal transection. The gastrotomy is closed in two layers, using interrupted sutures for both layers.

The anesthesiologist then passes a nasogastric tube across the line of transection into the stomach. Bleeding from the anastomotic line is checked by gastric lavage, using cold saline. Hemostasis should be verified at this time.

Finally, pyloroplasty is performed to prevent postoperative gastric retention, since the vagal nerves are usually divided in the process of esophageal devascularization. A silicone rubber drain is inserted in the left infraphrenic space, and the abdomen is closed.

Esophageal transection and resuture may be performed manually or by using autosuture (EEA). Until 1976, when the use of stapler devices was introduced in Japan, the transection procedure was always performed manually. There are both advantages and disadvantages to using stapler devices in esophageal transection. The advantages are as follows: (1) division and resuture of the esophagus can be performed quickly, with one action; (2) a uniform anastomosis is obtained; (3) all layers of the esophagus are divided, so that blockade of the collaterals within the wall is complete, whereas with manual transection, the muscle layer on right side of the esophagus is left intact; (4) the esophagus is not opened, thereby minimizing contamination of the operative field; (5) damage to the esophageal wall is avoided, since esophageal clamps are not applied; (6) visualization of the gastric muscosa for the presence of gastric varices, ulcers, or gastritis is possible through the gastrotomy; and (7) histological examination of the esophageal wall within the ring resected by the autosuture is possible.

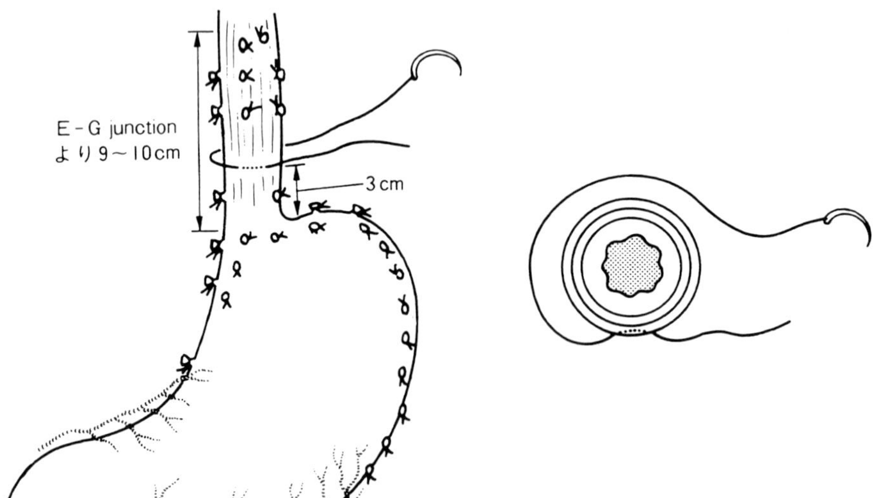

Figure 34.2. After devascularization, a suture is placed around the esophagus.

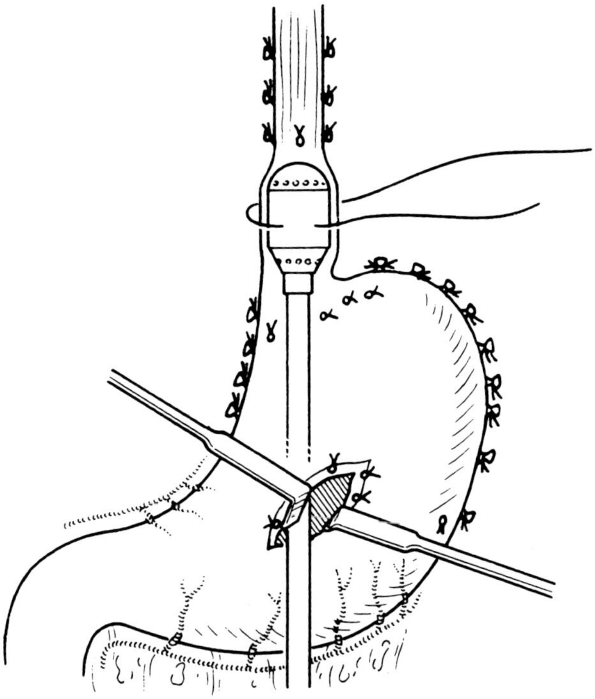

Figure 34.3. The EEA stapler is inserted into the esophagus through the gastrotomy.

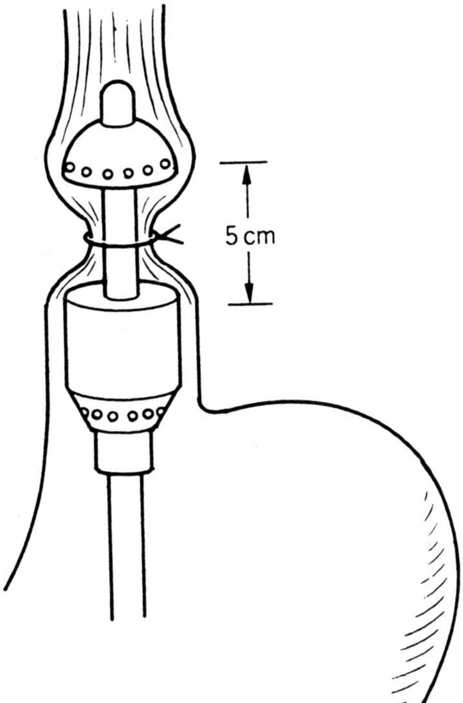

Figure 34.4. The suture is tied securely to the rod, and then transection and reanastomosis are performed in one action.

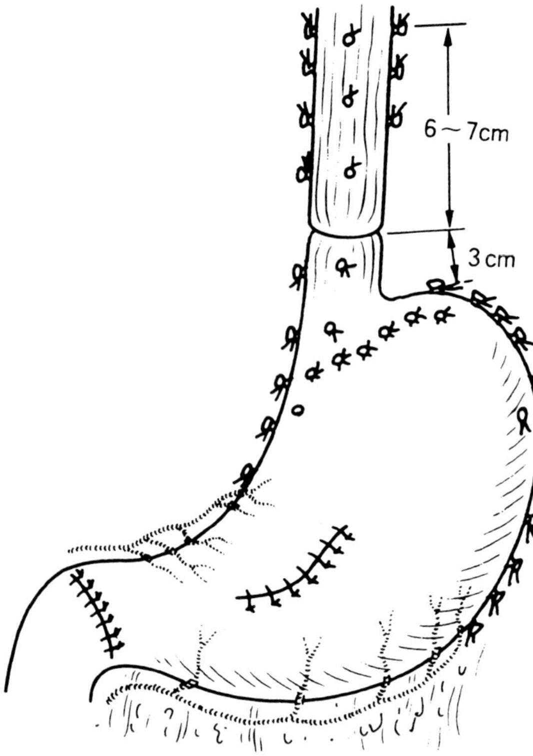

Figure 34.5. The gastrotomy is closed and a pyloroplasty is performed.

The disadvantages of using the EEA stapler are as follows: (1) the size of the cartridges is fixed so that the autosuture cannot be used in small children; (2) when pathological changes (inflammation, tears, or scar tissue) exist, the risk of anastomotic leakage is high, since the autosuture is applied to the ischemic region, which has undergone extensive devascularization; (3) gastrotomy is necessary to make sure that a 25- or 28-mm cartridge can be inserted into the esophagus without difficulty and that the wall thickness of the esophagus is normal, without edema, inflammation, scar formation, muscular layer tears, or other pathological changes; and (4) sclerotherapy immediately prior to operation may cause edema and inflammation of the esophagocardiac region, thereby making transection and stapling risky. When possible, this Sugiura procedure is delayed for three months in patients previously treated by sclerotherapy.

RESULTS

This type of nonshunting direct operation has been performed in over 500 patients with esophagogastric varices during the past quarter of a century. Our experience confirms that this procedure is effective for both elective and prophylactic operations and also for the emergency treatment of bleeding varices.[12] A recent nationwide survey of the treatment of esophagogastric varices in Japan has shown that stapler esophageal transection and devascularization is by far the most popular operation for varices in Japan. The operative mortality rate of 7.7%, and the cumulative survival rates of 65.9% and 50.6% at 5 and 10 years, respectively, confirm the efficacy of this approach. More detailed results of this nationwide survey will be reported elsewhere.[13]

The occurrence of postoperative stricture of the esophagus is higher in stapler-transected patients compared to manually transected patients; the occurrence rates of postoperative stricture are 20% and 13%, respectively.[13] The higher occurrence of stricture in EEA transection may be due to complete division of all the layers of the esophagus. Fortunately, these postoperative strictures can be treated successfully by bougienage or endoscopic dilatation, using laser or cautery. Major surgery is seldom needed.

Anastomotic leaks and abdominal discomfort are other postoperative complications observed after the transection procedure. Major anastomotic leaks may become fatal complications in patients with advanced cirrhosis of the liver but, fortunately, operative mortality due to major anastomotic leaks has been very low (0.5%). Abdominal discomfort is often caused by deformity of the stomach due to extensive devascularization and gastric retention of meals in spite of pyloroplasty. Abdominal discomfort is observed in about one-third of the patients after the transection and devascularization procedures. Usually, this disappears spontaneously within three months. Despite these drawbacks, the esophageal transection and devascularization procedure, using the EEA stapler, has proved to be a safe and dependable method of treatment for esophagocardiac varices.

REFERENCES

1. Blain AN: Ligation of the splenic artery for Banti's disease. Report of a case, experimental studies. *Surg Gynecol Obstet* 26:660–664, 1918.
2. Pemberton JDJ, Kiernan P: Surgery of the spleen. *Surg Clin North Am* 25:880–889, 1945.
3. Walters W, Rowntree LG, McIndoe AH: Ligation of coronary veins for bleeding esophageal varices. *Proc Staff Meet Mayo Clin* 4:146, 1927.
4. Womack NA, Peters RM: The significance of splenomegaly in cirrhosis of the liver. *Ann Surg* 153:1006–1112, 1961.
5. Dumont AE, Berman IR, Stahl W: Significance of an enlarged S.A. in patients with bleeding varices. *Ann Surg* 175:466–470, 1972.
6. Keagy BA, Schwartz JA, Johnson G Jr: Should ablative operations be used for bleeding esophageal varices? *Ann Surg* 203:463–469, 1986.
7. Walker RM: Transection operation for portal hypertension. *Thorax* 15:218, 1960.
8. Walker RM: Esophageal transection for bleeding varices. *Surg Gynecol Obstet* 118:323, 1964.
9. Idezuki Y, Sugiura M, Sakamoto K, et al: Rationale for transthoracic esophageal transection for bleeding varices. *Dis Chest* 52:621–631, 1967.
10. Sugiura M, Futagawa S: A new technique for treating esophageal varices. *J Thora Cardiovasc Surg* 66:667–685, 1973.
11. Iwatsuka M, Kobayashi S, Takasaki K, et al: Esophageal transection using autosuture. *Shujutstu Operation* 30:489, 1976. (In Japanese)
12. Idezuki Y, Sanjo K: Twenty-five-year experiences with esophageal transection for esophageal varices. *J Thorac Cardiovasc Surg* 98:876–883, 1989.

13. Idezuki Y: Present status of sclerotherapy and surgical treatment for esophageal varices in Japan. (Japanese Research Society for Portal Hypertension and Japanese Research Society for Sclerotherapy of Esophageal Varices.) To be published in *World J Surg*.
14. Idezuki Y, Sanjo K, Bandai Y, et al: Current strategy for esophageal varices in Japan. *Am J Surg* 160:98, 1990.
15. Beppu K, Inokuchi K, Koyanagi N, et al: Prediction of variceal hemorrhage by esophageal endoscopy. *Gastrointest Endosc* 27:213–218, 1981.
16. Koyanagi N and the Cooperative Study Group of Portal Hypertension in Japan: Prognostic blue varices as a discriminant factor of findings of esophageal varices. *Jpn J Surg* 18:142–145, 1988.

INDEX

C

F

G